Karate-do Master Reference

空手道選集

An Anthology
Volume 2

COMPILED BY
MICHAEL A. DeMARCO, M.A.

VIA MEDIA PUBLISHING | ARTICLES FROM THE JOURNAL OF ASIAN MARTIAL ARTS

Disclaimer

Please note that the author and publisher of this book are not responsible in any manner whatsoever for any injury that may result from practicing the techniques and/or following the instructions given herein. Participation in martial arts activities can be dangerous and can lead to serious injury. The material presented in this book is intended for reference only, and the reader assumes all risks associated with attempting to perform any of the activities described herein. Before attempting any of the physical activities described in this book, the reader should consult a physician for advice regarding their individual suitability for performing such activity.

All Rights Reserved

No part of this publication, including illustrations, may be reproduced or utilized in any form or by any means, electronic or mechanical, including photocopying, recording, or by any information storage and retrieval system (beyond that copying permitted by sections 107 and 108 of the US Copyright Law and except by reviewers for the public press), without written permission from Via Media Publishing Company.

Warning: Any unauthorized act in relation to a copyright work may result in both a civil claim for damages and criminal prosecution.

Copyright © 2025
by Via Media Publishing Company
941 Calle Mejia #822
Santa Fe, NM 87501 USA

Book and cover design
by Via Media Publishing Company
Background texture ID 114599087
© Naokikim| Dreamstime.com

ISBN 979-8-9922430-3-1

www.viamediapublishing.com

Dedication

To all those who have contributed to the
Journal of Asian Martial Arts (1992–2016)
providing articles of high academic standards
that will continue to inspire research and practice.

Table of Contents

Preface — ix

- Karate Pioneer Yabu Kentsu, 1866-1937 — 388
  Joseph R. Svinth, M.A.

- An Analysis of Parallel Techniques: — 397
  The Kinetic Connection Between Sanseru and Shishochin
  Robert Toth

- Isshin Kempo: Isshin-ryu's Missing Link to the Internal — 404
  Christopher Goedecke, B.S.

- Koshin-ryu: The Rebirth of Okinawa's Kojo Family Martial Arts — 428
  Richard B. Florence, M.A.

- Incorporating the Main Principles of Kata Training — 447
  Marvin Labatte

- Kobudo: Okinawan Weapons are Not All Flash — 462
  Mary Bolz, B.A.

- Robert M. Dalgleish: "The Father of Canadian Goju-ryu Karate" — 473
  Robert Toth

- The Lost Secrets of Okinawan Goju-ryu: What the Kata Shows — 482
  Giles Hopkins, M.A.

- Basic Foundations in Okinawan Karate: — 500
  Interview with Canadian Tsuruoka Masami
  Olga Toth and Robert Toth

- The Shape of Kata: An Enigma of Pattern — 513
  Giles Hopkins, M.A.

- Yagi Meitatsu Discusses the Not-So-Secret — 522
  Techniques of Okinawan Goju-ryu Karate
  Robert Toth

- Steve Arneil and the British Kyokushinkai: An Interview — 532
  Graham Noble

- The Teaching of Goju-ryu Kata: A Brief Look at Methodology and Practice — 554
  Giles Hopkins, M.A.

- The Five Katas of Yagi Meitoku — 568
  Perry Campbell, B.Sc.

- The Legacy of Dr. Richard Kim: An Interview with Brian Ricci — 579
  Robert Toth

- George Dillman and the Influences in Pressure Point Theory and Practice — 591
  Peter Hobart, J.D.

- Kaho: Cultural Meaning and Educational Method in Kata Training — 599
  John J. Donohue, Ph.D.

▸ Masaru Shintani: The Making of a Modern Canadian Karate Master 607
Robert Toth

▸ The Stories of Meibukan Gojyu-ryu Karate as Told by Yagi Meitatsu 624
Robert Toth

▸ Politics and Karate: Historical Influences on the Practice of Goju-ryu 636
Giles Hopkins, M.A.

▸ A Preliminary Analysis of Goju-ryu Kata Structure 654
Fernando Portela Câmara, Ph.D. and Mario McKenna, M.S.

▸ Defending to the Four Directions: 661
Evolving Uechi-ryu's Hojoundo Exercises for Advanced Students
Ihor Rymaruk

▸ Kata and Bunkai: 676
A Study in Theme and Variations in Karate's Solo Practice Routines
Giles Hopkins, M.A.

▸ Evaluating Makiwara Punching Board Performance 694
Paul K. Smith, Ph.D. Timothy Niiler, Ph.D. and Peter W. McCullough, B.S.

▸ Attention, Sit, Meditate, Bow, Ready Position: 702
Ritualized Dojo Pattern or Character Training?
Marvin Labbate

▸ Nahate: The Old-School Okinawan Martial Art 711
and Its Original Four-Kata Curriculum, Part I
Mario McKenna, M.S.

▸ Nahate: The Old-School Okinawan Martial Art 725
and Its Original Four-Kata Curriculum, Part II
Mario McKenna, M.S.

▸ Issues Concerning Board Breaking 743
Phil Davidson, M.A.

▸ Ryukyu Kempo and Small Circle Jujitsu 749
Will Higginbotham, B.A.

▸ Kata-Based Training of Goju-ryu Karate 752
Marvin Labbate

▸ Tekko: Ryukyu Kobudo Shinkokai's Knuckle Duster 755
Mario McKenna, M.S.

Sources of Original Publication 758

Index 760

Preface

Via Media Publishing was founded in 1992 in order to produce the peer reviewed quarterly *Journal of Asian Martial Arts* (1992–2012)—the first publication of its kind to focus on martial traditions in an academic format. Many of the authors were scholar–practitioners, who utilized their unique talents to present articles from various specializations, such as Asian Studies, kinesiology, history, anthropology, philosophy, and physical education.

Those who were serious about this field subscribed to the journal to read articles noted for their high academic and aesthetic standards. Most were in the United States, Canada, and Europe, but also in other areas of the world. Subscribers naturally included martial art schools and individual practitioners. There was a strong base among university and public libraries too.

As founder of Via Media, I've decided to assemble this anthology of articles relating to the martial arts associated with Okinawa. There are over a hundred million karate practitioners worldwide, drawn to the art mainly for self-defense and a form of exercise. Researchers can benefit from this handy anthology, particularly for the information and analyses presented, including the rich bibliographic listings. Karate practitioners will also gain insights to benefit their own practice, be it for health and/or self-defense.

A total of sixty-three chapters are conveniently compiled in this two-volume set. In addition to 1,780 illustrations, there are glossaries, maps, charts, and bibliographies. *Karate* is the term representing the general category of study, but it can be subdivided into its branches, from indigenous practices to styles influenced from Chinese systems from Fujian Province.

The variety of material in this anthology reflects in-depth scholarly research and the experience of master practitioners. It will be a valuable source for karate enthusiasts for future decades. By making this book available to individuals and libraries, we hope this rare material will greatly contribute to further research in this field and inspire many to learn karate with aspirations to mastery.

Michael DeMarco

Michael DeMarco, Publisher
Santa Fe, NM, January 2025

chapter 33

Karate Pioneer Yabu Kentsu, 1866–1937

by Joseph Svinth, M.A.

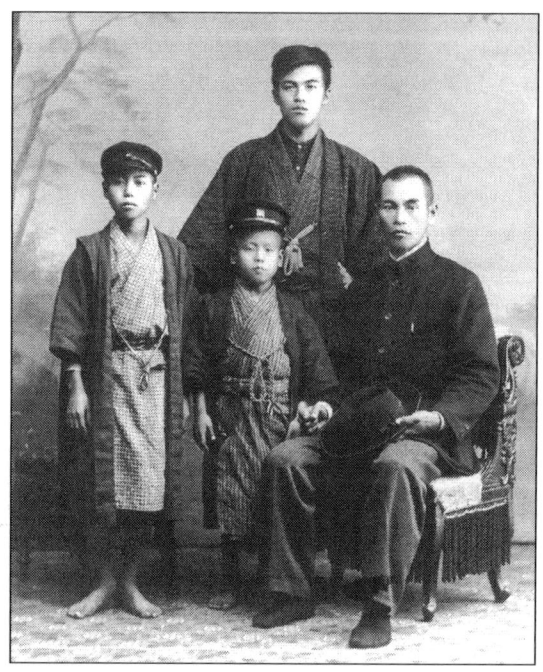

Yabu Kentsu with his three oldest sons in 1906. The standing youth is 18-year old Kenden.
On the left is Kenyu, who later shortened his name to Ken, and on the right is Kenshin.
This photograph, or any negatives derived therefrom, may not be copyrighted.
Courtesy of the Yabe/Yasui Family Collection.

Introduction

A couple years ago I was researching sumo and judo in Oregon before World War II, and during the research I started corresponding with Homer Yasui. One day Homer asked, "By the way, are you interested in karate, too? My wife's grandfather did karate."

"Sure," I replied. "So who was grandpa?"

"Kentsu Yabu," replied Homer. "Ever heard of him?"

Actually, I had. He was a well-known Shorin-ryu karate teacher of the early twentieth century, a peer of Funakoshi and others of that generation. He was supposed to have introduced karate to Hawai'i during the 1920's, but so far as I knew, there weren't too many pictures or reliable English-language stories about him.

"Oh," said Homer. "Would you like some?"

•••

The eldest son of Yabu Kenten[1] and Shun Morinaga, Yabu Kentsu was born at Shuri City, Yamakawa-cho, Ni-chome #8, in 1866. Known in childhood as Kamadu, he had three brothers, three sisters, and three half-sisters: second brother Kencho, a graduate of the Medicine and Biology Institute (Ishi Isei Kyoshujo), died at age 25; third brother, Kenkyu, was a well-known painter and calligrapher whose pen names included Kinto and Muka Sanjin (Yabu, 1986:98–99).

The family was of mid-aristocracy (*pechin*), and had been ever since the Ryukyuan genealogical bureau was first established in 1689. As a group, the middle aristocracy worked in jobs such as civil administration and domestic law enforcement. So, besides often having acquired some proficiency in methods of physical restraint, male members of this class typically received training in calligraphy, politics, and Confucian pedagogy (McCarthy, 1994:1). What this meant for the Yabu family was that Kentsu's paternal grandfather, Ken'yo, was the archery instructor for Lord Ikegusuku, while his father was a court calligrapher (Yabu, 1986:98–99; Yasui, 1998 Sep. 6; Yasui, 1998 Dec. 12).

As a young man, Kentsu received training in what would become known as Shorin-ryu karate. Hokama Tetsuhiro says that Yabu's teacher was Matsumura Sokon (1998:35). On the other hand, Dave Lowry says that Yabu's teacher was Itosu "Ankoh" Yasutsune (1985:11). Since both Matsumura and Itosu were well-known Okinawan karate teachers, Yabu probably studied with each at different times.

When Yabu began this training is unclear. Dave Lowry says that as a child Yabu was bigger and stronger than his playmates, so was naturally attracted to karate (1985:11). If this is correct, then he probably started circa 1880. On the other hand, in *Karate-Do Nyumon*, Funakoshi Gichin wrote:

> During the Sino-Japanese War [of 1894–1895] a young man trained earnestly with [Ankoh] Itosu for several months before joining the army. When he was assigned to the Kumamoto Division, the division medical examiner, noticing his well-balanced muscular development, said, "I hear you're from Okinawa. What martial art did you train in?" The recruit replied that farm labor was all he had ever done. But a friend who was with him blurted out, "He's been practicing karate." The doctor only murmured, "I see, I see," but he was deeply impressed. — 1988:25–26

So perhaps Yabu only began his training after deciding to go into the service in 1891.

Despite being exempt from Japanese military service—Okinawans were not yet subject to Japanese conscription—and although he had married Takahara Oto around 1887 and the couple had a son, Kenden, in 1888, Yabu was still among the first Okinawans to voluntarily serve in the Japanese Army. His goal was evidently to prove to the Japanese that Okinawans could be every bit as good of soldiers as any home island Japanese (Yabu, 1986:98–99; Yasui, 1998 Sep. 6).

The Japanese Army sent Yabu to a school for noncommissioned officers. Upon graduation, he was promoted to sergeant. He was then sent to China, where he saw service during the Sino-Japanese War (Kim, 1974:64–65; Noble, n.d.:32; Yasui, 1998 Sep. 6).

There is a story told on Okinawa that Yabu was promoted to lieutenant before his discharge, and that his uniform and sword were subsequently kept in Shuri Castle (Kim, 1974:64–65; Noble, n.d.:32; Yasui, 1998 Sep. 6). However, family documents do not verify this, and Yabu's students often called him "sergeant." Research into Japanese military archives is probably required to resolve the question.

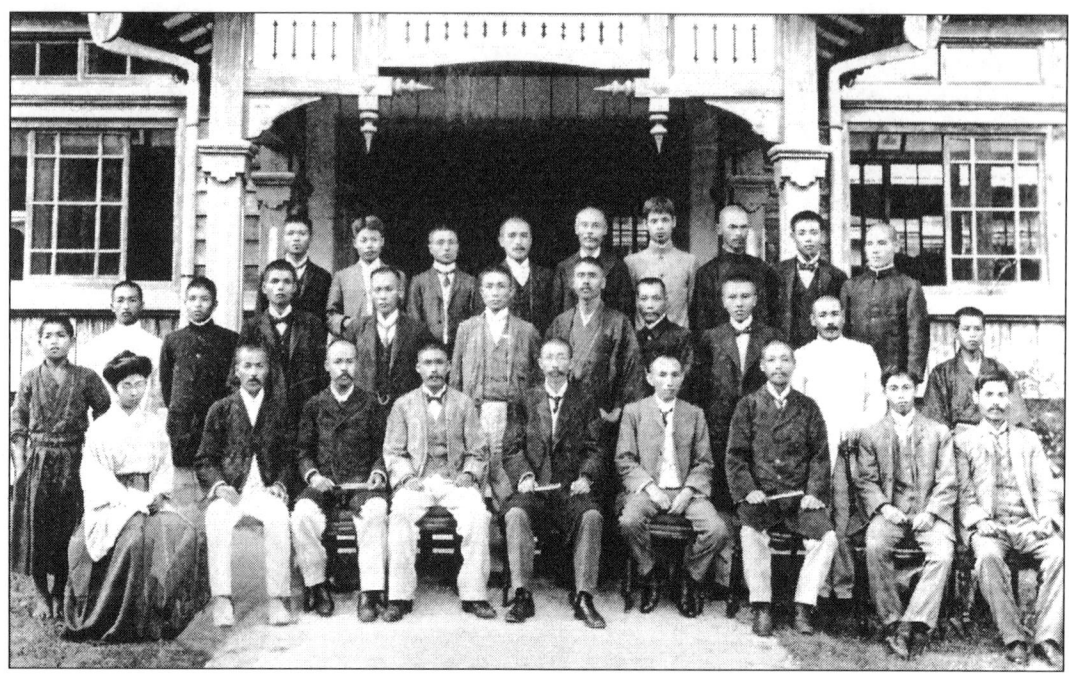

A group photo taken in 1908, in which Yabu Kentsu appears third from the right in the back row. The location is said to be the school where Yabu received his training as a teacher. If so, then the building was probably part of the Prefectural Teachers' Training College, where Itosu Ankoh taught karate from 1905. However, it could also be the Prefectural Number One School, where Yabu worked as a teacher. The original photograph belonged to a man named Nakahara Tetsushijo and is presently in the collection of Ryukyu University history professor Hiyane Teruo. Miyuki Yabe Yasui got her copy from her cousin Yohko Yabu Ikeda while visiting Shuri in 1993. This photograph, or any negatives derived therefrom, may not be copyrighted.

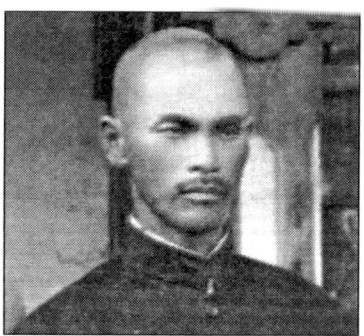

Detail from the above photo of Kentsu Yabu. He would
have been about 42 years old when this photo was taken.
Courtesy of the Yabe/Yasui Family Collection.

    I am unaware of any further information concerning Yabu's military career. However, at the speculative levels, Richard Kim has written that Yabu perfected his karate on the battlefield against the Chinese (Kim, 1974:64–65). George Alexander wrote that "Yabu [reportedly] fought over sixty lethal karate duels and was never defeated" (1991:64). But, men who knew Yabu recalled that he was someone who despised hyperbole: "When Kentsu Yabu came into the room, all the brag, all the talk, all the opinions, they stopped," Dave Lowry has quoted an unnamed source as saying. Such stories are probably heroic rather than factual (1985:13).

On a more plausible level, Graham Noble has cited hearsay evidence that one of Yabu's military subordinates died after Yabu struck him. During the subsequent inquiry, Yabu told investigators that he had struck the other man with his open palm, which was legal under Japanese military law, rather than with his fist, which was not.[2] The court accepted his statement after seeing him break some boards with his fist, and as a result dropped the manslaughter charge (Noble, n.d.:32). Again, this story is hearsay and needs corroboration.

Upon separation from the service, Yabu returned to Okinawa. After settling in, he began studying at Shuri's Prefectural Teachers' Training College. While there, he frequently helped Itosu Ankoh, who was then leading a campaign to have karate made part of the Okinawan public schools' physical education curriculum, by giving public demonstrations of karate katas, or practice forms. His favorite kata was reportedly Gojushiho, an old Chinese form distinguished by its use of open-handed palm-heel and finger strikes (Noble, n.d.:32-33). As for the way he did this kata, Dave Lowry cites an unnamed witness as saying that Yabu's version was unusual because "it was nothing at all like a dance, more like the motion of the surf, soft, soft, soft, as it comes in, then smash—hard like a rock" (1985:12).

In 1902, Yabu became a karate instructor at Shuri's Prefectural Number One School (Hokama, 1998:88). Former students recalled that his instruction stressed constant repetitions of Naihanchi kata. Toward that end, he liked to say that students should do 10,000 kata a year (Noble, n.d.:33). Probably the latter statement was hyperbolic; in Japanese when one says "ten thousand," one is not necessarily being literal, but it still gives an idea of the level of technical proficiency Yabu expected from his karate students.

Since Yabu was one of Okinawa's earliest public school karate teachers, the modern Shotokai karate teacher Harada Mitsusuke, who met various Okinawan teachers while living in Brazil, has speculated that modern karate's tendency toward doing things "by the numbers" may be attributable to Yabu (Noble, n.d.:33). But as Japanese scholars have since shown that all Japanese athletic training was heavily militarized during the 1930's and 1940's, that is probably exaggerating things a bit (Abe, Kiyohara, and Nakajima, 1990: 27-43).

During his life, Yabu's peers frequently honored him. For example, during the mid-1910's, he received the gift of a sword from Higa Toki, who had himself received the weapon from the Chinese leader Sun Yat-sen in appreciation for his service to China during the Chinese Revolution (History of the Okinawans, 1988:12-14).[3] In 1924, Yabu was asked to become a charter member of the Okinawa Tode Research Club, an organization dedicated to protecting and preserving tode, as Ryukyuans then called karate (Bishop, 1989:153). And in 1936, he was asked to join the council of distinguished karate teachers that ultimately agreed to change the name of karate from its old characters (*kanji*) meaning "Chinese hands" into its modern characters meaning "empty hands" (Funakoshi, 1973:3-4; Funakoshi, 1988:24-25; Hokama, 1998:36, 93).[4]

George Alexander and Richard Kim have written that Yabu once defeated the famous karate fighter Motobu Choki during a private contest held at Motobu's Okinawan estate (Alexander, 1991:64; Kim, 1974:64-65). Kim said that during their battle, "The air cracked with the sound of loud *kiai*,[5] feet shuffling, punches and kicks landing on human flesh, and the excited gasps of the few privileged viewers" (1974:64-65). However, less breathless researchers have been unable to find evidence proving that the two men ever fought, let alone such vivid descriptions of their contest (Noble, 2000; Silvan, 1998:93).

Dave Lowry has speculated that the contest between Motobu and Yabu was not in karate, but in *tegumi*, or Ryukyuan sumo (1985:13). That sounds plausible, especially since Yabu went out of his way to organize tegumi matches during the Okinawan celebrations held near Fresno in July 1921 and August 1922.[6] The *History of Okinawans* (1988:339) reports that:

> Sergeant Kentsu Yabe[7] was a great fan of sumo. In Okinawa, he had been so enthusiastic that he got involved in every match that came up. His talking of sumo fired up all the younger men, and they decided to hold a big match. Considering the absence of entertainment in the life of the issei immigrant, those who participated in the sumo returned home pleased and happy.

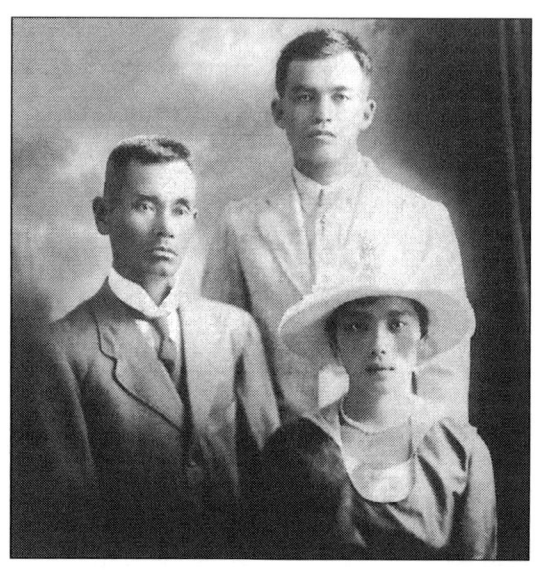

Yabu Kentsu with his son Kenden and daughter-in-law Mitsuye. The photo was probably taken in 1921–1922, when Mitsuye was pregnant with eldest daughter Emi. This photograph, or any negatives derived therefrom, may not be copyrighted. Courtesy of the Yabe/Yasui Family Collection.

Yabu was in Fresno visiting his eldest son, Kenden, who was then living in California. Although this visit is sometimes said to be the first visit of an Okinawan karate teacher to the US, this is not quite correct. According to the History of the Okinawans in North America, Nakaza Seijo, who moved to San Francisco around 1902, used karate during various physical confrontations with *hakujin* (European Americans) who enjoyed harassing Japanese. Neither did Yabu teach karate while in California. Instead, he was simply visiting his son, who had specifically asked his father to not "wear his sword" while visiting the United States (*History of the Okinawans*, 1988:341).

Yabu Kenden emigrated to Hawai'i around 1908. After four years, he moved to California. His "Certificate of Fact of Issue of a Passport" signed by the Japanese consul in Los Angeles in 1912 says that his purpose for coming to America was to study Western theology. However, in Hawai'i, he was an agricultural worker and, in California, he worked for many years as a gardener. He eventually became more interested in socialism than Christianity (Yabu, 1986:99; Yasui, 1998 Sep. 6; Yasui, 1998 Dec. 12).

In 1919, Kenden married a Japanese woman, Mitsuye Jyoko, and, by 1921, she was pregnant with the couple's first child. The family therefore believes that Kentsu's two visits to the United States were made in hopes that his eldest son would give him a grandson. Writes Kenden's son-in-law Homer Yasui (1998 Sep. 6):

Since Kenden was Kentsu's firstborn and a son at that—the *chonan*—it was very important that a male child be produced. It didn't happen that way, because their fourth child was also a girl. That child is my wife, Miyuki Yabe Yasui, who was born on September 18, 1926.

The story goes that it was Kentsu's intention—if the child was a boy—to take him back to Shuri to raise in a proper Okinawan fashion. Japanese fathers in those days were very powerful, so it wouldn't have been a bit surprising if Kenden and Mitsuye would have allowed that. Even in my generation, our fathers were powerful, and the chonans quite a bit less so, but still powerful nevertheless. Anyway, since Miki turned out to be yet another girl, Grandpa Kentsu returned home, probably disgusted, and certainly empty-handed.

The Yabes' oldest daughter, Emi, was born during Grandpa Kentsu's first visit and was about seven years old during his second visit. All she remembers of the second visit was that her grandfather dearly loved sweets and that her mother complained that Grandpa always wore shirts that were about an inch too big around the collar. Their other children (two of whom were still alive in 1998) were too young to remember anything of this visit (Yasui, 1998 November 7).

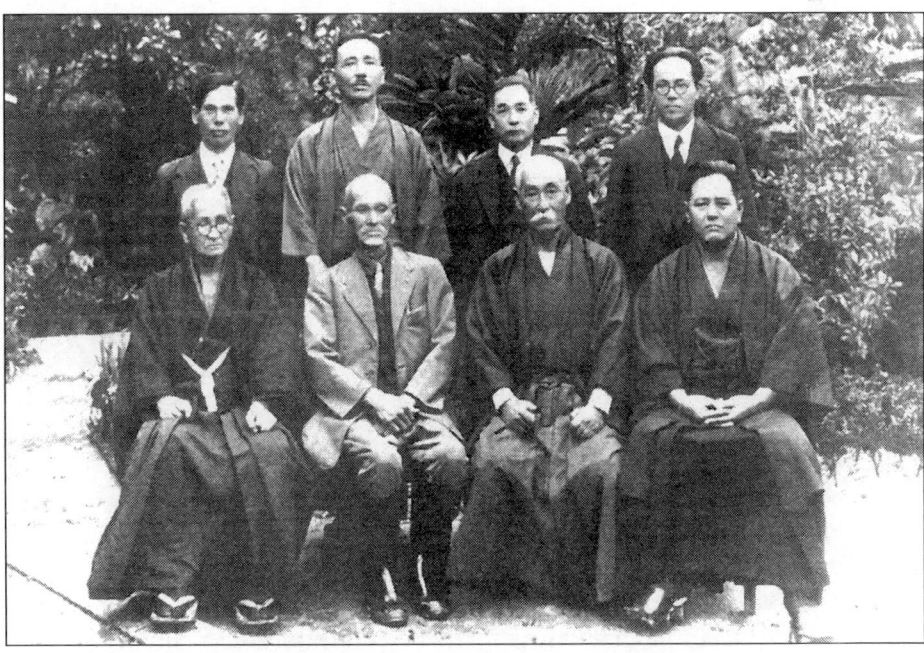

Eight of Okinawa's leading karate men. Back row, left to right: Shiroma Shinpan, Maeshiro Choryo, Chibana Choshin, Nakasone Genwa. Front row, left to right: Kyan Chotoku, Yabu Kentsu, Hanashiro Chomo, Miyagi Chojun. A frequently reproduced photo—it commemorates a major meeting hosted by an Okinawan newspaper in October 1936—its first known publication was in Karatedo Taikan in 1938. Photo courtesy of Graham Noble.

On his way back to Okinawa, Yabu Kentsu visited the Territory of Hawai'i. There, a local Japanese association had Yabu give Hawai'i's first public karate demonstration.

The demonstration took place at the Nuuanu YMCA, then located at Fourth and Vineyard in Honolulu, on Friday, July 8, 1927. Special guests included American Army and Navy officers and a visiting Waseda University baseball team (Nippu Jiji, 1927 July 6). Afterwards, a *Honolulu Advertiser* reporter wrote (1927 July 9):

Compared with jiujitsu, karate is more destructive. Jiujitsu is the art of throwing and holding and is slow compared to karate. No weapons of any kind are used and blows are struck with the clenched fist and aimed at vital spots such as the solar plexus, point of jaw, and other nerve centers. It enables a little man to successfully defend himself in hand-to-hand conflict with a larger adversary.

Lieutenant Yabe stated that boxing was being introduced into Japan but he doubted if it would ever be as popular or used as universally as karate. Legs as well as arms are brought into play.

The various holds and poses of karate were shown and described as follows: Kusanku, Gojushiho, Naihanchi, Sanchin, preparatory drill, Pinan... Passai, etc. The talk and drill were highly pleasing and instructive. The big crowd appeared to be duly impressed with the possibilities of this sport.

The latter statement was not simply hype. Yabu's demonstrations encouraged nisei (people of Japanese descent, born and educated in the US), such as Thomas Miyashiro, to subsequently establish karate dojo that offered instruction to anyone, not just people of Okinawan descent (Haines, 1968:119–121).

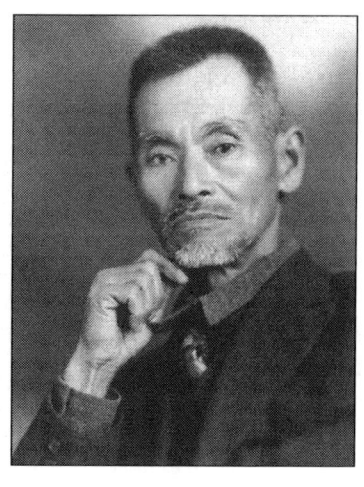

Yabu Kentsu circa 1927. This photograph, or any negatives derived therefrom, may not be copyrighted. Courtesy of the Yabe/Yasui Family Collection.

During this visit, Yabu also traveled to Kauai (Lowry, 1985:12). "Although we digress a bit," notes the History of the Okinawans in North America, "Yabe learned a great deal about *samisen* (the stringed musical instrument) and the performing arts in Hawai'i from one of his students there, Ryokin Nakama" (1988:341). Which is not surprising: apparently Yabu financed part of his trip by taking orders for Ryukyuan artifacts such as musical instruments and then mailing them to Hawai'i upon his return to Okinawa (Goodin, 1999 Apr. 9).

In 1936, Yabu visited Tokyo. Since he had terminal tuberculosis, it wouldn't be too surprising to learn that he was visiting physicians. Speculation aside, while in Japan, Yabu watched the young Nagamine Shoshin practicing karate. According to Mark Bishop, Yabu then warned Nagamine that karate's katas were undergoing rapid change in Japan and that it was up to Nagamine and other young men of his generation to preserve the Okinawan katas in their traditional forms (1989:86).

Less than a year later, Yabu was dead. While the ancestral home was destroyed during the fighting in 1945, second son Yabu Ken later rebuilt the house and Ken's widow, Emi, lives there to this day.

Notes

[1] "From early times until fairly recently," wrote Sakamaki Shunzo, "every [Ryukyuan] child was given a *domyo* (or *warabe-na*)—literally, his 'childhood name'. For a long time, it was generally his only name throughout his lifetime, since most members of

the upper classes did not have surnames and formal names (*nanori*) until after 1689, and commoners did not have surnames until the 1870s" (1964:13). In general, the oldest son took the same domyo as the paternal grandfather while younger sons took the names of relatives or friends. Although there were only about fifty individual *domyo*, suffixes ("Big," "Little," etc.) differentiated between grandfather and grandson while differences in pronunciation distinguished between aristocrats and commoners.

[2] The Japanese Army used to encourage its commissioned and noncommissioned officers to use corporal discipline as a form of what would today be called "tough love." Indeed, the usual euphemism for the practice was *bentatsu*, or "act of love." For an introduction to the topic, see Chang, 1997:217.

[3] Arriving in San Francisco in 1896, Higa is also known as the first Okinawan to have lived in the United States.

[4] Although the Okinawan karate teacher Hanashiro Chomo proposed the new name as early as 1905, it was not formally adopted until October 1936. The fact that Japan was at war with Russia in 1905 and China in 1936 undoubtedly had something to do with the timing of the name change.

[5] Literally, "a blending of vital energy," the word kiai properly refers to a manifestation of inner harmonics and discords transmitted directly from the psychic and physical center of the body. In a classic short story, "The Shout," English writer Robert Graves once wrote of an audible expression of such energy: "My shout is not a matter of tone or vibration but something not to be explained. It is a shout of pure [energy], and there is no fixed place for it on the scale." However, in North American and Japanese karate classes, the word is usually more narrowly defined as the noise that the athlete makes while executing a punch or kick.

[6] In *tegumi*, officials restarted bouts whenever one of the players was thrown to his stomach or knees. Also, judges only counted falls to the back. A typical outdoor tournament started about 10:30 a.m. and continued until dark. To give everyone a better chance of winning, American competitors were sometimes divided by age and weight. If so, then divisions were usually 150 pounds and over, 130–149 pounds, and 129 pounds and under. Hawaiian blue laws, by the way, required players to wear a pair of shorts under their wrestling belts (for further details, see Adaniya, et al., 1988:37–38).

[7] "Yabe" is the Japanese pronunciation of the two Chinese characters pronounced "Yabu" in the Shuri dialect of the Ryukyuan language. The change in pronunciation was made unilaterally by some individuals (including Yabu's son Kenden) during the 1910's and officially by the Education Society of Okinawa in 1937. However, the changes "in the reading of surnames were more effective in overseas areas than in Japan proper," noted Higa Shuncho. "The reason for this was that in Japan proper, although a person announced a change in the reading of his name, the written characters were not altered, and other people did not readily accept the changed reading. On the other hand, in overseas areas, names were spelled out in Roman writing and there was immediate acceptance of the pronunciation indicated by the Romanized version" (Sakamaki, 1964:38).

References

Abe, I., Kiyohara, Y., and Nakajima, K. (1990). Sport and physical education under fascistization in Japan. *Bulletin of Health & Sport Sciences*, University of Tsukuba, (13): 25–46; reprinted at http://ejmas.com/jalt/jaltart_abe_0600.htm. Downloaded September 26, 2000.

Adaniya, R., Njus, A., and Yamate, M. (Eds.). (1988). *Of andagi and sanshin: Okinawan culture in Hawai'i*. Honolulu: Hui O Laulima.

Alexander, G. (1991). *Okinawa: Island of karate*. Lake Worth, FL: Yamazato Publications.

Bishop, M. (1989). *Okinawan karate: Teachers, styles and secret techniques*. London: A&C Black.

Chang, I. (1997). T*he rape of Nanking: The forgotten holocaust of World War II*. New York: Basic Books.

Funakoshi, G. (1973). *Karate-do kyohan: The master tex*t. Tokyo: Kodansha International.

Funakoshi, G. (1988). *Karate-do nyumon: The master introductory text*. Tokyo: Kodansha International.

Goodin, C. (1999, April 9). Personal communication.

Haines, B. (1968). *Karate's history and traditions*. Rutland, VT: Charles E. Tuttle.

Kobashigawa, B. (Trans.). (1988). *History of the Okinawans in North America. Translation of Hokubei Okinawajin shi*. Los Angeles: University of California and the Okinawan Club of America.

Hokama, T. (1998). *History and traditions of Okinawan karate*. (C. Borkowski, Trans.). Hamilton, Ontario: Masters Publication.

Kim, R. (n.d.). The sergeant. *Karate Illustrated*, page unknown. (Xerographic copy courtesy Graham Noble).

Kim, R. (1974). *The weaponless warriors*. Burbank, CA: Ohara Publications.

Lowry, D. (1985). Yabu Kentsu, An Okinawan karateman. *Karate Illustrated*, (7):10–13.

Lum, S. (1999, April 2). Wanted: Hawaii karate 'pioneers', *Hawaii Herald*, A-13.

McCarthy, P. (1995). *Bubishi: The bible of karate*. Rutland, VT: Charles E. Tuttle.

McCarthy, P. (1987). *Classical kata of Okinawan karate*. Burbank, CA: Ohara Publications.

McCarthy, P. (1994). The sapposhi, pechin, and samurai. *The Ryukyuanist 24*, 1–3.

Noble, G. (1998, November). Letter to the author.

Noble, G., McLaren, I., and Karasawa, N. (n.d.). Masters of the Shorin-ryu, Part II. *Fighting Arts International*, 32–33.

Noble, G. (2000). Master Choki Motobu. http://ejmas.com/jcs/jcsart_noble1_0200.htm. Downloaded September 26, 2000.

Sakamaki, S. (Ed.) (1964). *Ryukyuan names: Monographs on and lists of personal and place names in the Ryukyus*. Honolulu: East-West Center Press.

Silvan, J. (1998). Oral traditions of Okinawan karate. *Journal of Asian Martial Arts, 7*(3): 72–95.

Yabu, K. (1986, May 31). Genealogy of the surname So family (from Kengi the founder): The Okushima family line, An annotated text. Translated with supplementary notes by Ben Kobashigawa and Yoko Fukumura. Both the Japanese original and the English translation are privately published. The Japanese original is in the Yabu Family Collection while the English translation is in the Yabe/Yasui Family Collection.

Yasui, H. (1998, September 6). Letter to the author.

Yasui, H. (1998, October 6). Letter to the author.

Yasui, H. (1998, November 7). Letter to the author.

Yasui, H. (1998, December 12). Letter to the author.

Acknowledgments

The following people provided assistance in completing this chapter: Michel Brousse, Charles Goodin, Richard Hayes, Eric Madis, Graham Noble, Robert W. Smith, Curtis Stanley, Homer Yasui, and Miyuki Yabe Yasui. The financial support of the Japanese American National Museum and the King County Landmarks and Heritage Commission is also gratefully acknowledged.

chapter 34

An Analysis of Parallel Techniques:
The Kinetic Connection Between Sanseru and Shishochin

by Robert Toth

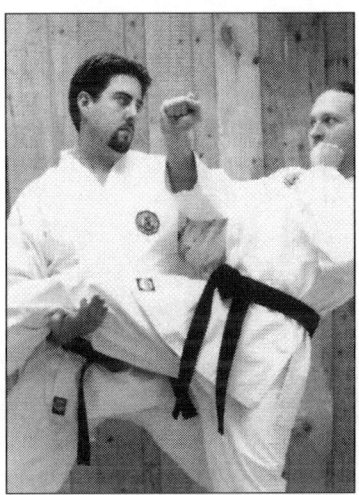

All photographs by Wai Hung Tang.

Introduction
Is there a secret connection between the traditional Goju-ryu routines (*kata*) called Sanseru and Shishochin? Has something been hidden from practitioners regarding them? Perhaps the key to understanding them better lies in the routines themselves. The purpose of this article is to look at the technical relationship between these two. The templates of both routines are very similar.

History
The founder of Goju-ryu, Miyagi Chojun, was born in Naha, Okinawa, on April 25, 1888. His family imported pharmaceuticals and was one of the wealthiest in Naha (Porta and McCabe, 1994:64; Higaonna, 1985:25). Miyagi began his martial arts training with Aragaki Ryuko when he was eleven years old. Three years later, Aragaki introduced his student to Higaonna Kanryo. As a youth, Higaonna had studied martial arts with Aragaki Seisho and Kojo Taitei (Hokama, 1998:36). Higaonna had also spent a number of years in Fuzhou, China, studying the martial arts with Ryu Ryu Ko (McCarthy, 1987:30; Higaonna 1985:22). Higaonna Kanryo's style has been called Nahate. Miyagi Chojun trained with Higaonna Kanryo until Higaonna's death in 1916. In that year, Miyagi also made his first trip to China to further his martial arts knowledge.

Miyagi Chojun used twelve routines (*kata*) as part of his training syllabus: Sanchin, Gekisai I, Gekisai II, Saifa, Shishochin, Sanseru, Seiunchin, Sesan, Sepai, Kururunfa, Suparinpei, and Tensho (Porta and McCabe, 1994:66). Of these, Miyagi was involved in the creation of four. Miyagi and Nagamine Shoshin created Gekisai I in 1940; Nagamine called it Fukyugata (Nagamine, 1976:104; Sells, 2000:227–228). Miyagi alone created Gekisai II. Miyagi revised the breathing exercise Sanchin that Higaonna Kanryo taught him. And the routine considered his masterpiece, Tensho, was based on the Rokkishu (Higaonna, 1985:26), which is found in the old Chinese martial arts text, *Bubishi* (McKenna, 2000:38). It is believed that the other Goju-ryu routines were passed down from Higaonna Kanryo, who had learned them from Ryu Ryu Ko in Fuzhou, China (Higaonna, 1986:15).

In 1885, Higaonna Kanryo brought Sanseru from Fuzhou (Sells, 2000:275), but its lineage after that is uncertain. In the postscript of the translation of Miyagi's "Outline of Karate-do," Kinjo Hiroshi states, ". . . the fighting tradition established by master Miyagi was based upon the southern *kung-fu* [*gongfu*] style which his teacher Higaonna Kanryo had brought from Fuzhou. . ." (Miyagi, 1934:26).

There is some question as to whether Miyagi learned Sanseru from Higaonna. It seems that Higaonna taught Sanseru to Kyoda Juhatsu, his senior student, but not to Miyagi (McKenna, 2000:39, 42). Miyagi learned a different version elsewhere, possibly during one of his trips to China or from an Okinawan source other than Higaonna.

Some historians also believe that Higaonna brought Shishochin back from China (Sells, 2000:274). But Richard Kim, in his article "Shorinji ryu: An overview of all karate kata" and in one of his lectures at Guelph University, Ontario, Canada, says that only the Goju-ryu students of Miyagi train in Shishochin (Kim, 1992:15).

If Miyagi Chojun did not learn Sanseru from Higaonna, then he might not have learned Shishochin from him either. Either both routines came from the same source (other than Higaonna), or Miyagi Chojun created Shishochin after learning Sanseru from that other source.

Over the years, the personal students of Miyagi Chojun have said little about their teacher and his teacher before him. Perhaps they also followed the attitude of Kanzaki Shigekazu, one of Kyoda Juhatsu's students, who thought that it was impolite to ask questions about Higaonna Kanryo (McKenna, 2000:54).

Miyagi Chojun, the only man who knew the origins of the Goju-ryu routines stated, "The only detail we can be sure of is that during the eleventh year of Bunsei [1828] a Chinese system from Fuzhou unfurled and was studied deeply, and from which Goju-ryu karate kempo ascended" (Miyagi, 1934:21).[1] With Miyagi's death in 1953, the origins of the Goju-ryu kata, and especially the relationship between Sanseru and Shishochin, will never be certain.

Comparing Techniques from Shishochin and Sanseru

Higaonna Morio has said that Shishochin was a favorite routine of Miyagi Chojun in his latter years (1986:113). Shishochin means "Four Directional Battle" and concentrates on four-directional fighting, consisting of open-hand strikes: spear-hand and palm strikes (Yagi, 2000:82).

Sanseru uses very strong attacking techniques. Written in Chinese characters, *Sanseru* means the number "36."

> The theme of the two routines is the same at the beginning.
> Both Shishochin and Sanseru start with three steps forward
> in an hour-glass stance (*sanchin dachi*).

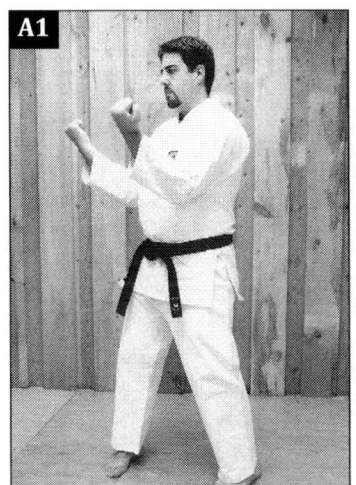 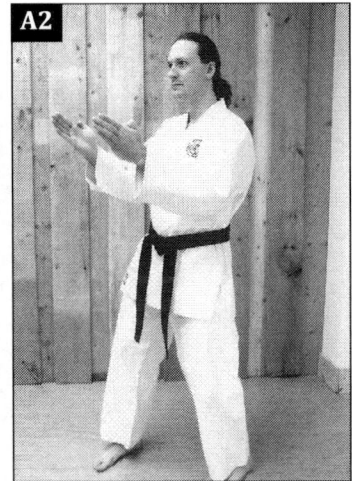

A1: Sanseru—uses closed fists. A2: Shishochin—uses open hand strikes.

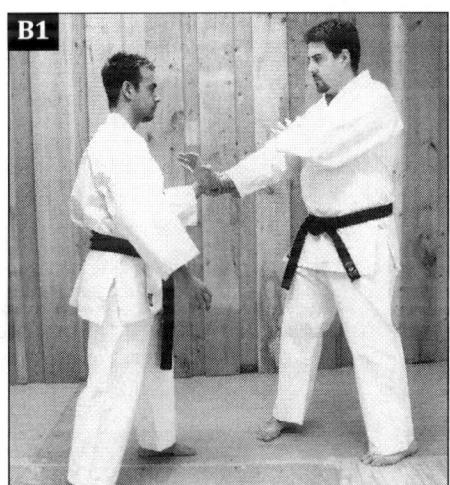 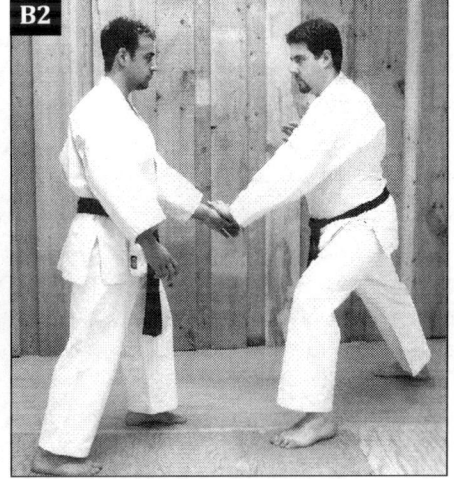

B1–2: Sanseru—a technique to release from a hand grab.

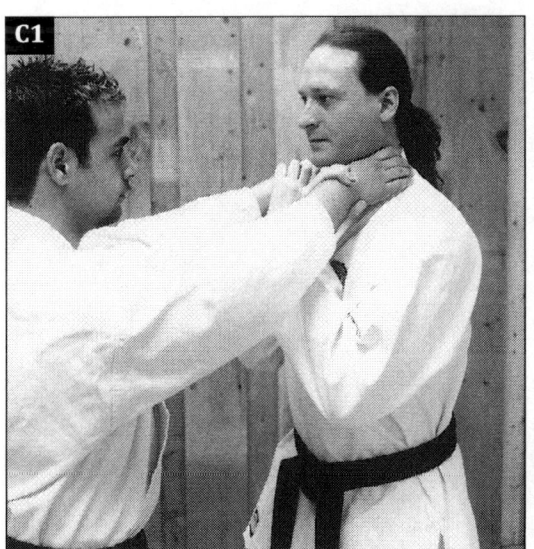 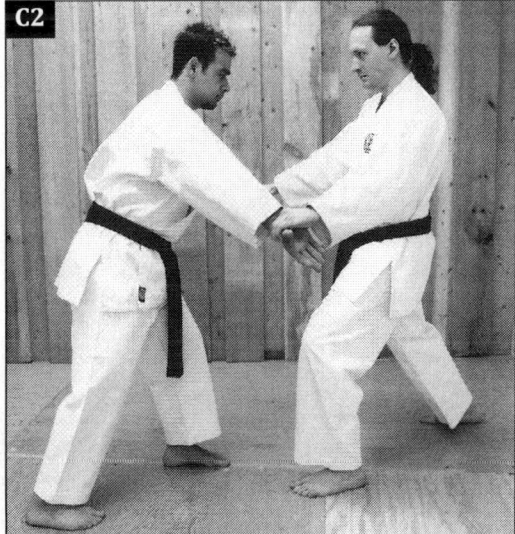

C1–2 Shishochin—a technique to release from a choke.

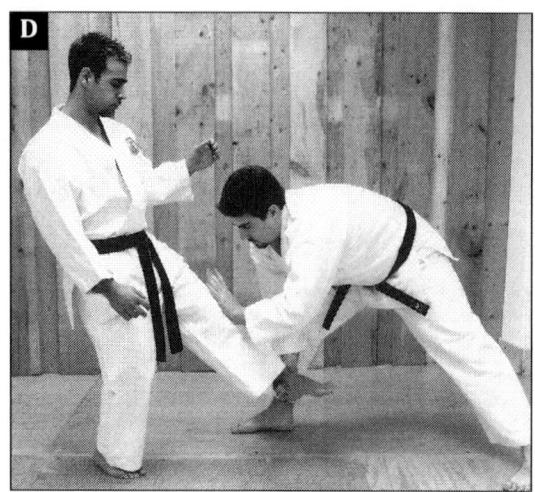
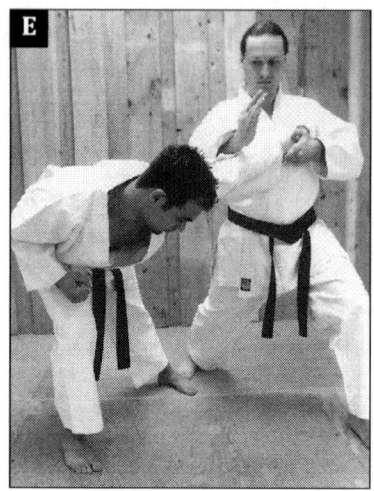

D: Sanseru—attacking an opponent's knee. E: Shishochin—attacking an opponent's elbow.

The next two Shishochin movements are not connected to the Sanseru routine, but they do not negate this chapter's premise. The Shishochin elbow attack is repeated on the left side using the left forearm. Then Shishochin brings the feet together and attacks with the right elbow (or punches over the shoulder, depending on the interpretation).

Now the routines work against each other. While Sanseru kicks north, Shishochin blocks and strikes south (F). Then Sanseru kicks south, and Shishochin blocks and strikes north. Sanseru turns and kicks east; Shishochin blocks and strikes west. Then, Sanseru kicks west, and Shishochin blocks and strikes east. If you could overlay diagrams of the Sanseru and Shishochin movements, and view them from above, you can see the connection.

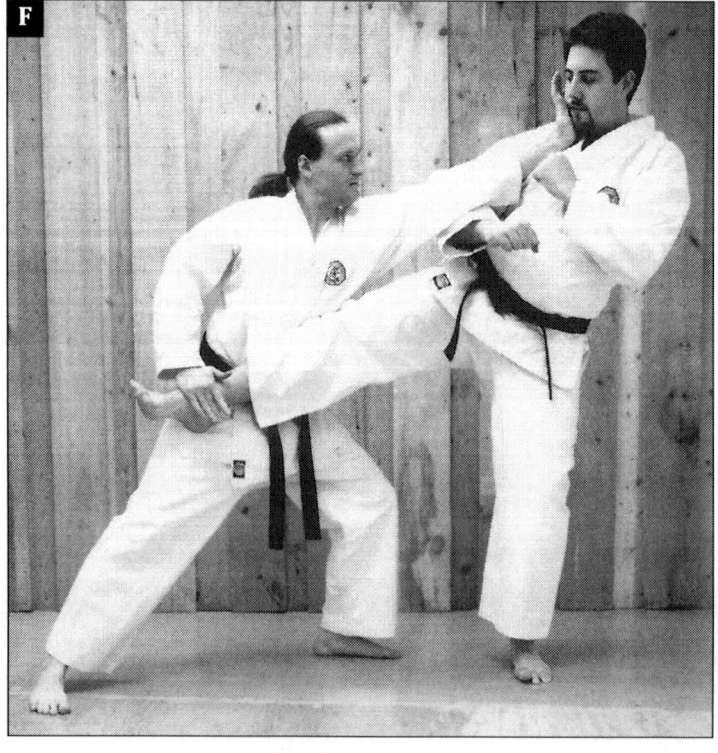

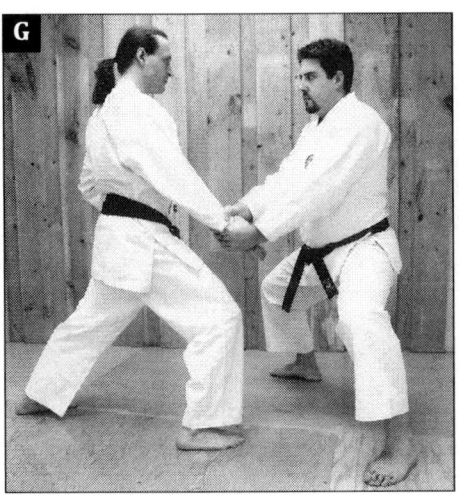 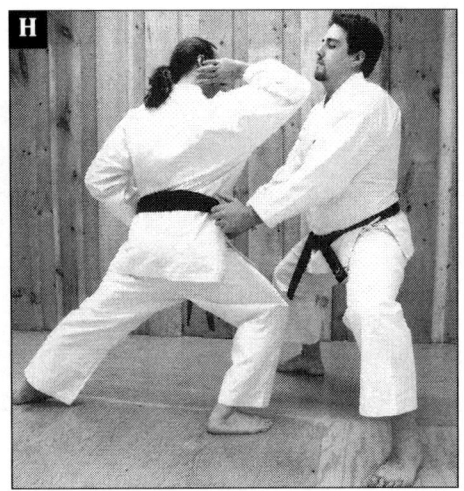

G–H: Shishochin's release and counter against Sanseru's double hand grab.

The next two movements are not in a complementary sequence, but are consistent as far as their application. After Sanseru's fourth front kick, the practitioner shifts into a modified horse stance (*shiko dachi*) with the hands crossed and down, facing south. The application of this movement could be a wrist grab against Shishochin's move facing north (G). Then, Shishochin's reaction to Sanseru's wrist grab is to pull the hand up and hit with the elbow (H). Sanseru's next movement is a lapel grab facing north in a horse stance (I). Shishochin then steps into a cat stance (*neko ashi dachi*) facing south, breaks the grip, and steps in doing a head butt (J).

I–J: Shishochin's release from a lapel grab and the head butt counter.

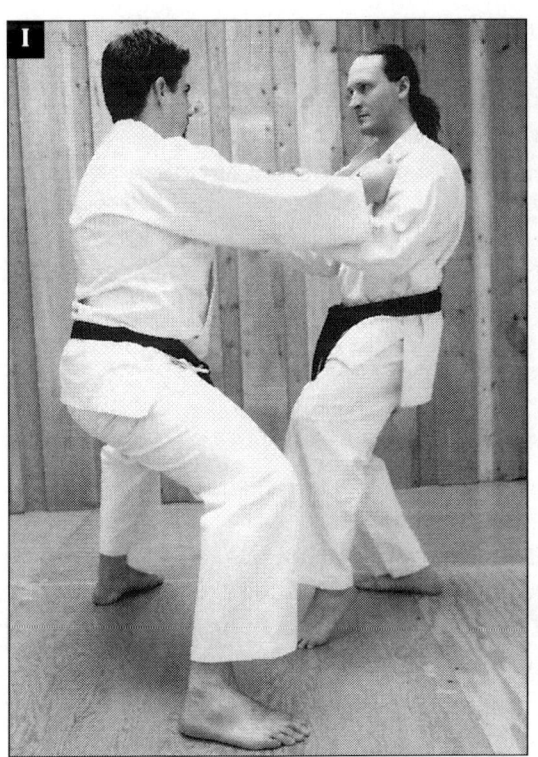 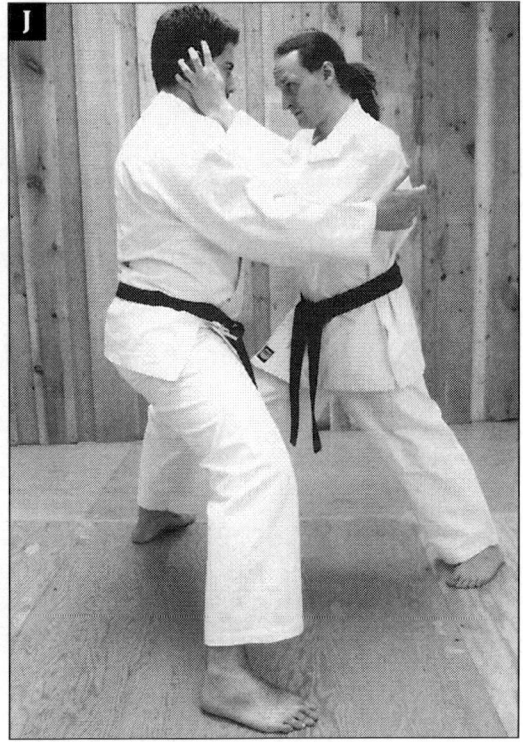

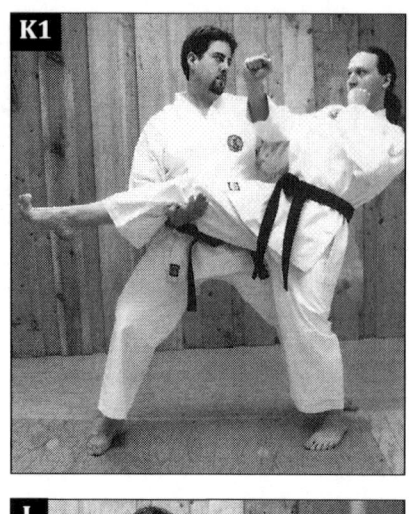
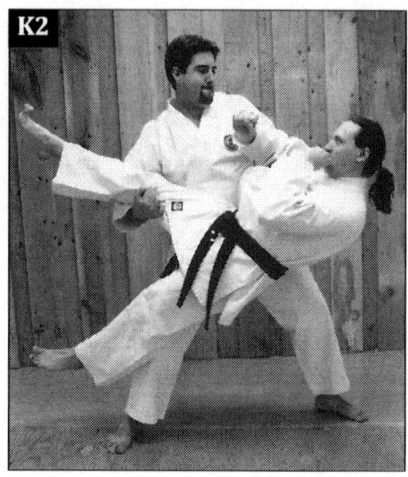
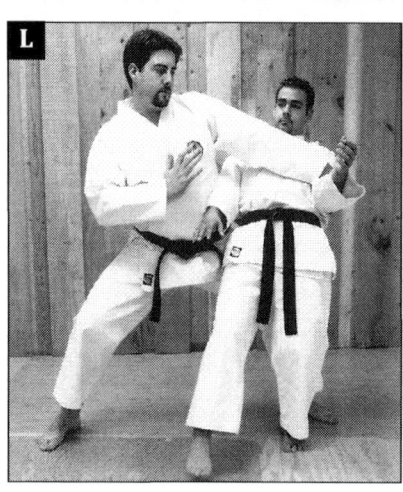
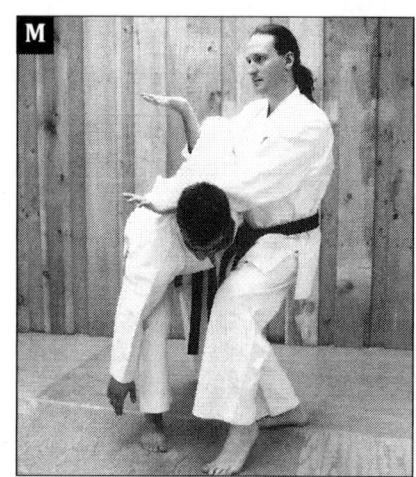

Shishochin then kicks to the east. Sanseru responds by grabbing the kicking leg (K1) and sweeping Shishochin's support leg to complete the throw (K2). Shishochin kicks again, and Sanseru counter with the same throw. Again, if you overlay these movements and view them from above, you can see the connection.

The two movements before the final movement of Shishochin are supplementary in that they are not connected to Sanseru, but serve to balance the routine. They do not affect the premise of this chapter. These movements are two more elbow breaks: one with the left forearm and one with the right, both facing south; then stepping into *musuba dachi* (heels together, toes apart) with a left elbow (or punch over the shoulder), again facing south.

The last technique in both Sanseru and Shishochin are throws (L–M).

Conclusion

Sanseru and Shishochin relate in two ways. First, we see that parts of one routine act as the application of the other. At some point perhaps that is what Shishochin was: a drill to practice some of the applications of Sanseru. Shishochin has also been supplemented with movements—such as the releases, joint attacks, and takedowns—at the beginning and end that are similar in theme to Sanseru. The similarities in Sanseru and Shishochin substantiate the idea that these two Goju-ryu routines are related.[2]

Notes

[1] Perhaps Miyagi was referring to Sakiyama Kitoku and Nakaima Kenri, both from Naha, Okinawa, who may have trained in China before Higaonna Kanryo (Sells, 2000:43).

[2] One of Miyagi Chojun's senior students, Yagi Meitoku, has created five additional routines. Tenshi can be split into two forms that work against each other; one is the application of the other. The pairs Byakko and Seiryu and Genbu and Shujakku work in the same way. Perhaps Miyagi also passed down the idea of one form holding the applications of another.

Bibliography

Higaonna, M. (1985). *Traditional karate do Okinawa Goju-ryu, Vol. 1*. Toyko: Minato Research and Publishing Co.

Higaonna, M. (1986). *Traditional karate do Okinawa Goju-ryu Vol. 2*. Toyko: Minato Research and Publishing Co.

Hokama, T. and Borkowski, C. (Trans.) (1998). *History and traditions of Okinawan karate*. Hamilton, Ontario: Masters Publication.

Kim, R. (1992, Fall). Shorinji ryu: An overview of all kata forms. *Budo Dojo*: 13–16.

McCarthy, P. (1987). *Classical kata of Okinawan karate*. Santa Clarita, CA: Ohara Publications.

McCarthy, P. (1995). *The bible of karate, Bubishi*. Rutland, VT: Tuttle.

McKenna, M. (2000), To'on-ryu: A glimpse into karate-do's roots. *Journal of Asian Martial Arts, 9*(3), 32–43.

McKenna, M. (2000) Kanzaki Shigekazu: An interview with To'on-ryu's leading representative. *Journal of Asian Martial Arts, 9*(3), 45–57.

Miyagi, C., and International Ryukyu Karate Research Society (Trans.) (1934). Karate-doh Gaisetsu: An outline of karate-doh. Yokohama, Japan: International Ryukyu Karate Research Society.

Nagamine, S. (1976). The essence of Okinawan karate do. Rutland, VT: Tuttle.

Porta, J., and McCabe, J. (1994). The karate of Chojun Miyagi. *Journal of Asian Martial Arts, 3*(3), 62–71.

Sells, J. (2000). *Unante: The secrets of karate*. Hollywood, CA: W.M. Hawley.

Yagi, M. (2000). *Okinawan karate do Goju-ryu Meibukan*. Dundas, Ontario: Yagi-Wheeler-Vickerson, L.T. Designs Ltd.

Acknowledgment

A special thanks goes to Corey Belliveau, Carry Smith, and Lawrence Macoretta for appearing in the photos; to Wai Hung Tang for taking the photos; to Olga Toth for setting up the photos and to Lisa Toth and Cam McGill for proof reading the article. Great appreciation also goes to Sensei Richard Kim for his guidance.

chapter 35

Isshin Kempo: Isshin-ryu's Missing Link to the Internal

by Christopher Goedecke, B.S.

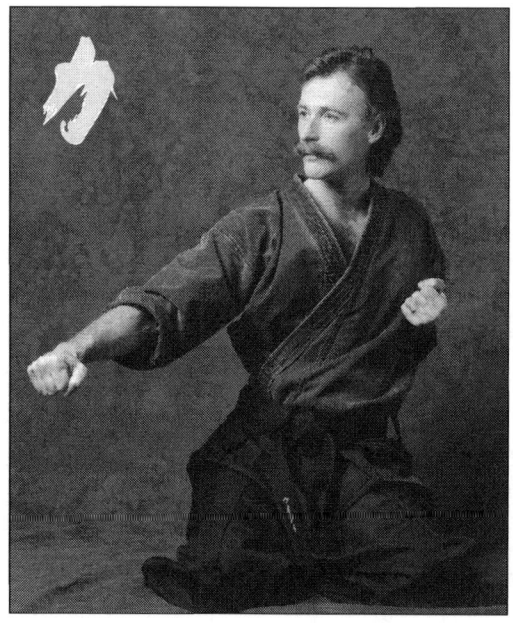

Set within the author's portait is the character *chikara* (energy, force, power) which is used as the logo on the Isshin Kempo promotional certificate.
Illustrations courtesy of C. Goedecke.

To understand the thirty-year history of Isshin Kempo, one needs to begin with three premises about the Okinawan system of Isshin-ryu karate formally introduced to the Ryukyu martial art community in 1956:

1) Shimabuku Sanchin, Isshin-ryu's founder, may not have completed his system. Thus, his unfinished business remains part of his legacy.
2) Isshin-ryu may have been under-interpreted by Shimabuku's early American disciples and hence their followers, perpetuating several martial generation
with blind spots of unrevealed and latent teachings.
3) Shimabuku Tatsuo may have invited only a select few Americans, if any at all, into the inner teachings of his style. This refers to the relationship of *ki* (internal energy) to kata and then, that of ki-infused kata to combat. Internal work is the art within and behind the hard surface performance of karate-do practice.

If any one of the above three premises is true, then Shimabuku left a large portion of the Isshin-ryu community to fend for themselves with a less than full deck of martial principles and ample room for growth.

For thirty years, Isshin Kempo has reflected upon these three premises searching for deeper insights into its own Isshin-ryu foundation.

In an interview with Frank Van Lenten – American Goju-ryu master and Goshin-do Karate Association founder and president (who Shimabuku also awarded high rank in 1970) – the imposing, ex-Marine stated that it was Shimabuku Tatsuo who first taught the young, buck sergeant about internal power when he studied at Shimabuku's Agena dojo in 1959 (Goedecke, 1992:50). When pressed during this interview as to what Shimabuku specifically revealed about internal energy, Van Lenten unhesitatingly replied that only his advanced black belts were privy to such knowledge (Van Lenten, 1988). Van Lenten and others lend credence to the idea that Shimabuku well knew of energy management methods (Lennox, 1980: 215). Van Lenten alluded only that he was instructed in how to alter his body temperature.

Closed door arts exist, particularly among the tighter-knit Asian family systems to guard such inner teachings. A system's quintessential teachings or family "jewels" are sometimes referred to as hidden teachings (*kuden*). Tomio Nagaboshi (adopted name of Terence Dukes), British martial scholar and head of the British Mushindo Kempo Association (a Buddhist-based classical martial arts organization), described the concept of kuden in a lecture at the Hakuren Temple in 1983: "Many teachings are not complete without kuden. A true kuden is a living interactive event which, because it can only be generated and transmitted from within the special relationship and experiential history developed between a teacher and his student, loses all significance to an outsider" (Tomio, N., 1983).

An unusual incident that occurred on the evening of February 18, 1998 illustrates the uniqueness of one level of kuden. Fifteen-year Isshin Kempo practitioner and former yoga instructor K. Smith relates that while in the locker room one day, his teacher mentioned Smith's black belt held a unique power. To demonstrate, Smith was requested to place his belt aside and assume a horse ridding stance (*kiba dachi*). His teacher directed an athletic brown belt to unbalance the black belt by pushing against his leg. With difficulty, Smith was forced several inches backward.

The instructor then requested Smith to put on a white belt and resist again. Surprisingly, the brown belt "easily" moved the black belt out of his stance. Asking for a retest, Smith was again summarily uprooted. The moment he placed his black belt around his waist, however, the brown belt could not budge him regardless of how hard he tried. When the two men asked for an explanation, Smith recalls being told that there were internal principles currently outside of his grasp.

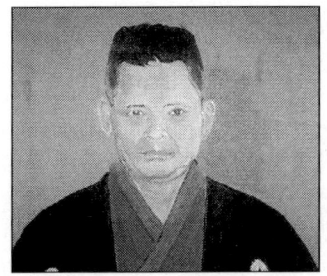 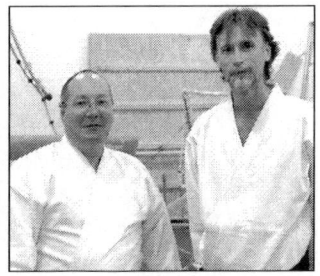

Left: The author's pastel painting of Isshin-ryu karate founder, Shimabuku Tatsuo.
Right: Tomio Arakawa and the author, September of 2000.

No matter how powerful the body or mind, without knowledge of the full spectrum of human potential, of the complex intertwining of the mental/emotional, physical, and spiritual energies, one is not using a full deck of martial principles. Though one may easily win battles against his opponents, this will often be the result of others holding fewer cards. Whether this incident was a result of a well-crafted mental suggestion, a hidden internal dynamic, or the actual effects of one's belt and/or mental attachments to it, the results unfolded as predicted. One man was weaker in the face of his adversary. A relevant and observable martial puzzle had been imparted to elevate their perceptions and consciousness.

Tomio Arakawa, Tenshin Ryushin Buddhist master, 7th-degree black belt, and head of the Mushindo Kempo Association, USA, offers an educated observation based upon his forty-three years of study that Shimabuku did not live long enough to complete what he had in mind for his not fully matured karate style. According to Tomio, "Why would a master of Shorin descent, already considered a great master, create another karate ryu almost the same as Shorin extraction but intensify its [technique] to a higher, more scientific tier? He did not need two arts, one in the same, but instead sought to present distinctive aspects of karate-do. Isshin-ryu was meant to become the hierarchy of the Shorin 'te' lines which he would elevate his black belts to study" (Tomio, A., 2000).

The Isshin Kempo system holds that the Isshin-ryu kata are masterful compositions that cannot be penetrated without intensive study and guidance. It is questionable whether any of the post-war, American military black belts walked away with a profound understanding of Isshin-ryu because the average tour of duty was only sixteen to eighteen months. Most, regardless of their intelligence, would have been hard pressed to extract the deeper lessons inherent in the Isshin-ryu kata syllabi in such a short time frame. Isshin-ryu itself was the culmination of Shimabuku's thirty-eight years of prior training. In addition, students need their instructor's keys to open the unfamiliar doors to knowledge. Such keys were not easily forthcoming from Okinawan instructors. Many obstacles prevailed, the least of which was breaching the language barrier.

This observation is further substantiated in a 1984 interview given by long term American Isshin-ryu disciple Arsenio J. Advincula with three of Shimabuku's former senior Okinawan students (Kaneshi Eiko, Shigema Genyu, and Kaneshiro Kenji). Kaneshi, who began training at Shimabuku's Tairagawa dojo in 1947, left Tatsuo because he indiscriminately gave out first-, second-, and 3rd-degree ranking to, "Americans who came and learned for six months" (Advincula, 2001). He disagreed with Shimabuku's rationale to rank the Americans since they were going home. Unable to reconcile their perspectives, Kaneshi and others quit the Isshin-ryu founder's dojo. According to Kaneshi, "It took five years for an exceptional student to get [4th-degree] in their dojo and fifteen to twenty years for [5th-degree] and [6th-degree]. You can't make 1st degree in a year" (Advincula, 2001). Kaneshi was further disgruntled that the Americans didn't even understand "karate seishin," referring to the mental, spiritual, and moral precepts in their training, "... yet they made black belts" (Advincula, 2001).

The high ranking of Americans is not the core issue but rather a questionable inequity between the knowledge and the rank that so embittered Shimabuku's Okinawan hierarchy. If high rank did not equate with advanced skills, what then did the Americans leave with?

Kaneshiro cited additional insight that altered the American rank equation: "Americans thought they were strong. They would push for rank higher than the Okinawans. To the Okinawans, Americans did not even know how to pronounce karate much less understand it. When Americans went back to the States, they would proclaim their prowess in karate and explain it wrong. Diploma has nothing to do with karate. . . . I received my *kyoshi* [expert instructor] certificate two years ago [1982, over 32 years after starting with Shimabuku]. We're not after certificates, we do it for health and heart. . . . In karate on Okinawa, there are few *judan* [10th-degree]. Americans think if you fight and win, you are an expert. If this is all there is to it then the strongest in the world are the best. Strength and power is not enough for judan. . . ." (Advincula, 1984).

American Isshin-ryu instructor Harold Long remarked in an interview about his personal study with Shimabuku, that although he received a high rank (6th degree) from Shimabuku in just nineteen months of intensive training, in his words, ". . .you will find that I had the equivalent of twenty years training during that time period" (Long and McGhee, 1977:279). Reasonable American pioneers the forefathers who set the standards for "future" generations of students?

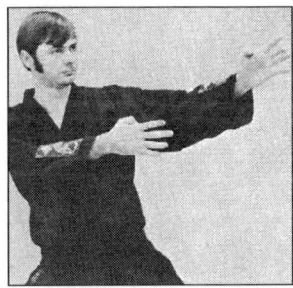
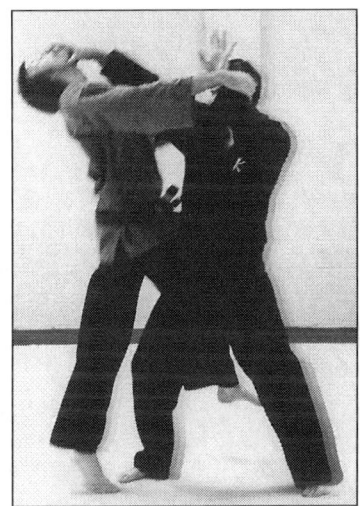
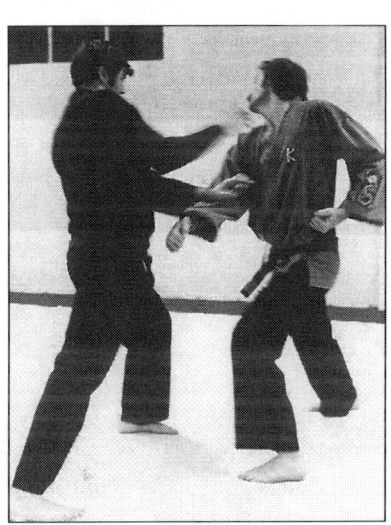

Above: Isshin Kempo founder, W. Scott Russell, in the early 1970's. Right: Russell demonstrates hand techniques on the author in the 1970's at the Livingston Isshin Kempo Dojo.

Those early pioneering black belts who became teachers, for better or worse, impacted their systems, often reshaping either the curriculum or the foundations upon which the teachings reside. A teacher's fundamental system of beliefs, techniques, teaching methods, strategies, and concepts form each martial arts style's unique expression. It is impossible for any martial artist not to put his or her particular spin on their system. In that spin, new perspectives are gained, some lost; techniques are polished, others dulled; and curiosities and questions naturally emerge. Realistically, the quest to advance is generally uneven. The martial arts themselves then enter into the fray of surviving their own founder, successors, and student body. It becomes a martial art "survival of the fittest."

Birth of a Martial Art

Isshin Kempo has entered that survival role. The fledgling system was founded in 1971 by a charismatic and controversial martial artist, William Scott Russell. Born in a tough New Jersey neighborhood, Russell was no stranger to street fights. He once confided to his senior instructor, Jay Austin, that he left most of his teeth on the streets. Russell's parents had him train as a youth with welterweight Golden Gloves boxer Dan "Danny Man" Sophman, who held an impressive 40–0 record. Coupling his street experience with supervised boxing training, Russell then pursued an interest in the growing popularity of martial arts by studying Okinawan karate. By the early 1970's, Russell had assumed the head instructorship of the pioneering Bank Street School in

Summit, New Jersey. This school saw several of the state's top martial teachers pass through its doors, including Bob Murphy, Isshin Shorinji-ryu; Gary Alexander, Isshin-ryu; Shimamoto Mamoru, judo; Edward Doyle, Isshin-ryu; Tony Franco, Hung Gar; and Tom Bisio, xingyi and taijiquan.

In evaluating his early martial roots, Russell had begun to make several observations about Isshin-ryu kata performance. It appeared over stylized, hence unrealistic and disconnected from actual combat rhythm. In addition, few Isshin-ryu men moved like their forms in free sparring (*jiu kumite*). Russell found this incongruous. He thought the Isshin-ryu system itself was well-constructed, but that the American comprehension lacked depth and dynamism. This was also Bruce Lee's observation about form in general, leading to his infamous comment that kata was nothing more than "organized despair" (Lee, 1975:14).

Rather than dismiss kata outright, as Lee did, Russell sought to bring kata and sparring closer together. Russell would often say that kata should reflect combat and combat should reflect kata. To compensate for the performance rigidity, he emphasized suppleness to generate a more relaxed and fluid torso motion aimed at overcoming Isshin-ryu's over-stylized, stiff, and staccato-like movements. Isshin Kempo tournament kata performers of the 1970's fared as well as other styles. But there was a distinctly different quality to the emphasis placed upon their kata moves that separated them from their Isshin-ryu counterparts. At one regional tournament this distinction was painfully obvious as one judge disavowed all three of the Isshin Kempo's top kata performers. Although their skills were duly noted and praised by both fellow competitors and spectators, they received perversely low scores. When questioning the central judge, he asserted that, "no one could pull off the moves that fast!"

Early Isshin Kempo training emphasized flat out speed. Controversy surrounded Russell's radical choice of training methods to encourage such high octane performance. The "gauntlet" was a grueling and barbaric rite of passage. Two columns of up to twenty men per side, standing several feet apart, would intercept a single defender whose task was to race down the center while deflecting or avoiding a barrage of kicks and punches. Some men were knocked unconscious or blasted through the living wall.

At another point in the early years of Isshin Kempo's training regime, Russell appeared on the mat with a cow prod. His goal was to stimulate adrenaline flow and switch on the sympathetic nervous system to expedite the fight response (flight was not an option). This was Russell's modern and most controversial version of the cold waterfall technique used by Asian masters to familiarize karate men with shocks to their central nervous system (Ratti and Westbrook, 1973:413). The objective was to simulate and acclimatize the body to the stressors of battlefield realities. The mere sight of the live voltage, steel baton was enough to mentally jolt most students into intensified knee-jerk reactions. Even the slow students found it in themselves to shave fractions off their reaction time when Russell stood behind them with the baton turned on.

Russell once commented that his goal to turn out competent fighters was to place as much stress upon the students that they could bear. Quoting from his book on generating power through martial arts, Russell stated, internal energy "is the product of stress. And the more intense the stress, the more chi [sic] is liberated for use. The more energy, or [ki], a man needs, the more he will have—assuming all systems function properly. This is a natural, normal phenomenon. There is nothing strange or mystical about it" (Russell, 1976:43).

After slowly rehearsing applications, Russell's students were expected to execute them with real time speed and intensity. During free sparring, it was not uncommon to see blood, and broken bones. These were the days just prior to the advent of protective gear. The school was tough and the training overall was grueling. Classes generally lasted two to three hours. The school was open six days a week. In one year alone the Bank Street school boasted of over 1,000 students in its yearly membership, which this author can verify.

As the charismatic Russell built up his following and his line of upper belts at the Bank Street School, he became particularly intrigued by Isshin-ryu's internal dimensions. He subsequently wrote, Karate, the Energy Connection (Dell, 1973), in which he began to outline the diverse benefits he saw from tapping into what he referred to as the Sanchin "supercharger." Russell likened the internal aspect of his art to a supercharged car engine. Where most karate practitioners were driving around with normal 4-6 cylinder engines, the hidden resources of internal training unleashed a souped-up V-8 power house of additional energy.

Through an affiliation with the late Shorinji Tetsuken style's successor, Albert C. Church, Russell was recognized founder of his evolving Isshin Kempo system. Russell spent the last two decades of his life further developing mental concepts and internal teachings under a system he later referred to as *kyodan* (best standards).

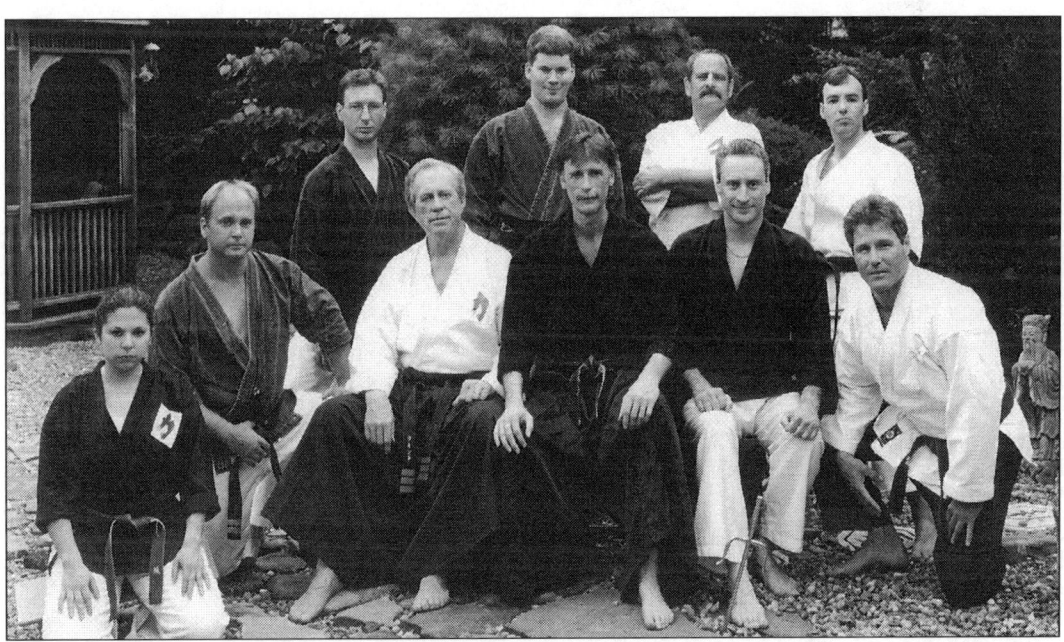

Depicted are senior members of the Isshin Kempo black belts. Each member has a minimum of 15–33 years of training, the most senior called the "Sanchin Seven." The name "Sanchin Seven" refers to the seven energy management principles permeating the three layers of human existence under one heart (accord). Left to right: Veronika Bellezza, Tom Lyons, Kevin Smith (standing, black jacket), Joe Noonan (seated, white jacket), Jeff Balbirnie (standing, black jacket), Chris Goedecke, John Kralovenec (standing, white jacket), Jay Austin (seated, white pants), Tim Smith (standing, white jacket), Ivan Geldzahler (kneeling). Photo by Bruce Berenson.

Sanchin Seven

That controversial first decade of training has given way to more sober-headed training methods and research over the last two decades. W. Scott Russell, who became more reclusive over the last decade of his life, passed away in late 1999. However, his work has continued to branch out with a seasoned group of senior black belts referred to as the "Sanchin Seven."

The basic premises about Isshin-ryu have been greatly illuminated through the Seven's on-going research. Isshin Kempo has cultivated its own family jewels and will follow in the footsteps of other closed door systems offering its deeper insights to select black belts.

The Three Spheres

Isshin Kempo has reached into classical martial art training (*budo*) values for solutions to the primary conflicts that exist both on the mat and in everyday life, for the dojo has always been viewed as a microcosm of the larger world and thus provides a well-equipped laboratory in which to study human nature. "True budo is about obtaining spiritual liberation over ego dominance, and scientific prominence over brute force on the battlefield," stated Tomio Arakawa (2000).

To accomplish these goals, the Isshin Kempo system encompasses three interlocking spheres of internal study. The first deals with training the perceptions to enhance awareness and to elevate practical combat skills. The second involves spiritual practices to help students comprehend the larger agenda and meaning of their actions. The third consists of specific inner energy development and manipulation to strengthen technique and to maximize control over conflicted engagements.

To continually remain "in the fight," that is, within a conflicted arena, is not the end point of martial training. The goal is to transcend conflict and friction whenever feasible. Looking into the martial past one can see that battlefield strategies, techniques and philosophical dilemmas had already been worked out to fine detail. Stripping down martial arts training to a bare minimum of strategy or techniques may have its place, however, it is a small one in the more comprehensive and life-centering martial arts study.

In an age of awakening spiritual potential, the United States is experiencing a growing movement of marital artists (still a minority) who are seeking out the spiritual wisdoms and the hidden technical dimensions within their disciplines. Classical martial arts study was and is a way of life because it enhances a way of being that leads to penetrating realizations about achieving both outer and inner peace. When balanced thought is transformed into action, obstacles and/or opponents can be re-moved toward achieving a deep and lasting harmony.

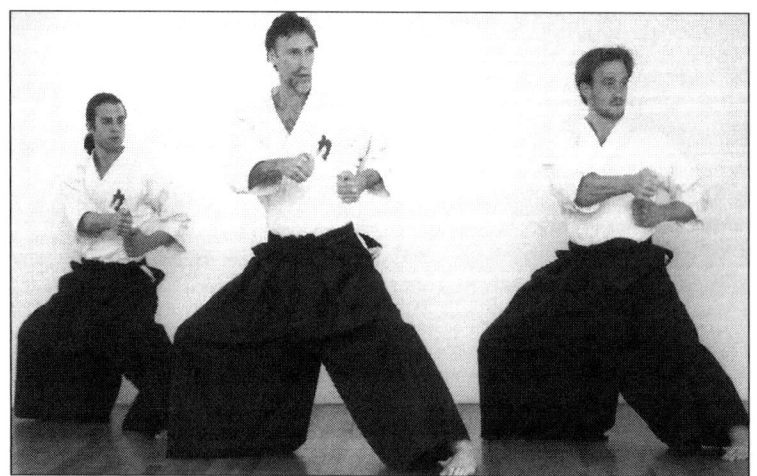

Chinto kata training.

A spiritually astute warrior understands that only when one is complete in one's self is the right energy signature left upon the battlefield. Injuring, or taking another's life is a "violation" that has far reaching consequences outside of the immediately vanquished or victorious combatants. People form an intricate web of energy exchange and relationships. To end or debilitate a life physically, or even emotionally, is to substantially alter a wider range of other lives. According to B.K. Frantzis, "Without morality, the true process of spiritual martial arts cannot begin" (Frantzis, 1998:12). One must have a correct spiritual attunement to injure or take a life, or one's karma is significantly altered. Americans have been too cavalier in determining martial value. Many romanticize their martial practice. These distorted, media-influenced perspectives make combat and death look appealing by glossing over the real anguish, intensity, damage, and trauma that occurs. This results in arts losing their way; becoming myopic; and serving only limited, one dimensional ends.

To avoid a short-sighted downfall, Isshin Kempo invites its student body into a broad, rounded perspective of martial life and training values.

Perception

The Japanese term different types of insight as ken. Kata work was designed to yield a type of insight called *jiken*, according to Tomio Nagaboshi, while kumite fostered another kind of insight called *taken*. Together, kata and kumite balance and fuse the initiate's insides with his outsides. Kata is the internal *kumite* (exchange). Free-form sparring is its external compliment. "*Jiken* refers to insights into one's own being. Taken refers to insights into other's being. Both of these are indispensable and they are likened to the right and left hands. Each has its own special provenance, particularities and relevance which works in different manners to pierce fictions of the ego, induce inner harmony and develop that confidence borne of a real self understanding. This is the only self understanding worthy of attainment" (Tomio, N., 1995).

Kata work is the paramount and core training focus in Isshin Kempo. The Isshin-ryu kata syllabus is the main teaching forum. The empty-hand forms are Seisan, Seiuchin, Wansu, Naihanchi, Chinto, Kusanku, Sunsu, Sanchin, and Tensho (the circular sister-compliment to Sanchin's linear principles).

By attending to kata detail at increasingly higher levels of performance, awareness and bodily strength is refined. Attention is first directed inward to the practitioner's own physical capabilities and sensations before an outward or opponent-focus is encouraged. Through repeated and mindful form practice, students learn to remain "in the kata" (i.e., in the present moment) without distraction and alert to all static and transitional changes. This prolonged focus over years eventually coordinates breath patterns, weight shiftings, torque, balance, and proximal relationships of the limbs. In this regard, kata work places a student in a meditative relationship with his body. This on-going dialogue between bodily sensations and mental cognitions, over time, redresses significant inequities between the two centers of head and center (*hara*). The resultant accord is the reason that hara is referred to as the psycho-physiological power center of the body (Ratti and Westbrook, 1973:410).

Furthermore, musculo-skeletal re-alignment and meridian flow rebalance is complimented with a Chinese kenpo yoga training regime. One's awareness is continually expanded by its ever-deepening entwinement with the details of the body postures leading to the development of a strategically advantageous meta-cognition. Improved concentration and focus also leads to a kinesthetic or "felt sense" of the body. This lays the groundwork of sensitivity necessary for advanced technical mechanics and an awareness of ki flow for later conscious manipulation.

Too often kata are overlooked or devalued due to a lack of apparent combat connectedness, relegated to dance or mere dojo decor. The late, respected Shorin-ryu master, Nagamine Shoshin, took a strong, pro-kata stance by stating bluntly, "If there is no kata, there is no karate, just kicking and punching" (2000:xvii). Homogenizing kata in the U.S. has caused an unfortunate shift away from what is then misperceived as flat, solo routines, refocusing instead on the growing modern trend of seeking kick-boxing, adrenaline highs. Free sparring has its place in martial arts practice but it is one of a triune of facets that comprise the complete Isshin Kempo path. The "Way" of karate study is about "getting whole," not getting high. Nagaboshi further states, sparring ". . . shows us how to sedate the body in order to see the mind whereas kata teaches us how to sedate the mind in order to see the body. If we can achieve this a different kind of seeing arises—one which is unrestricted by our physical or mental patterns and habits. Such a 'seeing' is often termed a 'flowing' insight" (Tomio, N., 1995).

Spiritual Training

In spiritual training, attitude takes precedence over behavior. A rightful, balanced attitude defines a person's actions. A cultivated mental composure often distinguishes the mediocre from the great student of the Way (*do-ka*). When a student's attitude is elevated or refocused upon acting out human virtues; when one is just, sincere, authentic, compassionate, and sensitive, the body complies with a superior and centered force of being. Attitudes also generate energy vibrations that influence immediate and future karmic outcomes in subtle ways.

Spirituality emerges from out of the stillness and silence of being through an internally active and dynamic meditative process. Isshin Kempo utilizes three spiritual-based techniques: still (seated or standing) meditation to cultivate an inner calm; moving meditation (*kata*), to cultivate an active, external calm; and psycho-spiritual based dialectic to challenge, delineate, reorganize, and integrate a student's physical, psychic/emotional, and spiritual layers.

Martial systems are controlled, to a large extent, by their teachers. Teachers set the tone and temper of a class and the direction of its teachings. A gentle, firm and alert demeanor is the hallmark of the true martial arts master. Martial schools are top-down organizations. If the top is grounded, the disciples will find their way with appropriately applied effort. If the top is dysfunctional, the way will be long, hard, and mostly obscured. Shimabuku was a spiritual man, a strict Zen Buddhist (Evseeff and Murphey, 1996:191). Isshin Kempo nourishes its spiritual roots by setting examples of maturity, composure, and responsibly applied power amongst its own hierarchy and by offering practices that provide both a mirror and a doorway for a deeper understanding and expression of one's human nature.

Internal Energy Work

Although the ground work is laid in the early levels of development, ki work in Isshin Kempo begins in earnest at 1st-degree black belt level, after the system's basic mechanical elements have been mastered. In deferring this insertion point for internal work to the black belt level grades, senior black belt Joseph Noonan explains, "It takes years to build up the appropriate sensitivity through the various bodily relationships of bone to muscle to nerves to blood to organs, and to overcome mental illusions to begin properly advancing in the internal dynamics of the Isshin Kempo system" (Noonan, 2001).

Paramount to Isshin Kempo is the kata Sanchin. Sanchin has been translated to mean "three conflicts" or "three battles" (Evseeff and Murphey, 1996: 124). This form was designed to work out a three-tiered matrix of internal and external combat variables existing within and between the physical, mental, and spiritual dimensions. By invitation, black belts enter the "Sanchin corridor," crossing over from training in the body's mechanical systems to their energetic or bio-electric (referring to direct ki manipulation) compliment. At the upper levels, Sanchin's outer skin is explored. First and naturally, surface moves are memorized, then follows a sequence of tension/relaxation drills to acquaint one to the body's dynamic power-to-weight musculo-skeletal relationships. At black belt level, one is then brought inside to the form's core teachings. Most skilled black belts admit that after two years plumbing Sanchin's internal depth, they are just skimming a vast interior and all, to date, unequivocally affirm, they can never perform their karate the same.

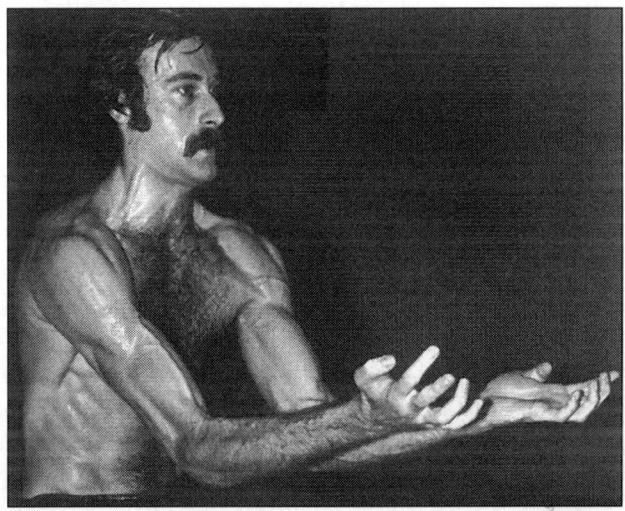

Author practicing Sanchin Kata in 1973 at the Livingston dojo. The Sanchin Kata has evolved as the primary training tool for the Issin Kempo black belts. Practitioners utilize the five element theory to unlock Sanchin's principles of the five directions, the three angles, the three attitudes or mental postures, the five categories of strikes and the eight tactical considerations.

Isshin Kempo's Sanchin departs dramatically from the "vein-popping," full-bore body tension of many Isshin-ryu stylists—a performance emphasis that has been criticized by some for damaging health (Bishop, 1999:36). We believe the Isshin-ryu community has grossly misunderstood Sanchin as a result of a prolonged indoctrination to its superficial lessons. Isshin Kempo has preserved the surface form of Shimabuku's kata but radically altered and expanded the understanding of its core purpose and internal execution.

Isshin Kempo black belts learn a natural progression of seven stages of energy management toward a self-mastery ideal. The first three levels comprise layers of concepts and techniques utilizing the principles of 1) direct confrontational forces, 2) yielding forces, and 3) complex torque forces. This is no small feat. Most of the world martial arts population rarely demonstrate skills beyond these three technical dimensions. Four additional internal levels dealing with specific ki manipulation are presented within Sanchin. Although to an outsider, Sanchin may appear a rather simple and direct martial pattern, internally, it is one of the most dynamic katas in existence today. According to British author Nathan Johnson, Sanchin "kata originated with the Shaolin tradition... where it remains simultaneously the primary and the most advanced boxing form for many Fukien-based systems" (Johnson, 1994:65).

Sanchin is virtually impenetrable to a karate practitioners with a conditioned consciousness. The Isshin-ryu community has summarily failed to penetrate its inner teachings. Rarely can one find more than a few pages written about this kata often described as the quintessential form without which no other form is necessary to understand the essence of karate. Tomio Nagaboshi further asserts that few, if any, Okinawan masters (let alone American masters, in the author's opinion) knew of or taught Sanchin's core lessons (1994:475-6).

No doubt, Sanchin was designed to both reference a complex of combat concepts and techniques and to camouflage its deeper spiritual rationale from a society too often conditioned to exclusively accept surface explanations.

Isshin Kempo avoids abstractions, generalizations, mystical or obtuse language. This does not contribute to either a system's or its kata's longevity. Within the Isshin Kempo kata hierarchy there are specific, empirical teachings about Sanchin currently unpublished and unknown to the general Isshin-ryu community.

Nourishing Roots

The inquisitive may be left with a cliffhanger. If closed door systems remain shut, how does one know if such higher level information exists at all? It's a justifiable challenge raising a central issue regarding the study of martial arts in general. Who should be privy to what knowledge and why? According to Tomio Arakawa, "The only [martial artists] who were graced with what is known in the martial arts world as 'closed door systems' were the 'discipled' students who had lived and serviced the master over many years and who were the numbered few, mostly not more than eight to ten students who rose through the ranks and were no less, masters in their own rights" (Tomio, A., 2000).

In evaluating the evolution of martial styles, we must factor in that there are those teachers who are not looking for more in their arts because they simply believe they already possess it! There are others whose political and financial gains have taken precedence over their advancement. Also, Americans tend to feel that if certain knowledge exists, then it's simply theirs for the taking whether they fully grasp its essence or not. Some Western and Asian counterparts hold opposing perspectives, contending in an age-old cliché that, "the ceiling only goes up after the walls." Quite simply, it is a universal common sense among the martial hierarchy that there is a time and place for advanced knowledge and it is often only for those who've prepared their walls.

Those early American pioneers of the 1940's and 1950's certainly had, tenacity, fighting spirit and adequate tools in their straightforward Isshin-ryu fighting system. But studying an art for a few years under a master's tutelage is never going to leave one with the insights resulting from twenty or thirty years of "guided" practice. The work to perpetuate the Isshin arts is now left up to those contemporary masters and their disciples, here and abroad.

Isshin-ryu has undergone multiple splinterings since the founder's death (Eveseef and Murphy, 1996:43). These splinters have left the Isshin-ryu community fragmented and handicapped with occasional personalities taking center stage over profound insights into their future. Isshin Kempo is restoring Isshin's core teachings by assimilating classical training values and methods. In this adventure, much has been learned about Isshin-ryu's vast potential. Our new branch, claiming sustenance from past insights, current research, and Buddhist-based martial alliances, is growing steadily.

In one of the more radical opinions of Tomio Arakawa, "The work begun by Isshin Kempo's founder, W. S. Russell and currently being pursued by its advanced [black belts] may be intuiting the spiritual essence of a Buddhist monastic temple art that existed in the 16–17th century, coincidentally known as Isshin Kempo" (Tomio, A., 2000). It is this very spirit that will reinfuse vitality and meaning into Isshin Kempo's future.

As superficial and popular values of the fast food martial mentality dilute the essence of serious martial arts training, the Isshin Kempo system reaches back into classical martial values, dharma teachings and philosophical insights into combat, to enhance its martial base regarding the complex nature of engagements. "The various combinations possible in different situations and in the face of differing forms and sequences of attack were worked out in great and intricate detail by the various masters of Kempo" (Tomio, N., 1983).

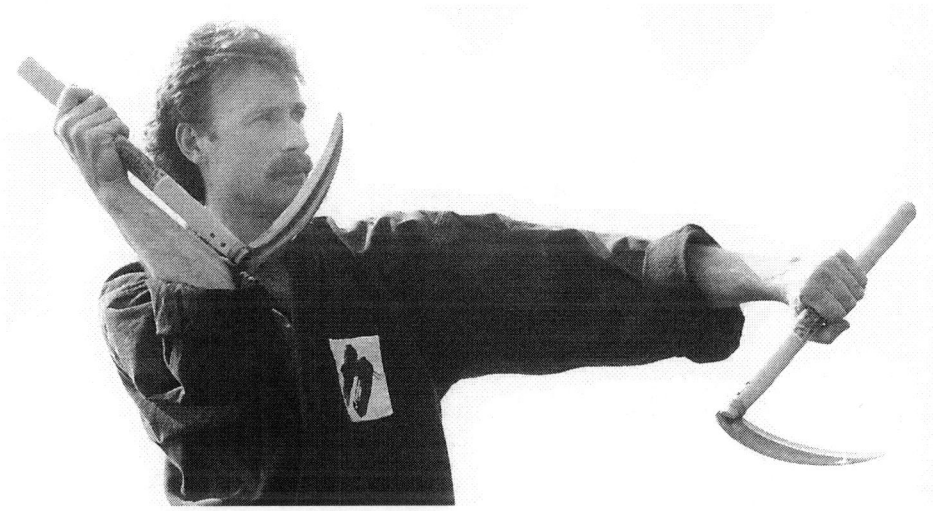

The author with double-sickle (*kama*). Photo by Rosemarie Hausherr.

Today's martial artists caught up in the competitive angle have sportified an art meant for scientific neutralization of the opponent when in dire straits and/or spiritual liberation from conflict's suffering in peacetime. The enlightened warrior's way is about accomplishing and strengthening one's spiritual fortitude using its technical skills to assert just causes when challenged. Profound martial practice is aimed at striking the target of one's own authentic self. Isshin Kempo is a tough, young system with a compassionate spiritual undertone and diligent black belts taking aim at these most worthy of martial targets.

Higher knowledge is powerful to those who possess it. Responsibility is greatest for those with the resources to dispense it. It is hoped such men and women exercise their wisdom by looking at the grander scheme of life and so do not cast their precious pearls to an insensitive and unprepared martial public.

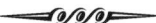

TECHNICAL SECTION

A1-2: Mudra of Inseparability
Often used in what appear passive or salutatory-like positions, unique hand formations (*mudra*) reveal an impressive depth of knowledge about subtle physical and mental effects upon the practitioner. In the case shown here, four men are trying to separate Joe Noonan's hands while in the Isshin Kempo Mudra of Inseparability. This mudra is unique to the Isshin Kempo system.

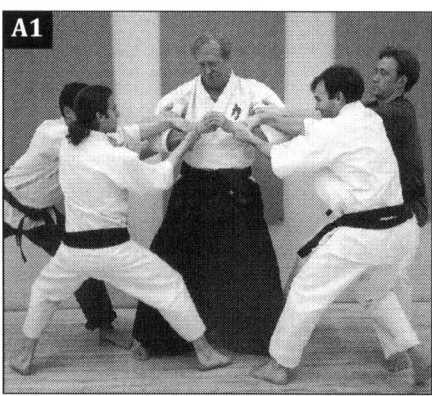
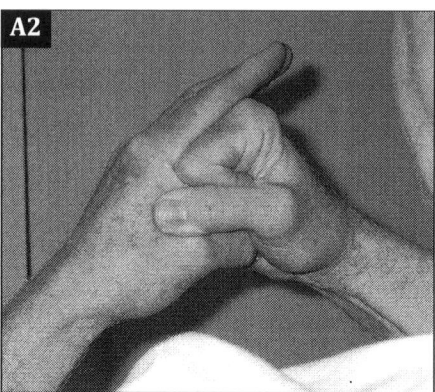

B1-2: Kempo Yoga Training
Goedecke and senior black belts maintain a stationary cat stance (*neko dachi*) as part of a lengthy Chinese kempo yoga training sequence. Later, a black belt assumes a meditative position.

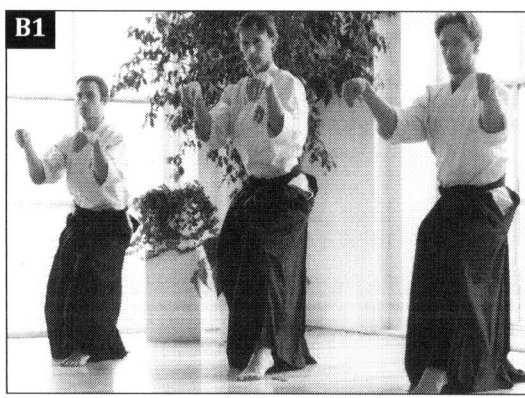

C: Three Sanchins Isshin
Kempo teaches three subtle variations of the kata Sanchin. Each variation begins with a base stance change: the Seisan, Seiuchin, and traditional Sanchin-stance versions. Note the slight degree of rotation of the feet.
C1: Seisan version, feet straight.
C2: Seiuchn version, toed out.
C3: Sanchin version, toed in.

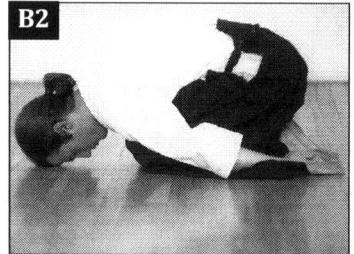
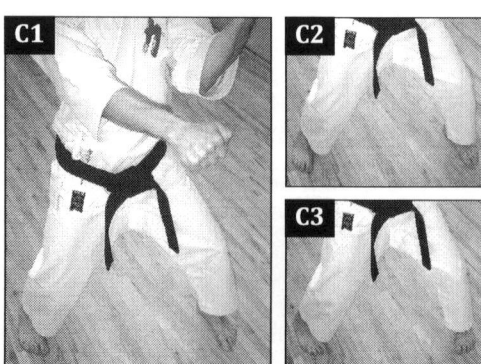

D: Okinawan Irony

There has been a gross under-interpretation regarding the specific reasons for most martial fist formations. An on-going debate into the bio-mechanical value of one punch over another to determine the best speed and alignment through scientific analysis has misdirected attention away from additional striking variables (Flanagan, 2000:83-91). The nature of a broader internal dynamic has been underestimated and the adversary's own internal organization, designed to alter the outcome of these variables, even when optimal, is often overlooked. In addition, Shimabuku's choice of placing the thumb on top of the fist extends its practical usage beyond the sole purpose of punching.

Internal fist formations offer superior weapons for offense and defense, not to be underestimated because of a practitioner's inability to penetrate their rationale. It should be noted that the primary limb, whether used as a strike or as a parry, has a specific proximal relationship to the rest of the body's posturing that can greatly enhance or weaken one's technique both mechanically and/or bio-electrically. Perhaps Okinawan masters have not yet revealed the full spectrum of knowledge in this regard.

Both internal and scientific principles are at work in many Okinawan-based fist positions. Among the Isshin Kempo advanced, internal hand postures are the superior "Cloud" and "Stone" fist formations.

The Isshin-ryu thumb-on-top vertical fist supports a rising punch. That being said, consider that the American servicemen, on average, towered at least a head over their Okinawan counterparts. If the shorter Okinawans were punching upwards in support of their fist strike, then the Marines had to punch downward! Who was truly getting the upper hand in that exchange?

F: Hand Formations

D1: Isshin-ryu fist (thumb on top).
D2-3: While little distinction is made in most schools in regard to these two traditional-fisted thumb positions, Isshin Kempo recognizes specific and separate functions for each position.
D4-5: The Cloud Fist and Stone Fist advanced fist formations.

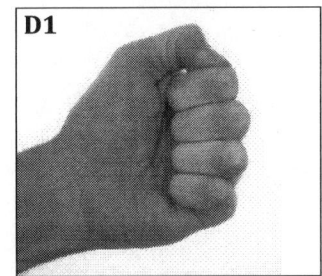

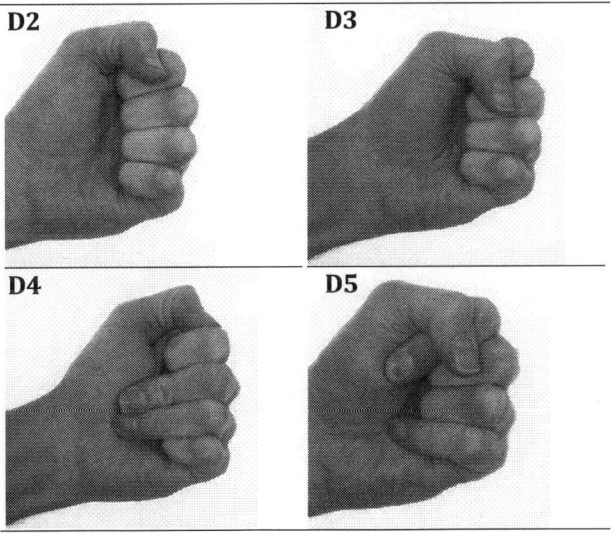

E: Deflections

On his 1966 U.S. trip, Shimabuku Tatsuo reportedly advised Don Nagle to maintain his use of the bent wrist middle block (Fitzgerald, 1984). Shimabuku implied that he had succumbed to pressure within his own camp to institute the straight wrist forearm block. Each blocking maneuver carries a particular purpose both in the immediate action as a deflection and in the setup for the next action. As found in the kata Seisan, the hooking palm block is utilized to both draw down the opponent's arm and, more importantly, to short circuit his ki flow, which sets the opponent's arm up for a succeeding grab and controlling lock. Kata moves are not separate or isolated events. Preceding and succeeding moves share a dynamic interdependence lost to most students of "modern" martial arts practice.

    E1: Forearm middle block.   E3: Hooking middle block.
    E2: Bent wrist forearm middle block.   E4: Follow up grab after the hook.

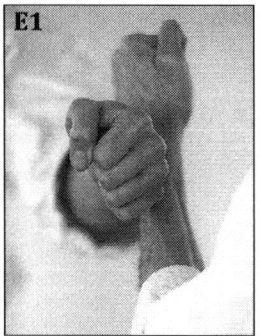 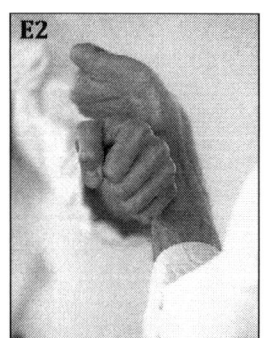 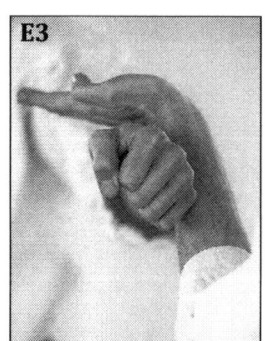 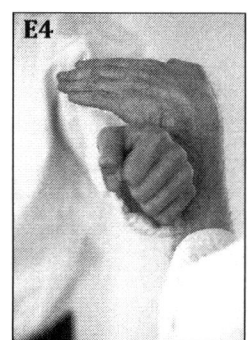

COUNTERING THE JAB — Eight Tactical Responses

Adaptable and spontaneous reactions require both a technical and conceptual knowledge base which encompasses skill in both body mechanics and internal power principles. Senior Isshin Kempo black belts demonstrate a variety of adaptive responses for neutralizing a committed, extended or quickly retracting jab. Competent fighters, like fine artists, learn to paint concise, finalizing reactions with speed and accuracy while exerting continuous control aimed at dismantling both an opponent's perceptive and physical defenses. One's martial personality, anatomy, strengths and skills will dictate the variety of responses. In each sequence, the opponent will attack with a lead-hand jab and the defender will deflect with a hooking palm followed by a counterpunch. Having first stunned the adversary, Isshin Kempo black belts will then demonstrate eight continuing tactical responses.

F1 SEQUENCE
F1.1: Set up.
F1.2: Hook.
F1.3: Stunning strike to face.
F1.4-9: Takedown with elbow lock.
F1.10: Close-up.

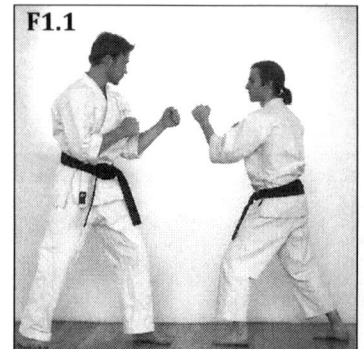 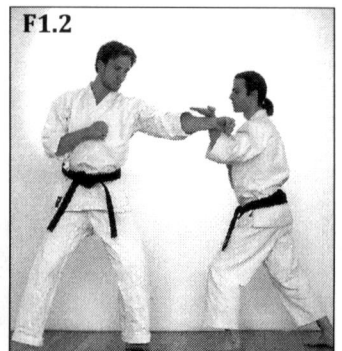

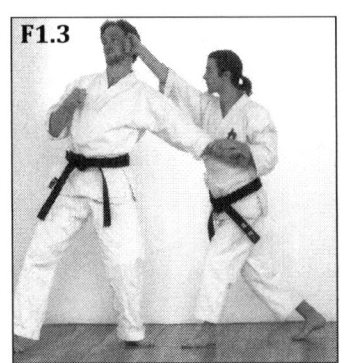

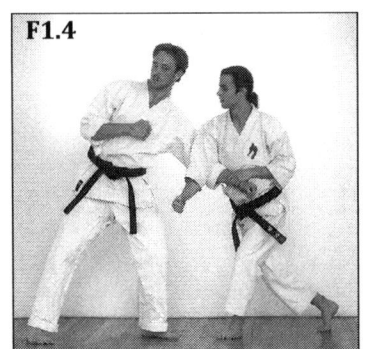

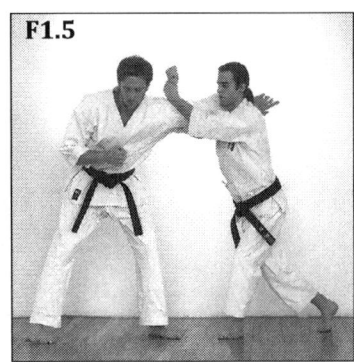

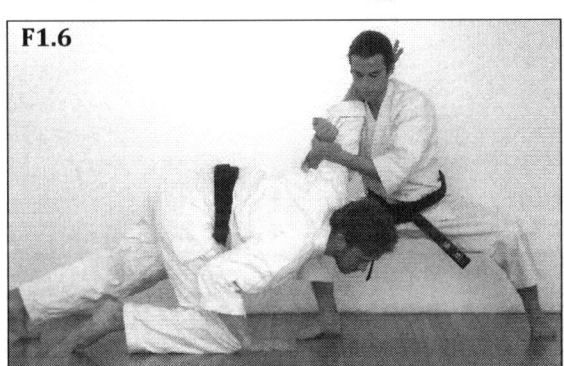

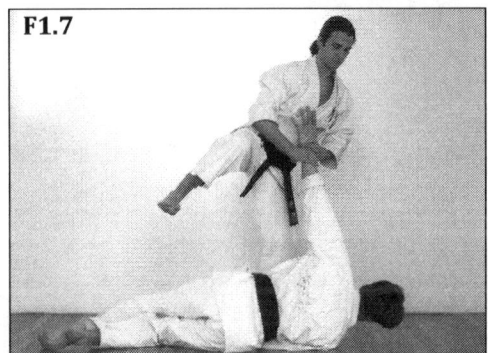

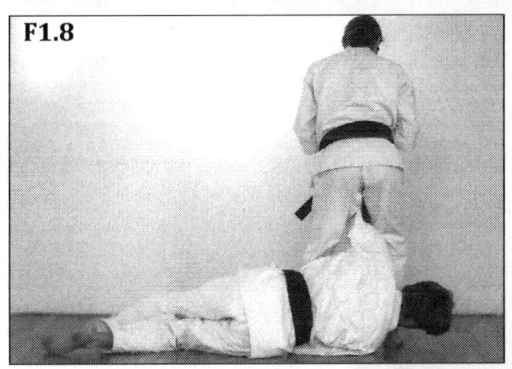

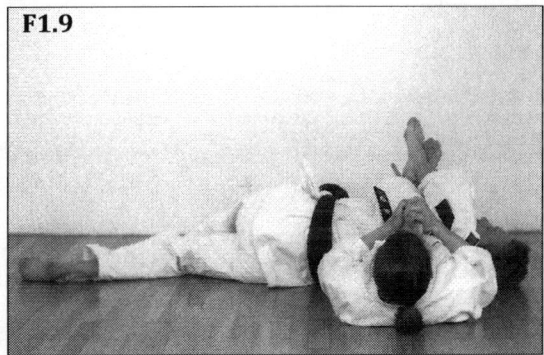

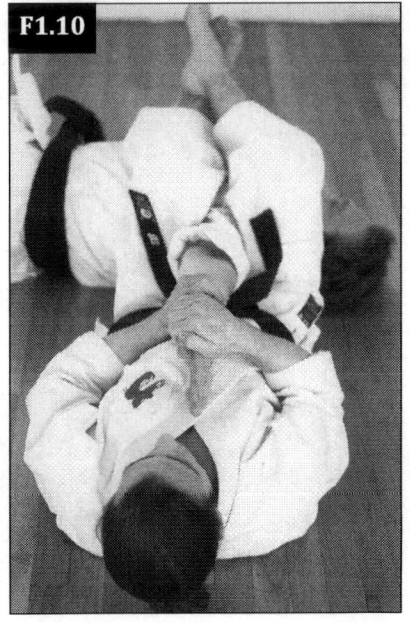

F2 SEQUENCE

F2.1: Same set up as above.
F2.2: Hook.
F2.3: Stunning strike to face.
F2.4-8: Strikes and neutralizing pressure point attack to the jaw.

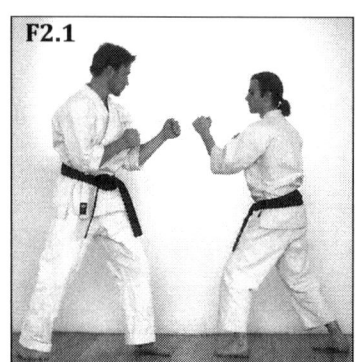
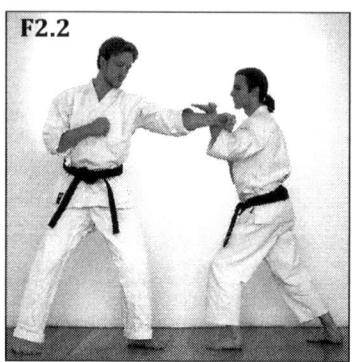
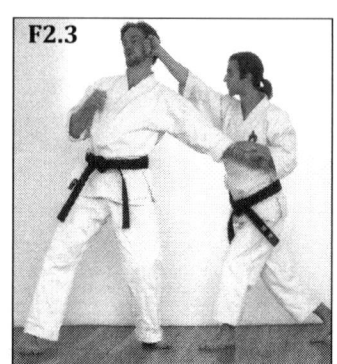
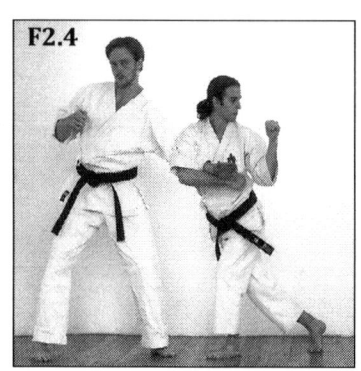
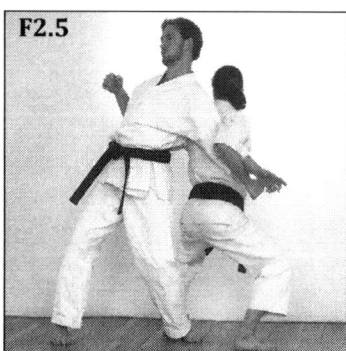
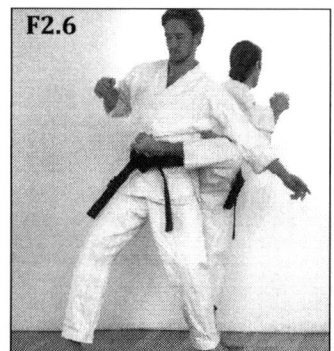
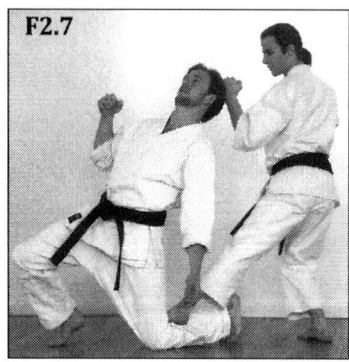
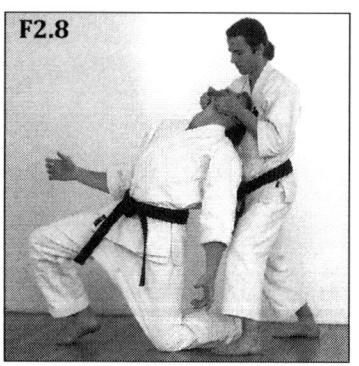

F3 SEQUENCE

F3.1: Set up.
F3.2: Hook.
F3.3: Stunning strike to face.
F3.4-6: Elbow to lower spine followed by a neck and elbow lock.

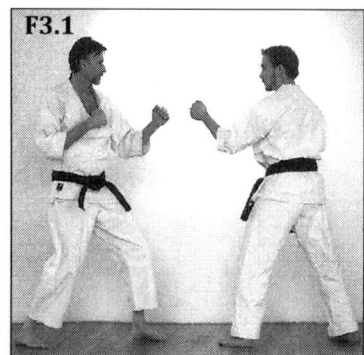
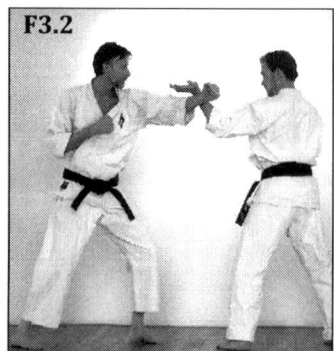

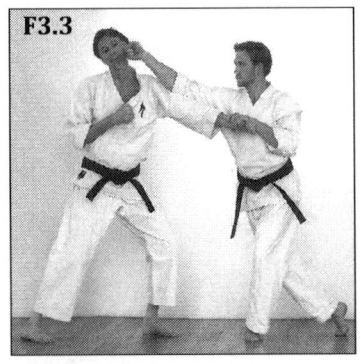
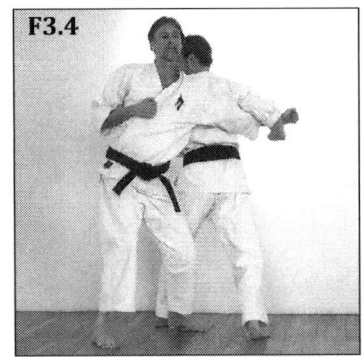
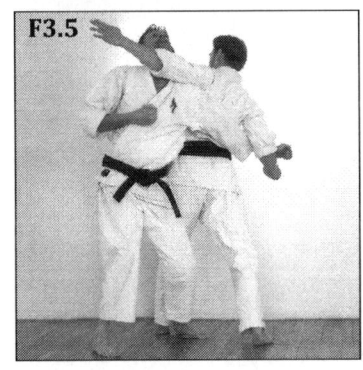
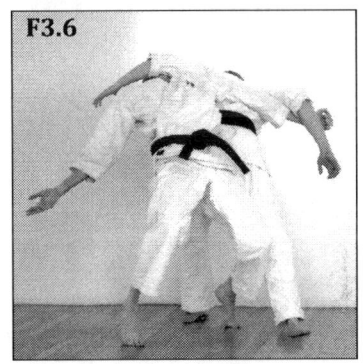

F4 SEQUENCE

F4.1: Set up.   F4.3: Opponent counters.
F4.2: Hook.   F4.4-5: Knee lock takedown with finishing elbow strike.

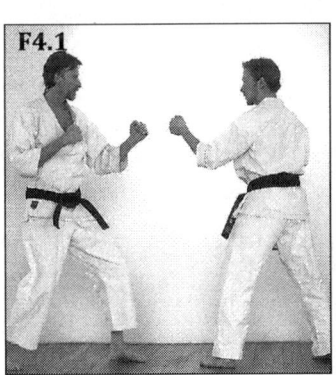
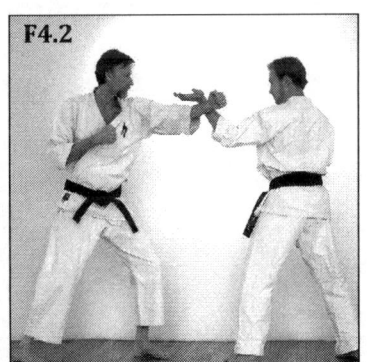
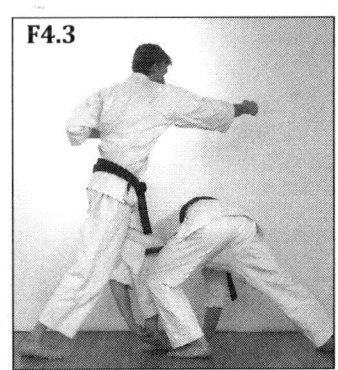
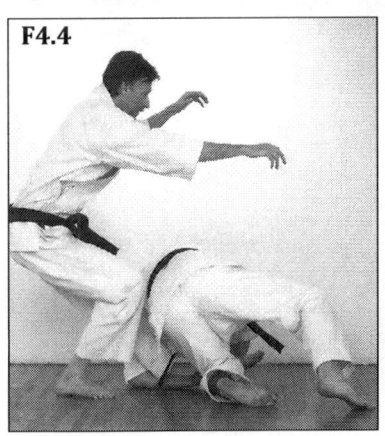
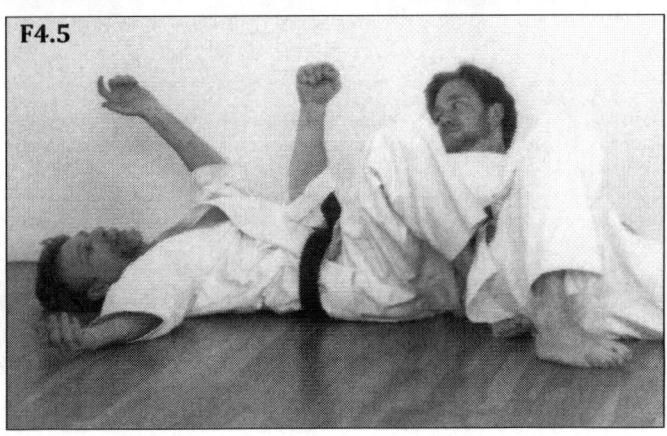

F5 SEQUENCE

F5.1: Set up.
F5.2: Hook.
F5.3: Strike to face.
F5.4-7: Single arm wrist lock control and takedown.
F5.8: Close-up.

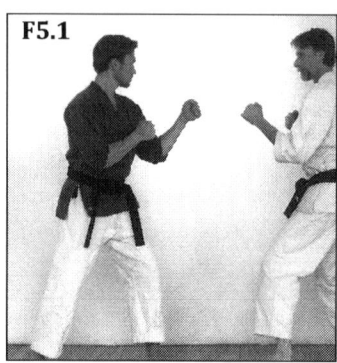
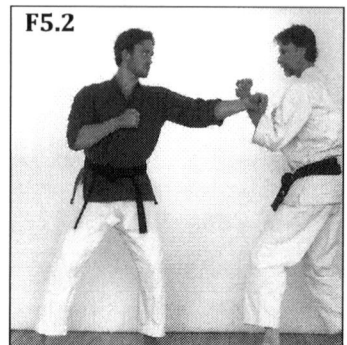
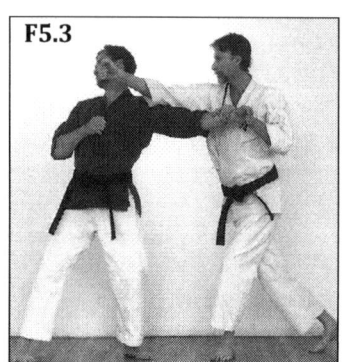
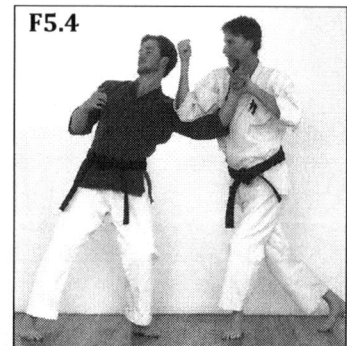
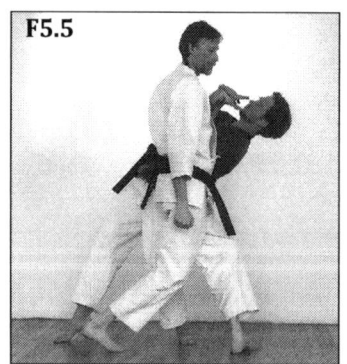
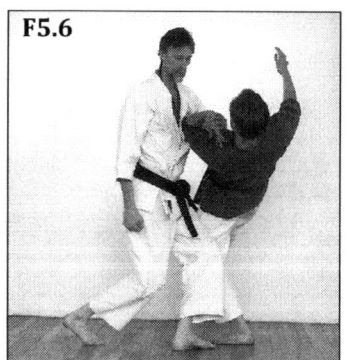
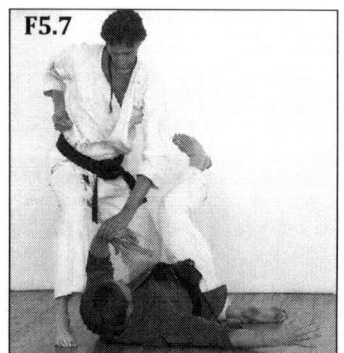
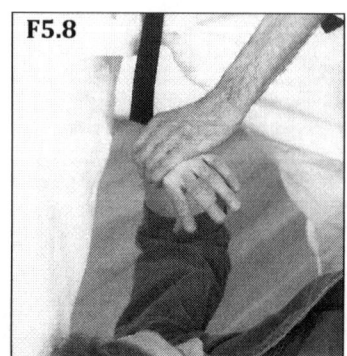

F6 SEQUENCE
F6.1: Set up.
F6.2: Hook.
F6.3: Strike to face.

F6.4-9: Elbow strike followed by shoulder lock.

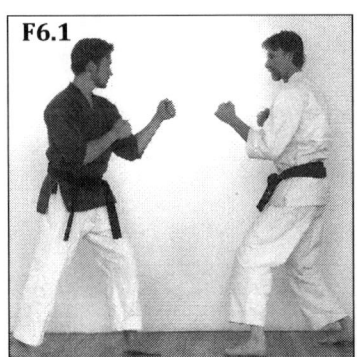
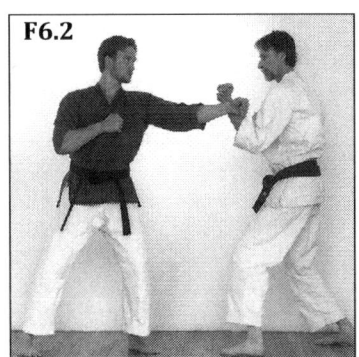
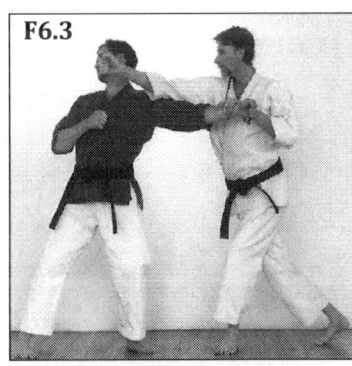
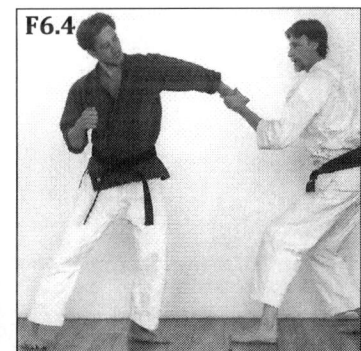
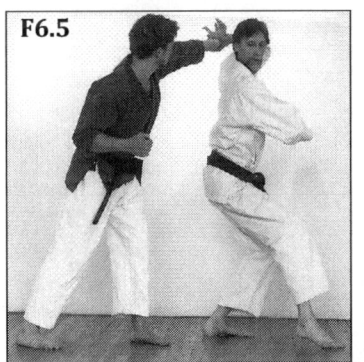
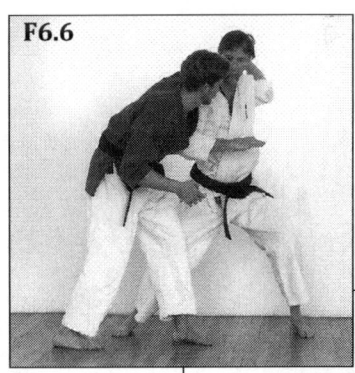
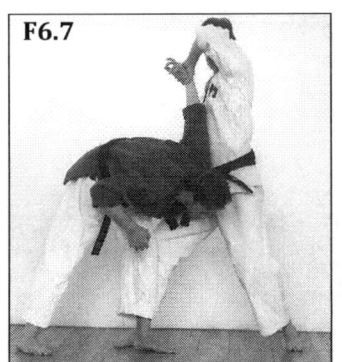
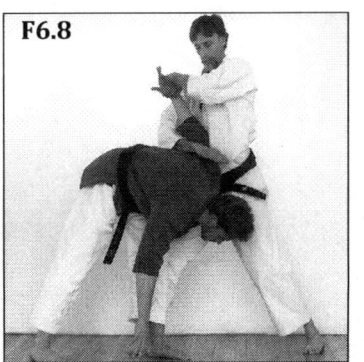
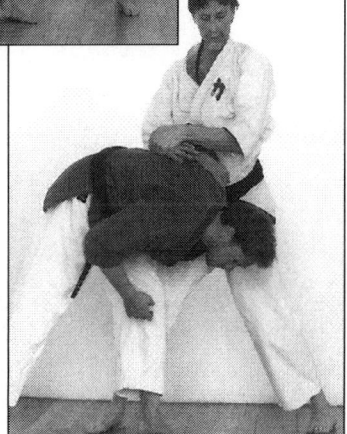

F7 SEQUENCE

F7.1: Set up.
F7.2: Hook.
F7.3: Strike to face.

F7.4-6: Shoulder manipulation followed by a step over, elbow lock applied with the leg.

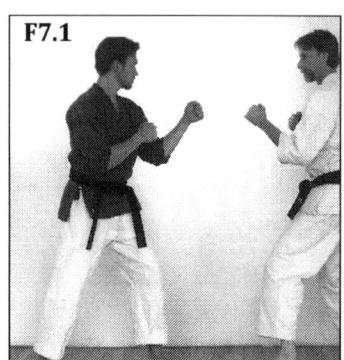
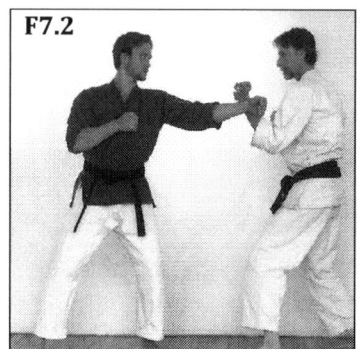
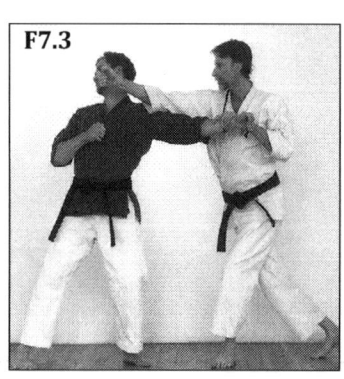
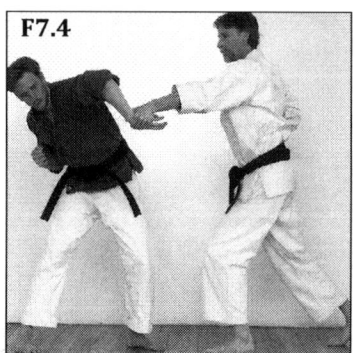
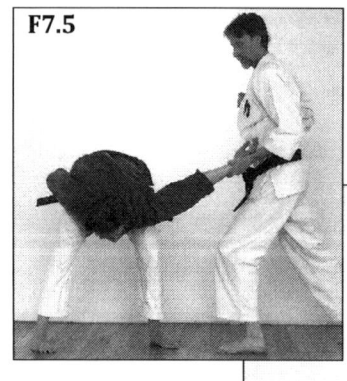
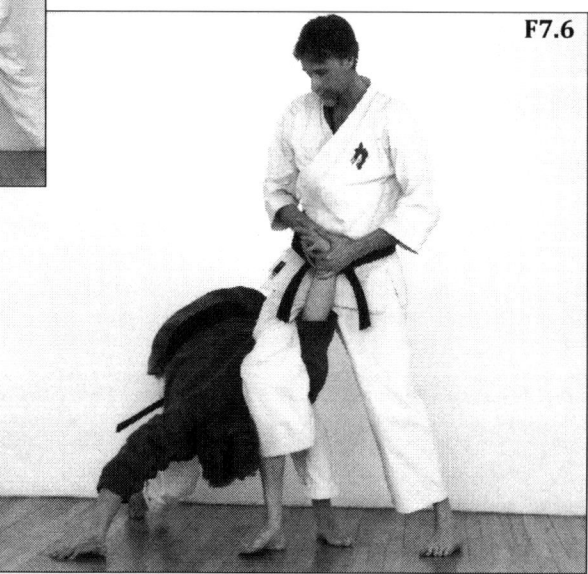

F8 SEQUENCE

F8.1: Set up.
F8.2: Hook.
F8.3: Strike to face.

F8.4-7: Knee and thigh leg strikes followed by a double knife-hand attack to the neck and spine.

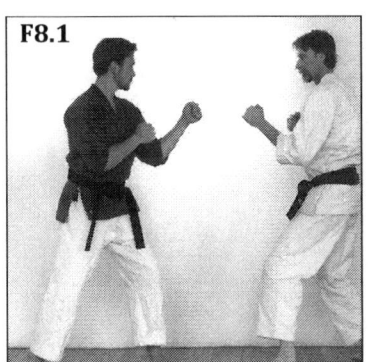
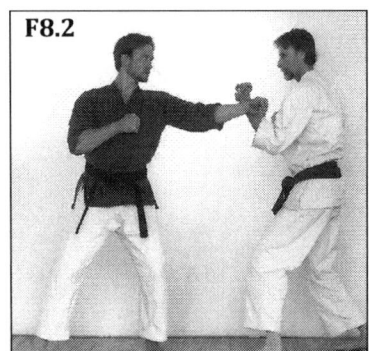
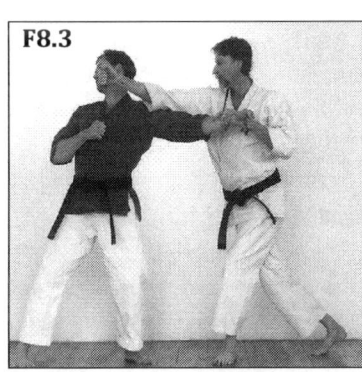
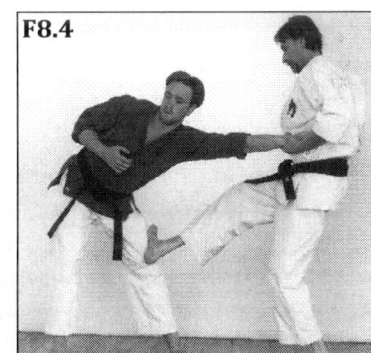
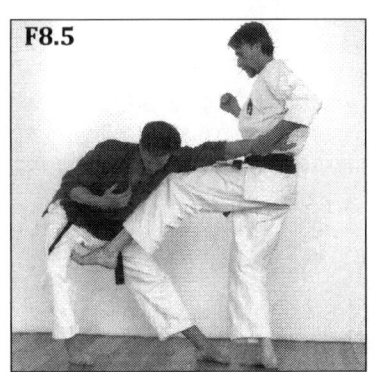
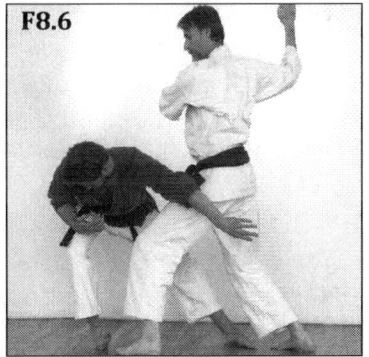
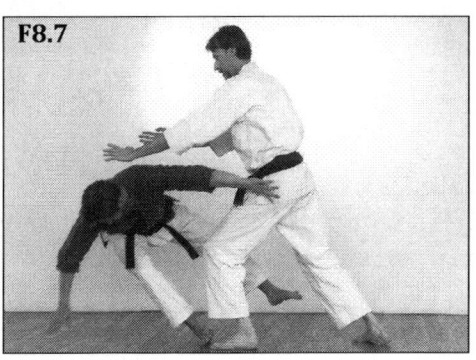

BIBLIOGRAPHY

Advincula, J. (2001). Excerpts from a December 24, 1984 interview with T. Shimabuku's senior Okinawan students: Kaneshi Eiko, Shigema Genyu, and Kaneshiro Kenjion. Personal communication.

Alexander, G. (1992). *Okinawa: Islands of karate*. Lake Worth, FL: Yamazato Publications.

Armstrong, S. (1984). *Isshin-ryu karate: The one heart method*. Tacoma, WA: DLAW Publications.

Bishop, M. (1999). *Okinawan karate: Teachers, styles and secret techniques*. Rutland, VT: Tuttle Publishing.

Dobyns, M. (1985). *History and philosophy of Isshin-ryu karate-do*. Colorado Springs, CO: Sanchin Publishing.

Dollar, A. (1996). *Secrets of Uechi-ryu karate and the mysteries of Okinawa*. Antioch, CA: Cherokee Publishing.

Donnelly, N. (1999). *The Isshin-ryu system*. Waterford, MI: Donnelly.

Evseeff, D. and Murphey, M. (1996). *Isshin-ryu karate-do.* Ellicott City, MD: One Heart Publishing.

Fitzgerald, B. (1984). Personal communication.

Flanagan, S. (2000). Use of the wrist in the vertical punch and the twisting straight punch: A biomechanical comparison. *Journal of Asian Martial Arts, 9*(1):83–91.

Frantzis, B. (1998). *The power of internal martial arts: Combat secrets of Ba Gua, Tai Chi, and Hsing-i*. Berkeley, CA: North Atlantic Books.

Goedecke, C. (1995). Sensei-do: The do and do not of martial teaching. In C. Wiley (Ed.), *Martial arts teachers on teaching*. Berkeley, CA: Frog Limited.

Goedecke, C. (1993). Okinawa revisited: The travels of Goju master Frank Van Lenten. *Inside Karate, 14*(1):34–39, 74; Vol. 14(2):50–55.

Goedecke, C. (1992). America's emissary to Okinawa's Goju: Up close and personal with Goju master Frank Van Lenten. *Martial Art Masters*, 50.

Goedecke, C. (1992). Moving mind: An exclusive interview with Goju's Frank Van Lenten. *Martial Arts Masters, 1*(5):45–52, 76.

Goedecke, C. (1990). Grasping the heart: The inner psychology of karate training. *Internal Arts, 5*(1):16–19.

Goedecke, C. (1983). Okinawa remembered. *Kick Illustrated Yearbook*: 33–39.

Goedecke, C. (1979). Kata and the art of war. *Offical Karate, 11*(84):22–27, 60.

Johnson, N. (1994). *Zen Shaolin karate: The complete practice, philosophy and history*. Rutland, VT: Tuttle Publishing.

Lee, B. (1975). *Tao of Jeet Kune Do*. Burbank, CA: Ohara Publications.

Lennox, J. (1980). *Isshin-ryu karate*. Farmingdale, NJ: Dolan Sports.

Long, H. and McGhee, T. (1977). *Isshin-ryu karate: The ultimate fighting art*. Mascot, TN: Isshin-ryu Productions.

Long, A. and Wheeler, H. (1979). *Dynamics of Isshin-ryu karate. Book 2*. Mascot, TN: National Paperback Books.

Long, A. and Wheeler, H. (1979). *Dynamics of Isshin-ryu karate. Book 3*. Mascot, TN: National Paperback Books.

Nagamine, S. (2000). *Tales of Okinawa's great masters.* (P. McCarthy, Trans.). Rutland, VT: Tuttle Publishing.

Nakkaya, T. (1986). *Karate-do: History and philosophy*. Carrollton, TX: JSS Publishing.

Noonan, J. (2001). Personal communication.

Ratti, O. and Westbrook, A. (1973). *Secrets of the samurai: A survey of the martial arts of feudal Japan*. Rutland, VT: Tuttle Publishing.

Rosenbaum, M. (2001). *Okinawa's complete karate system: Isshin-ryu.* Boston, MA: YMAA Publication Center.

Russell, W. (1976). *Karate: The energy connection.* New York: Delacorte Press.

Sells, J. (2000). *Unante: The secrets of karate.* Hollywood, CA: W. M. Hawley.

Tomio, A. (2000–2001). Personal communications.

Tomio, N. (1995). Kempo kumite: A Buddhist spiritual cathartic. Revised essay extract from the *Journal of Mushindo Studies*, London: England.

Mushindo Kempo Naha Dojo. http://www.mushindo.kempo.org.uk/kumite.htm

Tomio, N. (1994). *Boddhisattva warrior: The origins, inner philosophy, history, and symbolism of the Buddhist art within India and China.* York Beach, ME: Samuel Weiser.

Tomio, N. (1983). Chen Yen Shingon lecture, Hakurenji Temple, London. Edited by Shinsei Tomio, 1997, Kongoryuji Temple. *Journal of the British Shingon Buddhist Association.*

Tomio, N. (1982). *Chinese yoga – Healing movement.* London, England: The Kongosatta Chinese Yoga Dojo.

Uezu, A. (1992). *Encyclopedia of Isshin-ryu karate, book 1.* San Clemente, CA: Kiai Productions.

Van Leten, F. (1984). Personal communication.

Wheeler, A. (1986). Isshin-ryu: The one heart-one mind method. Knoxville, TN: National Paperback Books.

Acknowledgments

I'd like to thank Tomio Arakawa for sharing his personal correspondences; to Jim Advincula for insights into Shimabuku's senior Okinawan students; to teachers Noonan, Armitage, and DeMarco for their technical support; to the photo artists Bruce Berenson, Colin Goedecke and Rosemarie Hausherr; and to Jeff Balbirnie for his research aid and access to his extensive martial library.

chapter 36

Koshin-ryu: The Rebirth of Okinawa's Kojo Family Martial Arts

by Richard B. Florence, M.A.

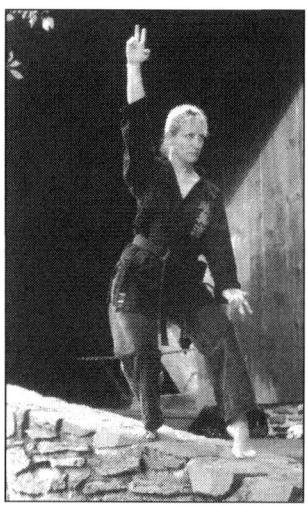

Koshin-ryu fifth degree Joyce Stech in the Dragon Posture.
All photographs courtesy of Chuck Chandler.

Introduction

The need for self-defense goes back to the beginning of time. As time progressed, these early archaic and unstructured techniques gained structure as human society gained structure. Self-defense or offense systems developed under two primary influences: the military and individual families. These trends can be seen throughout the world, no matter the continent or country. On the military side, such styles as taijiquan in China and numerous weapons styles were developed. More often than not, an individual, or individuals working together who were soldiers, developed these styles. Oftentimes, civilian families further refined them. In China and Japan, numerous styles were given the name of the family that developed them.

Of course, this doesn't mean that all family styles were named after the family. Other familial-inherited lines were passed on without direct reference to the family, for instance, Ueshiba Morihei founded the art of aikido, who passed it on to his son, Kisshomaru, who passed it on to his son, Moriteru. In fact, the history of any one art would show how convoluted these arts are. Eventually the students of all arts and styles affect the development and naming of the mother art.

The martial traditions on Okinawa are no different.[1] This chapter will introduce, or re-introduce, one of the family styles once thought to have died out, the karate and weapon arts of the Kojo family. The development of the Kojo style is obviously directly linked to Okinawa's history.

A Short History of Okinawan Karate

Although most histories discuss the development of an indigenous mother art called *torite, tuidi*, or just *te/ti/di* (hand),[2] there is little actual information on its beginnings. However, te eventually took on primarily empty-handed elements of Chinese civilian martial systems. The Okinawa Board of Education places the major impetus on Okinawan development of a civilian martial art on the need for sailors to defend themselves against pirates (1995:2). The flourishing trade with China and Japan brought about a large population of sailors to the Naha area. Of course, this influx of foreigners, as temporary as it may have been, did not preclude the need for self-defense throughout the island from local trouble makers.

Most karate styles can also trace their lineage to China[3] and the art called "Tang Hand." This term comes from the Tang Dynasty (618 CE–907), which came to mean China itself due to its cultural and political dominance, thus "China Hand" (Japanese: "*karate*"; Okinawan: "*todi*," also "*toudi*") originally.[4] However, Funakoshi Gichin, considered by some to be the father of modern karate, is uncertain if Okinawa ever actually adopted the "Tang" ideogram for karate (1988:24–25).

Okinawa's relationship with China goes back a long way. It is possible that Okinawa came into at least indirect contact with China as early as the later half of the 3rd century B.C.E. (Kerr, 1958/1980:29). Direct contact with China may have first occurred in 608 C.E., when a Chinese Sui Dynasty expedition looking for the fabled Land of the Immortals reached some Okinawan islands. In 1369, Chuzan[5] King Satto (r. 1422–39) accepted Chinese supremacy and sent representatives to the court of Chinese Emperor Hong Wu, founder of the Ming Dynasty (1369–1644). One result of this political relationship was that Okinawan "foreign students" (*ryugakusei*) were sent to Beijing and Nanjing to study Chinese culture and language. To further their education, young Okinawan scholars often traveled to Fuzhou, which was the closest large Chinese metropolis. Upon their return to Kume Village, these young men often became successful businessmen and pro-Chinese members of society.

In 1392, a group of Chinese businessmen, artisans, and officials arrived in Okinawa, which Okinawan history refers to as the "Thirty-Six Families."[6] The group lived in Kume Village, which became the nexus of Chinese culture in Okinawa. These Chinese taught Okinawan scholars their language and helped cement trade relations between Okinawa and China. Among families sent to Okinawa at this time was a branch of the Cai, who, by the 17th century, had become Okinawanized and adopted the family name of Kojo.

Left: Sign outside the Kojo Headquarters Dojo which reads —

"Kojo-ryu Koshinkan Karatedo"

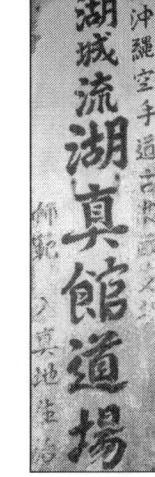

Right: Yabiku Takaya outside the dojo, which was opened in 1974.

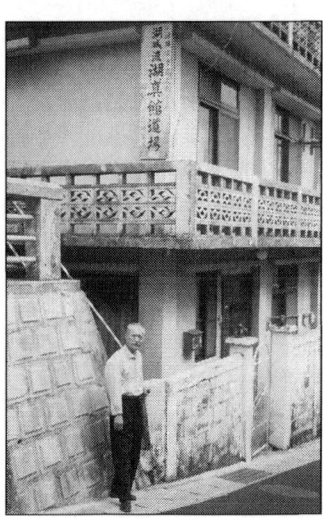

Along with the growth and evolution of Okinawan society, new laws were made to keep the society stable. It has long been believed, especially by the martial arts community, that Okinawa King Sho Shin-O (r. 1477–1526) outlawed the private ownership and stockpiling of weapons, the first of two such prohibitions. Part of this is based on George Kerr's seminal history on Okinawa. In the first edition (1958/2000:107), Kerr states this act came into effect when King Sho Shin-O ratified a decree in 1507 called "Eleven Distinctions of the Age." However, newer research refutes this. Sakihara Mitsugu says that the statement in question was found on a monument or stele erected in 1479 and called the Eleven Great Achievements of the Age. Sakihara explains that "(i)n 1926 Iha Fuyu misread the passage therein to mean 'this country used the armor for utensils,' and assumed that the king had confiscated all arms which were then made into practical tools such as farm implements. Thus originated the fallacy of a disarmed, peace-loving Ryukyu..." (1987:199). Tuttle Publishing chose Sakihara to revise Kerr's work. In the afterword, Sakihara retells the above story, although changes some of the facts. He notes that "the Momourasoe Balustrade monument of 1509 ... eulogizes King Sho Shin ... listing his achievements." He states that in 1955, Zenchu Nakahara pointed out the error in Iha's translation (2000:543–544).

Regarding the second widely believed myth that the Satsuma clan also imposed a weapons ban, Sakihara also provides an update. He notes that the clan conquered Okinawa in 1609; banned the importing of arms into the Ryukyus in 1639; and issued the "Prohibition of Those Who Travel to Ryukyu Carrying Arms," which allowed Okinawans to bring their arms to Satsuma for repair, but continued the 1639 ban on importing new weapons (2000:544).

As time progressed, the Okinawan martial arts developed along some roughly constructed stylistic lines; however, these were not as diverse as many have assumed. According to Tokashiki Iken, a noted karate historian and Tomari-te and Goju-ryu instructor, "There were no clear distinctions between te styles, each master had his own specialty" (Tokashiki, 18 February 1997). Until the 18th century, Okinawan martial arts had no set curriculum and no organizations, either domestic or international. There were no ranks, either by belt or licensing. A teacher taught what he knew without reporting to anyone else, except for maybe his own teacher. A teacher gained students through his reputation, since he was known as either a good teacher and/or fighter or not.

At one time, te/karate was described in a relatively generic form based on perceived stylistic differences centering in the urban districts of Okinawa's modern-day capital of Naha: Shuri-te, Naha-te, and Tomari-te (*te*, "hand").[7] Despite the long practice of martial arts in these areas, these geo-based names were not official designations. In fact, such a means of identifying the te arts did not exist until the winter of 1926–1927. In January 1927, judo founder Kano Jigoro made his third visit to Okinawa,[8] and was also the first time he saw tode on its native soil (McCarthy, 1994:3, 8). The Okinawan planning committee for Kano's visit decided it would be best if they called the Okinawan martial art, then known as "China Hand," something besides a name that reflected links to Japan's enemy, China. The group decided to give the arts style names based on the geographic areas where they were most commonly found: Shuri, Naha, and Tomari (McCarthy, 1994:3).

The next major stage in Okinawan karate was its development primarily along the so-called Naha-te, Shuri-te, Tomari-te models: Goju-ryu from the Naha-te lineage and Shorin-ryu from the Shuri-te[9] and Tomari-te lineages.[10] Two Okinawan styles that did not fall neatly within this model are Uechi-ryu, which was originally called Pangainoon-ryu (based on the Fujian dialect of spoken Chinese), but is sometimes considered a Naha-te style; and Kojo-ryu.

The Kojo Family

Like many other Okinawan families, the Kojo[11] family records only date back to the 1600's. Of those records, many were destroyed over time, including a large portion during the Japanese occupation and the Battle for Okinawa during World War II. The current family, non-practicing, head of the Kojo karate system, Kojo Yoshiaka, made many of these records available to Irimaji Seiji. These records link Kojo-ryu karate to Fuzhou through the Thirty-Six Families in Kume Village. Like much of the martial arts across Asia throughout the period of its development, Kojo-ryu remained pretty much a family style, handed down from father to son wherever possible. Occasionally, outsiders would get a glimpse of the style. This made sense since one's success in self-defense often depended on knowing something your opponent didn't, on the off chance that he was also a martial artist. Obviously, there is not strict secrecy in martial arts training, otherwise it would be nearly impossible to develop a viable system. The Kojo family system was therefore influenced by outside sources as well as the genius within the family.

Kojo Shinpo Uekata[12] appears to have been the first of a long line of Kojos to study Chinese martial arts. He was also known by the Sinified name of *Sai* (Mandarin: *Cai*) *Ko*. He was born in Kume Village in the late 1600's (family records are not specific as to the date). In the middle 1700's,[13] the records show that Kojo Shinpo studied gongfu (including weaponry and grappling) in Fuzhou, as a number of his family members and other Okinawans would do in later times. Kojo Shinpo may well have been one of the first martial artists to bring Chinese fighting arts to Okinawa. The art he taught to family members was simply called "fighting art" (*kumiaijutsu* or *kumiuchi*). As was the Kojo custom, he passed on what he knew to his eldest son, Shinunjo.

Kojo Shinunjo Peichin[14] (c. 1780–?) started martial arts training at a young age under Kojo Shinpo. In addition to his Kojo family training, he also apparently studied under Teruya Kanga, better known as *Tode* ("China Hand") Sakugawa, founder of Shurite.[15] He was sent to Fuzhou to further his studies. He added many new techniques to his father's system. In Kume Village, he was considered one of the finest Okinawan martial artists of his day. He seems also to have also used the name Matsu Higa, and was a senior Imperial guard at Shuri Castle (Sells, 1995:33). He was nicknamed "Born Warrior." Most karate historians credit him with the founding of the Kojo-ryu karate system. He passed down his system to his son, Saisho, in the late 19th century.

Kojo Saisho (1816–1906) is also referred to by the Sinified name, Sai Sho, Sai Shoi, and Sai Shoei. He studied in Fuzhou, bringing back a four-foot staff art (*jojutsu*) to Kume Village. Palace guards favored the staff because the ceilings were low and the standard six-foot staff (*rokushaku bo*) was too long to maneuver inside. Saisho was a famous Okinawan weapons art (*kobujutsu*) practitioner and maintained a very strong interest in weapons, especially the long and short staffs, to the neglect of his empty-hand skills. However, later in life, he perfected his empty-hand skills and passed them down to his son, Isei (also Isho). He was given the sobriquet "Wise Old Man" (Bishop, 1989:48). According to Bishop, he was stripped of his monetary privileges because he beat up two samurai who were attempting to rape an Okinawan woman. After such mistreatment from the Japanese authorities, he reportedly returned to Fuzhou, where he died (Bishop, 1989:48).

In 1848, Saisho took his son, Isei, and nephew, Taitei, to Fuzhou and introduced them to Iwah,[16] a noted Shaolin crane, tiger, and dragon gongfu teacher. As well as teaching Kojo Saisho, Isei, Taitei, and Koho, Iwah also taught Matsumura Sokon (founder of Shorin-ryu) and Maezato (Miyazato) Ranho (founder of Koho-ryu).[17] Upon his death, Saisho left his art to Isei.

Little is known about Kojo Taitei (1837–1917), Saisho's nephew, and his relationship to the Kojo family karate style is only minimal. Taitei also studied under Wai Xinxian. Like his cousin, Isei, he was known for his skill with the bow and arrow and the small spear (Bishop, 1996:115). He was given the sobriquet "Hard-Fisted Old Man." Taitei may have brought back a secret text that may be a version of the *Bubishi* (McCarthy, 1995a:42). Among his students were Kojo Saikyo; and Higashionna (Higaonna) Kanryo, who may have trained under Taitei for two years and then at the Kojo school in Fuzhou under Wai Xinxian and possibly even Iwah (McCarthy, 1995a:37).

In 1848, Kojo Isei (1832–1891)[18] went to Fuzhou with his father, Saisho, to study with Iwah. Reportedly, Isei quickly became Iwah's favorite student. A story passed down in the Kojo family notes that three of Iwah's students slipped into the dojo where Isei was practicing alone and attacked Isei. After Isei had quickly disarmed two of his attackers, the third one fled. These three Chinese may have been jealous of Isei's swift appointment as Iwah's assistant. Back in Okinawa, the story spread and became part of Kojo folklore as the saying, "One Kojo equals three others" (Bishop, 1989:47; Yabiku, 2000:40).

In 1862, at his teacher's request, Isei took over Iwah's dojo. This may have been the first time that a non-Chinese solely ran a martial arts school in Fuzhou.

During this period, Iwah was an imperial bodyguard. In 1868, he was apparently assassinated in the Chinese palace. In fear for his life, Isei returned to Okinawa believing that jealous imperial functionaries had killed his teacher.

When Isei returned to Okinawa in 1868, he taught his art to several family members. He brought with him three secret- or advanced-level katas: White Crane Fist, White Tiger Fist, and White Dragon Fist. Isei is also credited with preserving and bringing to Kumemura one of the several versions of the *Bubishi*. This textbook was carefully edited to fit the Kojo family's specific style of karate. Upon close examination, one can find the pressure point strikes and their correlation to the Kojo-ryu stances in this book.

Isei died suddenly of a blood clot in the brain, which left the art in the hands of his son, Koho.

Kojo Koho (also Kojo Kaho; 1849–1925) was born in Fuzhou, China. In addition to being the fourth headmaster of the family martial arts system, he was also a skilled calligrapher and government translator. In 1855, he began studying gongfu under Iwah and his father, Isei, in Fuzhou. On his family's return to Okinawa in 1868, he continued to train and perfect his father's art.

In 1880, he returned to China and located his father's old dojo. Two Chinese teachers, Wai Xinxian[19] and Ko Ryuryu, were now running it. Because he was a Kojo, Koho was allowed to rejoin the school. Wai Xinxian taught Koho two more Crane katas, Nepai and Hofa, which Koho did not teach to anyone else. In 1889, Koho took over the dojo. This made him the second non-Chinese to operate a dojo in China, who just happened to be a Kojo as well. He called his martial art, "Kogusuku." His assistants are listed as Udon Makabe and Matsuda Tokusaburu, Okinawan friends of the Kojo family in Kume. In 1900, Koho returned to Okinawa.

Koho completed the format of the Kojo family system. He created Kojo-ryu's three staff, two sai, and three empty-hand katas from the upper-level katas of the White Tiger Fist, White Crane Fist, and White Dragon Fist. The three Koho-created empty-hand katas are Tenkan, Kukan, and Chikan. Each of these forms contain four different stances, which are to be used to fight an opponent at different times of the day, much in line with the meridian theory discussed in the *Bubishi*: Tenkan stances are theoretically used to strike vital areas of the body from 6 to 10 am; Kukan stances are used between 10 am and 2 pm; and Chikan between 2 and 6 pm.

In Okinawa, Koho's system became known as Kojo-ryu Jutsu. In addition to teaching his grandson, Yoshitomi, to whom he left the system, Koho also taught his son Saikyo; his brother, Koshiro Shuren (1883–1945),[20] one of the first Meiji Era (1868–1912) native Okinawan police inspectors in the prefecture; and Matsuda Tokusaburo (Nakaya, 1986:51).

Kojo Saikyo (1873–1941) was known as the "King of Kume" because of his wealth. He studied the Kojo system under his grandfather, Kojo Isei; his father, Kojo Koho; and Kojo Taitei. Saikyo's business concerns may have precluded him from learning the entire system and thus taking over the family system from his father, Koho. Saikyo taught his son, Yoshitomi.[21]

The fifth generation headmaster, Kojo Yoshitomi, (also Kojo Kafu; 1909–1995) began training in his family's karate and weapons system in 1921 under his grandfather, Koho. There is very little written about Yoshitomi. The only extensive information available is an oral history from his eldest living son, Yoshiaka, and one of his senior martial arts students, Irimaji Seiji. Yoshitomi began training under his father, Saikyo, and uncle, Shuren, soon after his grandfather's death in 1925. In the late 1930's, Yoshitomi was drafted into the Japanese Army and became a highly decorated soldier while fighting in the Philippines.

In 1958, Yoshitomi and his eldest son from his first marriage, Shigeru, opened a dojo in Naha and began teaching Kojo-ryu karate and weaponry. Among their first students were two sons from his second marriage, Kaoru and Tatsumi, and Shigeru's brother, Yoshiaka. Yoshitomi's first non-family student was Irimaji Seiji. Two non-family, mainland Japanese members, Hayashi Shingo, a dentist in Totori, Totori Prefecture, Japan, and Sokomoto (first name unknown) would begin study under Yoshitomi later on.

In the later 1960's, Yoshitomi was a nominal member of Higa Seitoku's (b. 1921) All-Okinawa Karate and Kobudo United Association (Bishop, 1996:140). In 1974, Yoshitomi closed the Naha dojo because Shigeru was diagnosed with cancer. He decided not to reopen it because he liked the quiet living and few students were willing to undergo the harsh training (Silvan, 1993:78; Bishop, 1996:116; Yabiku, 2000:42). Sometime before 1980, Yoshitomi and his two sons, Shigeru and Tatsumi, self-published ten textbooks on Kojo karate and weaponry. And with the help of senior students of Go Kenki, Yoshitomi reconstructed and brought back into the Kojo-ryu system the katas Nepai and Hofa, the two Crane katas that were lost when his grandfather died. He also created the sparring versions of katas Hakukoken, Hakutsuruken, and Hakuryuken (Yabiku, 2000:42).

Yoshitomi built a very large family home in Naha that resembles an American ranch-style house. This house has several wings that housed his sons and guests. His son, Yoshiaka, now lives in and owns the house.

Yoshitomi often practiced alongside his students in his rigorous training regime. Classes were three to five hours long. Although known as a strict teacher, he was apparently well liked (Irimaji, 2000 August).

In November 1991, Yoshitomi promoted Yabiku Takaya to 8th-degree. In 1995, he promoted Irimaji Seiji to 9th-degree and gave him a full instructor's license, which authorized him to teach the Kojo family system. Since Shigeru died before Yoshitomi, the Kojo system was left to Kojo Yoshiaka as headmaster and Irimaji as chief instructor. Also in 1995, Yoshitomi awarded Yabiku his instructor's license.

Kojo Shigeru (1934–1993) began training under his father, Yoshitomi, in 1948. In 1958, they opened the first commercial Kojo-ryu dojo in Okinawa and began teaching family members and a select few non-family members, although Shigeru depended primarily on his job as a taxi driver for living expenses.

His right hand and arm were severely injured in a teen-age accident. Because of this, Shigeru become an expert in the use of his legs. Irimaji Seiji and Yabiku Takaya note that Shigeru performed over three hundred kicks with each leg during a training session (Chandler, 2000). Among Kojo Shigeru's few students was Yabiku Takaya, who trained under Shigeru from 1973 until his first retirement in 1975.

When Shigeru was diagnosed with cancer in 1975, the Kojos closed the dojo and turned the building into a chicken coop to make money. In 1980, with his health seemingly restored, he taught a few private students on a part-time basis. However, the cancer eventually killed Shigeru.

As the eldest surviving son of Kojo Yoshitomi, Yoshiaka remains the headmaster of Kojo-ryu karate and kobudo, although he does not practice or teach the art himself.

The Next Generation: Kojo-ryu Reaches Outside the Family

Irimaji Seiji (b. 1941) was born to an Okinawan couple in Iceland. After World War II, his family moved back to Okinawa and bought a home in Naha. In 1958, he enrolled in Kojo Yoshitomi's dojo, becoming the first non-Kojo family member to be fully instructed in the art.

From 1965 to 1968, as a 3rd-degree, Irimaji was the all-Okinawa full-contact champion. He stopped competing because he kept winning, thus proving, at least within the confines of the punch-kick arts in Okinawa, his claim that the style was able "to overcome any and all other types of martial arts" (Yabiku, 2000:v).

Before 1974, Irimaji taught at the Kojo-ryu headquarters dojo in the morning. At night, Irimaji, Yabiku, and Shigeru would train together in their free time at the taxi company where all three worked.

In 1974, Kojo Yoshitomi made Irimaji the first non-family member to be awarded the senior teacher's certification (*kyoshi*) in the style and also named Irimaji the Kojo-ryu chief instructor. Because he had nowhere to train after Kojo Yoshitomi closed the Naha headquarters dojo in 1974, Irimaji asked Yoshitomi for permission to open another dojo in Naha, making him the second person, and first non-Kojo family member, to open a Kojo-ryu dojo in Okinawa. Called the Kojo-ryu Koshinkan, Irimaji's school served as the official Kojo-ryu headquarters until he retired from teaching in 1990. In 1990, Irimaji closed this school and became a nighttime manager for a taxi company. Irimaji has taught only one private student, Yabiku Takaya, who became his student in 1976.

Irimaji is well known for cutting chopsticks in two with a playing card, which has been filmed a number of times. To perform this feat, someone holds a pair of chopsticks between the thumb and index fingers of each hand at chest level. Irimaji takes a standard playing card and cleanly slices the chopsticks in two. He is the only one known who can perform this feat and says that Yoshitomi taught it to him (Yabiku, 2000:44).

In 1995, Kojo Yoshitomi promoted Irimaji to Kojo-ryu 9th-degree, and, as the style's chief instructor (Yabiku, 2000:53). He is the senior most Kojo-ryu instructor in the world and is recognized as such by the current headmaster, Kojo Yoshiaka.

After the death of his teacher in 1995, Irimaji founded the Koshin-ryu Kohokan Karate and Kobudo Organization in honor of Yoshitomi; therefore, Irimaji is the headmaster, 10th-degree grandmaster for Koshin-ryu. As is often the case with a family-named style, when the family-member headmaster dies and the style is left to someone outside the genetic line, the new chief instructor will give the style a new name, using elements of the old name. In this case, Koshin uses "Ko," the first character of the Kojo family name and the character "shin," for "original methods." Kohokan means "yellow mountain peak house/hall" or "Koho's Hall," and was named in honor of Kojo Koho.

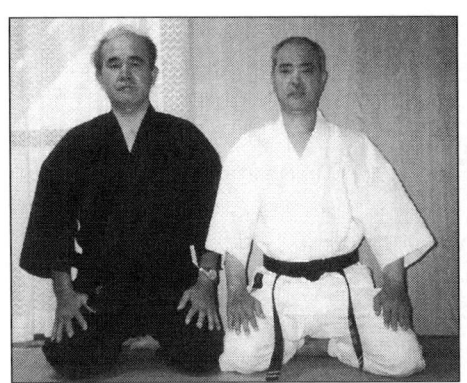 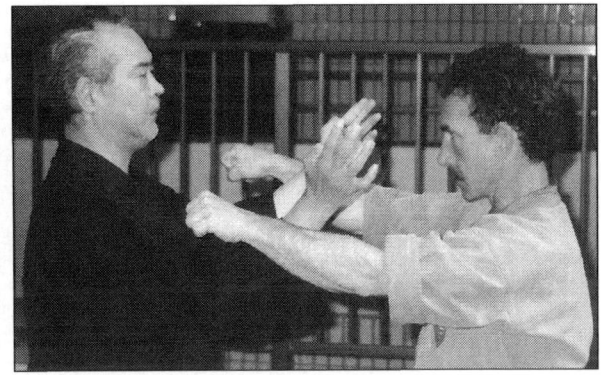

Left: Irimaji Seiji (L.) and Yabiku Takaya, Directors of the Koshin-ryu Kohokan.
Right: Yabiku Takaya demonstrating a technique from the Nepai kata
with Koshin-ryu Kohokan U.S. Director Chuck Chandler.

Irimaji lives with his current wife, Mieko, in rural Naha and continues to teach Kojo-ryu karate to his senior student, Yabiku Takaya. In October 1999, he appointed Yabiku Koshin-ryu Kohokan chief instructor, chief examiner, and vice chairman. In August 2000, he promoted Chuck Chandler, a senior student of Yabiku, to 7th-degree. Chandler is the first non-Oriental to train in Kojo-ryu and the first to be awarded a 7th-degree in the style—apparently Kojo Yoshitomi did not like Americans. Chandler is the international director, an international examiner, and chief instructor in the U.S. for the Koshin-ryu Kohokan (as well as for Yabiku's Okinawa Konan-ryu Kohokan Karate and Kobudo Kyokai).

On 5 August 2000, during the Obon Festival, Messrs. Yabiku and Chandler participated in a historical event. During the Thirty-Fifth Karate and Kobudo Festival in Honor of Kinjo Takashi, they and Mr. Irimaji were presented to the public as the next generation of Kojo-ryu. It was also announced that Yabiku was opening up the Koshin-ryu system to the public (as Irimaji has retired from public teaching). Messrs. Yabiku and Chandler also presented to the public the Kojo-ryu kata Hakukuken and Tenkan, respectively (Yabiku, 2000:iv).

Yabiku Takaya (b. 1945) was born in Kumamoto City, Kumamoto Prefecture, Japan. He is a descendent of Gosamaru, the Okinawan noble who built Nakgusuku Castle in the 15th century. Like many Okinawan karate and weapons masters of his generation, Yabiku studied a number of styles under a number of instructors before deciding to concentrate on the Kojo family system. He started his journey in the martial arts in 1951, under Sakihama Seijiro (1903–1997), a cousin of his grandfather and founder of Goju Shizen-ryu karatedo (in 1945); and his father, a Shorin-ryu practitioner. From 1960 to 1978, he was a private student of Soken Hohan, third grandmaster of Matsumura Seito Shorin-ryu karate and weaponry. From 1960 to 1990, he studied Yamane-ryu weaponry under Kochinda Saburo (1904–1998), a student of Chinen Masami. He studied Kojo-ryu under Kojo Shigeru from 1973 to 1975 and then under Irimaji Seiji from 1976 to the present. Yabiku is a taxi driver for the same company where Irimaji is a supervisor and Kojo Shigeru worked. Yabiku has also made an extensive study of Uechi-ryu and China's White Crane.

In August 2000, Irimaji said: "I trained and taught as teacher Yoshitomi taught me. I've had many students come and go. I believe my training methods were too hard and severe for those who wished to train there. Maybe six months and they were gone. Only one [Yabiku Takaya] stayed for the duration of my 15-years teaching at this dojo" (Yabiku, 2000:44).

Kojo-ryu is seeing a rebirth through the Koshin-ryu. Its founder, Irimaji Seiji, was the chief instructor of Kojo-ryu after the death of Kojo Yoshitomi and Shigeru. He created the Koshin-ryu because a Kojo family member, Yoshiaka, is still alive, although he doesn't train or teach.

Two mainland Japanese, Hayashi and Sokomoto (first name unknown) trained on Okinawa for two to three years in the early 1970's. Hayashi returned to Totori City, Totori Prefecture, to work as a dentist and to teach what he had learned of the Kojo-ryu. He apparently has not been back to Okinawa since then, although Irimaji Seiji has maintained contact with him. Further information regarding Hayashi and the enigmatic Sokomoto would be a great boon to the history of Okinawan karate.

THE SYSTEM

Fighting Postures

One of Kojo-ryu's, and thus Koshin-ryu's, hallmarks is its emphasis on twelve somewhat stylized fighting postures, much like the postures or stances familiar to practitioners of swordsmanship and those who watch Japanese sword movies. Each posture is related to one of the Chinese zodiac signs.

Sparring is often initiated from these postures. The intent is that the practitioner sets up his opponent who will "run into" the practitioner's technique, much like a spider trap. Below are the characteristics of these stances (Yabiku, 2000:57-80):

- **Front or Forward Stance** (*Seishin*): The primary sparring stance. The practitioner stands in a cat stance (heels on a line, one foot in front of the other, one stride in length, front heel up). The arms are held straight out in a relaxed manner. The hands are held palms down, wrists straight, and fingers slightly curled. It is linked to the Rat Zodiac sign and is emphasized in kata Tenkan.
- **Immovable Stance** (*Fudo*): Done with the feet about two fists apart, one foot in front of the other, and both heels planted (rooted or grounded); the arms are held hanging down, hands open, and fingers straight like sword hands. It is used for resting, quick changes of body postures, awareness of the environment and the opponent, and facilitates counter techniques. It is linked to the Ox Zodiac and is emphasized in the kata Tenkan.
- **Wind Hands Stance** (*Jinpu*): Done much like a cat stance, only the front heel rests lightly on the ground; both hands are open, palms out, the back hand is held above brow level (looking much like a military salute), and the front arm hangs down so that the lower arm and open hand protect the thigh. It is an aggressive posture used primarily against quick opponents. It is linked to the Tiger sign and is emphasized in kata Tenkan.
- **Cross Stance** (*Jumonji*): Done from a cat stance. One arm is held straight resting atop the wrist of the other arm, the hand in the spear-hand position. The other arm is bent and held parallel to the ground, the hand is in the spear-hand position, perpendicular to the other hand. It is linked to the Rabbit and is emphasized in kata Tenkan.
- **Cloud Dragon Stance** (*Unryu*): Done from a cat stance. One arm is held forward, palm open and facing the opponent, as though feeling for movement. The other hand is held above the ear, palm open in a 45-degree position to the front. It is linked to the Dragon and is emphasized in kata Kukan.
- **Blending Stance** (*Aiki*): Done from the cat stance. The arm above the front leg is bent, parallel to the ground, palm open and facing the ground, covering the body's

centerline. The other arm is held forward, slightly bent, parallel to the ground, palm facing down. It is considered an aggressive stance, making body transitions and quick hand attacks easier. It is linked to the Snake sign and is emphasized in kata Kukan.

- **Sword in the Eyes Stance** (*Seigan*): Done from the cat stance. The arm above the front leg is held straight, parallel to the ground, with the palm facing down. The other hand is held in a fist above the fist in the classic ready-to-punch position. It is considered a good stance to use when facing an opponent with a weapon. It is linked to the Horse sign and is emphasized in kata Kukan.
- **Moving Rock Stance** (*Dogan*): Done from a one-leg kneeling position. The hands are held as in the Front Stance position: arms held straight out in a relaxed manner; hands held palms down, wrists straight, and fingers slightly curled. It is considered a good stance against kicks. It is linked to the Sheep sign and is emphasized in kata Kukan.
- **Heaven and Earth Stance** (*Tenchi*): Done from is done with the feet about two fists apart, one foot in front of the other, and both heels planted, as in the Fudo Stance. The arm over the front leg is held forward, elbow bent at a 45-degree angle, palm open and facing the opponent, also at a 45-degree angle. The other hand is held above the ear, but not above the head, palm open in a 45-degree position to the front. It is considered a good stance for quick attacks. It is linked to the Monkey sign and is emphasized in kata Chikan.
- **Blowing Down Stance** (*Fukiroshi*): Also called the Crane Method (*Tsuru Ho*). It is done with the feet about two fists apart, one foot in front of the other, and both heels planted, as in the Fudo Stance. The hands are held somewhat similar to the Jinpu stance. However, in the Blowing Down Stance, the back arm is bent at approximately 90-degrees, the forearm pointing to the heavens, the palm open and facing forward. It is linked to the Rooster sign and is emphasized in kata Chikan.
- **Pointing at the Ground Stance** (*Chi Seigan*): Done with the feet about two fists apart, one foot in front of the other, and both heels planted, as in the Immovable Stance. The front arm hangs down so that the lower arm and open hand protect the thigh. The back arm is bent, parallel to the ground, crossing the body's center line; the palm is open and facing down. It is considered a good stance from which to defend against kicks. It is linked to the Dog sign and is emphasized in kata Chikan.
- **Number One Stance** (*Ichimonji*): Done from the cat stance. The front arm is bent, the fist resting a little bit above the solar plexus area. The back fist is held above the waist in the ready-to-punch position. It is linked to the Boar sign and is emphasized in kata Chikan.

KATA	STANCE	CHINESE ZODIAC ANIMAL
Chikan	Ground (Chiseigan)	Dog
	Number One (Ichimonji)	Boar
	Blowing Down (Fukioroshi)	Rooster
	Heaven and Earth (Tenchi)	Monkey
Kukan	Blending (Aiki)	Snake
	Forward (Seigan)	Horse
	Moving Rock (Dogan)	Sheep
	Cloud Dragon (Unryu)	Dragon
Tenkan	Immovable (Fudo)	Bull
	Wind Hands (Jinpu)	Tiger
	Cross (Jumonji)	Rabbit
	Front (Seishin)	Rat

Use of Open-Hands

In addition to the emphasis on fighting postures, another unique feature of the Kojo system is its preference for open-handed techniques rather than the classic karate punch.

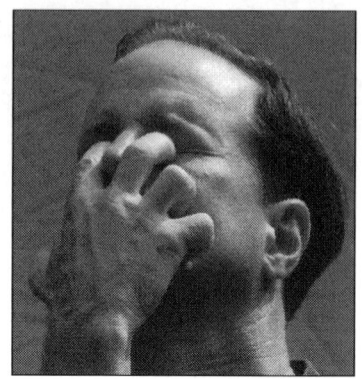

In hand-to-hand combat, a Kojo-ryu fighter likes to slide in close to his opponent, lock the opponent's leg with his own leading leg, and strike, generally with an open hand. As he is striking, the Kojo-ryu fighter will often use the locking leg to sweep his opponent to the ground.

The importance of grappling and open-hand strikes is best symbolized by the three higher-level, animal katas created by the Kojo family: White Crane, White Tiger, and White Dragon. The Crane arts emphasize grabbing and open-hand strikes, usually with the finger tips. The Tiger arts emphasize striking with harder parts of the still open hand, such as the thumb, and dividing and ripping muscles and ligaments. The Dragon arts are predominately grappling oriented.

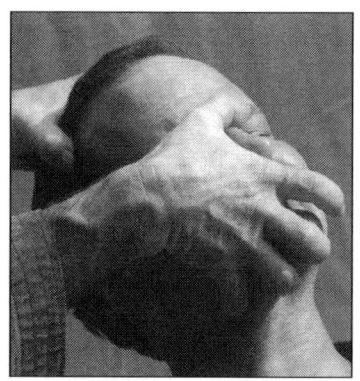

Kojo-ryu and Uechi-ryu are the two Okinawan karate styles that most emphasize open-hand strikes over close-fisted punching. Both styles' techniques reflect the same three animals: crane, tiger, and dragon, emphasizing of the shared Fuzhou training hall. In Kojo-ryu, there are eleven primary open-handed strikes:

- **Tiger Claw:** The hand looks somewhat like a tiger's claw and is used for grabbing, tearing, and ripping.
- **Tiger Thumb**: The protruding thumb joint in the Tiger Claw position is used to strike soft tissue areas.
- **Tiger Paw Strike:** Also called the four-knuckle punch. The thumb is laid across the palm and the four fingers are bent at the second knuckle.

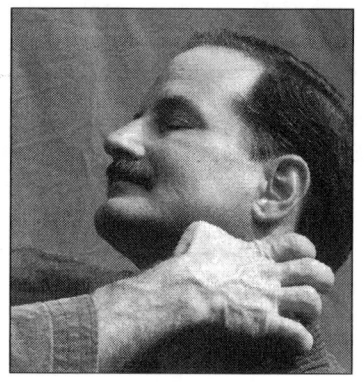

- **Tiger Palm Heel:** The palm heel of the Tiger Claw position used as a strike against harder targets, such as the chin.
- **Crane Beak:** The fingertips are held folded together and used in pinpoint strikes.
- **Crane Wing:** The fingertips are held together but flat, as opposed to the Crane Beak, and generally held with the palm facing the ground, striking soft tissue areas.
- **Dragon Claw:** A position similar to the Tiger Claw, and also used for grabbing, tearing, and ripping.
- **Cobra Strike:** The middle finger crosses over the ring finger, with the pointer finger lying atop of the

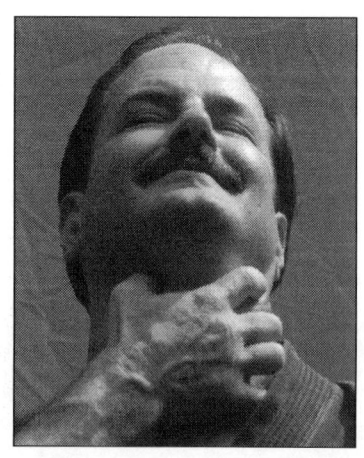

ring finger and next to the middle finger, used for supported, pinpoint striking to penetrate soft tissue areas, such as the spot behind the collar bone. It was also taught in the Tiger, Crane, Dragon school of Shushiwa, the Chinese teacher of Uechi Kanbun, the founder of Uechi-ryu, who took the strike out of his style because he considered it too dangerous and replaced it with the Crane Beak strike (Dollar, 1996:66).[21]

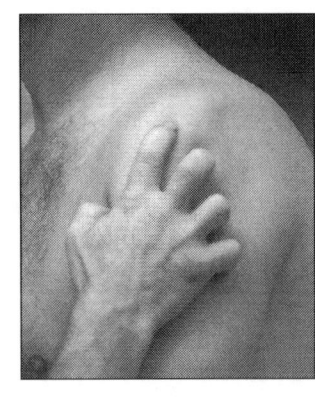

- **Iron Palm:** The hand is open and the fingers tensed backward. The striking area is the set of small bones at the top of the palm, right below the last segment of the fingers. In such a position, the Iron Palm is much like an Iron Bar.
- **Sword Hand:** Also called the Spear Hand. The wrist and fingers are held straight, with the fingertips doing the striking. The classic "karate chop" position.

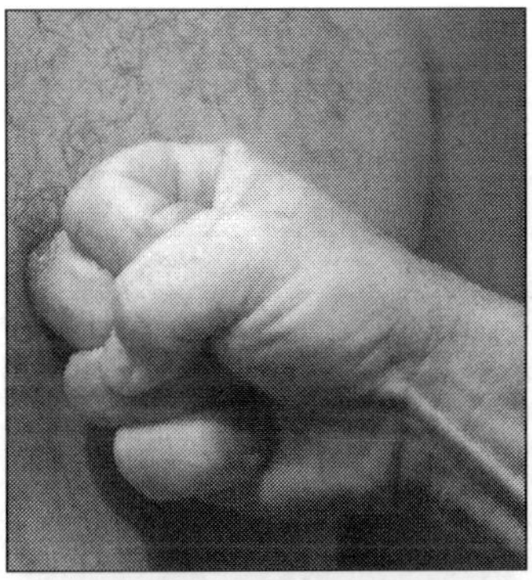

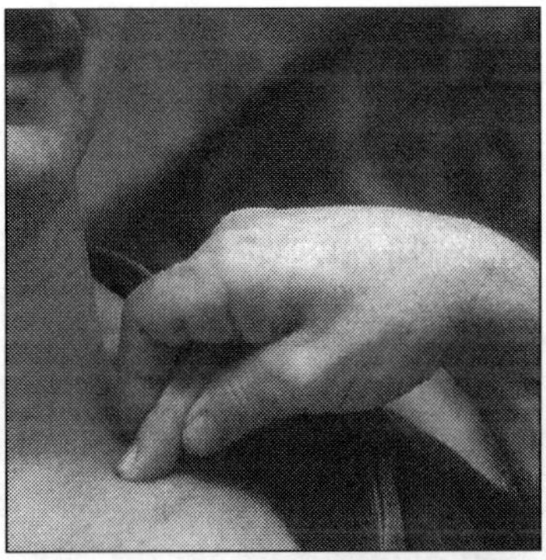

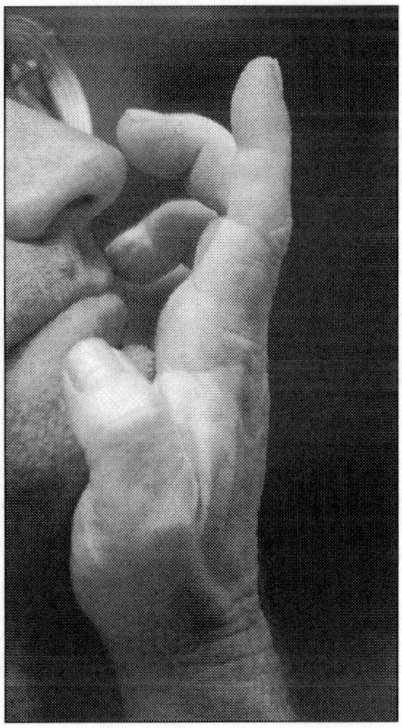

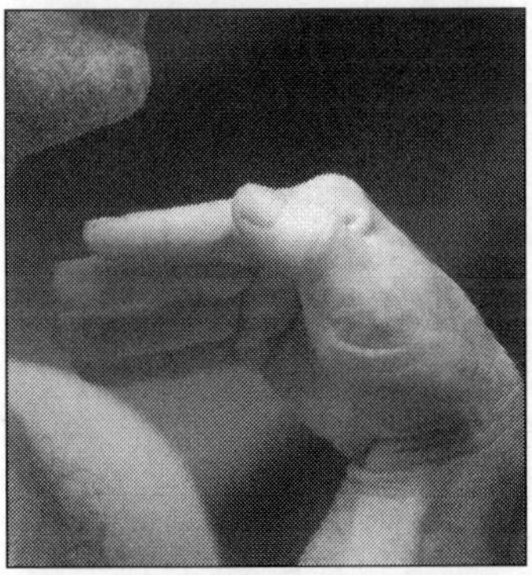

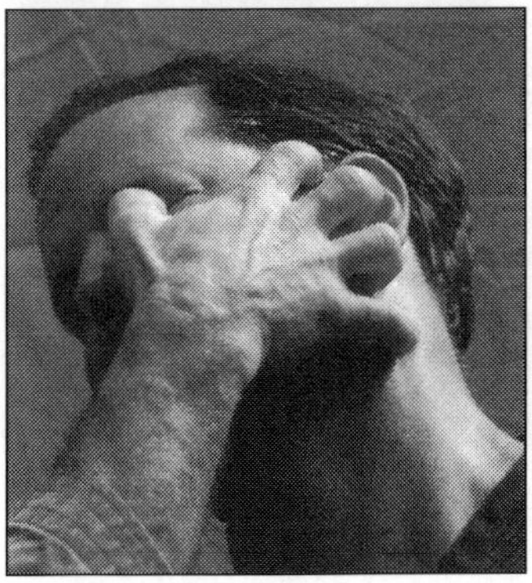

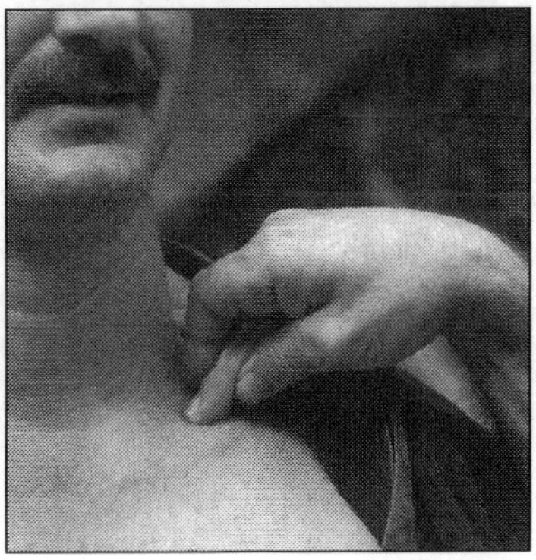

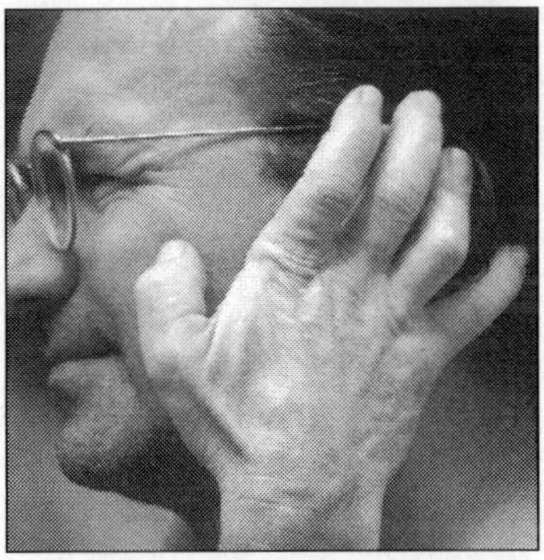

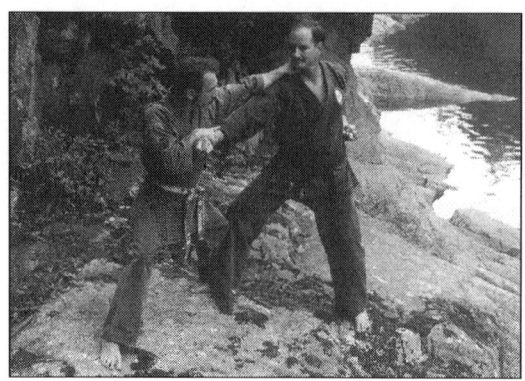
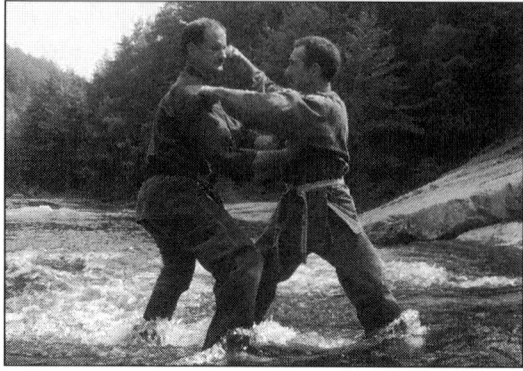

Katas

The Kojo-ryu katas reflect the history of Okinawan karate. They include Chinese forms learned in southern China, family-created forms based on the Chinese forms, traditional Okinawan (Shorin-ryu) katas adopted in the 20th century to serve as a bridge for outsiders, and modified family katas to help introduce the system to the next generation. These katas are:[23]

Empty-Hand Katas

- **Pinan Shodan:** A kata from the Shuri-te/Shorin-ryu lineage. Kojo Yoshitomi learned this kata while in elementary school and brought it into the Kojo-ryu.
- **Pinan Nidan:** A kata from the Shuri-te/Shorin-ryu lineage. Kojo Yoshitomi learned this kata while in elementary school and brought it into the Kojo-ryu.
- **Naihanchi Shodan:** A kata from the Shuri-te/Shorin-ryu lineage. Kojo Yoshitomi learned this kata while in elementary school and brought it into the Kojo-ryu.
- **Passai:** A kata from the Shuri-te/Shorin-ryu lineage. Kojo Yoshitomi learned this kata while in elementary school and brought it into the Kojo-ryu.
- **Chinto:** A kata that originally came from the Tomari-te tradition. Kojo Yoshitomi learned this kata while in elementary school and brought it into the Kojo-ryu.
- **Tenkan** (Heaven): One of three Kojo-ryu katas created by Kojo Koho based on the teachings of Iwah and principles found in the *Bubishi*. The other two are Chikan and Kukan. "Tinkan" in Okinawan.
- **Kukan** (Sky): One of three Kojo-ryu katas created by Kojo Koho based on the teachings of Iwah and principles found in the *Bubishi*. The other two are Chikan and Tenkan.
- **Chikan** (Earth): One of three Kojo-ryu katas created by Kojo Koho based on the teachings of Iwah and principles found in the *Bubishi*. The other two are Kukan and Tenkan.
- **Hakutsuruken Kumite** (White Tiger Fist Sparring): A Kojo-ryu kata that extracts non-lethal sparring principles from kata Hakukuken. Kojo Yoshitomi created this kata for his son, Shigeru, to teach the public the basic concepts without danger of hurting the student. It can also be called "Hakukuken Kumite."
- **Hakutsuruken** (White Crane Fist): Also called Hakukuken. A Kojo-ryu kata created by Kojo Shigeru. It was created as the international version of Hakukuken for competition. Shigeru taught it to Irimaji Seiji, who taught it to Yabiku Takaya.
- **Hakukuken** (White Crane Fist): One of the three Kojo-ryu higher-level katas. It is also called "Hakutsuruken." The others are Hakuryuken and Hakukoken.
- **Hakukoken Kumite** (White Tiger Fist Sparring): A Kojo-ryu kata that extracts non-lethal (ie., sans pressure point applications) sparring principles from kata Haku-

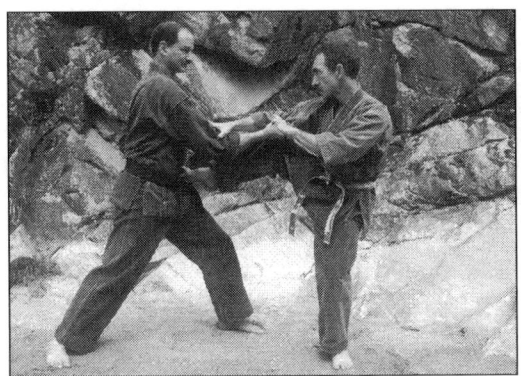
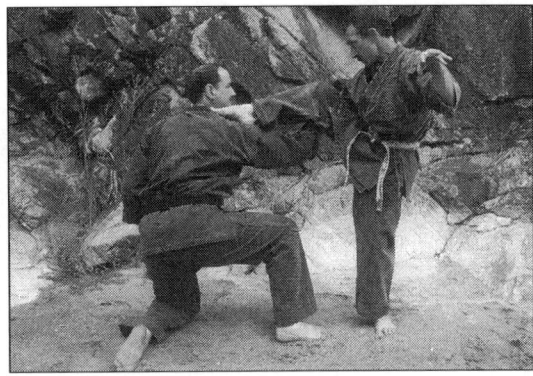

koken. Kojo Yoshitomi created this kata for his son, Shigeru, to teach to the public the basic concepts without danger of hurting the student.
- **Hakuryuken Kumite** (White Dragon Fist Sparring): A Kojo-ryu kata that extracts non-lethal sparring principles from kata Hakuryuken. Kojo Yoshitomi created this kata for his son, Shigeru, to teach the public the basic concepts without danger of hurting the student.
- **Hakuryuken** (White Dragon Fist): One of six primary Kojo-ryu katas. The others are Hakakuken, Hakutsuruken, Chikan, Kukan, and Tenkan.
- **Nepai:** One of the 13 forms taught at the Wai Xinxian gongfu school in Fuzhou. It is based on Hofa.
- **Hofa or Houfua:** One of the thirteen forms taught at the Wai Xinxian gongfu school in Fuzhou. It is also called Nipaipo. It is the base from which the kata Nepai is taken.
- **Nunfa:** One of the 13 forms taught at the Wai Xinxian gongfu school in Fuzhou.
- **Paichu:** One of the 13 forms taught at the Wai Xinxian gongfu school in Fuzhou.
- **Paishi:** One of the 13 forms taught at the Wai Xinxian gongfu school in Fuzhou.
- **Pachin:** One of the 13 forms taught at the Wai Xinxian gongfu school in Fuzhou.
- **Tanchin:** One of the 13 forms taught at the Wai Xinxian gongfu school in Fuzhou.
- **Nijikken:** "Twenty Fists." One of the 13 forms taught at the Wai Xinxian gongfu school in Fuzhou.
- **Sodenkan:** One of the 13 forms taught at the Wai Xinxian gongfu school in Fuzhou.
- **Gogiho:** "Five Skills Way." One of the 13 forms taught at the Wai Xinxian gongfu school in Fuzhou.
- **Shitenkan:** "Four Points Fist." One of the 13 forms taught at the Wai Xinxian gongfu school in Fuzhou.
- **Suiken:** One of the 13 forms taught at the Wai Xinxian gongfu school in Fuzhou.
- **Shimonken:** "Four Gates Fist." One of the 13 forms taught at the Wai Xinxian gongfu school in Fuzhou.
- **Kokukakuken:** "Royal Crane Fist." Kojo Koho may have created this kata.

In the 20th century, Kojo Yoshitomi reconstructed the two crane-based kata, Nepai and Hofa, that were lost when his grandfather, Koho, died in 1925. In the kata names, Hakutsuruken/Hakukuken, Hakukoken, and Hakuryuken, "*haku*" (white) is added to the animal names to indicate that they are the pure, original methods of the crane, tiger, and dragon.

Because the three elemental katas (Tenkan, Kukan, and Chikan) are so difficult for beginner-level students to understand, in 2000, at the request of Chuck Chandler, Irimaji Seiji and Yabiku Takaya put their mark on Kojo-ryu by adding two katas:

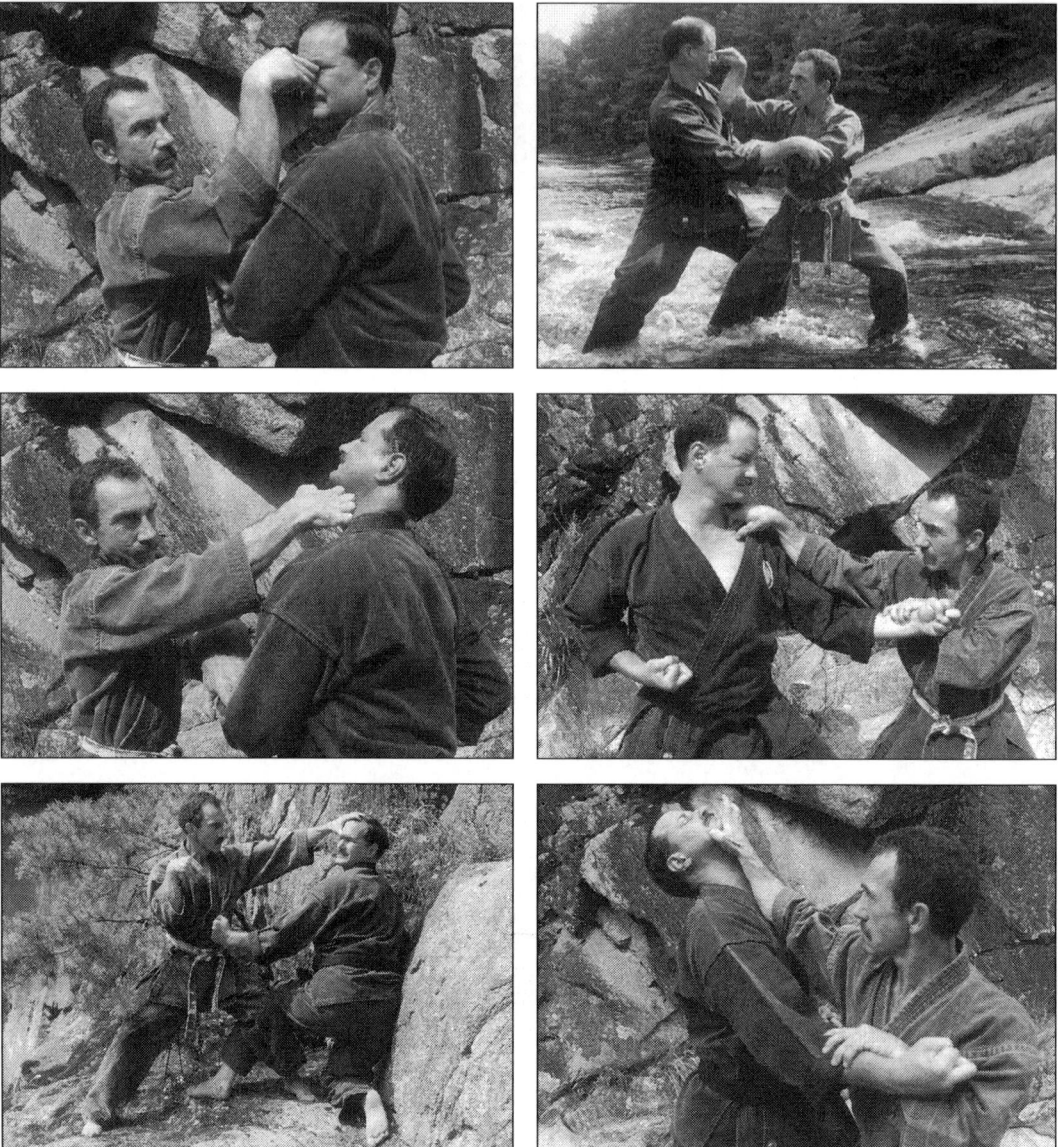

- Tenkan Kihon Ichi: "Heaven Basics One." A Koshin-ryu kata created by Irimaji Seiji and Yabiku Takaya.
- Tenkan Kihon Ni: "Heaven Basics Two." The second of two Koshin-ryu katas created by Irimaji Seiji and Yabiku Takaya.

In 2001, Irimaji and Yabiku developed three basic-level katas for the Kukan series. Eventually, they will develop a series of basic katas to help learn kata Chikan as well.

Weaponry

There are three weapons taught, with a total of five weapons katas in Kojo-ryu:
- Bo Shodan: The first staff kata created by Kojo Koho.
- Bo Nidan: The second staff kata created by Kojo Koho.
- Sai Shodan: The first sai kata created by Kojo Koho.
- Sai Nidan: The second sai kata created by Kojo Koho.
- Jo: Kojo Saisho brought this 4' staff form back from Fuzhou.

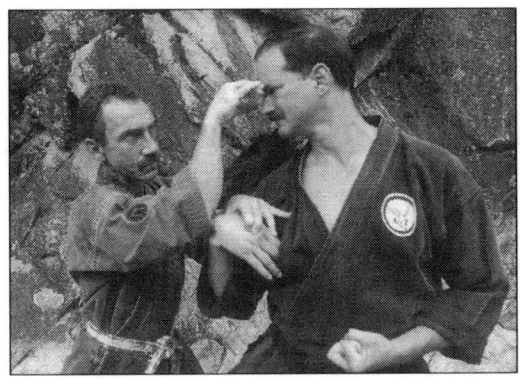
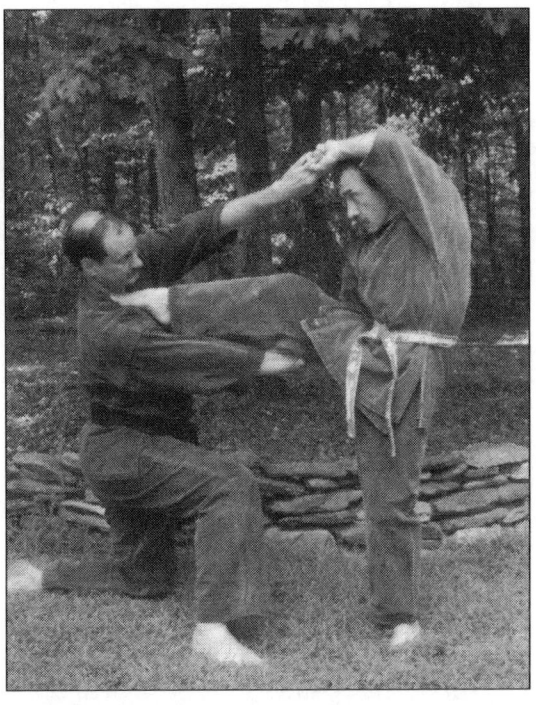

Conclusion

In this day and age when many seem to be searching for the origins of the martial arts, and Okinawa karate in particular, the Kojo family system may be an answer. It is one of the oldest of the Okinawan systems still practiced today. As noted above, the system is a good paradigm of the evolution of Okinawan karate, reflecting the various stages and influences that describe those systems: it has strong ties to the Chinese martial arts, both historically and stylistically; it provides its own unique touch in the six family-created katas; a touch of traditional Okinawan karate, adopting some Shorin-ryu katas to provide a more familiar transition to outsiders; and has changed with the times with the contributions of Irimaji and Yabiku. The Kojo family is intimately linked with many of the better known names of Okinawan karate: among others, Kojos trained under Iwah, Ko Ryuryu, Wai Xinxian, Tode Sakugawa, Matsumura Sokon; Kojos trained alongside Maezato Ranho and Go Kenki; and Kojos trained Higashionna Kanryo.

Koshin-ryu is the continuation of the relatively unknown but often spoken about Kojo family karate. There is a direct historical link to the Kojo family arts through Koshin-ryu's founder, Irimaji Seiji, who is the most senior ranking Kojo-ryu practitioner and was personally selected by the last practicing family member to be the style's chief instructor.

There is no question that Irimaji Seiji and his Koshin-ryu are the legitimate heirs of Kojo-ryu. However, like all things historical, there is much yet to uncover about Okinawa karate in general, and Kojo-ryu in particular. For instance, since the Kojos trained in China with Chinese instructors who taught other Okinawans who became well-known and because the Okinawan martial arts world was relatively small and its members knew each other and often shared techniques with each other, how did Kojo-ryu remain out of the public for so long? When Mark Bishop came around to research his book, *Okinawan Karate: Teachers, Styles and Secret Techniques* (1989), why didn't Kojo Yoshitomi note that Irimaji was his senior student?

In any case, the Koshin-ryu Koshinkan is a good place to start this search.

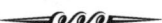

Notes

1. Okinawa is the main island in the chain of islands called the Ryukyus. Today, the entire chain is a Japanese prefecture using the main island's name.
2. In Japanese and Okinawan, words are Romanized differently when appearing alone and when in combination with other words/sounds. For instance, the Okinawan term "ti" and the Japanese term "te" use the initial "t" sound when appearing alone; however, when appearing as the second or later syllable of a word, they sound more like "di" and "de," respectively. I have tried to reflect this dichotomy throughout the chapter. I have also adopted the Japanese pronunciation over the Okinawan because it is the more readily recognized.
3. Nagaboshi Tomio (adopted name of Englishman Terence Dukes; 1994:456) believes that the major influence on any indigenous Okinawan martial arts was Chinese Buddhist monks and traders.
4. In Korea, Hwang Kee chose to name his Shotokan-based art "Tang Soo Do," which also means "China Hand Way."
5. Okinawan legend says that the Tenson ("Heaven") Dynasty ruled over a unified Okinawa for 1500 years until 1314, when Tamagusuku succeeded his father, Eiji. Because of Tamagusuku's weak character and abilities, Okinawa broke up into three "kingdoms": *Nanzan* ("southern mountain"), *Chuzan* ("central mountain," ruled by Tamagusuku), and *Hokuzan* ("northern mountain)." Chuzan King Sho Hashi conquered Hokuzan in 1416. With Sho Hashi's conquest of Nanzan in 1422 (or 1429), Okinawa was again unified. And much as the Tang Dynasty came to signify all of China, Chuzan then became synonymous with all of Okinawa (Sakihara, 1987:9, 82; Kerr, 1958/2000:60, 86).
6. The number thirty-six does not mean literally only thirty-six families went to Okinawa at this time. It was a symbolic term meaning a large number of Chinese, with their families, moved to Okinawa, at least temporarily.
7. Today, Shuri ("first village" or "head village"; Sui in the Okinawan dialect) and Tomari ("port"; Tumai in Okinawan) are districts of Naha, the Okinawan capital. Before Okinawa became a Japanese prefecture in 1879, Shuri was the royal district housing the king's castle; Tomari was the port district; and Naha (Nafa in Okinawan) was the business and residential district. There were, and are, other, lesser-known districts of Naha.
8. Kano lectured on judo at the Okinawa Teacher's College in 1922 and in the summer of 1926. See McCarthy, 1994:8-9.
9. Tomari-te is said to have been much like Naha-te, which would explain their marriage in Tokashiki Iken's Gohakukai, a combination of Goju-ryu and Tomari-te. However, Tomari-te kata are quite frequently found in the Shorin-ryu styles as well. For more information, see my "Where Goju-ryu and Tomari-te Meet: Tokashiki Iken and the Gohakukai," *Bugeisha*, Summer 1998.
10. In Okinawa karate systems, it is actually more common for a senior student to give his interpretation of the original style a new name without reference to the founder's name, often the name is based on the name of the new founder's school, such as Shorin-ryu Kenshinkan, Shorin-ryu Shorinkan, Goju-ryu Meibukan, and Goju-ryu Jundokan. Then there are cases in which a founder has studied several arts and gives the art a name that in some way reflects those arts, such as Higa Seitoku's Bugeikan Te ("Martial Arts Place/Hall Hand," based on Shorin-ryu, Motobu-ryu Udun-di, and Yamane-ryu kobujutsu), and Kyoda Juhatsu's To'on-ryu (a variant reading of the "Kanryo" in Higaonna Kanryo, founder of Naha-te/Nafa-di).
11. In Okinawa, "Kojo" can also be pronounced "Koshiro," "Kogusuku," "Kugushiku," and

"Kogushiku." In Chinese Mandarin, the characters for the name are pronounced "Hucheng" and mean "lake wall" or "lake city."

12. The *oyakata* (or *uekata*) were the third highest class in Okinawa, coming beneath the royal family and the *aji* (or *anji*), feudal-type lords, often the sons of the king's brothers and uncles (McCarthy, 1995:48, citing Douglas Haring, *Okinawan Customs: Yesterday and Today*, 1969, Rutland; VT: Charles E. Tuttle).
13. Sells says Shinpo went to China in 1665 (1995:23).
14. Peichin were the fourth class in Okinawa, under the royal family, aji, and oyakata.
15. Sakugawa was a student of Wai Xinxian and/or Ko Ryuryu (Nagamine, 2000:61).
16. Iwah taught other Okinawans, including Matsumura Sokon.
17. Upon his return to Okinawa, Ranho settled in Kume Village, where the Kojo family also lived.
18. These dates are based on family records available to Irimaji Seiji and provided to Chuck Chandler. Bishop (1996:115) gives the dates as 1839–1891.
19. Like most history of this period, little is known about Wai Xinxian. He may have been senior to Ko Ryuryu, or a practitioner of equal skill in another style. He may have taught Higaonna Kanryo and did teach Aragaki Seisho, who did teach Higaonna; and Uechi Kanbun for a short time (McCarthy, 1996:34–35, 60).
20. Shuren also studied under Maezato Ranho, who was another student of Iwah in Fuzhou.
21. There are unsubstantiated rumors that Kojo Saikyo taught Maezato Ranho's grandson, Miyazato Eiko. However, the current Kojo-ryu headmaster, Irimaji Seiji, says that Kojo Yoshitomi was Saikyo's son and inherited the system from his grandfather, becoming the fifth-generation headmaster.
22. This book is poorly produced, with no editing, a poor index, and no footnotes. However, I use it here because its main source, the opus Uechi-ryu karatedo (1975) by Uechi Kanbun and Takamiyagi Shigeru, is a font of information regarding Okinawa history, culture, and karate. It has also been replicated in other self-promoting books such as *The 100 Year History of Shorin-ryu Karate* (1986) by Frank Hargrove.
23. The series Shoshingata, Fudogata, Chinpugata, Jumonjigata, Unryugata, Aikigata, Segangata, Domyogata, Techigata, Suikagata, Ichimonjigata, listed in Nakaya (1986:86), Silvan (1993:78), and copied onto the Internet at Paranto (1996) are not Kojo-ryu katas. They are actually the twelve stances taught in the katas.

Bibliography

Bishop, M. (1989). *Okinawan karate: Teachers, styles and secret techniques*. London: A&C Black.

Bishop, M. (1996). *Zen kobudo: Mysteries of Okinawan weaponry and te*. Rutland, VT: Charles E. Tuttle Co.

Chandler, C. (2000, September). Personal conversation with the author.

Dollar, A. (1996). *Secrets of Uechi-ryu karate and the mysteries of Okinawa*. Antioch, CA: Cherokee Publishing.

Florence, R. (1998, Summer). "Where Goju-ryu and Tomari-te meet: Tokashiki Iken and the Gohakukai." *Bugeisha* 6:46–54.

Funakoshi, G. (1973). *Karate-do kyohan: The master text*. Tokyo: Kodansha.

Funakoshi, G. (1975). *Karatedo: My way of life*. Tokyo: Kodansha.

Funakoshi, G. (1988). *Karate-do nyumon: The master introductory text*. Tokyo: Kodansha.

Haines, B. (1995). *Karate's history and traditions: Revised edition*. Rutland, VT: Charles E. Tuttle Co.

Irimaji, S. (2000, August). Personal interview conducted by Chuck Chandler in Naha, Okinawa.
Jones, C. M. (2001, August 31). Personal correspondence with the author.
Kerr, G. H. (1958/1980). *Okinawa: The history of an island people.* Tokyo: Charles E. Tuttle Co.
Kojo, Y. (nd). *Kojo family records.*
McCarthy, P. (1995a). *The bible of karate: Bubishi.* Rutland, VT: Charles E. Tuttle Co.
McCarthy, P. (1995b). When masters meet: The 1936 meeting of Okinawan karate masters. *Furyu, 1*(4):10–17.
Nagamine, S. (2000). *Tales of Okinawa's great masters.* Rutland, VT: Charles E. Tuttle Co.
Nakaya, T. (1986). *Karate-do: History and philosophy.* Carrollton, TX: JSS Publishing Co.
Okinawa Prefecture Board of Education. (1995). *Okinawa karate "kobudo" graph.* Naha: Okinawa Prefecture Board of Education.
Paranto, N. (1996). http://www.kojosho.com/kata.html; International Kojosho Karate Federation (IKKF) home page; downloaded: 8 Oct. 2000.
Sakihara, M. (1987). *A brief history of early Okinawa based on the Omoro soshi.* Tokyo: Honpo Shoseki Press.
Sells, J. (1995). *Unante: The secrets of karate.* Hollywood, CA: W.M. Hawley.
Silvan, J. (1993). *Okinawan karate: Its teachers and their styles.* New York: Vantage Press, Inc.
Tokashiki, I. (1997, 18 February). Personal interview; oral. Bank of Japan; Naha, Okinawa, Japan.
Yabiku, T. (2000, September). *Ryukyu hiden karate-do: The pathway to Okinawa's secret karate—My 50 years as a karateka.* Summerville, SC: Resources Unlimited.

Acknowledgment

I would like to express my appreciation to Chuck Chandler who provided me with the results of his own research and Kojo family information from his instructors, Irimaji Seiji and Yabiku Takaya.

chapter 37

Incorporating the Main Principles of Kata Training

by Marvin Labbate

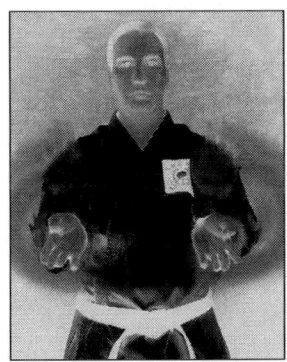

All photos courtesy of M. Labbate.

Introduction

This is the fourth in a series of chapters that describe the core principals of Okinawan Goju-ryu karatedo. Previous articles focused on hard principles of structure, movement, and breathing (Labbate, 1999); intermediate principals associated with building, controlling, and transferring internal energy (Labbate, 2000); and soft principals associated with making contact, following, and controlling an opponent (Labbate, 2001). This article builds upon these ideas and incorporates them into a general set of kata training principals. Kata are stylized fighting forms, or sequences, developed over the centuries and based on actual combat experience. Here the ideas are illustrated through the study of Kata Seiunchin. However, each Goju-ryu kata can be developed with the same ideas.

Every kata exists at many levels of sophistication and can be studied from a broad variety of viewpoints. At the most basic level, a kata is simply a pattern of movements that train typical fighting scenarios. At the most advanced level, a kata is a sequence of dangerous vital point strikes that can cause paralysis, unconsciousness, or death. Between these extremes are levels of development to which the masters of old tightly controlled access. The highest levels were transmitted orally to only a chosen son, or in the absence of a son, to a top student. This control was not simply to provide an advantage in combat: it provided safeguards to ensure that the information was transmitted to only those who proved to be of the appropriate spiritual and moral background, people who would exercise social responsibility in their teaching and use of the ideas. In modern times, these controls have been sadly undermined for commercial gain. A number of books and seminars have appeared that teach extremely dangerous techniques without integrity or an appreciation of the concepts' medical implications. This article takes some techniques from the Seiunchin kata that have recently become well known, and explores their devastating significance to underlie the importance of responsible teaching methods.

Basic Kata Training

At its heart, every kata contains a sequence of basic moves that must be memorized by the student. For example, the opening movements of Seiunchin are shown in Figure 1. Initially, the right foot moves forward 45 degrees into a straddle-leg stance (*shiko dachi*) and both hands are chambered (1a). Once in shiko dachi, both hands move straight up simultaneously to a spear-hand strike (*morote sukui uke*) and are placed back-to-back as they reach chin level (1b); the elbows in this position should be about a fist distance from the ribs, the fingertips are at chin height and are pointed upwards. Remaining in the straddle-leg stance, both hands then perform an augmented downward block (*morote gedan uke*) (1c). Both hands then make a right upward scooping block (*sukui uke*), the right hand palm faces upwards while performing the block while the left hand moves into an open handed chambered position (1d). While keeping the left hand chambered, a right hand hooking block (*kaki uke*) is then performed (1e). Finally, the left hand performs a finger thrust (*hira nukite tsuki*) as the right hand draws back to a chamber position facing downward (1f).

FIGURE 1— *Kata Seiunchin*

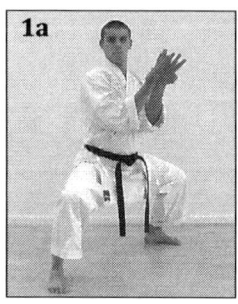
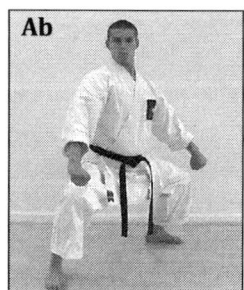
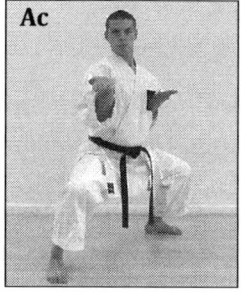
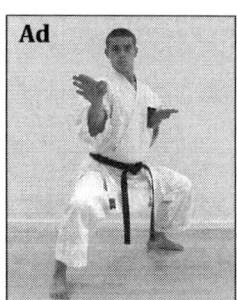
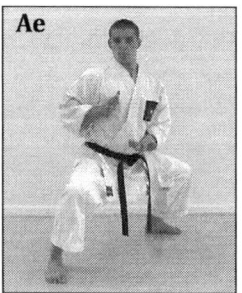
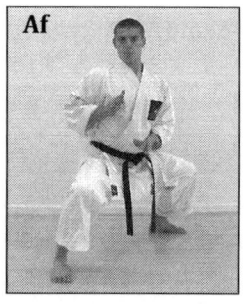

The constant repetition of this basic pattern over a period of years, consisting of literally thousands of repetitions, perfects the basic motor movements associated with the pattern and develops concentration and focus. The kata should be performed in every direction, beginning by facing north, south, east, or west. Eventually, from any given starting position, the student should be able to complete the kata, ending at the original starting position, facing in the starting direction. As a result of this training process, muscle memory develops such that in a real combat situation, the associated response to an attack occurs automatically and without thought.

Intermediate Kata Training
There is a significant difference between learning a kata, and training one-self in kata. Every student is endowed with a level of endurance, strength, and speed that form the primary abilities for performing kata. Endurance is the ability to continue working despite the onset of fatigue and is directly tied to cardio-respiratory performance and correct breathing. Often students may hold their breath while performing a kata leading to fatigue, tension, and sloppy technique; upon completion they may stand gasping for air. Alternatively, due to nervousness or tension, they may breathe too quickly and are thus susceptible to hyperventilation. There are several methods to improve endurance, including repetitions of kata and cross-training with other activities such as running, cycling, or skiing.

Strength is the ability to overcome resistance. It can be improved by weight training with a variety of traditional Okinawan training implements or modern equipment.

Speed is the ability to move quickly. Studies of world-class athletes indicate a higher level of twitch muscles. Thus speed is tied directly to genetic makeup. To increase speed, the student must utilize economy of motion to reduce wasted energy. Therefore, speed is directly tied to improved quality in performing karate techniques, such as in reducing the motion of the shoulder muscle groups during blocks and punches.

Students typically memorize a kata at a given level and then use repetition to improve these primary abilities. However, there are several alternative training methods that can be incorporated into practice to not only improve physical performance but also to achieve harmony between mind and body. These methods systematically isolate and improve a particular aspect of the kata. They allow the student to step back and assess weaknesses in need of additional practice. Each method emphasizes and develops a core set of principals from the Goju-ryu system.

Hard Principles
Initially, the kata is performed using the hard principals associated with the Sanchin kata (Labbate, 1999). This isolates and develops the principals of structure, movement, and breathing. The kata is performed slowly, with strong tension, and paying close attention to transitioning and positioning. Each blow is supported from the entire shoulder muscle group and locked down at the end of each motion. Movement between stances is accomplished at the same level, without causing the body to bob up and down, or move from side to side. Mental focus allows the weight of the body to be lowered into the stance such that each technique is performed with the body firmly rooted to the ground and supported by correct positioning. In a straddle-leg stance, the legs and feet are positioned at 90 degrees to each other, and the foreleg is at 90 degrees to the ground. The back remains straight and supported, the feet move through an arc that bisects the stride. Breathing is coordinated with movement: inhalation occurs between techniques in Seiunchin, and exhalation occurs on each technique. All of these concepts

arise directly from the study of Sanchin.

The hard principals are then developed further through exaggeration with weight resistance to enhance both speed and strength. The kata can be performed with traditional training implements such as weighted shoes (*geka*) and dumbbells (*sashi*) as shown in Figure 2a, or straw grips shown in Figure 2b. Modern wrist and ankle weights and weight vests, shown in Figure 2c, can also be used to provide additional resistance. It is important when training with these implements that full power is not put into each technique, this can lead to pulled muscles and strains. Instead, the student reduces power to focus on positioning and strength. When the weights are removed, speed will increase naturally.

FIGURE 2 — Resistance Training

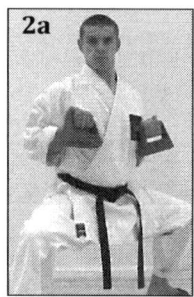 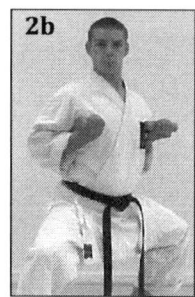 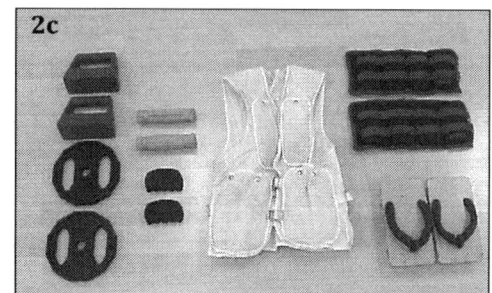

Speed Training

In speed training, the kata is performed as fast and explosively as possible without attention to form or technique. No power or tension is applied in this method, and the techniques are allowed to flow continuously into each as fast as possible. This method deliberately isolates and improves kata performance speed.

Form Training

The goal of form training is to develop perfect technique. The kata is performed slowly with no power or speed. At every movement, stance, position, and form are carefully examined and corrected. Distancing and angles on stances are adjusted, hand techniques are adjusted for correct positioning, and transitions are performed with circular motions. Breathing and movement are carefully coordinated and at the conclusion of each technique the body should be centered and aligned correctly (Labbate, 2000).

Rhythm and Tempo

Every kata has a prescribed cadence or rhythm by virtue of the order of techniques in each fighting sequence. For example, in Seiunchin, the motions from the entry to sumo stance (Fig. 1A) through to the spear-hand strike (Fig. 1F) correspond to a single sequence. Each movement in the sequence is performed slowly on a slow count of four, except for the movement in Figure 1E, which is performed on a slow count of two. The complete sequence is repeated three times at the beginning of the kata, first to the right, then to the left, and finally to the right again. There is a slight pause designating the transition between sides and each sequence should be performed symmetrically: a movement on the left, corresponding in length and speed to the same movement on the right. Rhythm training focuses attention on consistency and the balance of timing throughout the kata.

The tempo at which the kata movements are performed is dependent on the student's capabilities. Every student is endowed with a level of strength and speed that improve naturally as training proceeds. Most students exert either too much power or too much speed in their practice. This results in poor form, balance, and symmetry, or over exertion and fatigue. By focusing on tempo, the student learns to harmonize speed and power. The kata is performed as fast a possible, while attempting to maintain form, deliver maximum power in each strike, and correctly lock down the muscle groups at the end of each movement. If the speed is too fast, there is a noticeable sloppiness in form, and as a result strikes lose their power and are ineffective. Conversely, if the kata is performed with too much power, then it will cause jerky and slow motions that will result in fatigue. Tempo training aims to push the boundary of this relationship.

Power Training

Power training is an advanced method based on the "karate drum." In this technique, energy is transferred into techniques from the abdomen (*tanden*) through a subtle shaking motion at the hips (Labbate, 2000; Labbate, 2001). This allows the student to load energy into a technique, transfer it, lock down the technique using Sanchin style structure, and rebound into a countering movement. Figure 3 shows how the movements in Figures 1a, 1b, and 1c are adapted in this method. The guiding principal is that the reverse hand moves first. Notice in Figure 3 how the left hand and hip (reverse in the stance) lead the right. This movement sets up the correct motion to load energy such that subsequent movements rebound into an opponent.

FIGURE 3 — Power Training

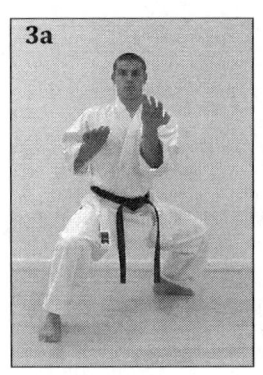
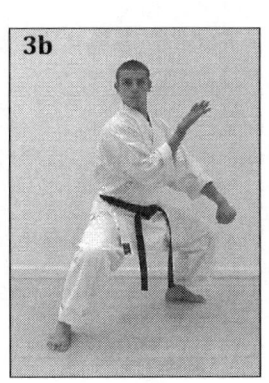
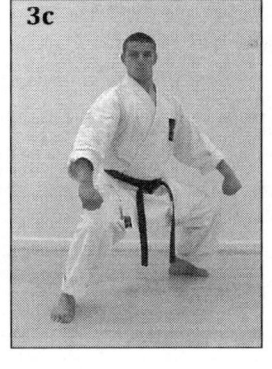
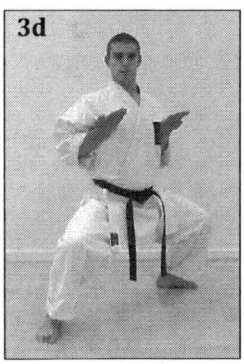

Focus Training

All of the previous training methods are on the physical level. Unfortunately, a kata performed simply as a sequence of moves is like a book with blank pages. To breathe life into the kata, it is necessary to visualize the fighting movements. Focus training harmonizes speed, power, and technique at normal speed by developing intent. Each movement in a kata is designated a basic level application; for Seiunchin, two such applications are developed later in this paper. The masters of old specifically chose the basic application to allow students to visualize an opponent but protect the kata's more dangerous secrets. In this manner, students were kept at a particular level until their social responsibility and humility were established and they were trusted.

Meditation Training

Meditation isolates and develops the mental aspects to create mind-body harmony and enhance fighting intent. It allows a student to learn about him or herself and assess their strengths and weaknesses. This training method aligns intent with physical training on a subconscious level, so that each movement has a clear purpose.

Meditation can be accomplished in any location or position, for example in the kneeling position (*seiza*) at the training hall (*dojo*) or when simply lying in bed. The student clears the mind and imagines him or herself in an attractive location, perhaps on a beach, at a park, or in the dojo. Then the student mentally performs the entire kata as if watching a video. Any of the intermediate training methods can be adopted during meditation to focus on a specific aspect of kata training. The result of this meditation is that the kata's physical performance is enhanced by the understanding and awareness developed through meditation.

Partner Training

All of the previous training methods focus on independent development and improvement, intended to give a student an understanding of their own level and ability. Partner training is intended to develop an understanding of an opponent: their speed, strength, and ability. It also allows new concepts to be developed such as timing, balancing, and distancing. Generally, sequences from each kata are taken separately and practiced using a variety of positions with the attacker standing in front, behind, or to the side, or with the defender placed at a disadvantage against a wall or on the ground. The intent is for the students to understand the different modes of attack a particular kata sequence is able to deal with, and to be able to recognize a given situation in combat. Having first made contact, it is also valuable for the defender to close their eyes and follow the movements of the attacker through contact, attempting to stick, redirect, and counter their movements (Labbate, 2000; Labbate, 2001).

Partners are joined in friendship and collaboration to help each other improve their skills, timing, and reflexes. It is the instructor's responsibility to ensure that this perspective is transmitted to students. If partner training is allowed to degenerate into a contest, then the value is lost and it becomes simply an issue of winning and ego, rather than an exercise to elevate skill.

Advanced Kata Training

Advanced kata training is focused around the designation of targets and the development of applications to attack them. There are two additional components to the applications: the first involves a variety of joint and wrist locks, arm bars, chokes, and throws; the second involves vital point striking (*kyushojutsu*). The intent is to apply force to carefully chosen points of weakness by understanding the opponent, overcoming their strength or speed, undermining their balance, or smoothly and effectively countering their movements. This is significantly different from blindly performing a given set of movements, in a preset order, toward a general area of the body, such as the head or chest. Like all elements of training, applications have several levels of sophistication. These levels are examined and their medical impact assessed here.

BASIC LEVEL APPLICATION 1

Figure 4 shows how the opening sequence from the Seiunchin kata can be used to counter an opponent that attempts to grab both hands (4a). The counter move is to escape the grab by raising both arms upward in a middle-block fashion (4b). The defender then counterattacks by grabbing the attacker's wrists and (4c) performing a knee strike to the groin (4d).

FIGURE 4 — Attacker Attempts to Grab

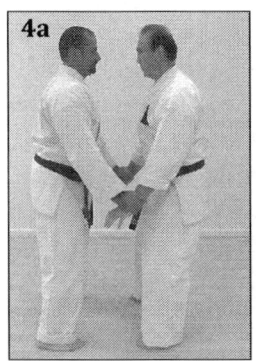
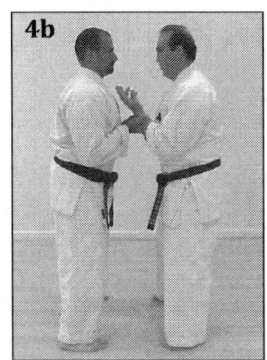
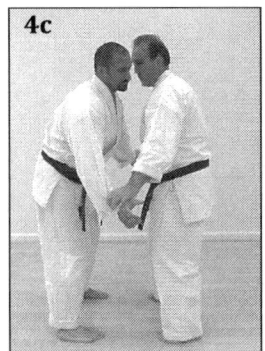
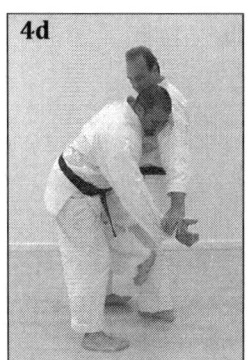

Medical Implications

The knee strike to the groin will cause immense pain and be debilitating. The attacker will experience any or all of the following: pain, shock, nausea, vomiting, and loss of breath or consciousness. A solid strike can fracture the pubic bone and rupture the bladder. The weakest area is the center of the pubic bone. Once the bone is fractured, the opponent will be rendered in a prone position due to the nauseating pain. Once injured, blood and urine will collect in the abdominal cavity causing tenderness and pain. Typically, the individual will experience an inability to urinate more than a few drops of bloody urine. If untreated, infection may occur. A direct strike can crush the testes and scrotum against the pubic bones resulting in castration.

BASIC LEVEL APPLICATION 2

An alternative kata application can be used if the attacker attempts to grab at the lapels, as shown in Figure 5A. The attackers' hands are covered and grabbed with the defender's left hand. While the defender's left hand applies a wristlock on the opponent's left hand, the defender's right performs a palm-heel strike into the attacker's groin (5B); this corresponds to Figure 1d in the kata. While the defender's left hand continues to maintain a wristlock on the opponent, the defender's right hand grabs the attacker's lapel (5C); this corresponds to Figure 1E. Finally, the defender pulls into a chamber position while applying a left knife-hand strike (*shuto*) to the ear (5D); this corresponds to Figure 1F.

FIGURE 5 — Attacker Attempts to Push

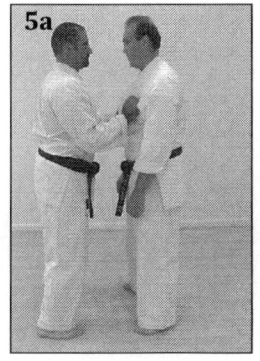
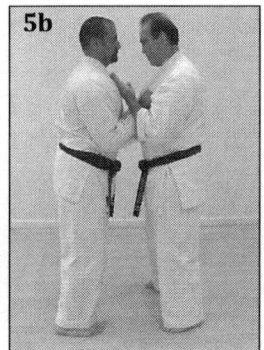
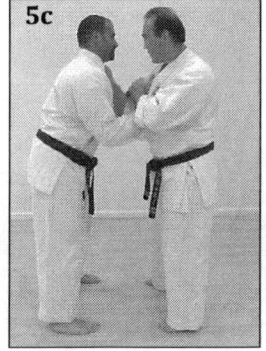
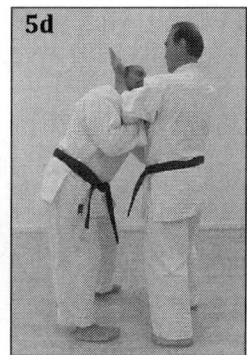

Medical Implications

As explained earlier, a severe blow to the testicles will cause the attacker to experience any or all of pain, shock, nausea, vomiting, and loss of breath or consciousness. The attack in Figure 5d directly strikes the ear. A percussive type shock to the eardrum (tympanac membrane) expands the auditory canal and eustachian tube with compressed air. The impact by such a blow will cause the small blood vessels and capillaries of the outer ear to rupture, thus swelling the ear. Because the air expands in volume as it travels through the narrow eustachian tube, the capillaries inside the canal, and even the eardrum, can rupture and swell. This will cause the eustachian tube to swell completely shut. The sensory nerves inside the auditory canal and eardrum contribute to hearing and balance. The locked air pressure inside produces severe pain, dizziness, and even unconsciousness. Permanent hearing loss can result.

Intermediate Application

Figure 6 shows an intermediate application in which the attacker grabs the defender with a bear hug from behind (6a). The defender grabs the attacker's fingers by moving both hands upwards (6b); this corresponds to Figure 1b. The defender then counters by grabbing the attacker's fingers in a downward fashion (6c); this corresponds to Figure 1c. While maintaining a finger lock on the opponent with the left hand, the defender takes a right step forward and moves back around to the left (approximately 270 degrees). The defender then pops the back of the elbow and grabs the triceps with the right hand (6d); this corresponds to Figure 1d. Finally, while maintaining a finger lock with the left hand, the defender shifts the right hand toward the back of the opponent's elbow and steps toward the left; the right hand then moves up and inward, while the left hand snaps in an outward fashion thus dislocating the elbow and fingers (6e); this corresponds to Figures 1e and 1f.

FIGURE 6 — Elbow Application

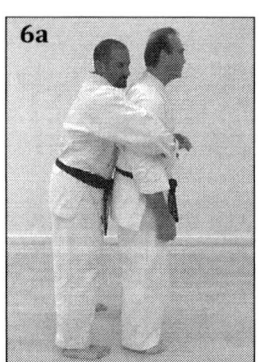
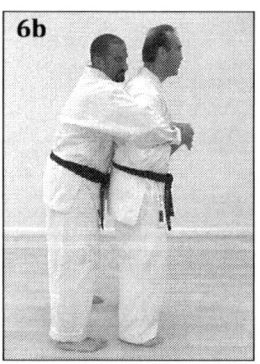
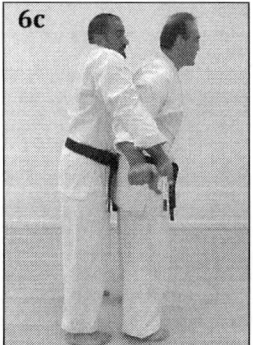
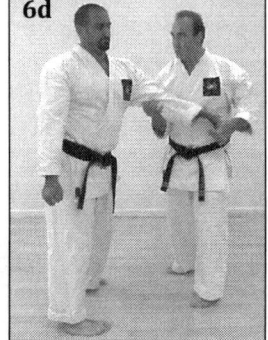
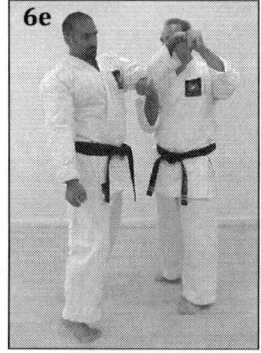

Medical Implications

Figure 7 shows a schematic of the elbow manipulated in the latter parts of this application. A strike to the superficial branch located on the forearm, approximately three inches down from the top of the elbow will cause the arm and hand to suffer a dull aching pain. Since the radial nerve is affected, the opponent will have difficulty making a fist because the muscle is weakened. Popping the elbow joint located at the back of a straightened arm can dislocate the elbow (ulna from humerus) and break the arm. If the blow is strong enough, it will affect the ulnar nerve in approximately 25 percent of cases (Haymaker, 1953:133-184). The ulnar nerve runs distally (away from the point of origin) and crosses the elbow joint to the forearm. The affected area, commonly referred as the "funny bone," will cause the opponent to experience a pinprick-like shock down the forearm and hand.

If a supracondylar fracture at the humerus' distal end shown in Figure 7 occurs the opponent will experience diffuse swelling in the elbow region and intense pain, thus disabling the arm. The bicep and tricep muscles can be torn if the resultant trauma is severe. The radial nerve is most commonly injured from fractures (Haymaker, 1953). The individual may experience nerve compression or bone fragments can even sever the nerve. Pain, loss of sensation, and possible paralysis of parts of the arm and/or hand may result with this type of injury. If the brachial artery is pinched or severed, tissue damage will occur and may develop into gangrene in extreme cases.

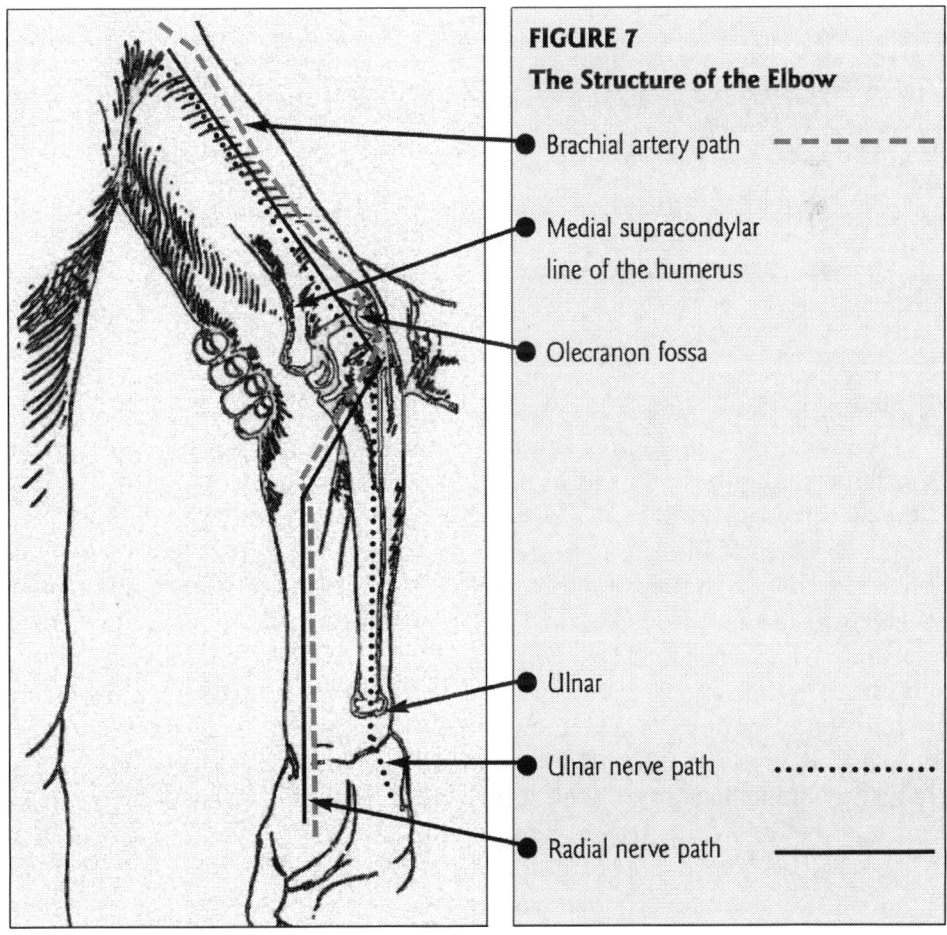

FIGURE 7
The Structure of the Elbow

- Brachial artery path `- - - - - - -`
- Medial supracondylar line of the humerus
- Olecranon fossa
- Ulnar
- Ulnar nerve path `. . . . . . . . . . . . .`
- Radial nerve path `_____`

Figure 8 shows the structure of the human wrist and hand manipulated through a wrist-lock or finger-hold in this application.

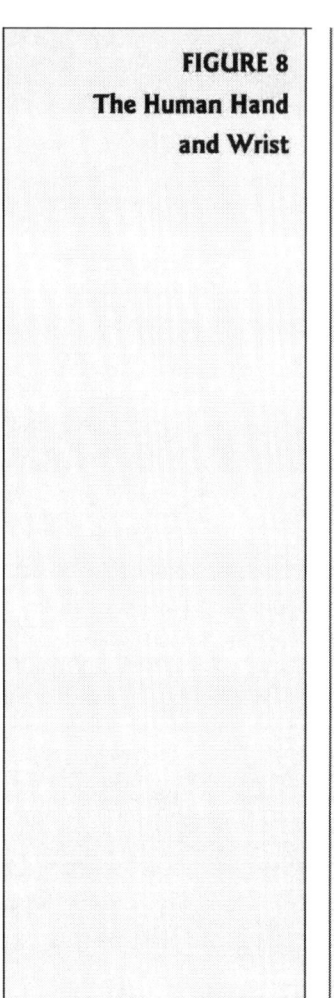
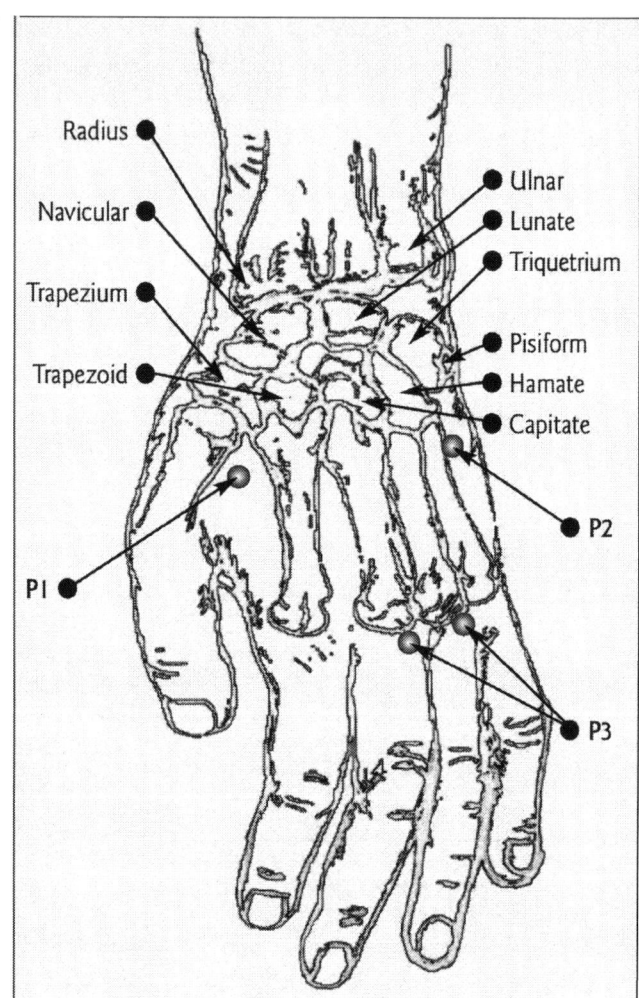

**FIGURE 8
The Human Hand and Wrist**

The fingers are particularly vulnerable to being sprained or broken, which can make it difficult for the opponent to make a fist. The radial artery, flexor tendons, and medial nerves are reachable in the inner side of the wrist. If the defender digs their fingers or knuckles centrally in this area at the median nerve, it will produce a sharp pain in the forearm and a weakened feeling in the hand. Grabbing the back of the hand can produce severe pain in the opponent's hand and arm. The key pressure points depicted in Figure 8 are: between the thumb and the index finger (P1), where the radial nerve is exposed against the side of the second metacarpal bone; along the little finger side of the fourth metacarpal (P2), where the ulnar nerve is exposed; and between the knuckles of the middle and ring fingers (P3). Finger holds in any of these areas can be used to control the opponent's movement and weaken the grip. The wrist is composed of eight carpal bones in two rows. The navicular (scaphoid bone) is the most commonly fractured bone and is located on the radial side of the carpus (above the radius near your thumb). The lunate located proximal to the capitate (above the radius near the middle finger) is the second most commonly fractured bone. The triquetrium is located distal (opposite) to the ulnar styloid process (above the ulnar near the pinkie finger) and is also vulnerable to injury and the third most commonly fractured bone (Hoppenfeld, 1976:65-71). Once the wrist is fractured, the hand is useless.

Advanced Level Application

Figure 9 shows an advanced application in which the attacker grabs at the chest (9a). The defender moves both hands simultaneously upward and traps both forearms (9b); this corresponds to the beginning of the movement in Figure 1b. The defender then applies a right and left knife-hand strike to the neck (9c); corresponding to the conclusion of the movement in Figure 1c. The defender then thumb rakes the eyes downward (9d–e); corresponding to Figure 1c. While the attacker tries to maintain a hold on the defenders lapel, the opponent's left hand is trapped and a right knife-hand strike to the side or back of the head is performed (9f); corresponding to Figure 1d. The back of the attacker's neck is grabbed with the right hand, while striking the chin with the left hand (9g). A quick pull with the right hand and a push with the left snaps the attacker's neck (9g). This corresponds to Figures 1e and 1f.

Figure 9 — Application Resulting in Severe Injury

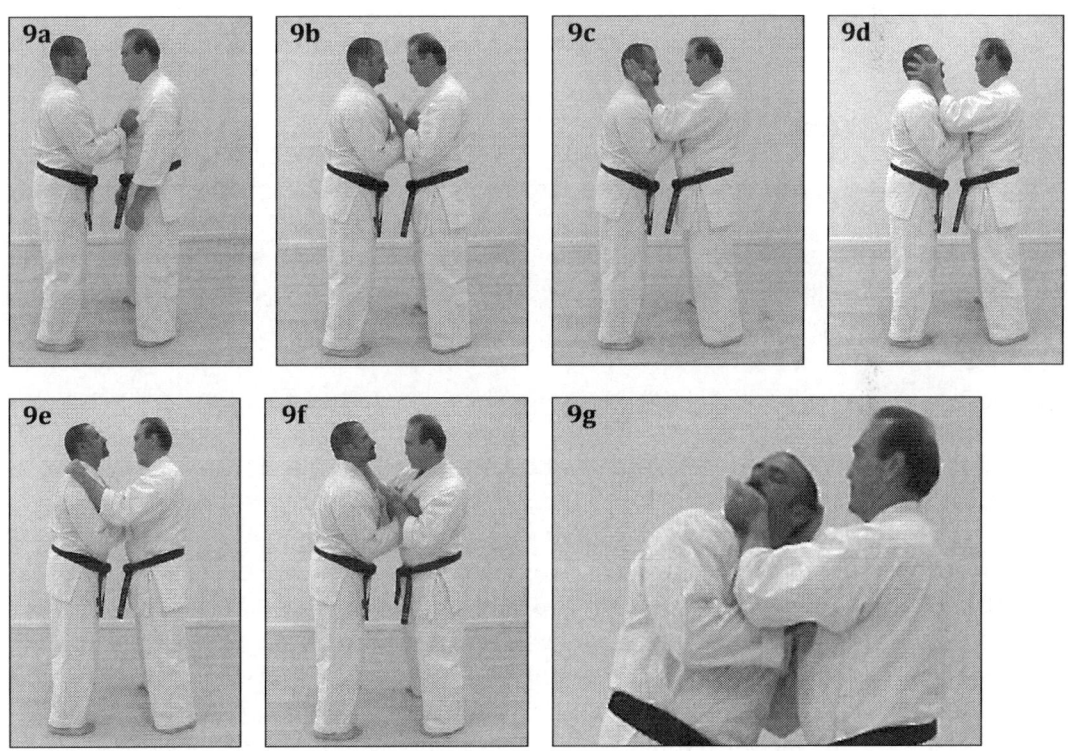

Medical Implications

The thumb rake to the eyes can cause hemorrhage and loss of sight. Disruption of the cornea, lens, and rectus muscle results. The eyelid may be vulnerable to a tear by the striking fingers, thereby increasing the risk for infection. If the strike is severe, the optic nerve may be injured. Jennett et al. (in Bailes et al, 1989:137–156) reported this was the most common cranial nerve injury seen in head injuries. Retinal detachment occurred in 7 percent of martial arts related injuries (Rabadi, Birrer, Jordan, 2000:297–303). In both scenarios, emergent surgical intervention is required as treatment.

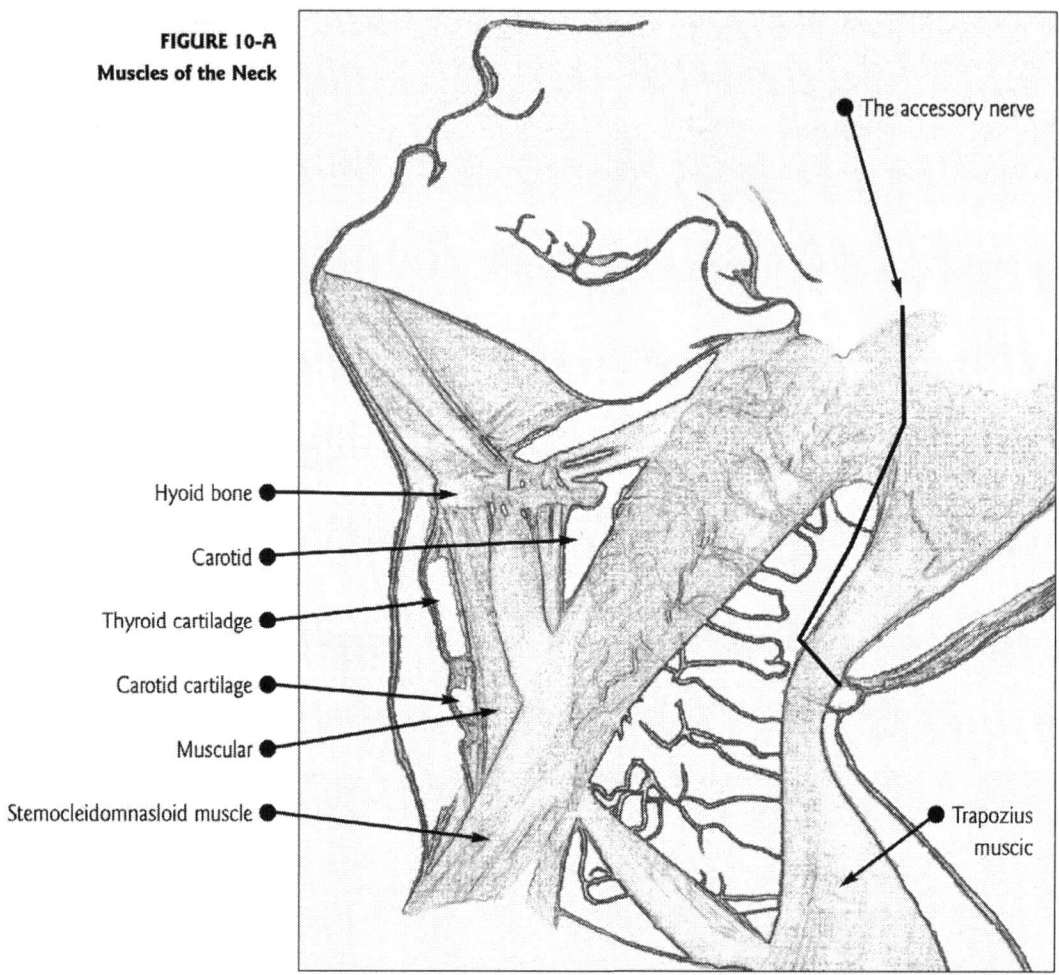

FIGURE 10-A
Muscles of the Neck

Figure 10-A shows a schematic of the head and neck manipulated in Figures 9F and 9. Neck and head injuries are the result of three distinct types of stresses generated by a force applied to the head (Cantu, 2000:137–156). The first two are compressive and tensile or linear forces. An example would be an athlete who is standing still and struck by a moving object. Focal injuries are produced such as brain contusions or intracranial hematoma. The third force is a rotational or shearing force. This creates diffuse brain injuries from a concussion to coma. These injuries can result in other deficits such as cognition, memory, attention, language, and psychosocial adaptation and even death. The most common acute traumatic brain injury in martial arts is cerebral concussion (Rabadi, Birrer, and Jordan, 2000:297–303). This injury can become cumulative. The chronic traumatic brain injury results in Parkinsonism or progressive difficulty in ambulation, coordination, and display of cognitive dysfunction (Jordan, 2000:339–346).

The sternocleidomastoid muscle and trapezius shown in Figure 10-A share a continuous attachment along the base of the skull to the mastoid process where they split and have a different attachment along the clavicle. They share the accessory nerve (cranial nerve XI). A strike approximately an inch below the angle of the jaw will bruise both the sternocleidomastoid muscle and accessory nerve. This causes pain and partial temporary paralysis of the neck and shoulder area. The carotid artery and jugular vein shown in Figure 10-B runs along the carotid tubercle of C6. A blow in this region can cause occlusion, dissection or even a thrombic emboli into the intracranial vessels and resultant stroke (Rabadi, Birrer, and Jordan 2000:297–303) and (McCrory, 2000:200–209). There is a documented case where a 26-year old sustained a carotid dissection and resultant hemispheric infarction after sustaining a knife-hand strike to the carotid artery (Fig. 10-B). There are also documented cases with vertebral artery dissection. A strike to the vagus nerve produces an inhibitory effect, slowing the heart rate and lowering the blood pressure. A severe strike in this region can produce loss of consciousness (Gott, 1997:110–113) and a deep contusion.

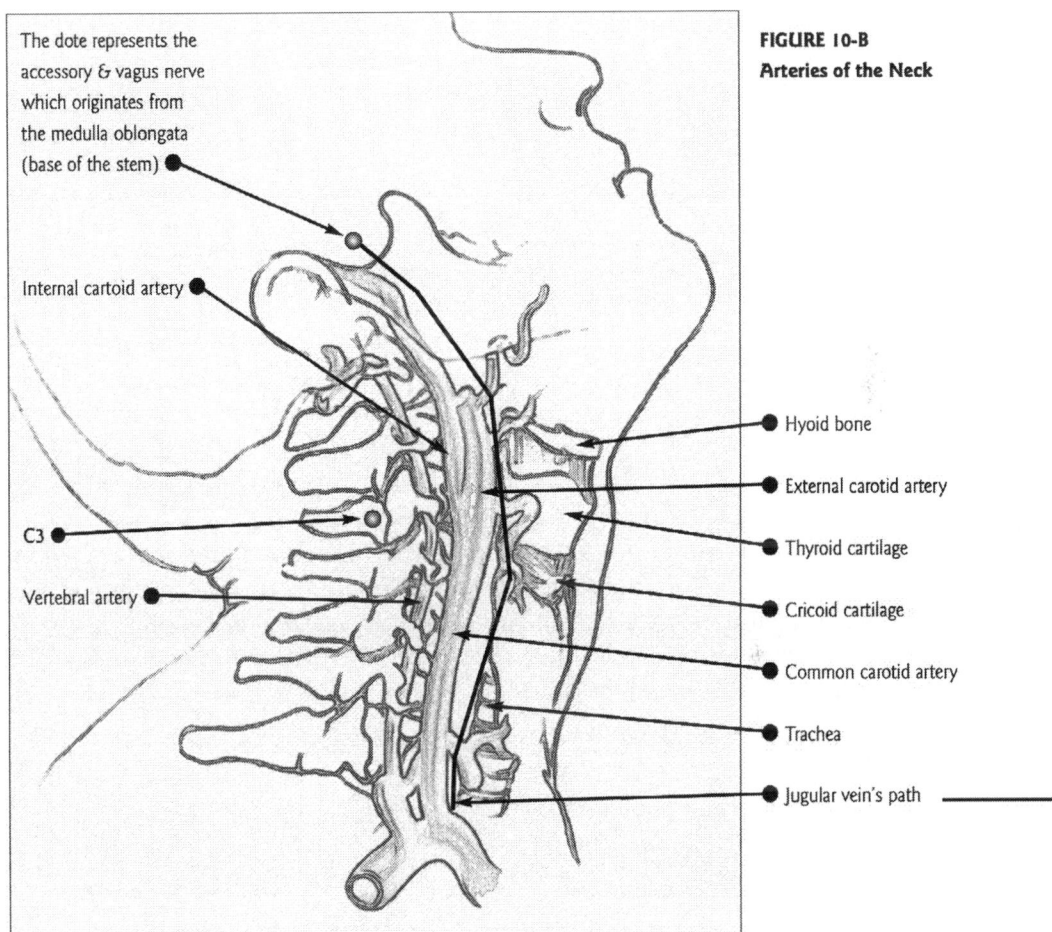

FIGURE 10-B
Arteries of the Neck

A dislocation to the thyroid cartilage or the tracheal ring (Fig. 10-B) can occur by snapping the neck. Suffocation typically results due to the windpipe swelling shut. A severe blow to the back of the neck or disruption to the C3 vertebrae results in spinal cord injury. The individual may need to be ventilated since respiratory dysfunction occurs (Bailes, Cerullo, and Engelhard, 1989: 137–156). Cervical spine injuries can be as simple as soft tissue injuries (whiplash) to actual fractures or dislocation of the cervical spine. Although rare, neurologic injuries can be very debilitating and can cause death. Extreme awareness and education is needed to fully understand the medical implications. Medical authorities advise that preventive guidelines need to be followed to make the martial arts safer (Rabadi, Birrer, and Jordan, 2000: 297–303). As noted in "Article 3: Advice on Correct Etiquette" in the *Bubishi*:

> Regardless of whether people study quanfa for health, recreation, or self-defense, everyone must understand that it is not to be misused. Therefore, teachers should have their disciples swear an oath. In this oath disciples must pledge to never intentionally hurt anyone or do anything unjust.
> — McCarthy, 1995: 68

Conclusion

This chapter has described a variety of principals that can be employed in kata training to elevate skill level and improve self-awareness and focus. The techniques allow a student to understand their strengths and weaknesses and to focus on areas where improvement is needed. At the most basic levels, these techniques gradually breathe life into a kata and aid the student. At the advanced levels, this chapter has shown that there are dangerous consequences.

Over the last few decades, techniques that were formerly passed down by oral tradition, from father to son or a cherished student, have been published openly for commercial gain. For example, the *Bubishi*, once a carefully guarded secret text, is now widely available through a variety of publishers. Details of vital point striking have appeared in numerous books. Thus the controls that the masters once exerted, carefully picking worthy students, with impeccable character and social responsibility, to carry forward the art have now been compromised. In recent years, this process has degenerated into shameful demonstrations and seminars where students have been struck, and in some cases made unconscious, to illustrate the ideas. An attack on an unwitting student requires no skill, and serves no purpose other than to inflate the instructor's ego. These actions set the wrong example entirely: there is no honor, integrity, respect, or courtesy that can be learned from such irresponsible behavior. This chapter has shown that there are serious, unpredictable medical risks associated with vital point striking. The real challenge to an instructor is not to demonstrate the effects, but rather to advance students through the levels of teaching at a pace that is consistent with responsible behavior and student safety.

Bibliography

Bailes, J., Cerullo, L., and Engelhard, H. (1989). Neurologic assessment and management of head injuries. In Paul Meyer, Jr. (Ed.), *Surgery of spine trauma* (pp. 137–156). New York: Churchill Living Stone, Inc.

Cantu, M. (Ed.) (2000). *Biomechanics of head injury in neurologic athletic head and spine injuries*. Philadelphia: W. B. Saunders Co.

Gott, V. (1997). The heart. In George Zuidema (Ed.), *The John Hopkins atlas of human functional anatomy* (pp. 110–113). Baltimore: John Hopkins University Press.

Haymaker, W., and Woodhall, B. (1953). *Peripheral nerve injuries: Principles of diagnosis*, 2nd edition. Philadelphia: W. B. Saunders Co.

Hoppenfield, S. (1976). *Physical examination of the spine and extremities*. New York: Appleton-Century-Crofts.

Jordan, B. (2000). Head and spine injuries in boxing, (pp. 297–303). In Robert Cantu (Ed.), *Biomechanics of head injury in neurologic athletic head and spine injuries*. Philadelphia: W. B. Saunders Co.

Labbate, M. (1999). Elements of advanced karate techniques. *Journal of Asian Martial Arts,* 8(2), 80–95.

Labbate, M. (2000). Developing advanced Goju-ryu techniques: Illustrated in the rising block. *Journal of Asian Martial Arts,* 9(1), 56–69.

Labbate, M. (2001). Tensho kata: Goju-ryu's secret treasure. *Journal of Asian Martial Arts,* 10(1), 84–99.

McCarthy, P. (1995). *The bible of karate: Bubishi.* Rutland, VT: Charles E. Tuttle.

McCrory, P. (2000). Strokes in athletes, (pp. 200–209). In Robert Cantu (Ed.), *Biomechanics of head injury in neurologic athletic head and spine injuries.* Philadelphia: W. B. Saunders Co.

Rabadi, M., Birrer R., and Jordan, B. (2000). Head and spine injuries (pp. 297–303). In Robert Cantu, (Ed.), *Biomechanics of head injury in neurologic athletic head and spine injuries.* Philadelphia: W. B. Saunders Co.

Acknowledgments

The author would like to thank Ken Yonemura, M.D., and Grace Noda, medical consultant, for their aid in describing the medical implications of the karate principals in this paper. The author would like to thank Marc Gervais and Michael Egnato for performing the kata movements and applications for this paper.

chapter 38

Kobudo: Okinawan Weapons are Not All Flash

by Mary Bolz, B.S.

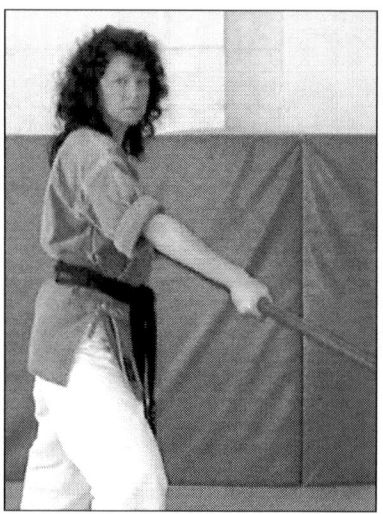

All photographs courtesy of Mary Bolz.

Introduction

People who practice martial arts do so for a variety of reasons. An often touted reason is to obtain self-defense skills. Another reason often given for studying a martial art is for cultivating self-discipline and building self-confidence. Yet, anyone experienced in the fighting arts will declare that these arts are more flash than useful self-defense. In actuality, what is usually seen is some sort of aerobic workout based on "punching and kicking," sometimes with music played in the background. If we wish to study a martial art for true self-defense and character development, we should utilize some guidelines to help us distinguish which practice methods realistically offer these benefits. Hopefully, this chapter will offer some practical information in this respect by looking at the "ancient martial art methods" associated with the Okinawan weapons (*kobudo*).*

> * *Notice: Anyone who wishes to practice with weapons, such as the nunchaku, should be aware of any local laws governing their use. Please check with local authorities.*

Weapons: "Flash" v.s. Realistic Self-Defense

What is involved in turning choreographed movements into practical self-defense? And, what manner of practice can guarantee character-building that is commonly associated with Asian martial traditions? Additionally, how does weapons practice fit in to these goals?

To answer the first question, the techniques taught must be of practical use—they must work when used against a real attack by a physically and mentally powerful opponent. Much of today's weapons practice is awe-inspiring with its associated acrobatics, speed, and beauty. However, such practice is usually of little use against a serious attacker.

An argument regarding weapons practice is that, in modern society, nobody carries weapons with them: defensive training with weapons is useless when facing any assault on the street. However, the practicality of weapons practice goes beyond this apparent limitation. The physical and mental skills obtained through weapons practice can be applied in the street by adapting and utilizing common everyday objects in place of the traditional weapons. For example, staff (*bo*) techniques can be easily be applied with a broom or mop. A frying pan can be used as a shield and a spoon used as a *tinaka* or *shuchu*.

If fighting techniques are practiced without realism and without active visualization of an attacker, either a false sense of self-confidence will develop, or certain physical and mental skills necessary for self-defense will not develop at all. Practice geared for health, for aerobic fitness, or performing routines to music is simply not enough. Although Okinawan kobudo may seem ancient and outdated, it can be very useful for developing real fighting skills and the mental toughness required in our modern world.

The following section presents a few Okinawan kobudo techniques and looks at a few training methods that bring out the proper physical skills and mind-set necessary for realistic self-defense. The drive to practice solely for flash, fun, and ego is a great obstacle to overcome. We can make our practice more realistic if we wish. The key is in how the practice is done.

TECHNICAL SECTION

Two-Person Drills

Distancing: Two opponents square off. The distance between two people (*maai*) is an extremely important aspect in all fighting arts, especially with weaponry. Here, in preparation for an actual attack, the distance between the two opponents should be such that neither of the two can reach the other with their weapon without having to step closer. This is a relatively safe distance at which to square off. The positions shown below are typical postures taken prior to practicing any technique.

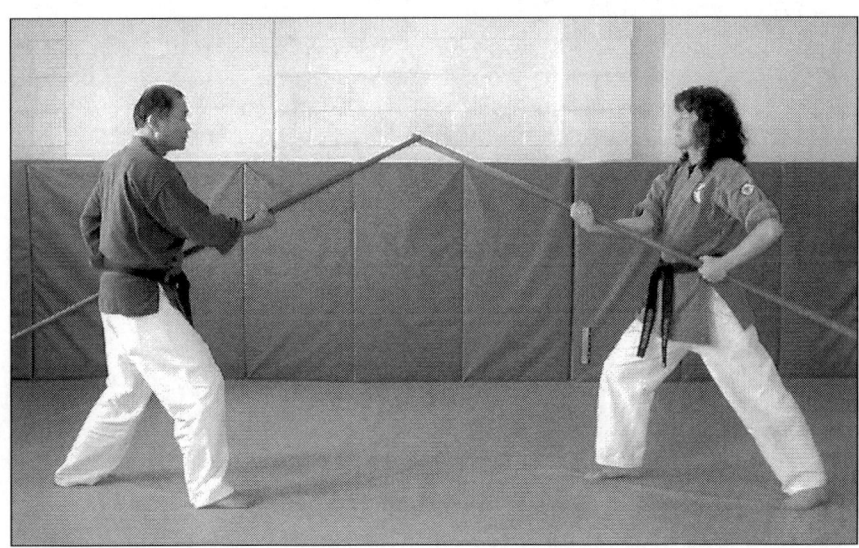

Staff vs. Staff

1a The aggressor advances.
1b He attempts a strike to the neck. The defender counters while slide-stepping to the outside.
1c The defender raises the right end of her staff, sliding it along the opponent's staff and then flipping her staff over his into a pressing maneuver. Note that it is the lower body, the hip and the legs, that lead this movement. Her body has turned to an even greater side-position by the movement of her hips and the sliding of the rear leg.
1d The defender slide-steps even more to the right, leading with the hip and forcefully pressing down on her opponent's staff with a twisting action of the wrist. Notice the direction of the defender's navel, compared to the previous photos.
1e The defender counter-attacks to her opponent's face with the staff's tail-end. The hips lead all of these movements and is the leading force in propelling the staff at maximum force.

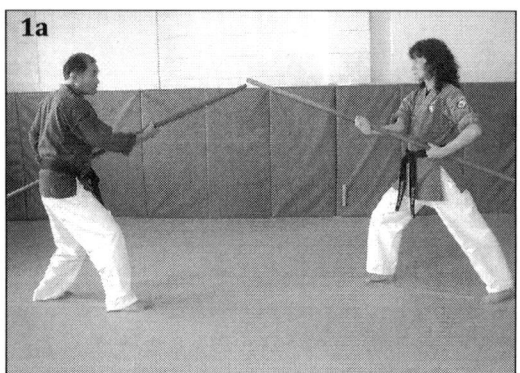
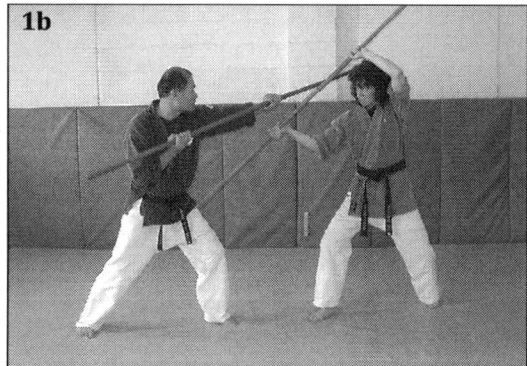
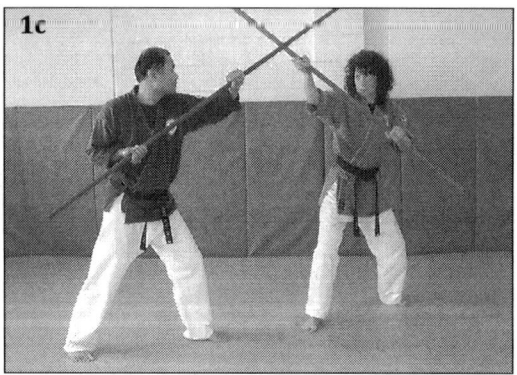
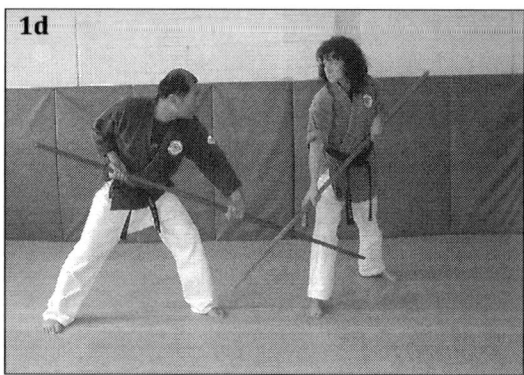
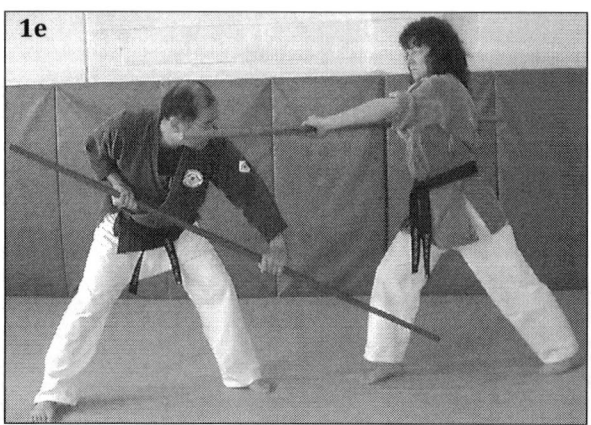

Staff vs. Staff

2a The opponents square off.
2b The attacker moves in with a thrust to the throat.
2c Leading with her hips, the defender steps forward and slightly to the right to simultaneously execute a full-force block with the side of her staff.
2d The defender sharply turns her hips and simultaneously twists her wrist upwards, causing a powerful counter-attack to the attacker's head at the temple.
2e Detail of the grip used in the beginning block (2b).
2f Detail of an incorrect grip to use while pressing.
2g Grip used for a properly executed press.

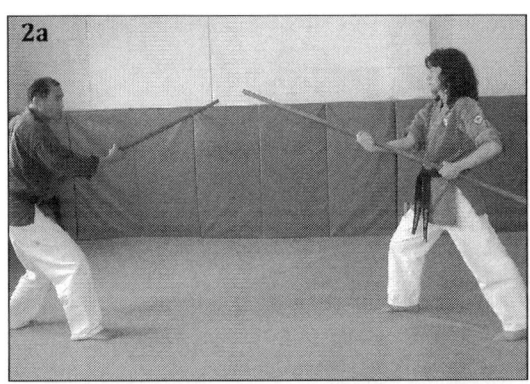
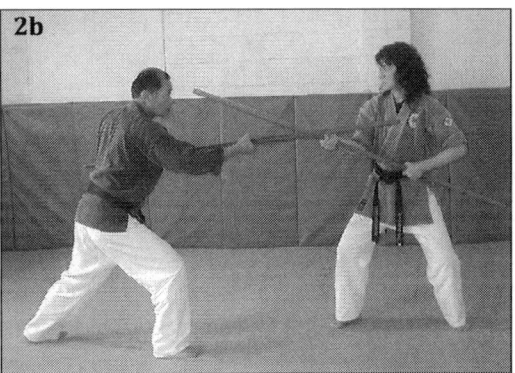
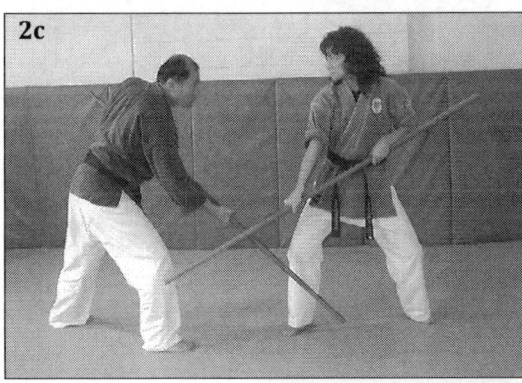
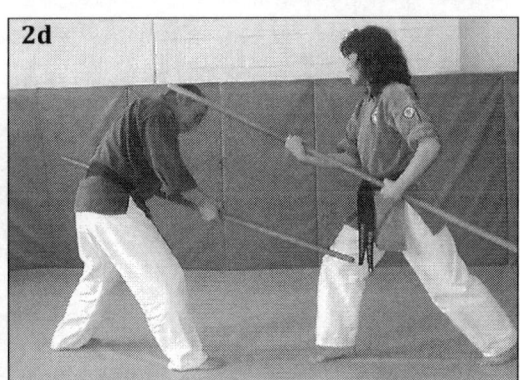
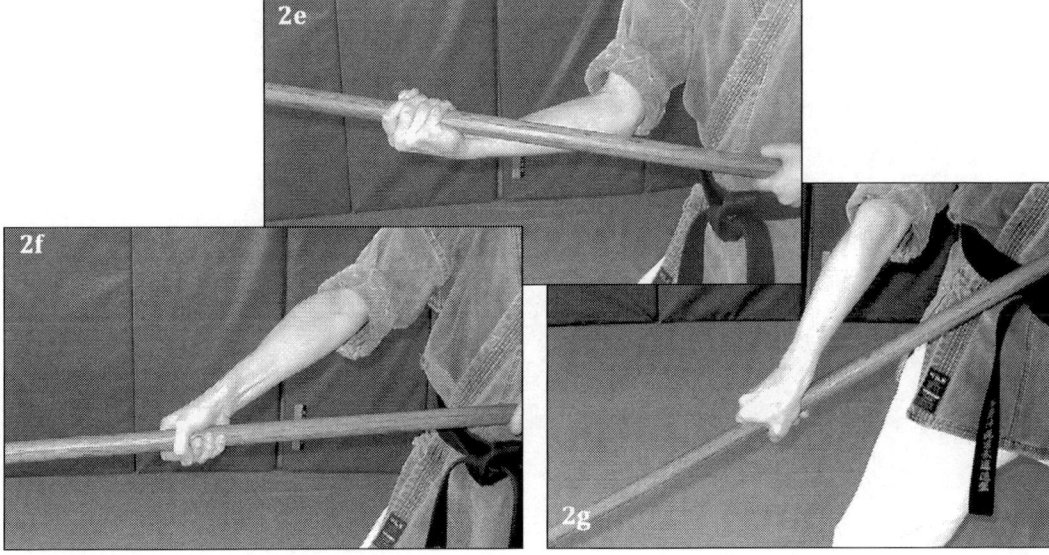

Nunchaku

3a A would-be attacker facing a defender with a nunchaku hidden behind her back that is tucked through her belt .
3b As he reaches to grab her, she reaches for the nunchaku.
3c As he grabs her collar, she starts to swing the nunchaku over his arm.
3d She prepares to "choke" his wrist.
3e Detail of the nunchaku being swung over the arm.
3f She catches the other end of the nunchaku and begins the choke.
3g The nunchaku is slid down the arm to the wrist. The defender twists forcefully, causing the nunchaku to choke the attacker's wrist. This brings pain and immobilizes the attacker.
3h The defender is now in control and can bring the attacker to the ground where she can follow-up with another technique if she wishes.

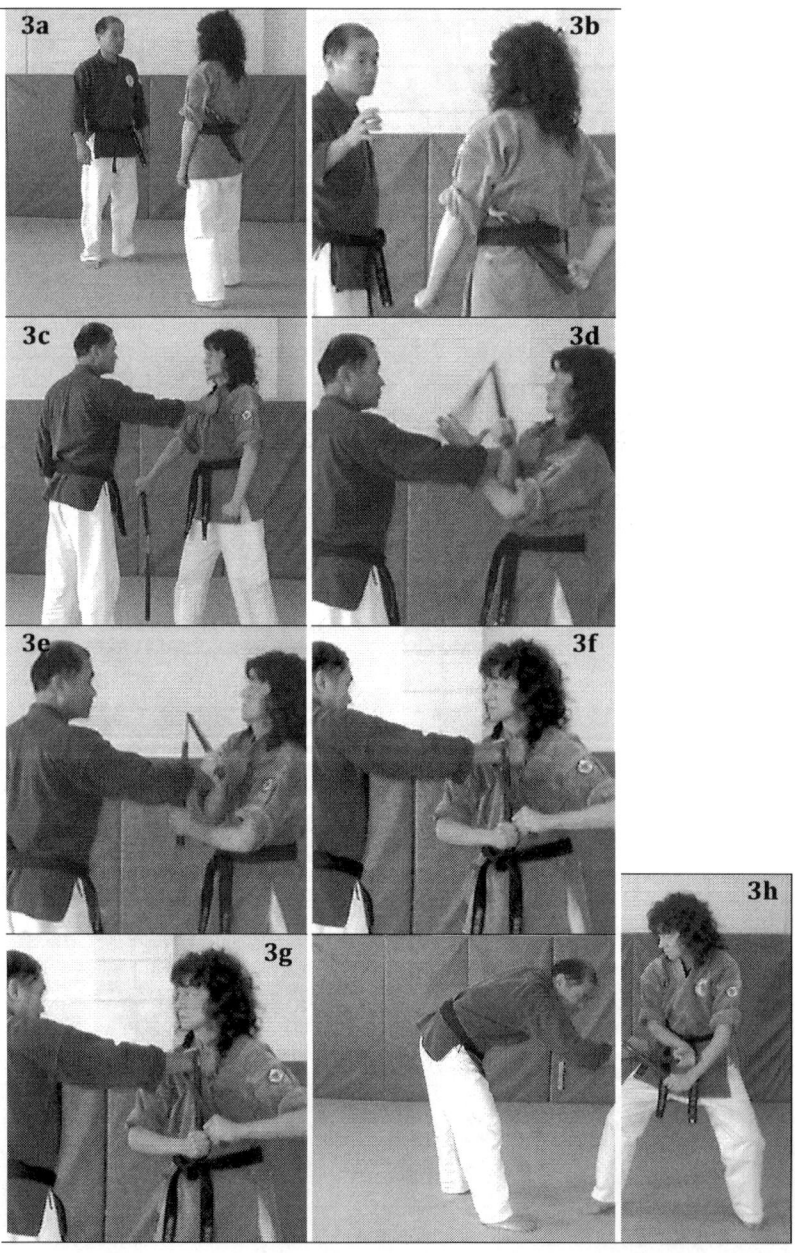

Nunchaku

4a A would-be attacker approaches.

4b He comes in closer to punch toward the face. To avoid the punch, the defender quickly drops and prepares to counter.

4c-d The defender drops further and prepares to wrap the nunchaku around the attacker's ankle.

4e She snares his ankle and tightens the grip, causing the attacker excruciating pain and leaving him immobile. He can not attack and she can follow with another technique if she wishes.

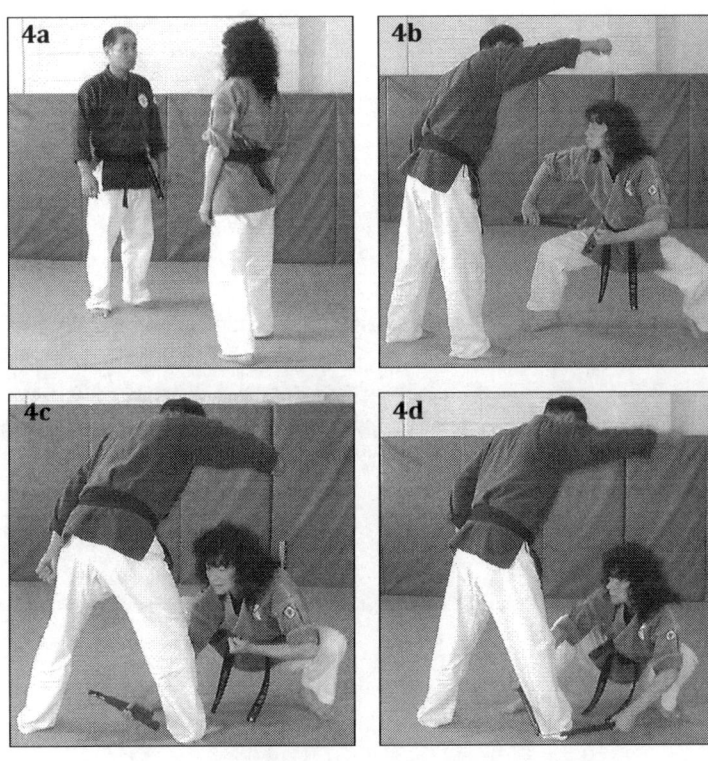

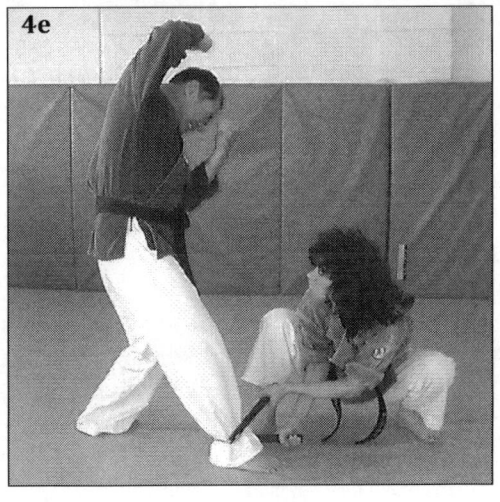

Nunchaku

5a A would-be attacker approaches.
5b He moves in closer, reaching out with both hands to grab.
5c The defender has the nunchaku in her right hand and, as the attacker grabs, she lifts both her arms to the outside and above his arms. In one fluid motion, she releases one handle and immediately catches it in her left hand.
5d She then pulls the nunchaku down over his wrists.
5e The defender entraps both of the attacker's wrists to immobilize him. She can follow-up with another technique if she wishes.

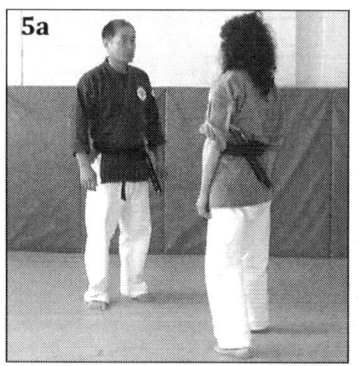
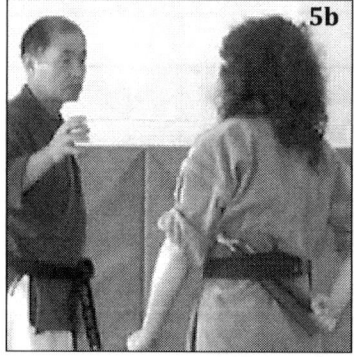
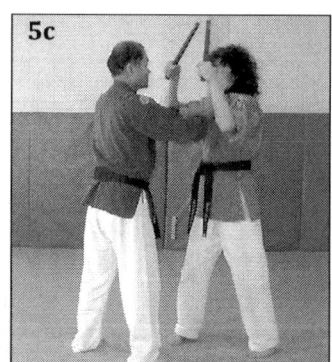
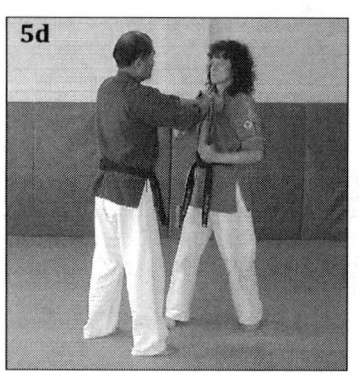
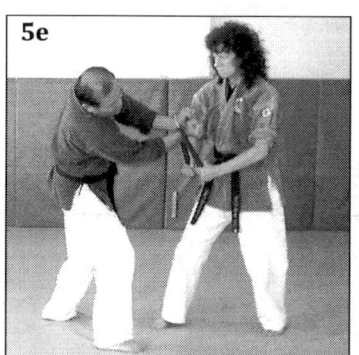
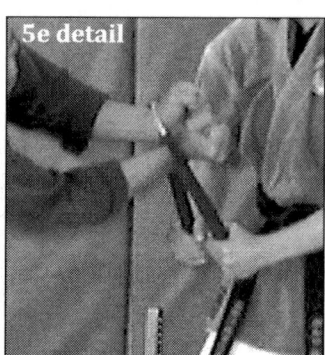

Staff vs. Nunchaku

6a Attacker/defender square off.
6b The attacker strikes toward the face. Side-stepping, the defender executes a powerful block and presses the nunchaku down forcefully by using the hips to turn the whole body.
6c She begins to flip the nunchaku underneath his right wrist.
6d The flipping action brings the free handle underneath the staff and into her left hand.
6e She executes a wrist choke.
6f After stunning the opponent with the painful wrist choke, the defender quickly initiates a throat choke.
6g-h Tightening the hold. Additional pressure is given on the neck.
6i Finishing the technique by securing the nunchaku under the jaw and pressing firmly upward.

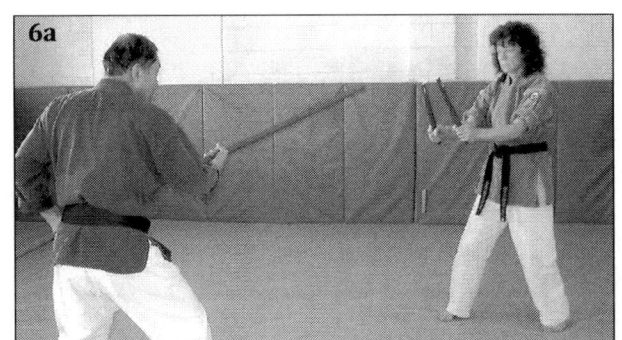

469

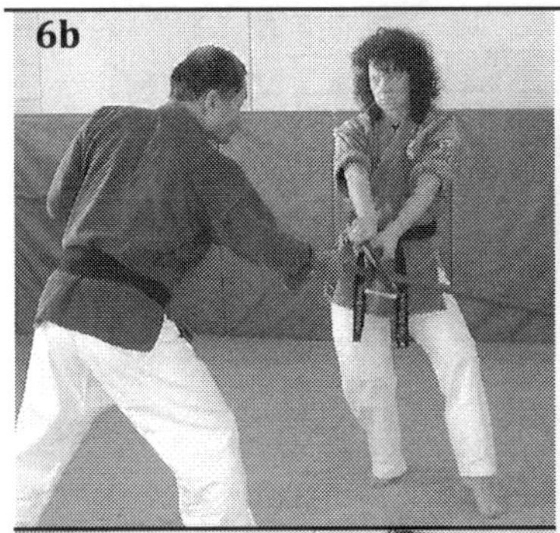

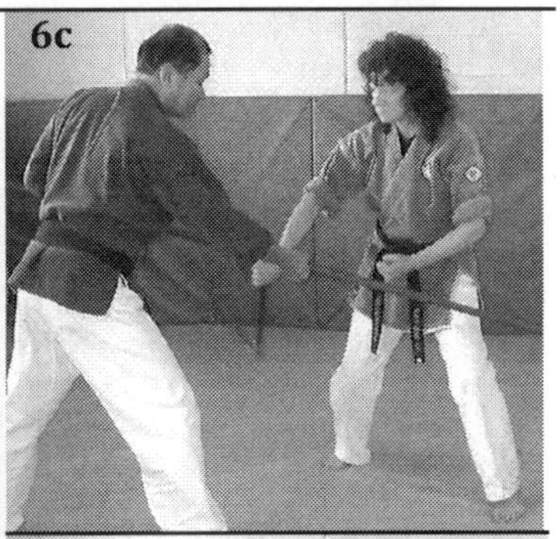

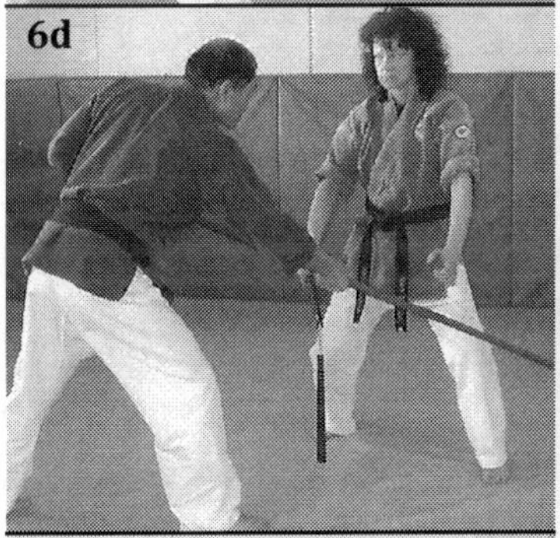

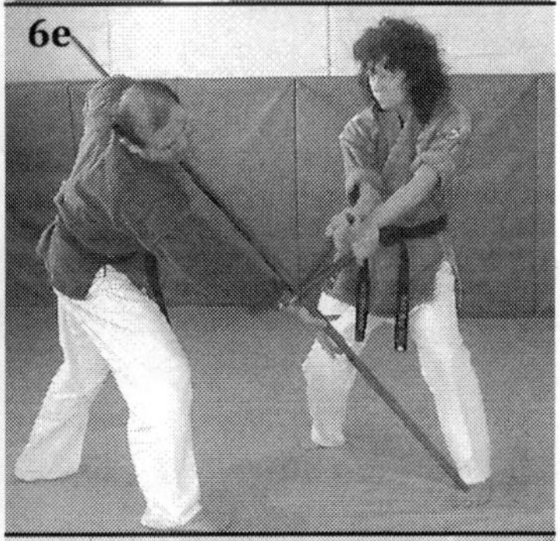

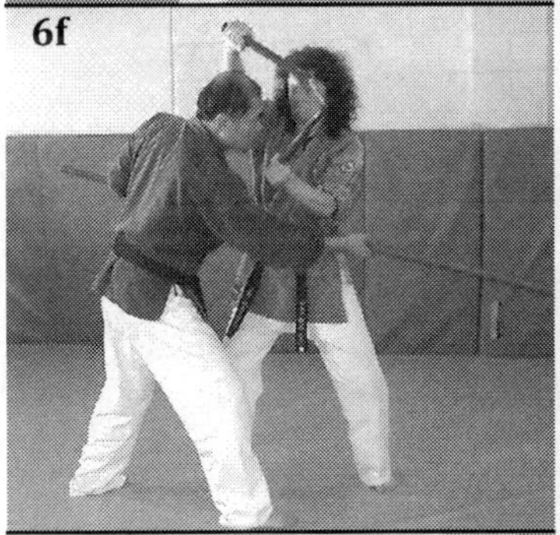

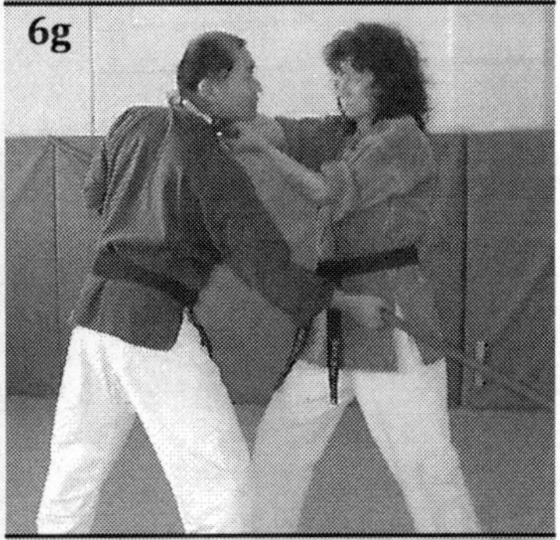

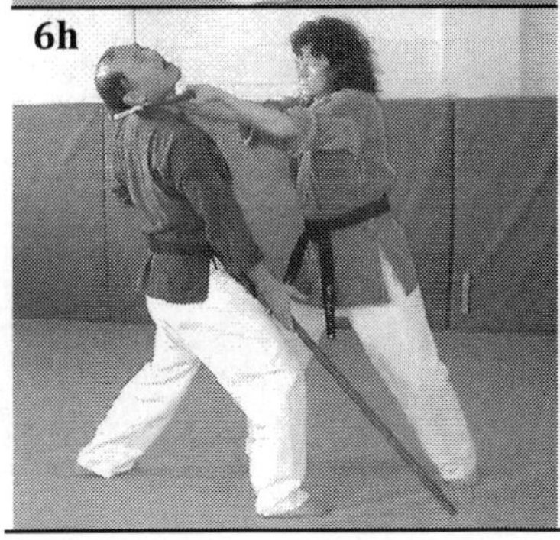

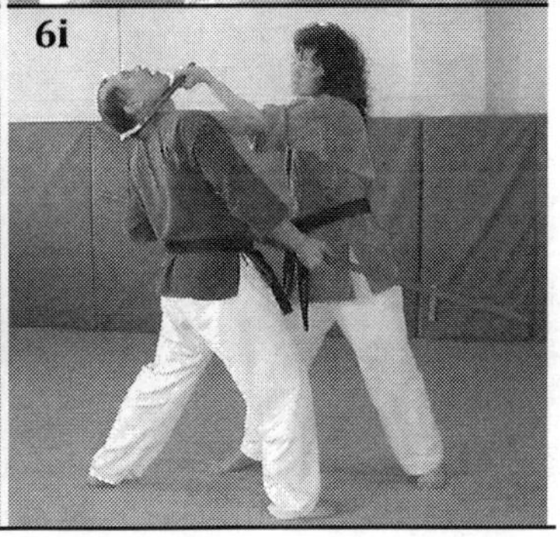

Single-Person Training Drill: Strike

7a Ready posture.
7b Starting to throw the butt-end of the nunchaku to its target.
7c Strike to the eye.
7d Alternate strike to the throat area.

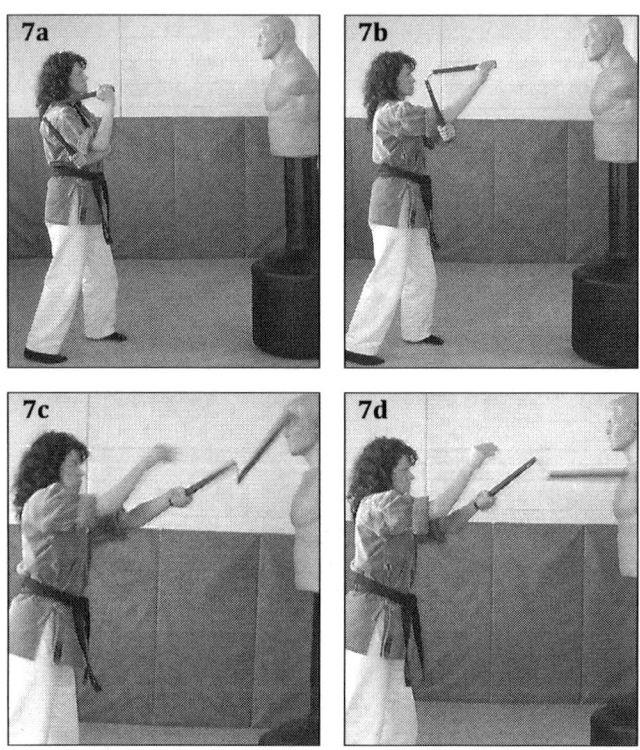

Single-Person Training Drill: Throat Choke

8a Incorrect position of nunchaku for a throat choke.
8b Correct position.

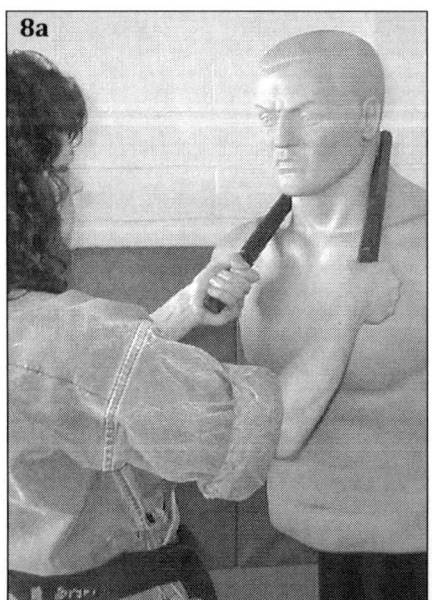
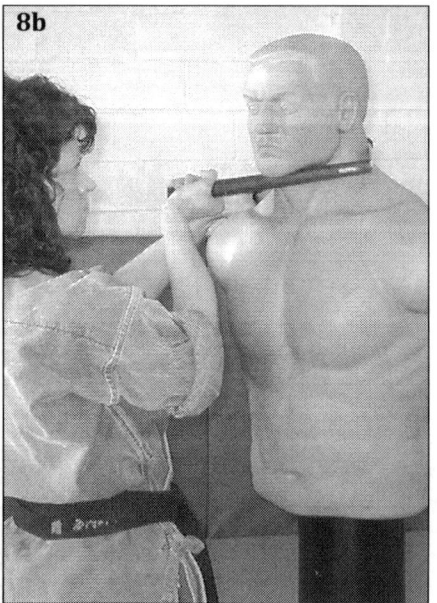

GUIDELINES FOR REALISTIC PRACTICE*

In order for self-defense techniques to be truly practical and effective, the mode of practice must be closely scrutinized. Constant practice develops habits—habits which can be valuable or totally useless, depending on whether practice drills are effective or not. Important guidelines are provided below which should be helpful when practicing with a partner.

* Editor's Note: The theories presented in this chapter are not universal, but are expressed as the main themes of this particular school.

1) At advanced levels, real weapons must be used. Practicing only with weapons of rubber or wood do not provide the true "feel"of a real weapon, or the mental alertness required wielding a lethal weapon as a sharp bladed sword.

2) Do not look at the opponent's limbs or his or her weapon. Gaze at the opponent neutrally and objectively. Serious practice required serious focus.

3) Do not start a technique over again if a mistake is made by either party. Keep on going! There are no second chances in the real world.

4) In defending, use side-stepping and parry. Never remain head-on with the opponent. Try to move forward, to the side, or circle, but not back. Side-stepping or circling is ideal, but going forward in response to an attack is highly discouraging to an attacker. Moving forward must be regulated by the reach of the technique you intend to try with your weapon. Don't let aggression interfere with proper distancing!

5) The best form of self-defense is to attack. In our particular style, we try never to step back from an attack. A block is only the first part of an attack. The best form of self-defense is often in attacking. In our particular style, we rarely step back from an attack. A block is only the first part of an attack.

6) Keep the mouth closed by keeping the lips and teeth together and the tongue touching firmly to the roof of the mouth. This produces focus, spirit and concentration of mind. It also lessens any probability of damage to the face and head if a blow of less than full-force is received. It also presents a stronger image. When the lips are apart and the mouth open, a weak countenance is shown. But you can breathe. Fighting is an aerobic activity, or should be!

7) While practicing with a partner, do not converse. Too much socializing and casual practice can be seen in many martial art classes. This type of practice will not produce true defensive fighting ability. Remember that a partner is an opponent and enemies do not casually talk or smile while fighting each other.

8) Always move from the hips. The hips lead the rest of the movement. Many martial art practitioners move their hands first. This is limiting in power and effectiveness. For beginners, make a habit of moving the hips and feet first, then the hands. The movements will become unified as training progresses. If the habit of moving one's hands first is not corrected, one's technical ability will never improve.

9) "Upper empty and lower full." Relax the shoulders and keep them down. Make the feet, legs, and hips bear the responsibility of stability, power, and speed of movement, i.e., the hips should be low and more contracted and does more muscular work than the upper body in a ratio of 70/30. Keeping the hips low and square in training is conducive to this.

10) Realistic distance (*maai*) in prearranged sparring is very important. If the attack does not reach the opponent, he or she should not block. Conversely, if a proper attack is made and it is not blocked, the defender should be hit! . . .within the limits of what is safe, of course.

Self-Defense as a Unified Effort

For many, the study of a martial art is a quest for spiritual and mental development and is not separated from the physical aspects of the art. The previously mentioned points will go far to develop the mental side. For the sake of clarity, we can treat these aspects separately.

How can one apply martial training to one's personal life and somehow "better" one's mental and spiritual side? And, why should anyone even try? Can't spiritual/mental training best be developed by practices solely designed for that purpose, such as zazen and other forms of meditation? There are many methods for forging the spirit. However, in the martial traditions, a fundamental thought is of duality, in Japanese called *in-yo* (Chinese, yin-yang). These represent the complimentary and seemingly contradictory aspects found throughout all of nature. Since they are inseparable, can each be trained in isolation by themselves? It seems logical that both in and yo be trained simultaneously in a united effort. One way to do this is through martial arts practice, such as those with Okinawan weapons (*kobudo*). Here are some specific reasons why kobudo practice can develop the spiritual and mental aspects:

1) Fighting is very demanding physically, more so than non-fighting activities because of the fundamental associations it has with survival. The risk of injury is high. The intensity of the practice forces the "whole person" to participate in the practice. Thus, for spiritual development and mental discipline, one must practice kobudo as a fighting art, not merely as exercise or for fun.

2) Physical practice (*yo*) has an effect on the spiritual and mental (*in*), so the elements listed above should not be ignored.

3) To develop spiritually as well as physically, a person must train regularly, at least three times a week, several hours during each session. Otherwise, in and yo become lazy!

4) To go beyond the basics of practicing useful techniques, a growing awareness of the mental aspects involved in martial arts training is required. This can be achieved through serious practice, especially weapons practice with a partner which brings you closer to reality.

chapter 39

Robert M. Dalgleish:
"The Father of Canadian Goju-ryu Karate"

by Robert Toth

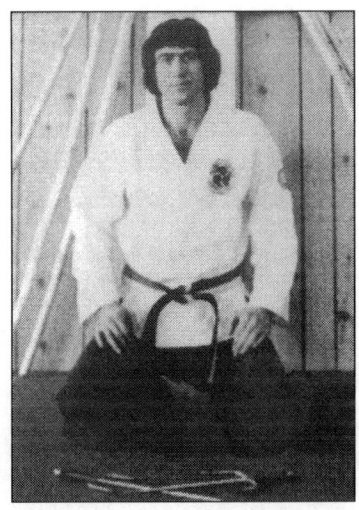

Photographs courtesy of Robert Toth.

Robert "Bob" Marshall Dalgleish was born on November 28, 1941, and died less than 37 years later. During his lively and highly misunderstood lifetime, he became a Canadian icon.[1]

Dalgleish was a martial arts gypsy, a nomad who traveled all over North America training in the martial arts with some of the most acclaimed instructors of his time.[2] This was at a time when travel was not as convenient as it is today and yet Dalgleish thought nothing of heading out to the West Coast, Florida, or New York and staying away for several months at a time. He had connections everywhere. He would train and then return to Canada to share what he had learned with just about anyone who was interested. It is the collecting and sharing of martial information that established Dalgleish as an essential character in Canadian martial arts history.

Dalgleish's Combative Studies

Dalgleish was born in Thunder Bay, a small city in northern Ontario. He moved to Toronto in 1958 with his mother. In the early 1960's, he began training in the only karate school in the city was a Chito-ryu school, which Tsuruoka Masami opened in 1956 (Ward, 1994:21–23). It was a predominantly male-oriented class and the bamboo sword (*shinai*) was used liberally to make corrections to the student's techniques.[3] Tsuruoka's formula for karate training was lots of forms and basics (Ward, 1994:24).

During this time, Dalgleish traveled to New York City to train in Goju-ryu ("Hard-Soft Style") with Peter Urban. Urban had been stationed in Japan when he was 18-years old while in the United States Navy (Petras, 1974:8) where he trained with Richard Kim, Yamaguchi Gogen, and Oyama Masutatsu. Urban introduced Japanese Goju-ryu to the United States in 1959 (Corcoran and Farkas, 1993:389).

The Goju-ryu system taught by Urban was very different from the style that Dalgleish had studied under Tsuruoka. The Goju-ryu style was a blend of the strong snap techniques of the Okinawan style blended with the dynamic and free techniques of the soft Chinese (Urban, 1967).

In the mid-1960's, Dalgleish had done a two-year stint in the Royal Canadian Navy. While in the Navy, he would travel to California to train with Yamaguchi Gosei.[4] Gosei is the son of Yamaguchi Gogen, who had been authorized by Goju-ryu founder Miyagi Chojun to promote the style on mainland Japan. In the early 1960's, another of Gogen's sons, Gosen, had moved to the United States and was attending San Francisco State University. He also brought the Yamaguchi brand of Goju-ryu karate to the United States. Yamaguchi Gosei replaced Gosen as the instructor of the school in 1964 (Castinado, 1995:35–36). Gosei taught punching, striking, and kicking with their applications to free fighting, which could be seen as the style's "hard" aspect. On the other hand, the forms represented Goju-ryu's aesthetic or "soft" side (Smoke, 1991:32).

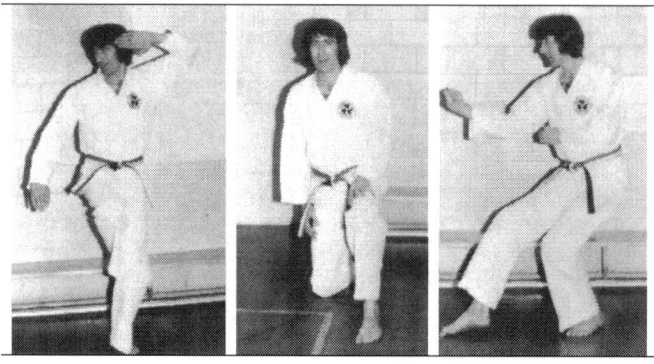

After he left the Navy, Dalgleish returned to Toronto and became involved with several local karate schools. He trained and taught at David Chong's Canadian Karate/Kung Fu Club and at fellow Tsuruoka alumni Benny Allen's Eastern Karate Club.[5] He shared the Japanese Goju-ryu he had studied under Peter Urban and Yamaguchi Gosei with his fellow Canadians. Allen allowed Dalgleish to take the class at the Club and gave him permission to show what he had learned on his latest travels.[6]

This program of traveling, learning, and teaching provided a comfortable lifestyle for Dalgleish. He again traveled to New York, then across middle US to California.[7] One of the instructors Dalgleish trained with on these trips was Chuck Merriman, who had originally taken up judo in 1960 (Liedke, 1990:50). Later, he trained in Shito-ryu karate and eventually in Goju-ryu with Peter Urban in New York. Although Urban broke away from his instructor Yamaguchi

Gogen, Merriman stayed with the Yamaguchi organization, training with Yamamoto Gonnoyoe (Simpkins and Simpkins, 1994:15–16). Yamamoto would eventually split from the Yamaguchis as well to form his own group, the International Karate Organization (IKO). Merriman stayed with the IKO until 1972. Dalgleish studied under both Merriman and Yamamoto.[8]

Dalgleish also trained with Daniel K. Pai, who taught White Dragon (Pai Lum) gongfu in Florida (Corcoran and Farkas, 1993:393). Later, Pai would visit Canada for seminars and demonstrations at Dalgliesh's invitation.[9]

In Phoenix, Arizona, Dalgleish trained with Robert Trias in Shuri-ryu (Corcoran and Farkas, 1993:318). Trias was reportedly the first to introduce karate in the United States.[10] Dalgleish was also a member of Trias' organization, the United States Karate Association (USKA) (Corcoran and Farkas, 1993:318). Trias would also visit Dalgleish in Canada.[11]

In California, Dalgleish trained with Shotokan instructor Nishiyama Hidetaka[12] and Shorinji kobudo and karate instructor Richard Kim.[13]

Teaching: The Way of the Wolverine

After his travels, Dalgleish was able to share his new knowledge with even more karate people. He continued to teach at the karate schools in Toronto and expanded to Benny Allen's satellite school in Hamilton, Ontario, the "Steel City." Dalgleish and Allen would make the 70-kilometer trek to Hamilton to teach on a regular basis. Tim Collingwood, a student at Eastern Karate, remembers Dalgleish coming to the Hamilton school: "When Bob would drop in, you'd appreciate him coming and you'd learn something new."[14] Eventually, several of the Hamilton students took over running the club but kept the name "Eastern Karate." By that time, Dalgleish was teaching at other Hamilton karate schools as well. "If you were a martial artist, he'd be glad to share with you," said Ken Hayashi.[15] Dalgleish's feeling was that if you wanted to learn, just give him a phone call, set it up, and he'd be there.[16] With this kind of attitude, Dalgleish's sphere of influence expanded rapidly.

In 1970, Dalgleish accepted a position as a draftsman at the International Nickel Company (INCO) and he and his wife Ruth moved to Sudbury, Ontario, about 390 kilometers from Toronto.[17] In this northern Ontario community, they opened a karate school that would become a Mecca for students training in karate.

Though the school would move several times as enrollment swelled, the first one was in a community center. The Sudbury Goju Kai Karate Dojo would eventually settle on Regent Street. It was in the front of the building and the Dalgleishs lived in the back. His father, Slim, was living with them.[18]

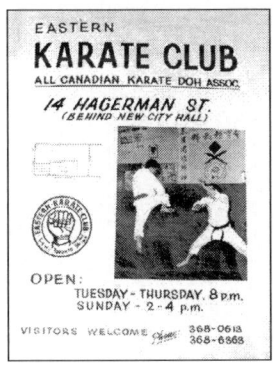 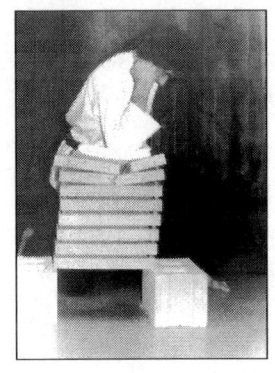 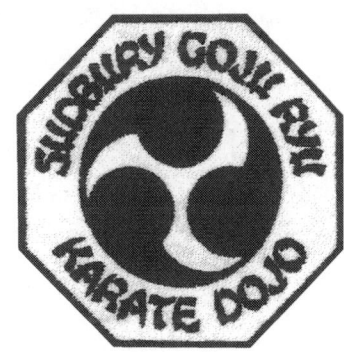

Dalgleish taught Japanese Goju-ryu karate and Okinawan weapons. He called it Canadian Goju-ryu because he was Canadian and was the Goju representative for Canada.[19] The new students stood at the back and mimicked the blocks and strikes of those in front and hoped that they were doing them properly. Notes taken from "The Sudbury Goju Kai Karate Outline of Classes" shows that, along with basics and forms, there were many different kinds of sparring drills taught: one-, two-, and three-step sparring;

circle sparring; gauntlet or special reflex sparring; and blindfold sparring. Students were also taught grabbing techniques, board breaking, jujutsu, "sticky hands" exercises, and resuscitation techniques. Most of the students were intimidated by Dalgleish's six-foot five-inch height and by the intensity of the workouts. This did not discourage serious martial artists, who often came from great distances to train at Dalgleish's school. Training was regular at the school, and if Dalgleish wasn't available, a number of his senior students took over.[20]

Dalgleish's philosophy is expressed in the "Cycle of Karate-do":

Every *karate-ka* (follower of the art of karate) must go through the cycle by doing basic blocking, punching and kicking techniques, then advance accordingly. When a black belt is going through a particular set of exercises or techniques and finds difficulty in part or all of them, he or she simply returns to the beginning of their cycle and reviews the basics until proficiency has again been achieved. The karate kata or formal exercise is a prime example of the importance of realizing and understanding the cycle. In the first kata one learns a block and a punch. Later on he or she advances to intermediate kata where kicking is involved, and much later the karate ka is taught the most advanced kata of that particular system. This also contains the same blocks, punches and kicks previously learned. If at that time the student experiences any difficulty with the various techniques of that advanced kata it means one of two things. He has not done his basics properly, or has not been taught properly. To perform advanced kata effectively, he or she must then start yet another cycle and return to the basics. – Dalgleish, 1975:16

While maintaining the operation of his school, Dalgleish began traveling to karate tournaments. His students were consistently winners at these tournaments and Dalgleish was in demand as a referee and martial arts demonstrator. Eileen Dennis remembers seeing Robert and Ruth Dalgleish in 1970 demonstrating a form at a tournament in Ottawa, Canada. At that time it was pretty special to know any weapons forms, and an especially rare talent to be able to demonstrate them to a crowd. Dalgleish was also remembered for his impressive board-breaking demonstration. He would do a finger-tip strike through four inches of pine boards.[21]

It was during this time in Sudbury that Dalgleish created what was to become his masterpiece: a true Canadian karate kata he called "The Way of the Wolverine." Dalgleish felt strongly about being Canadian, so he wanted to give something back to the martial arts that was Canadian. It was Dalgleish's desire that the "Way of the Wolverine" kata would distinguish Canadian Goju-ryu from traditional Japanese Goju-ryu. The kata is a mixture of Shotokan, Chito-ryu, Goju-ryu, Shaolin gongfu, and Wing Chun.[22] It is a definite reminder of the many different masters Dalgleish trained with.

The kata is still practiced throughout most of Canada. Frank Clayton in British Columbia taught the author "The Way of the Wolverine." Clayton had learned it from Ken Tallack, who had been a student of Dalglelish. Dalgleish will always be remembered by this kata. Though there are different variations, the kata can still be recognized even 24 years after his death.

Unfortunately, in the mid 1970's, there were problems. Despite all the students, the school did not do well financially because Dalgleish was not a businessman.[23] And there were personal problems. The Sudbury Goju Kai Karate Dojo closed and Dalgleish

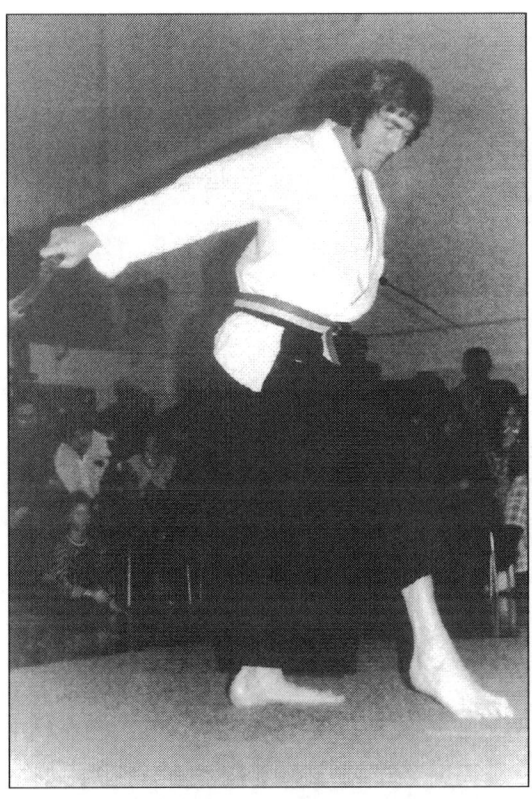 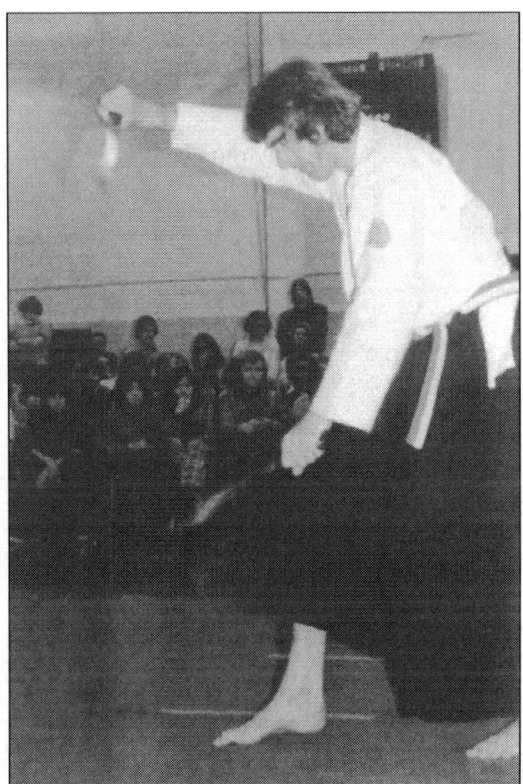

Over the next few years, Dalgleish would pop-up and disappear just as fast.[24] He stayed with Pat McCarthy for a while. McCarthy was the karate instructor at a local fitness club at the time.[25] Then he stayed at Ken Hayashi's karate school. Hayashi had been only 14-years-old when he first met Dalgleish at Dave Chong's Canadian Karate/Kung Fu Club. Dalgleish stayed in Hayashi's school and taught some of the classes. He also taught at seminars around the city. Dalgleish was invited to become a part of the karate organization that Hayashi was working on with Ron Yamanaka.[26] This was an attempt to gather a group of different schools under one umbrella organization. Dalgleish also saw it as a way of establishing potential income. He helped to teach seminars and demonstrate for the organization.[27] And he continued to travel.

For awhile, he was in London, Ontario, helping to open a karate school for one of his students and teaching karate. He then went down to the United States visiting friends, still taking on seminars and attending tournaments everywhere he could. Karate absorbed his every waking hour.[28]

Sparking an Interest in Canadian Goju-ryu

According to his friends, Dalgleish was definitely a "city guy." He liked being a part of downtown and Chinatown. And for periods of time, people took him into their homes and looked after him.[29] He helped to build karate schools and martial arts organizations, and taught Canadian Goju-ryu Karate wherever he could.

The weekend of July 6, 1978, Dalgleish canceled a planned seminar in Timmins, Ontario, because he felt that he had to visit his mother in Thunder Bay.[30] While at his mother's, Dalgleish died of heart failure.[31] He was buried in his karate uniform and belt.[32] Several years after his death, his students purchased a marker for his grave.[33] Twenty-four years later, some of his students still visit his grave site in Thunder Bay.

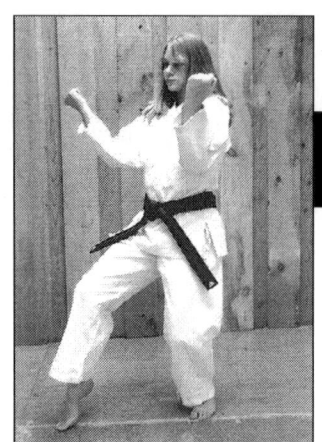

The Way of the Wolverine

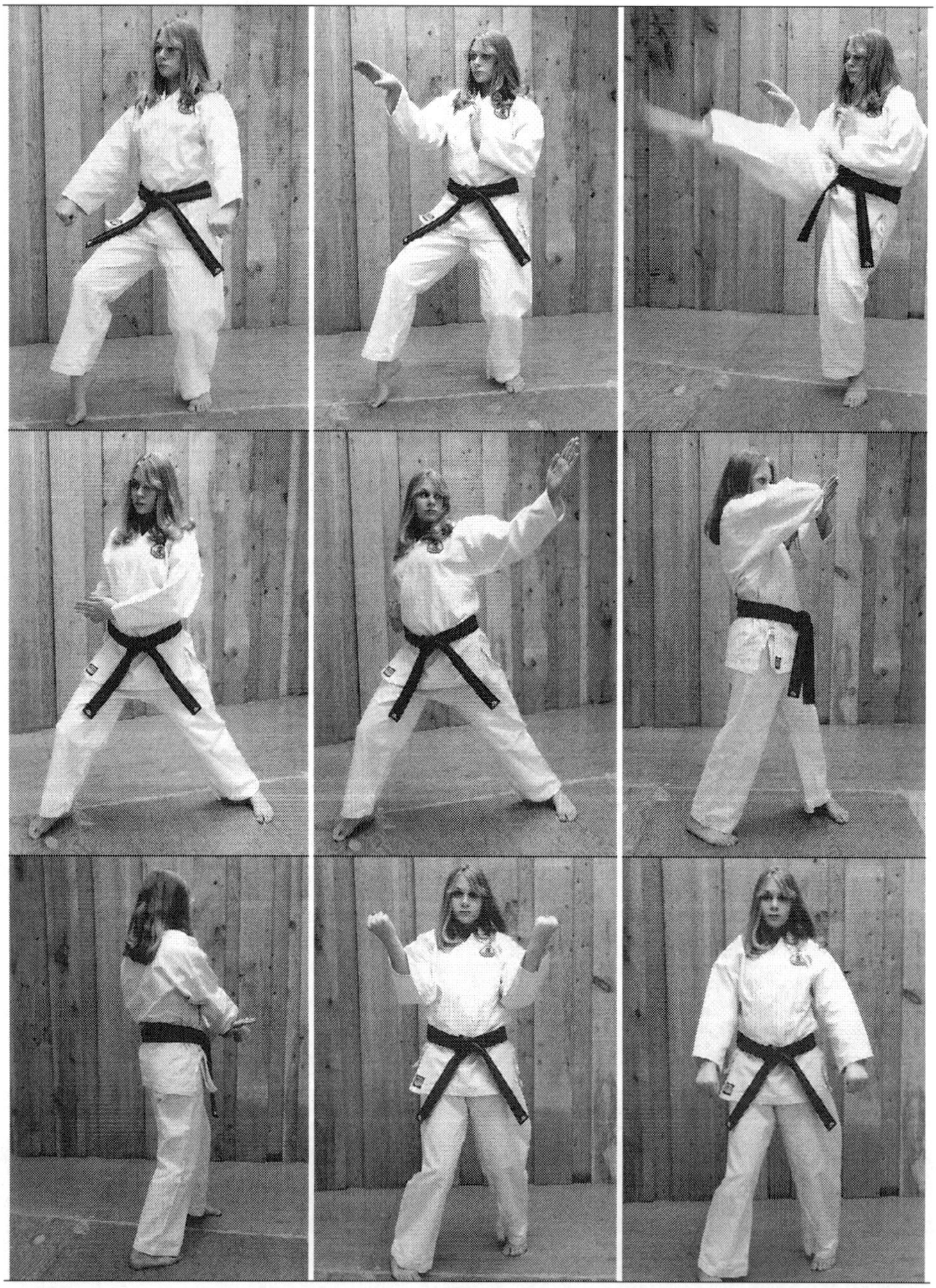

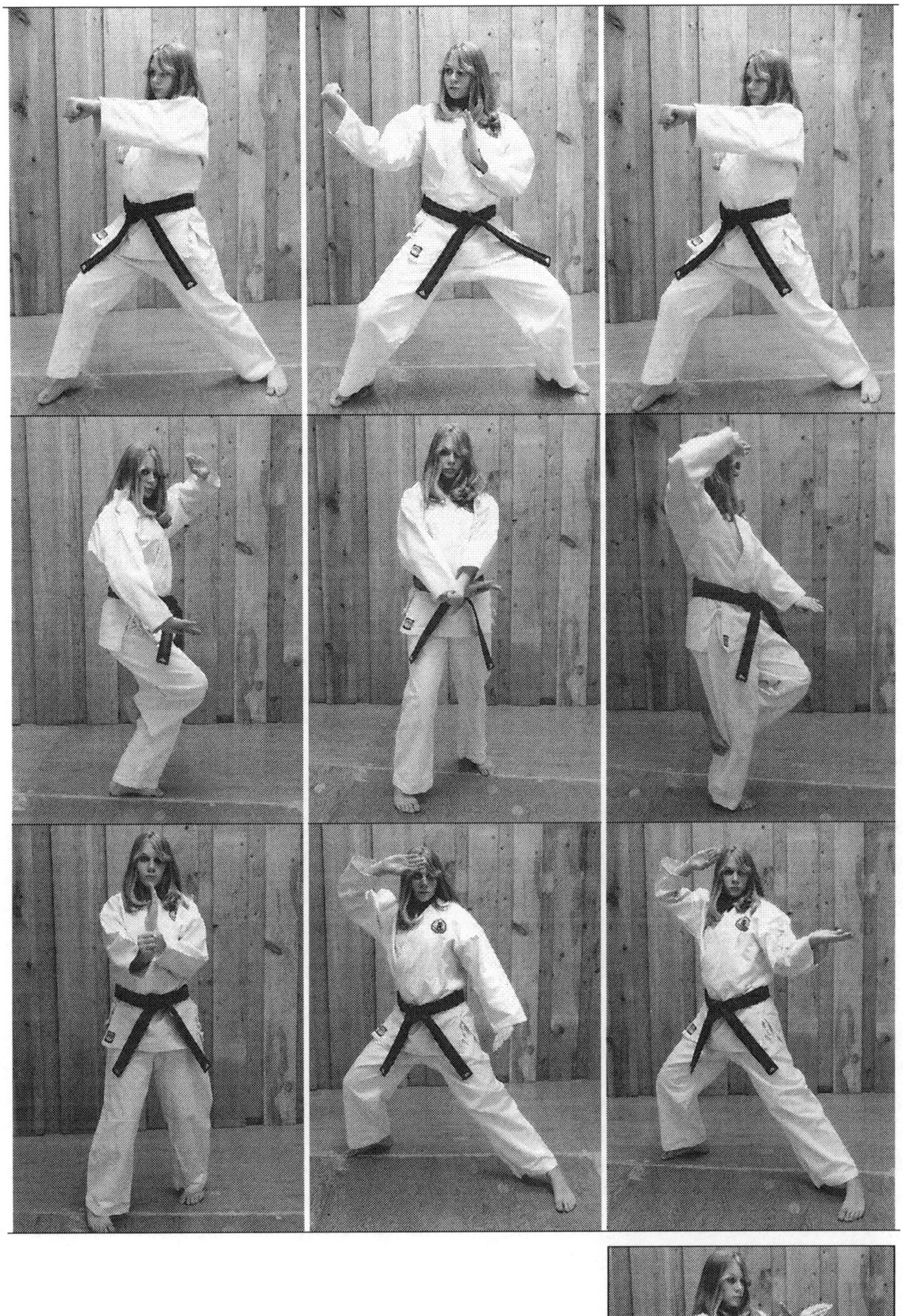

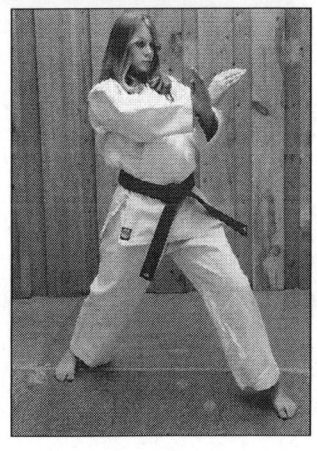

Desiree Felice demonstrating
some movements from the kata.

Bob Dalgleish is responsible for the majority of the Goju-ryu karate in Canada today. There are now fourth-generation instructors with full-time karate schools who owe Dalgleish a debt of gratitude. It is because of his efforts that so many Goju-ryu schools exist today. Dalgleish was also an innovator. A man who gathered information from Oriental and American instructors, then structured it for re-release to a Canadian audience. As well as his knowledge and teaching skills, his personality and character attracted many people.

Dalgleish touched a great many lives with his knowledge, and stimulated in his students a thirst for information. After his death, many of these students made the pilgrimage to Okinawa and Japan to research karate at the source. And although they may claim loyalty to Okinawan and Japanese instructors or organizations, they cannot ignore that initial spark that started their interest. That spark was the man that they called their teacher, Robert Marshall Dalgleish, "Father of Canadian Goju-ryu."

ACKNOWLEDGMENTS

If I have missed mentioning anyone who was involved in my research on for this article, I apologize. I have tried to form a true picture of the man's life and his legacy based on the information that was presented to me by those who knew him. Thank you, all. I would also like to thank: Desiree Felice for appearing in the photos; Hung Tang for taking the photos and Olga for setting up the photos; Adam Kieswetter for proof reading; and Joubert for his help in Thunder Bay. Photo credit is also given to the following individuals for the initial eight illustrations: Monty Guest, Michael McGuire, and Guy Ranger.

NOTES
Personal Communications and Website References

[1] M. Guest, January 21, 2002; K. Hayashi, January 17 and February 7, 2002; M. McGuire, January 13 and 27, 2002.

[2] M. Guest, January 21, 2002.

[3] Tsuruoka had been born in Cumberland, British Columbia, in 1929. Because of their Japanese decent, Tsuruoka and his family were confined to a Canadian internment camp during the World War II. After the war, the Tsuruoka family moved to Japan. Here Tsuruoka would begin karate training with Chitose Tsuyoshi, the founder of Chito-ryu. After attaining the rank of 2nd-degree, Tsuruoka returned to Canada in 1956 to settle in Toronto. There he opened the first karate school in Canada (M. Tsuruoka, January 17, 2002).

[4] K. Tallack, January 17, 2002.

[5] M. Guest, January 21, 2002; K. Hayashi, January 17 and February 7, 2002; B. Hind, January 30, 2002.

[6] B. Hind, January 30, 2002.

[7] Ibid.

[8] K. Hayashi, January 17 and February 7, 2002; K. Tallack, January 17, 2002.

[9] K. Tallack, January 17, 2002; E. Dennis, January 23, 2002.

[10] Shuri-ryu website.

[11] K. Tallack, January 17, 2002; M. Guest, January 21, 2002.

[12] Nishiyama had begun his karate training in Japan with the great Funakoshi Gichin in 1943 at the Shotokan headquarters. Nishiyama was a co-founder of the Japan Karate

Federation. In 1952, he had been selected as a member of the martial arts combat instruction staff for the US Strategic Air Command Combat Training Program. In 1961, he was invited to the United States to organize the All America Karate Federation (later renamed the American Amateur Karate Federation) (Corcoran and Farkas, 1993: 361–362). Richard Kim, whose mother was Japanese, was a native of Hawai'i. He had moved to Japan prior to World War II. Kim had trained in judo and karate since he was a boy and had boxed as a young man. While in Japan, he was admitted to the Butokukai where he was able to learn many forms of jujutsu, karate and Okinawan kobujutsu (Sells, 2000:135). He also had studied taijiquan and baguaquan in China. Dr. Kim settled in San Francisco in 1959 (Zen Bei Busen web site).

[14] T. Collingwood, January 26, 2002.
[15] K. Hayashi, January 17 and February 7, 2002.
[16] M. Guest, January 21, 2002.
[17] D. Gauthier, January 14 and 30, 2002.
[18] G. Ranger, January 23, 2002.
[19] G. Ranger, January 23, 2002.
[20] M. McGuire, January 13 and 27, 2002.
[21] W. Avery, January 21, 2002; K. Hayashi, January 17 and February 7, 2002.
[22] K. Tallack, January 17, 2002.
[23] M. McGuire, January 13 and 27, 2002; M. Guest, January 21, 2002.
[24] K. Hayashi, January 17 and February 7, 2002.
[25] P. McCarthy, November 15, 2001; February 7–8, 2002.
[26] K. Hayashi, January 17 and February 7, 2002; R. Yamanaka, January 17, 2002.
[27] P. McCarthy, November 15, 2001; February 7–8, 2002; K. Hayashi, January 17 and February 7, 2002.
[28] K. Tallack, January 17, 2002.
[29] M. Guest, January 21, 2002.
[30] G. Ranger, January 23, 2002.
[31] G. Ranger, January 23, 2002; M. McGuire, January 13 and 27, 2002.
[32] M. McGuire, January 13 and 27, 2002; I. Segarra, January 30, 2002.
[33] G. Ranger, January 23, 2002.

References

Castinado, M. (1995, December). Yamaguchi: The consistent innovator. *Budo Dojo*, 34–38.
Corcoran, J., Farkas, E., and Sobel, S. *The original martial arts encyclopedia*. Los Angeles: Pro-Action Publishing.
Dalgleish, R. (1975, August). Cycle of karate. *Oriental Fighting Arts*, 16.
Liedke, B. (1990, April). Chuck Merriman: The early days of karate. *Karate and Fitness International*, 50–52.
Petras, H. (1994, October). Peter Urban: Godfather of American Goju. *Masters of Self Defense*, 8, 58, 60.
Sells, J. (2000). *Unante: The secrets of karate*. 2rd edition. Hollywood, CA: Hawley Publications.
Simpkins, A. and Simpkins, A. (1994, March). Tournaments and their transcendence. *Secrets of the Masters*, 13–20.
Smoke, S. (1991, April). Goshei Yamaguchi son of the famous cat. *Meet the Masters*, 3–33.
Urban, P. (1991). *The karate dojo: Traditions and tales of a martial art*. Rutland, VT: Charles E. Tuttle Company.
Ward, R. (1994, Spring). Risen suns. *Canadian Martial Arts, 1*(3):21–24.

chapter 40

The Lost Secrets of Okinawan Goju-ryu: What the Kata Shows

by Giles Hopkins, M.A.

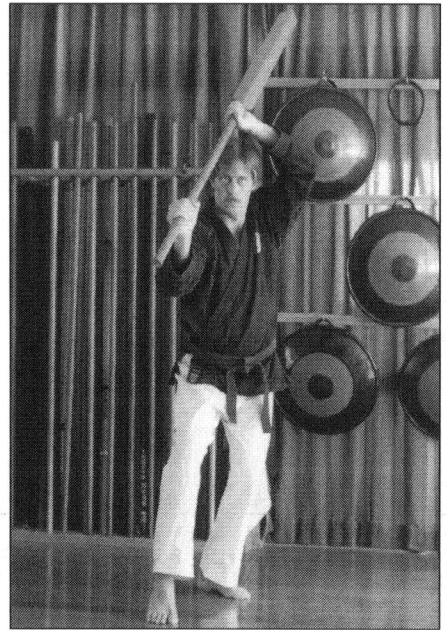
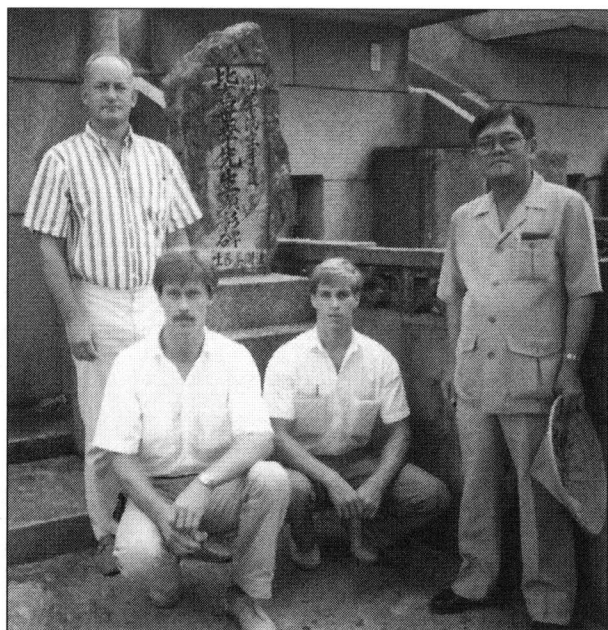

Left: The author training with the oar (*eku*) at Matayoshi Shinpo's dojo.
Right (L. to R.): Kimo Wall, the author, Paul Gorter, and Matayoshi Shinpo at Higa Seiko's grave site.
All photos courtesy of G. Hopkins.

Introduction

On a hot July evening in 1986, I was standing in the martial arts training hall listening to Matayoshi Shinpo explain one of the postures of kata Kakuho, a Kingai-ryu system form (*kata*). We had been walking up and down the floor in crane stance, toes of one foot curled under ready to throw small pebbles or sand into attacker's face, arms out to the side like wings. Matayoshi had come down earlier to watch *kobudo* (ancient weapons art) training. When we had finished, we began training some of the empty-hand katas of Matayoshi's family system and our own Goju-ryu. It was already late in the evening. Sometimes Matayoshi would stop and try to explain something with the few English words he knew and then laugh.

"You no show," he would say. "Okay?" That summer, sitting in an ice cream shop in downtown Naha, Matayoshi had heard a particularly blaring American pop song. The singers' voices were harsh and nasal as they repeated the chorus, "Show me, show me." Matayoshi had asked what the words meant, and from then on, he used the words frequently, and laugh.

At the moment, however, he was trying to explain how one of the moves in the kata was used. Though the application was obvious, we couldn't figure out what he was trying to get across. With Matayoshi's peculiar collection of a couple dozen English words or phrases and our handful of Japanese words, it was like some hilarious game of charades. Matayoshi would bend down and pretend to pull up clumps of imaginary grass (we later realized). Then he would rear back with both arms up in front of his body, elbows in, forearms vertical, wrists bent so that the hands, held above the head, formed claws. Then he would stop and hold one hand up with index finger and thumb spread apart.

"You know?" he would ask. Of course we didn't.

Finally, someone went for a small pocket dictionary.

"Mushi," Matayoshi said, pointing to the word, "Insect."

"Midori."

We all laughed. Matayoshi had only been trying to explain that it was a praying mantis technique. Nothing more. It made me wonder how many other things we had missed in translation that summer, and how situations not so different from this one may have affected the Okinawan martial arts in general and Goju-ryu specifically. Were secrets lost in translation? What sorts of things had other students misunderstood along the way?

Interpreting the Meaning of Katas

The history of Goju-ryu has been researched, second and third generation teachers have been interviewed, and, most importantly perhaps, the katas themselves have been scrutinized and analyzed. Each new journal article seems to have another theory about katas. Every teacher seems to have a new and different explanation of kata applications (*bunkai*). Internet discussion groups abound with imaginative discoveries of kata's meaning.

However, all of this discussion raises a far more perplexing question: How could so many practitioners be at odds about the meaning of things so fundamental to their art, to what they practice on a daily basis? Why do so many of these articles and books seem to be archeological treasure hunts in search of the Rosetta Stone—in search of something to unlock the key to Goju-ryu as a system? In other words, why don't we know what kata movements really mean? Why are we still debating applications, looking for what the original intent of the various Goju-ryu katas must have been?

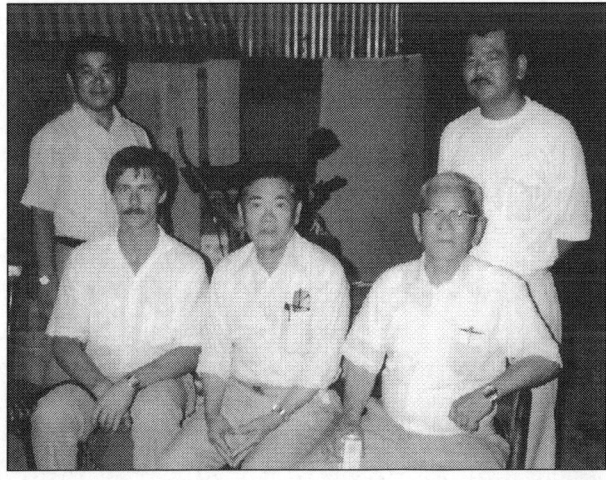

Seated, left to right: the author, Matayoshi Shinpo, and Kina Seiko.
Standing: Oshiro Zenei and Miyazato (Matayoshi's brother-in-law).

As it stands now, the kata applications mean whatever a "legitimate" instructor says they mean. And there is considerable disagreement. Every school seems to have its claim, well-established through various lineages, to authenticity. In the spirit of equanimity and brotherhood, students and teachers alike will argue that there are an almost infinite number of applications. So, if there is not one "right" application for each move, there would seem at least to be no wrong answers. Or, to rectify the disparity, some suggest that there are multiple levels of understanding. But these are not answers; they're rationalizations and only serve to confuse the issue. In the *Journal of Asian Martial Arts,* a Goju-ryu practitioner forwarded the theory that Shisochin was an answer to Sanseiru: that if you superimpose one kata over the other, the techniques of one seem to show counters to the other (Toth, 2001).

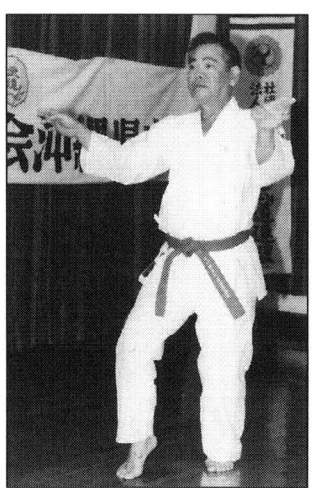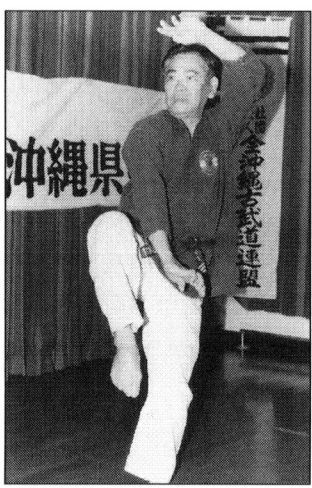

Matayoshi Shinpo demonstrating Kakuho
kata from his family system, Kingai-ryu.

Though the origins of katas are certainly lost in a distant past—as are the legendary creators of these katas—I find it hard to imagine that whoever made and formalized kata movements could have been so intentionally cryptic. It is as if the katas themselves were some elaborate Rorschach test, where different people see different things. At the very least, this kind of analysis serves to illustrate the dilemma.

Without becoming too philosophical, it isn't difficult to see how this can happen. It is easy to assign meaning, to rationalize an interpretation however idiosyncratic. After all, man is the great signifier. We can and do find meaning in the seeming randomness of nature, the chaos of the universe, the rantings of madmen, or the brush strokes of an elephant with a paintbrush. Why not kata?

The sad thing is that given this state of confusion with katas, some have, lamentably though I suppose understandably, "thrown out the baby with the bath water" and chosen to point an accusatory finger and shout, "the emperor has no clothes!" as Nathan Johnson does in *Barefoot Zen* (2000:125). That is to say, long time practitioners will throw their hands up in frustration—and Johnson is certainly not alone here—exclaiming that the katas don't mean anything, the movements are just movements and there is no system to be understood. As Johnson puts it: "People looking for a systematic or progressive development of attack and defense techniques in the traditional forms will be disappointed" (2000:122). It's an understandable frustration—a radical belief born out of confusion—but also mistaken.

Katas in Historical Perspective

I would suggest that the reason there is such debate about katas and their applications may lie in the turbulent nature of the 20th century or, in Goju-ryu's case, in Miyagi Chojun's untimely death at the age of 65. But in reality, I think it may have more to do with the very nature of karate training today and how it developed over the past 100 years.

Consider the direction that karate had taken in Okinawa in the early 20th century. Karate had already become a part of the Okinawan school system as early as 1909 (Toguchi, 1976:13–14; McCarthy, 1999:48). Whatever the reasons for this move, it would have far-reaching consequences. A martial art practiced by schoolchildren is necessarily very different from the system of self-defense trained by the Okinawan warrior class (*bushikaikyuu*) or the monk-warriors of China who may have developed the original katas.

With Gekisai I and Gekisai II—and various other "training" subjects added later by other teachers—Miyagi Chojun created "generic" katas that could more safely be taught to young people, to students. A beginner's curriculum based on these training subjects would be less lethal and a teacher would not be giving away the art's "secrets." But one would also not be studying the essence of Goju-ryu. This is apparent from the opening move of Gekisai I. The upper-level block as it is done in this kata is not found anywhere in Goju-ryu's "classical" katas. The Gekisai katas and basic training (*kihon*) may have served to popularize karate and improve its image—one of the goals that Miyagi seems to suggest in his 1934 *Outline of Karate-do* (McCarthy, 1999)—changing the public perception of the martial arts from the pugilistic occupation of warriors and street toughs to a systematized activity of physical conditioning. But a dojo curriculum based on these exercises would only serve to mask the real techniques, the essence, of the classical katas.

This seems to have been a goal that many Okinawan karate masters shared: not intentionally to hide real karate, but to popularize a version that would be more acceptable to the public. Katas were preserved but applications received less emphasis. Group exercise and physical conditioning replaced traditional application of technique because teachers like Itosu Ankoh considered the techniques "too dangerous" for schoolchildren. As McCarthy notes, "the emphasis shifted from a self-defense art to a cultural recreation for physical fitness" (1999:106). This shift in emphasis was further solidified in a 1936 meeting of Okinawan karate masters. Although Miyagi clearly states that "the classical kata must remain," there is a not-so-subtle push from some quarters to standardize technique and separate it from its Chinese roots. In line with his earlier interests in changing the public's perception of karate, Miyagi even suggests that "suitable kata, with both offensive and defensive [sic], for students from elementary school to university level should be developed" (McCarthy, 1999:65).

This shift in emphasis continued in the post-World War II years. Dan Smith, a long-time Shorin-ryu teacher, argues that the spread of karate to mainland Japan led to teachers who "did not stay with the Okinawans long enough to learn and the karate that was taught in the beginning was *kihon* [fundamentals]."

The same thing affected karate in Okinawa after the war, Smith goes on to say, for a variety of reasons. The older teachers in Okinawa—those that knew the "secrets"—far from any intentional effort at hiding technique, Smith writes, were merely responding to "the changing times." Smith suggests that they "designed their instruction to meet the perceived needs of the day. . . .[E]mphasis was put on kihon, kata and *jiu kumite* [free sparring]" (Smith, Letter 1).

Others have not been so charitable. Anthony Marquez, writing in the now defunct *Bugeisha* magazine, argues that even second generation Okinawan teachers didn't know the old applications. Marquez writes that Masanobu Shinjo told him that the "old techniques died with the past generations" (Marquez, 1996:13). So, for whatever reason, Okinawan karate underwent a significant change in the 20th century, whether this was due to an effort to popularize karate or because many younger teachers were ill equipped to teach the classical curriculum or that the older teachers didn't really know or were merely being accommodating.

In any case, this is the karate that we see practiced today—both here and in most Okinawan dojos. It is not real Goju-ryu. It is schoolboy karate. Certainly it can be effective, both for self-defense and physical conditioning, but it is not the same karate that we find in the classical Goju-ryu katas. It is also important to remember that the lessons of one do not necessarily translate into an understanding of the other.

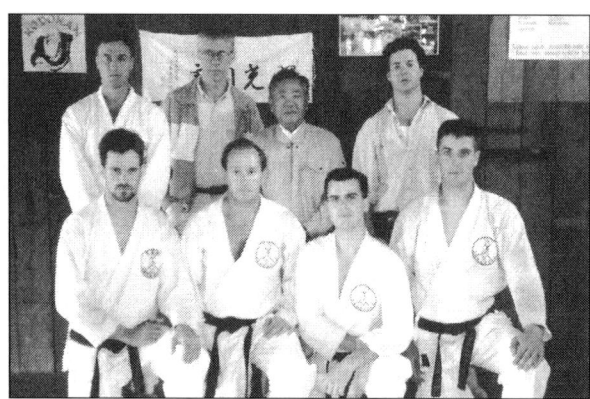

Matayoshi Shinpo visiting the author's dojo.

As evidenced from early demonstrations, Miyagi Chojun's karate consisted of "throwing and grappling techniques." According to Higaonna Morio's research, Miyagi was renown for his "pulling down techniques . . . *sabaki* (body movement) . . . and *muchimi* (sticky hands)" (Higaonna, 1985:28–29). This gives us some clue as to the real nature of Goju-ryu and techniques found within the classical katas.

Sadly, the training tools, like the Gekisai katas, shed little if any light on the meaning of classical katas and their self-defense applications. In fact, the training subjects and the two-person sets developed by Toguchi Seikichi and others work contrary to many of the principles found in the classical katas. And it is for this reason, I believe, that the real meaning of the Goju-ryu katas has remained a mystery to so many people for so long.

Seeing Katas for What They Are

However, the mystery can be unraveled by the katas themselves. Everything the traditional karate practitioner needs to know about Goju-ryu as a system is contained in the classical katas: Saifa, Seiunchin, Shisochin, Sepai, Sanseiru, Sesan, Kururunfa, and Suparinpei.

The only thing one needs to do in analyzing the katas—in studying applications correctly—is to apply martial principles to the movements, and this is exactly what has not been done. We have looked at katas as if they were arbitrary collections of techniques—so many contained in each kata, we are told, that it would take a lifetime to master just one—ignoring the lessons contained in the patterns themselves. Or, we have attempted to explain the movement as an imaginary battle against multiple attackers. Both of these explanations—while seemingly plausible—are at the very least misleading. Again, one need only apply the principles to see the katas as they were originally meant to be seen. If we don't, we are left with a generic art of punching and kicking—not much better than schoolboy karate. As the Chinese classics put it: "If we do not practice according to the applications of the principles, we can work forever without developing a superior art" (Wile, 1983:71).

The principles are basically simple. Always move off the centerline whenever possible. As the Chinese classics state: "We must quickly evade by withdrawing our center and attacking from the side" (Wile, 1983:67). Smith states this a bit more colloquially when he says, "Get out of the way" (Smith, Letter 3). This is the first principle. If the various katas were not meant to demonstrate this principle, then all of the katas would be done in a straight line. But they are not. The steps and turns—indeed, most of the direction changes within a kata—show where the attack is coming from, and, consequently, how to get out of the way of the attack or how to step off the centerline.

Repeatedly, what one will notice in practicing kata is that one turns to step off the centerline that the attacker is advancing along. If one applies this principle to the first move of the Sepai kata (see illustration, 1A and 1E), one can see that contrary to what is commonly taught—that the attack is a frontal attack and one is merely stepping back along the line of attack—the attack is really from the west. The step back into a horse stance side-steps the attack and removes one's center, placing the defender in a 90 degree relationship to the attacker.

The first movement in Goju-ryu is often to side-step the opponent, whether this is to the outside (usually) or the inside. But so often, dojo training seems to emphasize Goju-ryu's hardness. We train doing the Sanchin kata or arm-toughening drills (*koteikitai*) with the idea that we will stand squarely in front of an attacker and be able to take whatever he doles out.

However, what katas more often show is that Goju-ryu is initially soft, using angles and stepping to avoid the attack, blocking and hooking in circular motions, tying the attacker up, using his own momentum against him, redirecting the attack. As the Chinese classics remind us, we should "meet hardness with softness" (Wile, 1983:91). Goju-ryu is first soft, then hard.

Another principle one should keep in mind is, in a sense, more historical. Karate, and martial arts in general, was not originally intended as a sport or a casual pursuit restricted to the dojo or community center. It was a deadly martial art meant to be used in combat, intended to protect or save one's life. It was not intended for competition, a later modification or 20th century innovation when "the Butokukai required that there be a measurement of skill of the new martial art, 'karate'. . . . With this innovation karate introduced a new scenario . . . mutually agreed upon combat" (Smith, Letter 6). In traditional karate, the important point is that the attacker was fully committed to his attack, and this should be remembered when one looks at any application.

By the same token, the defender was fully committed to preserving his or her own life. The techniques were not intended to give the attacker a second chance. They were meant to be used only as a last resort. If we keep this idea in mind when looking at katas, we tend to see a different level of brutality for lack of a more euphemistic term—techniques that don't merely fight the arms of the attacker but go straight to more vital body parts. The classical katas teach one to block the arms, but attack the head. If we begin to look at katas in this way, the katas become much more lethal, and, I believe, more historical, truer to the original intent of the katas and their applications. At the same time, all of the techniques will begin to fit together and the combinations of moves will begin to make sense.

To illustrate, I will try to show how the techniques of the Sepai kata demonstrate these principles. The applications adhere to the kata's movement, but the rhythm at which the techniques are executed may vary considerably from what one usually practices in solo kata. What should become immediately apparent is that the kata is a collection of sequences or techniques done in combination against one attacker, not multiple opponents. Stepping and directional changes generally show where the attack is coming from and provide the defender with a graphic illustration of how to step off the centerline or how one should block and enter. Each sequence begins with a block and entry technique, and ends with the opponent on the ground. This is what is meant by the Okinawan saying, "*karate ni sente nashi*" ("in karate there is no first attack"). However, it is not just the kata that demonstrates this idea, but each sequence within the kata.

TECHNICAL SECTION

Sepai Kata (Sepai = eighteen)

First Sequence: Facing north, the kata begins with two circular arm movements, stepping back with the left foot into a horse stance with feet at 45-degree angles (*shiko dachi*) (1a). Take two steps forward in the basic stance, followed by a series of palm-to-palm grasping techniques (1b and c). Drop into a horse stance as the right elbow and forearm is brought up (1d).

Application: The attacker is coming from the west, stepping in with a right punch. By stepping back with the left foot into a horse stance, the kata is showing lateral movement, stepping off the centerline. The defender is sidestepping the attack and blocking with the left open hand. The right arm is brought over the attacking arm behind the opponent's head, coming down on the back of the neck (1e). Stepping up with the left foot, the left hand is brought underneath to the opponent's chin, the right hand is on top of the head (1f). Bring the opponent's head around with the right hand and secure with both hands, advancing with the right foot (1g). Step in behind and drop into a right-foot forward horse stance with a neck break (1h).

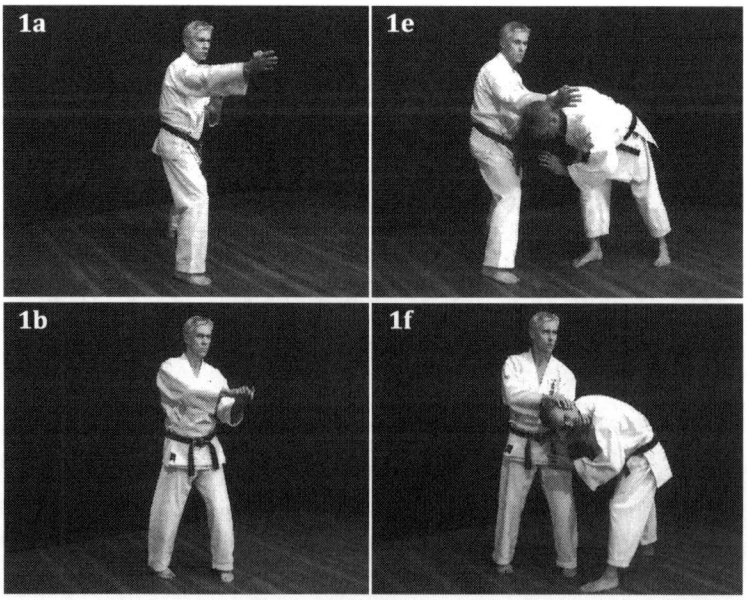

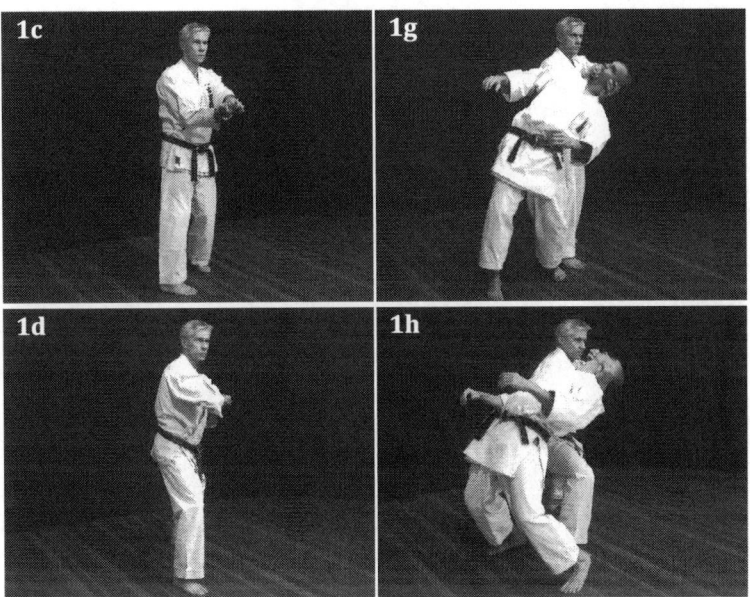

Second Sequence: The next series of techniques, done from a back stance (*kokutso dachi*), begins with what appears to be a left open-hand downward strike, while the right open-hand and forearm is held at chest level, palm down (2a). This is followed by a hooking block and a *shuto* (knife-edge attack) in a front stance (2b). The next technique is a front kick (2c) and grabbing technique, returning to a horse stance (2d), followed by a downward elbow or forearm strike (2e).

Application: Step in to the north with a sweeping left open-hand block in a clock-wise direction. The attacker is stepping in with a right punch that is blocked by the left sweeping block (2f), carrying the attack down in a clockwise direction and then, sticking to the attacking arm, carrying it up to the left in a trapping block. Pivoting to a left-foot forward front stance, the left hand opens the target as it is brought up. At the same time, a right knife-hand (*shuto*) attacks the opponent's head or neck (2g). The arms should move in unison here. The knee and foot are then brought up into the attacker's stomach and groin (2h). Stepping back into a horse stance, the attacker is pulled down with both hands (2i) and a downward elbow attack is used to finish him off (2j). It should be noted that the hands begin in the open-hand position to attack and then close to indicate a grab or grasping of the opponent.

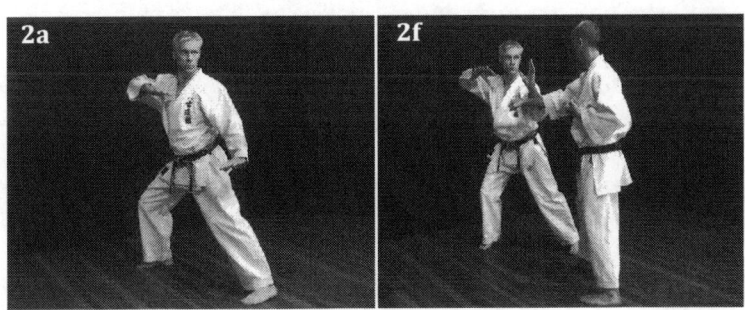

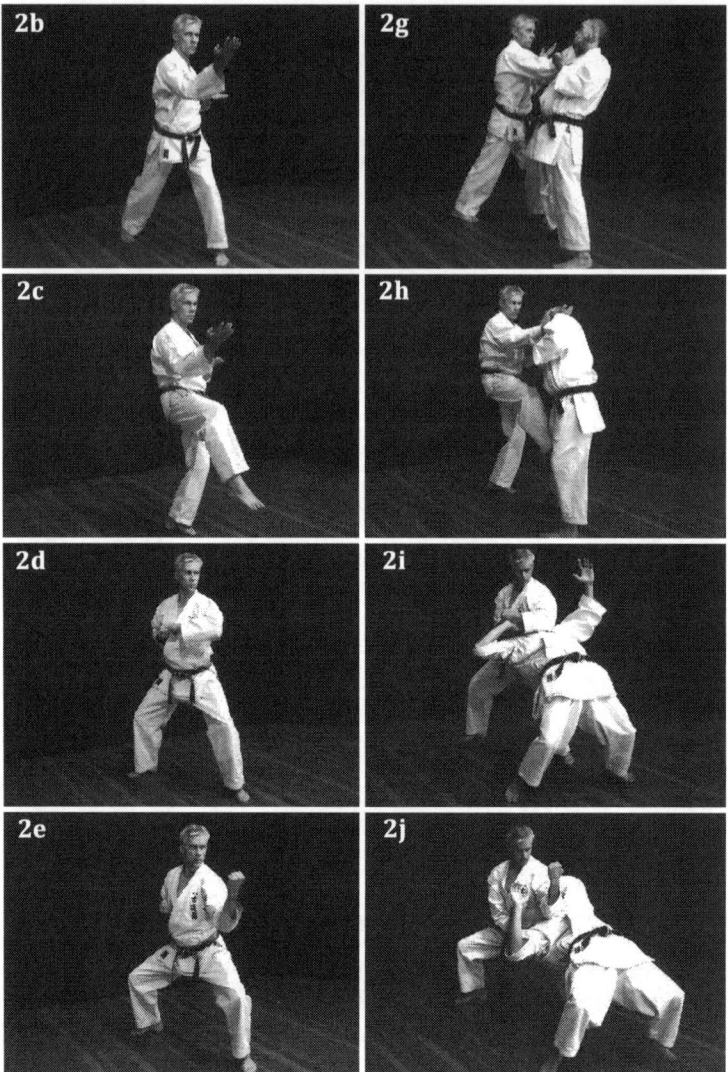

Third Sequence: The next series of moves begins in a front stance (*zenkutsu dachi*) and pulls back into a cat stance (*neko ashi dachi*), while executing what appears to be middle-level block. The left open-hand sweeps across the body, closing into a fist, and comes to rest beneath the right elbow (3a). The right arm, with closed fist, sweeps across the body, ending in lower-level position (3b). The right arm is then brought up into a middle-level blocking position as the weight shifts back into a cat stance. The right hand then opens (3c). The next move is a step and turn to the original front into a basic stance while the left arm is brought up and over the right, both arms finishing in front of the chest with closed fists (3d). The next technique—an upper-level circular arm movement and a lower-level open-hand attack—is executed with a turning step to the rear into a basic stance. The left arm circles counterclockwise to the ribs while the right hand follows the right foot, attacking with the palm, fingers down, palm forward, at thigh level (3e).

Application: Turning to the south into a right-foot-forward front stance, block the attacker's punch with the left open hand, while hooking and grabbing the arm. The attacker is stepping in to attack from the east with a right punch. The right arm is brought around the attacker's head, bringing the attacker's head down into the right knee of the front stance (3f–g). As the attacker is "released," the defender shifts back into a cat stance, pulling the opponent back by grabbing the head or hair with the right open hand, while maintaining control of the opponent's punching arm (3h). The right knee may be employed here as the shift into a cat stance indicates. Then, stepping in behind the attacker, the left arm is brought around the opponent's neck and thrust up in an attack to the throat (3i). The left hand then opens, to control the attacker's chin, and, turning to the left, the opponent is thrown to the rear. The right hand continues in a lower-level attack to facilitate the throw (3j).

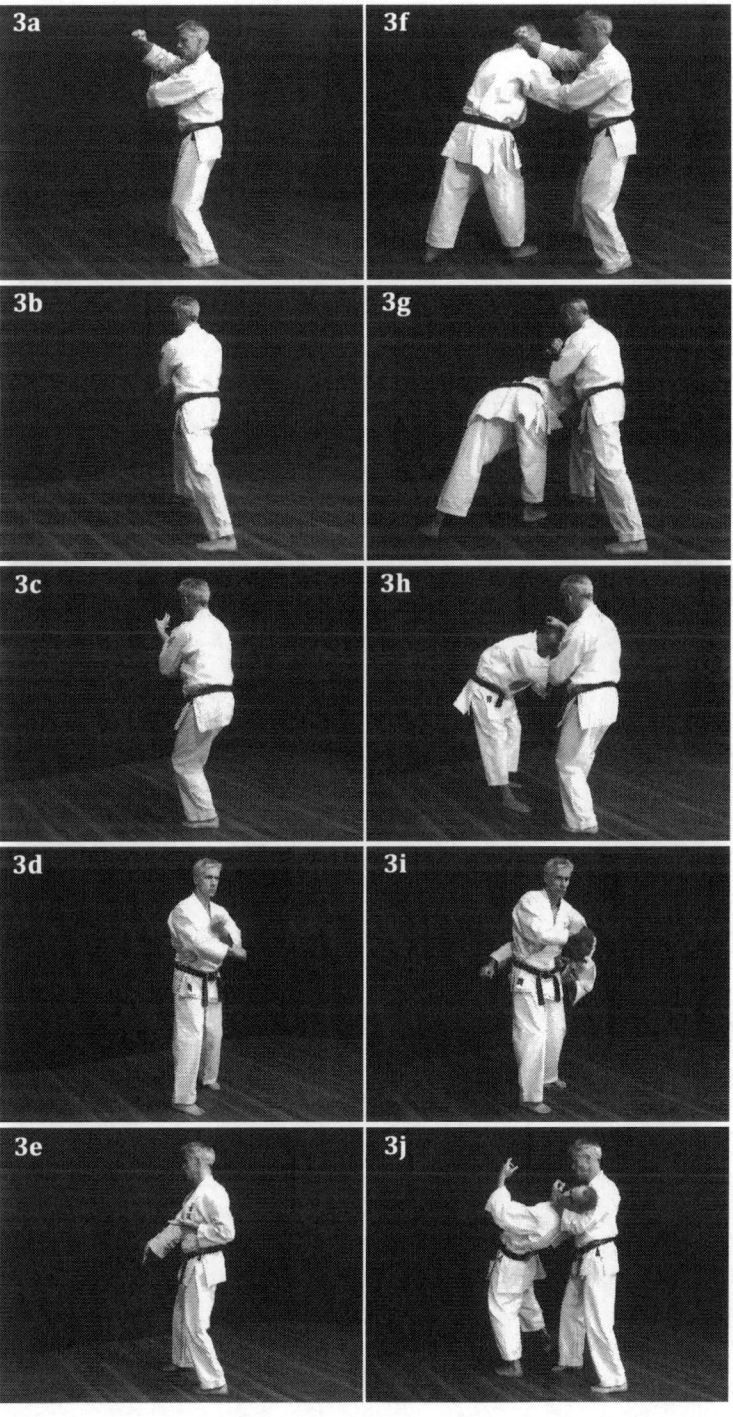

Fourth Sequence: The next series of movements is repeated to both the left and right sides, using an advancing natural stance (*renoji dachi*) (4a), followed by a step into a horse stance (4b), a throw, and a double attack, dropping into a low horse stance (4c).

Application: Step in to the southeast corner with the left foot while executing a circular sweeping left open-hand block in a clockwise direction (4d). The opponent is attacking with a right punch, from the southeast. As the sweeping block opens the target, the right open hand attacks the opponent's face. Continue the attack as the right foot steps in behind the attacker's right leg and hip (4e). Bring the right knee up and throw. Finish with a double punch or using both hands to drive the opponent into the ground (4f).

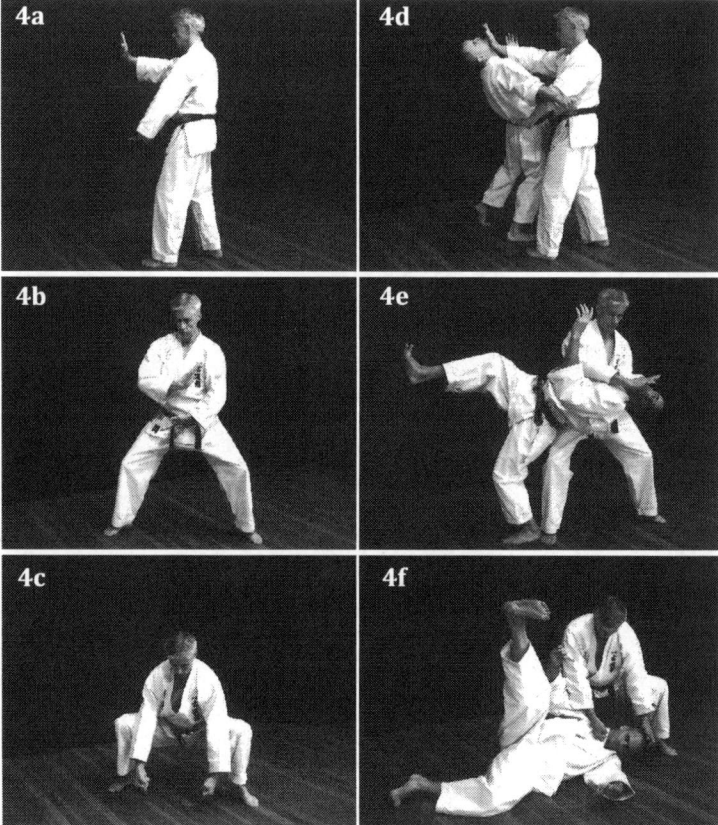

Fifth Sequence: Step back into a horse stance, executing a lower-level block (5a).

Application: The attacker is coming from the east, attacking with a right punch. Looking to the east, step back into a horse stance to block and grab with the right hand, as the left forearm is brought down on the attacker's neck and head (5b–c). Here the fourth sequence is repeated to the southwest corner, reversing the sides. This is followed by a repetition of the fifth sequence to the west, reversing the sides.

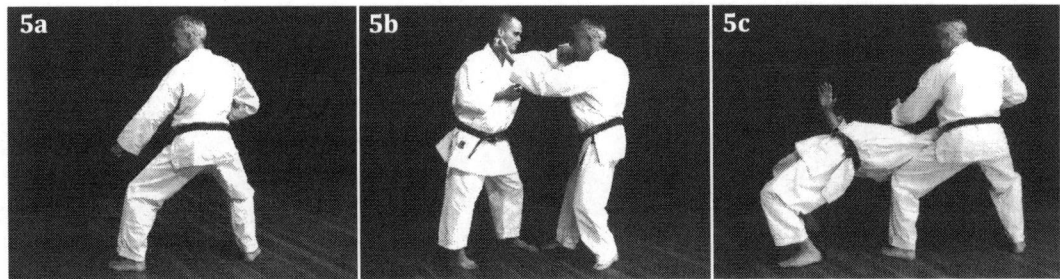

Sixth Sequence: The next technique involves a step into a cat stance with a middle-level block and upper-level hooking punch (6a). This is followed by a pivoting of the body wherein the weight is transferred to the other foot and the hands are brought down to the side (6b). This is followed by a jump or step to the front, landing in a cross-legged stance with the left foot behind the right, and the hands in reverse position to the previous middle-level and upper-level block and attack (6c). This is followed by a counter-clockwise pivot to end facing the east (6d).

Application: With a left-hand attack coming from the east, step off the centerline to the south with the right foot. In a left foot forward cat stance, block the opponent's attack with the left arm and attack to the head with the right (6e). The right arm is then brought down onto the attacker's left arm (6f) and hooks the arm as the "jump" is executed. The right foot then steps in to the north, behind the attacker. The left punch then attacks to the opponent's head as the left foot is brought in behind the right foot (6g). Then, pivoting sharply to the left, as the feet unwind, in a counter-clockwise three-quarter turn, the attacker is thrown to the east (6h), the original direction of the opponent's attack. This entire sequence should be done in a single flowing motion without stops. It will be noted that this throwing sequence is the reverse of the sequence that ends the kata.

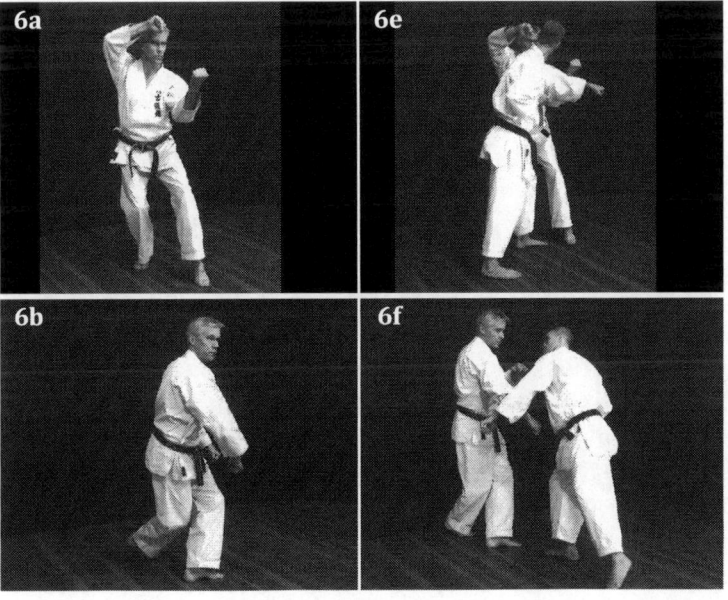

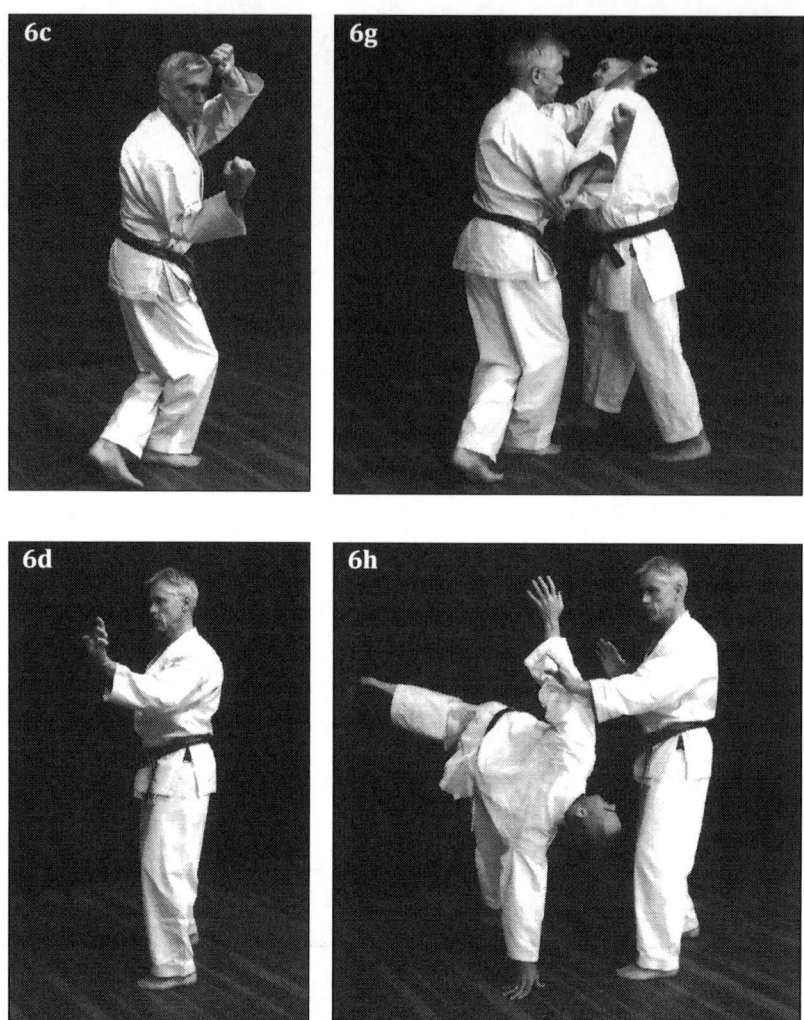

Seventh Sequence: This sequence is repeated on both the right and left sides after pivoting from the cross-legged stance into an open-hand block in a basic stance (7a). After again pivoting the body, execute a downward motion or strike with the left arm (7b), followed by back-fist (*uraken*) or a forearm attack (7c). Again, the stance pivots, while executing a middle-level block (7d). The next move involves an open-hand grabbing block, front instep kick (7e), and undercut attack (7f), ending in a horse stance.

Application: The final position of the previous throw and the initial technique of this next sequence almost overlap. Block the opponent's left punch with the right palm. The left hand simultaneously attacks to the opponent's head or neck (7g). Pivot in place, using the left arm to bring the opponent's head down in a clock-wise direction (7h). Attack to the back of the neck with the left forearm (7i). Pivot back toward the east and use the right forearm to come under the opponent's neck or to attack and control the other side of the neck and head (7j). The right hand then grabs the opponent, as the right knee lifts to strike the groin or midsection or as an instep kick (7k), and then the left undercut is used to attack (7l).

The seventh sequence is repeated to the left side or west.

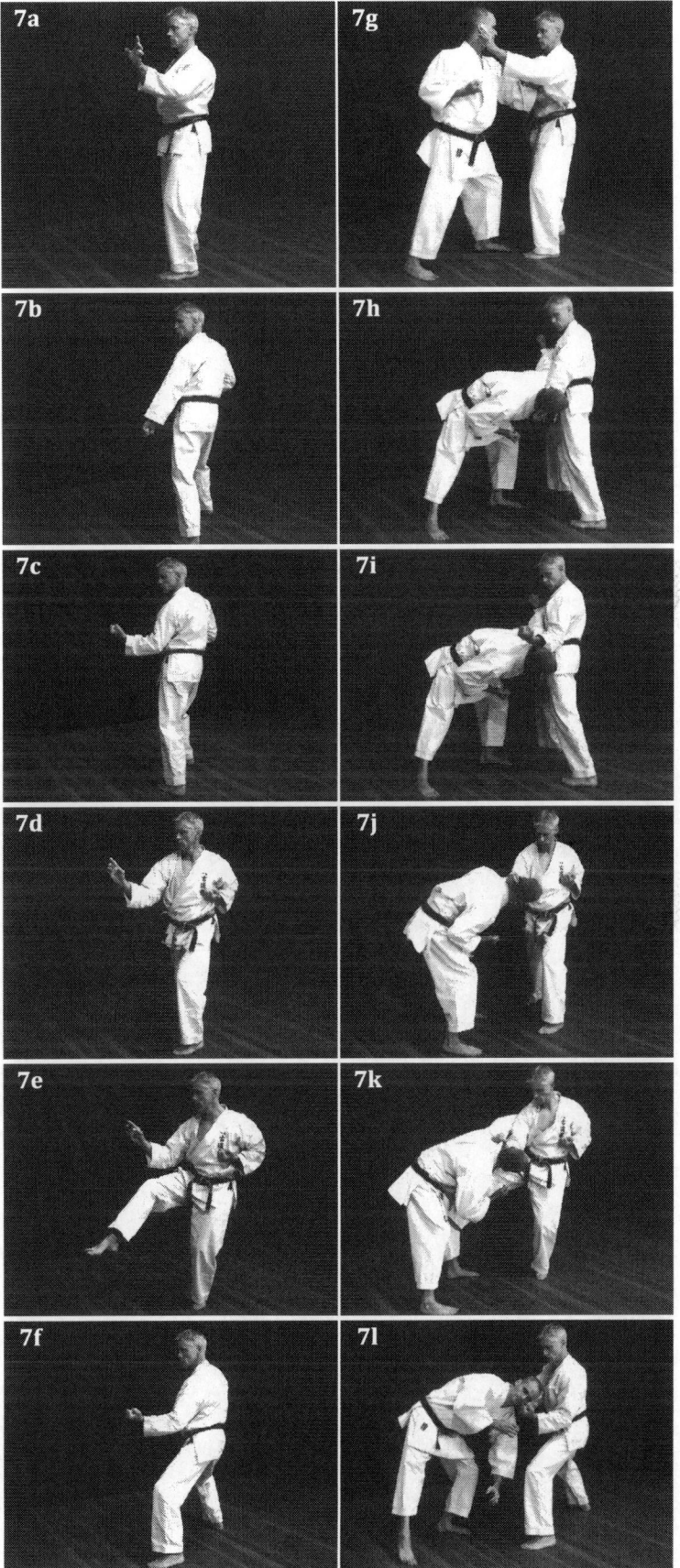

Eighth Sequence: The final series of techniques begins with a step and turn into a curious stance that has the heel of the right foot in contact with the left toes at roughly a 90-degree angle. The hands are brought into the body, palms facing each other, one above and one below the solar plexus (8a). Retreating into a cat stance, a throw is executed with the hands rotating in a clockwise direction (8b), followed by a hammer-fist strike (8c).

Application: With a right hand attack coming from the west, step off the centerline to the south with the left foot, while blocking the right punch with a left open-hand block (8d). The left-hand block comes to rest, palm up, on the top of the attacking arm. Stepping up into a cross-footed stance, right foot in front of left, the right hand, forearm, and elbow are brought across the attacker's face (8e). Now facing north, step back into a left-foot-forward cat stance, as the attacker's head is brought down and the left arm is brought up in a clockwise direction (8f). This series is completed as the left hand grabs the attacker's head and the right hammerfist attacks (8g). As in many other katas, the final position is in a cat stance to show that the front knee may be used to attack. This completes the kata.

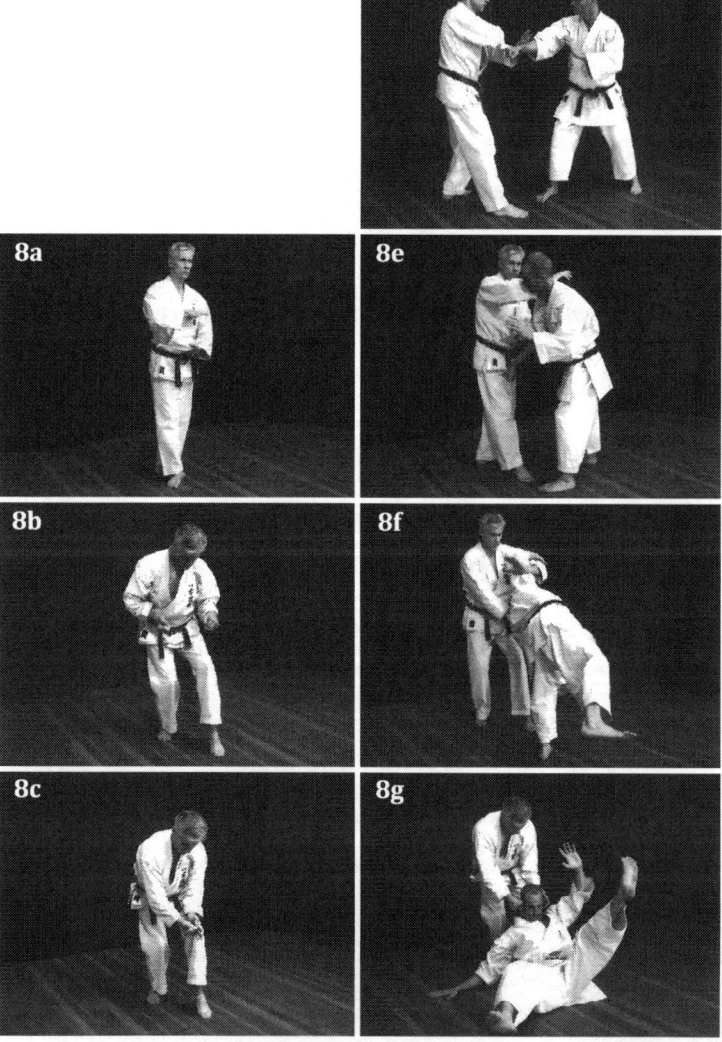

Conclusion

It has taken me many years to get to a point where I can see katas in this way. This was not an instant realization. However, what should be immediately apparent to any Goju-ryu practitioner is that the applications are different when one applies these principles to a study of katas. The paradigm that has informed—or misinformed—the study of kata applications in the past, taken from basic dojo drills or the Butokukai construct of mutually agreed upon combat for contest or testing purposes, actually affects how one looks at the techniques of kata even when applied to the classical subjects. One cannot study the applications of classical katas as if one is standing squarely in front of the opponent, feet planted, doing basic drills. One must take into account the katas' patterns and what they are attempting to show us. In other words, the applications of the hand techniques must also employ side-stepping and angular movement. Once this is done, and the blocking and entry techniques have been found, then the katas will be seen as collections of combinations. It will also reinforce the notion that the katas' original intent was to show specific martial principles and applications, not a multitude of possible interpretations.

I have used the Sepai kata to illustrate just a few of these principles. The same lessons, of course, can be applied to any of the classical forms. And certainly there are other principles that are also helpful. But there are some caveats as well. Great care should be taken to let go of preconceived notions of what Goju-ryu is and what it is not. As I have so often heard from my teacher, one should always train with an "open mind." However, one of the difficulties is that the formalities of training, or what we are used to, get in the way. The execution of the kata moves—particularly when it is performed within the dojo alongside others—sets up a rhythm that is at once metronomic and robotic. For teaching purposes, we regulate the speed within the kata and establish stopping points. All of this is artificial and, in fact, arbitrary to some extent.

Kata is dynamic. If the techniques are done against an attacker, they will flow in a continuous and uninterrupted stream. As the Chinese classics suggest, movements should be "continuous, circular and unending. Continuity without interruption" (Wile, 1983:13). This is the manner in which the various sequences in the Goju-ryu katas are meant to be done. Each has a distinct beginning and ending, but within the sequences themselves the movements should "not allow gaps" (Wile, 1983:102). Pauses and gaps in technique provide openings for an attacker. And though we may realize this, when it becomes ingrained in katas, we tend not to see the connections between techniques in application —we tend not to see the techniques as combinations.

However, altering the kata's rhythm is not the same as altering the moves themselves. I am not suggesting that kata form is at all arbitrary. That would be a particularly egregious misreading. While the altering, however slight, of kata movement can lead one down a number of interesting paths, discovering all sorts of unique applications, this is not what I am suggesting. To discover the original intent of the techniques in any kata—what I would suggest is the real application—an application should adhere as closely as possible to the kata's movement. The attempt is to discover what the kata is trying to show us. In most cases, this is hidden only if we don't apply the principles.

So often we simplify things to teach them or we standardize techniques that may only be similar. Both of these are dangerous shortcuts. To investigate kata movement, we must constantly keep in mind the art's principles—principles of movement that are often shared by a broad spectrum of martial arts—and scrutinize our technique in light of these principles.

Does this mean that we should abandon the entire curriculum of training subjects, based as they are on the Gekisai katas? Not necessarily. But we should see it for what it is, separate and distinct from the classical katas—and the essence I would argue—of Goju-ryu. They are worlds apart. The principles found within the classical katas, when applied, facilitate speed and power—in general, martial effectiveness—and those techniques and interpretations that do not conform to these principles will readily be seen to be less effective, and, in a word, questionable.

The classical Goju-ryu katas, like Sepai, illustrate and teach these principles. The katas' patterns shows how to step off the centerline, that is, how to avoid the attacker. Second, the techniques are meant to show responses against a fully committed attacker. These are not sparring techniques. As Dan Smith notes, "Uchinandi [Okinawan karate] is a self-defense based solution and works best when the opponent makes the first movement of attack" (Smith, Letter 6). And last, the various classical subjects of Goju-ryu are collections of techniques that fit together as combinations. They show variations of a finite number of themes in the same way that a classical music piece shows themes and variations. The combinations may be taken apart and put together in a variety of ways, but the first step is to see them as combinations. Each kata contains only a handful of combinations of techniques against an attacker.

For the most part, traditional Goju-ryu practitioners have done a wonderful job investigating individual techniques, but we have been lost in this forest of technique, so to speak, unable to see the "system" for the trees. To see Goju-ryu as a complete system, one must see the katas' techniques as combinations. And the way to see the various combinations of techniques is to apply the principles of movement to the katas. The proof, of course, will not be found in reference books but on the dojo floor.

Finally, one should remember that it is a lifetime pursuit to develop one's own self defense. It shouldn't be impossibly difficult or require great amounts of strength. If either were true, one would be least able to use it just when one needed it the most. The way I am suggesting we look at Goju-ryu is, in a sense, more simplified. It shows Goju-ryu as a system that makes use of certain martial principles, then gives examples to illustrate these principles, and finally shows a finite number of variations of the same principles and techniques. An understanding of this does not necessarily make the journey any shorter—one must still practice until the bones and the muscles and the blood begin to understand the technique—but the idea is to get the feet planted firmly on the right road before setting out on the journey. This is just the first step.

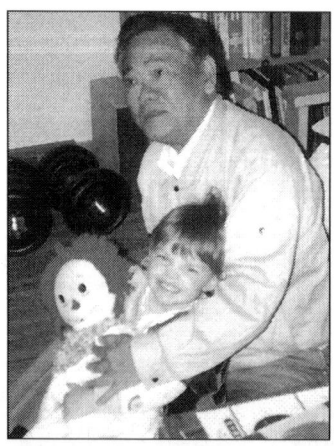

Matayoshi Shinpo with the author's daughter, Phoebe.

Most nights we would walk down the hill from Matayoshi's dojo late, with the smell of mosquito coils still in the air, tired and hungry. We would walk through Heiwa

Dori, feeling the soft tar on the roads, still hot from the day, looking for a late night soup shop or some place to sit and talk before turning in.

Nowadays, I find myself wishing that I had the opportunity to talk to Matayoshi one more time or wishing I had known then the right questions to ask. But Matayoshi died in 1997. I last saw him when he stayed at my house. It was another hot summer, this time in New England. My teacher, Kimo Wall, was taking Matayoshi on a driving tour of the United States, stopping to teach seminars along the way. That summer, Matayoshi had tried to explain to a friend of mine that there were really three kinds of karate. They were sitting at the dinner table. Matayoshi placed three forks on the table between them.

"Three kinds of karate," Matayoshi said, using Japanese this time. "There's what you teach to students," he said, picking up the first fork and setting it down again. "Then there's what you do for demonstrations," he said, picking up the second fork. "And then there's real karate," he said, pointing to the third fork. I think I know now what he meant. But I wish I could ask him a few more questions about real karate and how they did it in the old days.

Bibliography

Goodin, C. (1999). The 1940 karate-do special committee: The Fukyugata "promotional" kata. *Dragon Times*, 15.

Higaonna, M. (1985). *Traditional karate-do: Okinawa Goju Ryu: The fundamental techniques*. Tokyo: Japan Publications.

Johnson, N. (2000). *Barefoot Zen: The Shaolin roots of kung fu and karate*. York Beach, ME: Samuel Weiser.

Labbate, M. (2000). Developing advanced Goju-ryu techniques. *Journal of Asian Martial Arts, 9*(1), 56–69.

Marquez, A. (1996). Okinawan journey: Legacy of the past. *Bugeisha, 1*(1), 8–15.

McCarthy, P., and McCarthy, Y. (1999) *Ancient Okinawan martial arts: Koryu Uchinadi, Vol. 2.* Boston: Tuttle.

Smith, D. Letter 1—Kata and bunkai. Downloaded on September 22, 2001, from http://home.drenik.net/joemilos/sensei_dan_smith_letter1.htm

Smith, D. Letter 3—Are there blocks in Okinawan kata? Downloaded on September 22, 2001, from http://home.drenik.net/joemilos/letter_3.htm

Smith, D. Letter 6—About tegumi. Downloaded on September 22, 2001, from http://home.drenik.net/joemilos/letter_6.htm

Toguchi, S. (1976). *Okinawan Goju-ryu: The fundamentals of Shoreikan karate*. Burbank, CA: Ohara Publications.

Toth, R. (2001). An analysis of parallel techniques: The kinetic connection between Sanseru and Shishochin. *Journal of Asian Martial Arts, 10*(3), 84–91.

Wile, D. (1983). *T'ai-chi touchstones: Yang family secret transmissions*. New York: Sweet Ch'i Press.

Acknowledgment

Special thanks to John Jackson, fifth dan, for his assistance in demonstrating applications for this article and for his companionship along "the martial way." Also, a special thanks to Ivan Siff, fourth dan and training partner, without whom none of this might have come to fruition. And, of course, a very special thanks to my teachers, especially Kimo Wall, who set my feet on the correct path.

chapter 41

Basic Foundations in Okinawan Karate: Interview with Canadian Tsuruoka Masami

by Olga Toth and Robert Toth

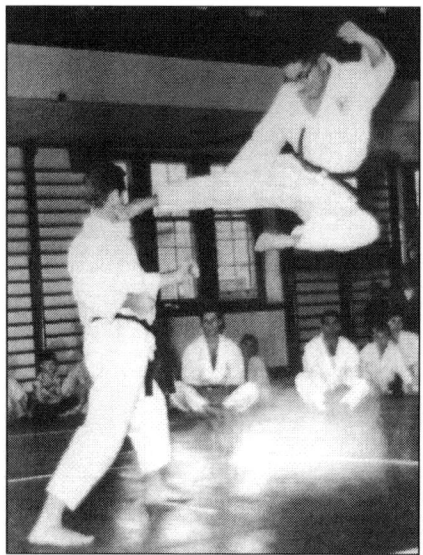
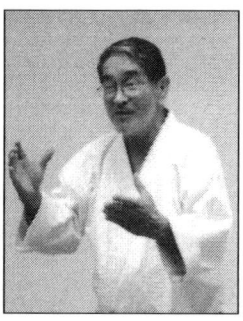

Left: Karate demonstration by a young Tsuruoka Masami.
Right: Tsuruoka Masami discusses fine points of karate practice during a recent seminar. Photos courtesy of Tsuruoka Masami.

Introduction

The first man to set foot on the moon was Neil Armstrong. The first person to break the four-minute mile was Sir Robert Bannister. Sir Edmund Hillary and Tenzing Norgay were the first to reach the summit of Mount Everest. Firsts have always been important to us: the breaking of new ground, standing above everyone else, and going where no one has gone before. Not following the pack, but leading it! Seventy-three-year-old Tsuruoka Masami is such a man in the karate world.

Born in Canada of Japanese parents in 1929, Tsuruoka's early life reads like an adventure story. Like many other people of Japanese ancestry living in North America, he was placed in an internment camp during World War II. Just after the war, Tsuruoka moved to Japan and trained with Dr. Chitose Tsuyoshi, a leading figure in modern karate. In 1958, Tsuruoka returned to Canada and opened the first karate school in the country, where he taught traditional karate at a time when most people had never even heard of it.

Today there seems to be martial arts schools on many corners of every major city in North America. But it was different forty-five years ago when Tsuruoka Masami was the first to introduce the Japanese art of karate to the Canadian public.

INTERVIEW • A CANADIAN BEGINNING[1]

■ Mr. Tsuruoka, could you start by telling us a bit about yourself?

I was born in Cumberland, British Columbia, in 1929. My dad immigrated to Canada in the early 1900's and brought my mum a little later. There was an influx of immigrants from Japan at that time. They were the young buckaroos. They wanted to make a fortune and then go back to Japan.

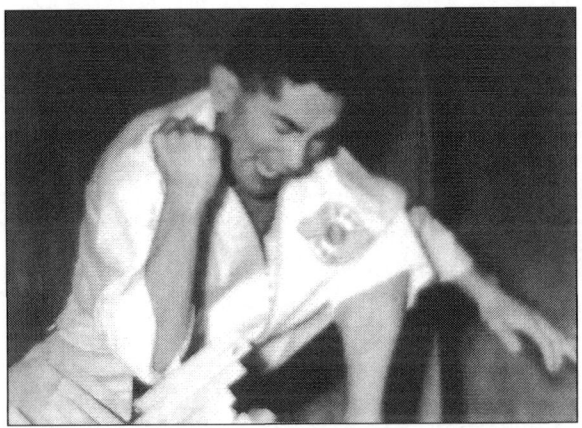

Karate demonstration by a young Tsuruoka Masami.
Photo courtesy of Tsuruoka Masami.

■ I've heard that your family was put in an internment camp during the Second World War. Could you tell us a little about that?

About a week or two weeks after the war began, they rounded us up and put us in the internment camp.[2] That was at Hastings Park, where they also kept the pigs and horses at the Pacific National Exhibition. We didn't know what we were getting into. It was very difficult. I'm sure that my parents and my brothers were devastated because they figured they were Canadians and would never be treated like that. They only gave us around twenty-four hours to prepare. So, we left everything behind . . . everything. The army people came with a big truck and just loaded us and we didn't know where we were going.

A lot of people went from the camp into the army. They volunteered for the Canadian Army and they were shipped to the Far East because they spoke Japanese.

IN JAPAN

■ I've read that after the war you moved to Japan. When exactly?

Yes. About eight months after the war. The Canadian government asked who wanted to go to Japan and who wanted to stay. And my dad wanted to see his mother before she died, so we moved to Kumomoto, Kyushu Prefecture.

You've never been to a country that lost a war. It's quite a sad thing, because there's no food. The only reason that we were okay was because we went to the country side, so we had enough to eat. A lot of people that went to the city had a hard time.

■ That was your first time in Japan. How did you feel about that?

Whenever you go to a foreign country that you've never seen before, you notice the atmosphere, attitudes, etc., are very different. Although I looked Japanese, they looked at me in a funny way, as if thinking to themselves: You look Japanese, but you're not Japanese.

■ Do you consider yourself Canadian?

I never really thought about that. Both my parents were Japanese, I spoke Japanese, I went to Japanese school so I had no problem in Japan. I was very fortunate because my dad sent me. I mean, he didn't send me, he forced me to go to Japanese school. When you're a kid, you were forced. I was very grateful for that.

MARTIAL ARTS TRAINING

■ When did you first start training in the martial arts?

In Canada, I first studied a little bit of judo. When I went to Japan, I was studying judo and a little kendo. Then I got mugged one time. I was mistaken for somebody else out on the street. I got left lying on the street because nobody wanted to help. Nobody intervened. I vowed to myself that nobody's going to do that to me again. When I was in Tokyo, I saw a demonstration of karate at a park. So, when I came back to my city, I started looking for a karate school and found my teacher.

Actually, I had a hard time finding him. There was a person that I knew who said that there is a karate master in the town. So, I went looking for him and found Dr. Chitose.[3] He had a small place on the outskirts of Kumomoto and about four or five students. At that time, right after the war, MacArthur said, "No martial arts."[4] So, they weren't allowed to teach openly. Chitose's *dojo* [training hall] wasn't even a dojo. He didn't have a dojo like the dojos here. It was his backyard. So when it rained, we were in the mud.

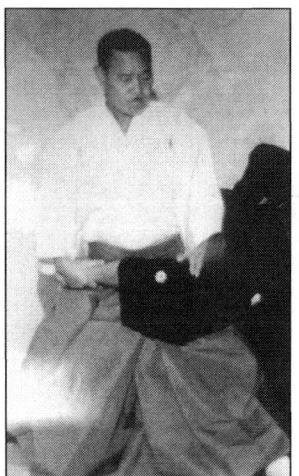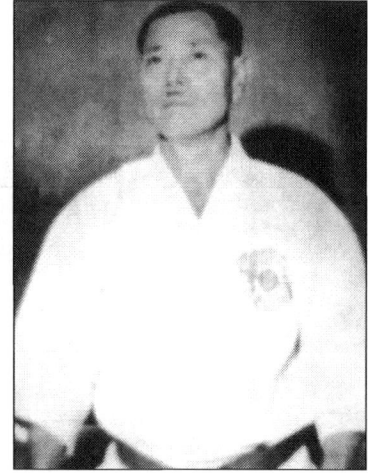

Dr. Chitose Tsuyoshi.
Photos courtesy of Tsuruoka Masami.

■ What was the training like under Dr. Chitose?

Well, I watched the other students and imitated them. It's not like over here. Here they take you by the hand and teach you. Over there you're on your own. Just don't open your mouth. You watch and imitate. That's all. We did basics, basics, basics, basics.

We didn't do *kumite* [free sparring] for awhile. Because if you did kumite and happened to get lucky and hit a black belt, you were going to get beat up. So you didn't do kumite.

Dr. Chitose always emphasized attitude in the training. And as a teacher he was a very kind man. During the war, Dr. Chitose was stationed in Tokyo. He was a doctor. His name was Chinen. But the name Chinen was very Okinawan and, at that time, many with Okinawan names wanted their names to be pronounced in standard Japanese. So, he changed it to a Japanese name.

- **DID HE EVER TALK WITH YOU ABOUT HIS TEACHERS?**

Not very much. He'd always say, I learned from him or I learned from him. You know, Naha-te and Shuri-te, and then the combination of both.[5] He learned both styles. Chito-ryu was a 50/50 combination of both.

- **DID YOUR TEACHER GIVE YOU A BLACK BELT TO WEAR?**

Oh, yes. And he gave a certificate, too. We had only white, brown, and black belt then.[6] I never even put a brown belt on. I just waited until I got a black belt. At the time, you had to register your name with the police in Japan. The master would register it for you. You wouldn't go to register yourself. Now it's all different. Black belts are a dime a dozen now. Don't forget in the old days karate had a very bad name in Japan. Kendo, judo, these were the Japanese arts that they cherished. So, when karate came, it was considered a foreign art.

KARATE IN CANADA

- **WHY DID YOU MOVE BACK TO CANADA?**

Well, I was born here. I always wanted to come back here. My brother was in Toronto. He didn't go back to Japan. I had to have a sponsor, so he sponsored me.

- **DID YOU START TEACHING KARATE AS SOON AS YOU MOVED BACK TO CANADA?**

No. I had no intention of teaching. I was happy. I was training in judo with a very good friend of mine. I used to go and help him teach judo. In Japan, judo is okay, but here there are many 6' 5", 250-pound guys. For a 129-pounder to move them, it is difficult to do. It's hard to throw them.

But somebody must have heard from Japan that there was karate here. Somebody came to me and said, "I heard that you know a little karate." I said, "I don't know karate enough to teach, but I did a little." And then they kept on bugging me. There was a body building place in Toronto and the owner found out I studied karate. At the time they used to have a body building contest and one year he invited me to go up there and put on a demonstration. The only demonstration we could do was to break bricks and boards because we had to show the difference between judo and karate.

When we came back after the demonstration, he had a big sign at his place advertising "Karate Training." I never even consented to it. However, I taught there for about two months. It didn't work out. But the people that were taking karate wanted me to continue teaching. So, they got the club going. The first dojo in Canada was on top of a bowling alley [laughs].

Things were quite difficult because people didn't know what karate was. All they wanted to know was how to break boards and bricks. A boxer would come in and I'd have to pull my punch, but the boxers train to hit, so they would hit you! Then I'd use my feet and they'd say: That's dirty fighting.

- **WHAT WERE YOUR CLASSES LIKE BACK THEN?**

Well, the students were in great shape. So, we did a lot of physical exercise. At that time, everyone used to work out hard. That's why the exercise part of a karate class that we still see today is for twenty-five or thirty minutes. You know, that's not necessary. For karate, you should do about ten to fifteen minutes of stretching exercises so you don't pull a muscle. But the trend at that time was to exercise for thirty minutes. Even if you were fit, you still had to do thirty minutes.

■ Did your Canadian students want to learn the same way that you were taught in Japan?
Oh, they did because my place was the only place. If they wanted to leave, I'd say leave. I didn't care. And I kept that trend up. That's why we had a lot of good champions coming out of our school.

Today, I try to keep the same way as much as possible. I still teach nothing but the basics. But now there's a lot of ladies and kids. I never used to teach kids. So, you have to kind of adapt your way of teaching. Right now, it's more sports orientated. There's more people practicing karate but they're getting away from the basics. That's why I have a very small class. My class is maybe, fifteen or twenty at the most. A lot of teachers have hundreds of students. But I just have my small group.

KARATE ORGANIZATIONS

■ What do you think is the most important thing in karate training?
If it's training, I say basics. Basic stance, basic block, basic punch, basic kick. Because once you can do your basics, the rest you can improvise yourself.

■ You were involved with organizing the National Karate Organization. How did that come to be? Why did you start that?
It was in 1964. At that time, there were so many associations coming into Canada, especially from the United States. So, I figured we must have one governing body. We were very fortunate, the government accepted us as the National Association of Canada. Now, whoever came had to join us. After we had the national association, we started forming provincial organizations. At that time we only had Quebec, Manitoba, Ontario, and New Brunswick. Only four provinces had karate at that time. Then it started spreading.

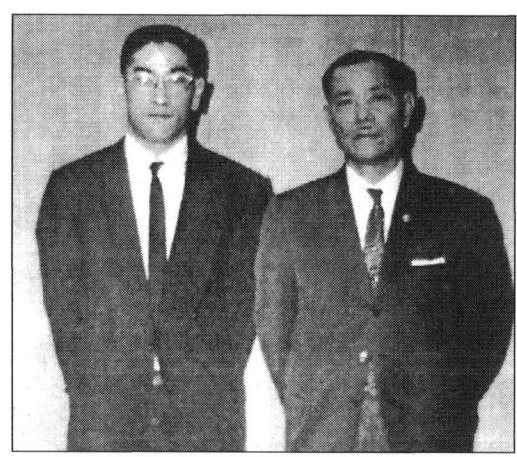

Tsuruoka Masami with Dr. Chitose Tsuyoshi.
Photos courtesy of Tsuruoka Masami.

■ Could you tell us about your leaving Dr. Chitose and the Chito-ryu federation?
It was all politics and I don't like politics. Like any master, Dr. Chitose got information from many people. So, he got all muddled up. I told him, I was the one that got karate out of Japan and made Chito-ryu known across the world. Then, the people from the United States, they started squabbling . . . and I said: OK, that's enough! Now, let me alone. Just let me teach my karate. I've got no time to spend on politics. I told Dr. Chitose that he'd be my only teacher. The last time I saw him was the year before he died. He and I had the opportunity to talk then.

After I left, Yamaguchi Gogen and Ohtsuka Hironri came to me and said: "Why don't you come to our organizations?"[7] But I said: "No, I have my teacher. I'll come and practice with you, but I have one master and I'll live with my master."

- COULD YOU TELL US ABOUT TSURUOKA KARATE?

It's a karate organization. That's it. We practice any style. I still practice Chito-ryu. I practice Shotokan. I practice Goju-ryu. Any opportunity to have a master come, I'll practice with him. I'll invite him to my club and let him teach, because my students must have some knowledge of different styles. I don't like that idea that "this is the only one good style." My master used to be very upset because I used to practice other styles. I said, I have to learn the other styles to be able to compete against that style.

People ask: Why don't you belong to Shotokan, because you claim to be Shotokan? I claim nothing. I say, I practice Shotokan. I practice Goju-ryu. I practice Chito-ryu. There's a difference between being part of an organization and practicing a style.

I think that the openness between different karate styles is important. Judo, at one time, had many styles. Now it's judo, which is one. So, karate . . . as long as the masters are alive, there will be styles. But after all the masters die, who's going to claim they're a master? Then there's no master and there's no organization. So, eventually, I think it will be like judo or swimming or basketball.

There will always be a traditional and a sports aspect. There should always be the traditional. I hope that will never die. Because once it's sport, rules dominate, and rules keep on changing every year. You should see the World Karate Federation rules. I can't keep up with them. In 1970, we were at the First World Championship [Tokyo] and we stuck to the rules printed then until 1978. Now it's completely changed. I mean, they have points after points. To me they do that [Tsuruoka demonstrates a back fist], it's a half a point. What? In those days we never even considered something like that because it was "one punch, one kill." And if you make a mistake, you're out [laughs]! Ten seconds. You traveled all the way to Japan to participate in a tournament for ten seconds?

TODAY AND TOMORROW

- WHAT'S THE BIGGEST CHANGE THAT YOU'VE SEEN IN THE KARATE WORLD?

Flashy people seem to get all the glory, and the people that are very dedicated get left behind. So, people that can go out in public and talk about how they are big heroes and are well-known, but the people that are at the grassroots, the ones that do all the work, they are not thought of like they should be.

- IF YOU COULD CHANGE ONE THING IN THE KARATE COMMUNITY WHAT WOULD YOU CHANGE?

I don't think that I'd change anything. When I go around the world or across the country I see little children. They are our future. They make me very, very happy. First of all, they learn discipline. They learn to respect. Their attitude is good and they're honest. I think that karate has given a lot to the country. If nothing else, it pleases me to see that. It doesn't matter what dojo it is. They are all trying their best. The black belt who teaches is teaching sincerely, and that's what I like about it.

You know, nobody has to belong to any big organization. Your student might open a club next door to you, but at least he picked up all the good points that you taught him and can pass it on to the little ones. At least he tries to emulate you and teach the children respect and discipline. When I see that, everybody's the same. There's no such thing as bad karate. Technically maybe you can say it is bad or good. But that doesn't matter, because your club is always the best anyway. If you see somebody else's technique, you think that they're no good [laughs]!...That's the way it is.

■ WHAT ADVICE WOULD YOU OFFER TO A YOUNG BLACK BELT WHO WANTS TO OPEN HIS OWN SCHOOL?
Keep the basics up. If you don't practice the basics, you won't be able to go forward. If you learn the basics, then you can create your own thing. Karate is about creation. It's not about copying one person. You must produce your own.

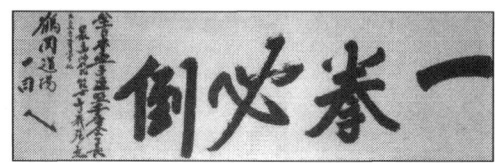

"All Your Spirit in One Punch"
Calligraphy by Dr. Chitose presented to Tsuruoka Masami and the
Tsuruoka Karate School. Photo courtesy of Tsuruoka Masami.

■ DURING SUCH A LONG CAREER, IS THERE ANY ONE THING THAT STANDS OUT IN YOUR MEMORY?
Not really, because I think that I've got a long ways to go yet [laughs], because everyday I learn something. I learn from the beginners. I learn more from my beginners than the black belts. Black belts have to go find their own way. If they don't want to work hard, that's not up to me.

■ IS THERE ANYTHING THAT YOU'D LIKE TO PASS ON TO THE NEXT GENERATION OF KARATE PRACTITIONERS?
As I said before, let the teacher teach the student discipline, respect and honesty. Try your best and teach with passion.

TECHNICAL SECTION

> To search for the old is to understand the new.
> The old, the new — This is a matter of time.
> In all things, man must have a clear mind.
> The Way: Who will pass it on straight and well?
> – Funakoshi Gichin, 1973

Tsuruoka Masami's advice to young karate instructors on what to teach students is to focus on perfecting basics. "If you learn the basics, then you can create your own personal style. Karate is about creation. It's not about copying. You must produce your own" (personal communication, 2 November 2002). The foundation for reaching this creative stage has always been strong basic techniques. Basic techniques are made up of balance and centering, stance and posture, the use of the hips to create power, and the use of the hands and feet as weapons (Nakayama, 1966:9). These traditional movements should remain as they were originally created by past generations. Many years were put into their development and each karate student should be sure that these techniques remain in their purist form to be passed on to the next generation (Bowerbank, 1997:75).

Scientific training of the basic techniques is essential. Faulty training methods can result in acquiring bad habits or even injury. But karate training can be considered scientific only if correct physiological principles are used. An examination of the techniques that past generations created reveals that the ideas agree with modern scientific principles (Nakayama, 1966:11, 15).

These basic techniques provide the foundation for all of the concepts that follow in karate training. For example, these same basic techniques are used to make up the forms that are a large part of traditional karate. As well, it is the basic techniques that are the most likely to score in free-sparring. This shows how the basic techniques play an important role in all parts of karate practice (Bowerbank, 1997:72).

To create a strong, balanced natural stance, one must stand up straight, straighten and tighten the legs, push out the stomach, and push the buttocks up, being careful not to concave the chest (Tsuruoka, personal communication, 2 November 2002). Stability depends on good balance. Without correct balance, it is impossible to deliver powerful techniques (Figures 1 and 2).

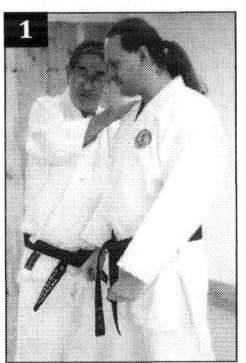
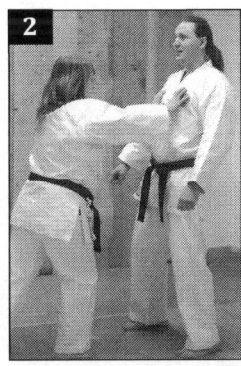
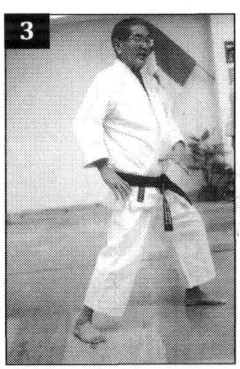

When standing erect, the body's center of gravity is located in the area slightly below and behind the navel (*tanden*). In Japan, the importance of the tanden has been taught from early times. This region of the body was emphasized because it was felt that it is where the human spirit is centered. This area also provides the basis of power and balance. A correct stance will enable the student to maintain the balance of both the upper and lower parts of the body.

If the power concentrated in the tanden is used in executing karate techniques, the interlocking support produced by the pelvic and hip bones supported by the thighs and the trunk by the spine will produce strong basic techniques (Nakayama, 1966:18). It is necessary to recognize the importance of the lower body as this is what provides balance and support and generates initial power through contact with the ground.

For a front leaning stance, maintaining posture is necessary to create stability. The front knee must be over the foot, but must not extend past the middle of the arch. The heel of the front foot, the knee, and the hip all line up (Bowerbank, 1997:51).

A front leaning stance is taught with a 60/40 weight distribution. But weight distribution is not what to look for. The pressure ratio is more important. It is the back leg that is going to hold the stance and that's where the pressure must be. Straighten the back leg to brace the stance, square the hips, shift the hip up, and tighten the buttocks (Tsuruoka, personal communication, 2 November 2002) (Figure 3).

The hip bone is where lower-body strength connects to upper-body movement. This is the largest bone in the body. If one learns to use the hip properly by contracting the muscles around it, one will be able to control movement of the entire body. All basic punches and blocks employ the use of the hip by rotating the pelvic bone (Bowerbank, 1997:64).

If the hips are correctly pushed forward, power travels through the thrusting leg to the hips. From the hips it continues to the backbone, the shoulder, and through the arm to finally end in the fist. To transmit this power effectively from the hips to the arm, a proper connection must exist between the hips and the upper body. To achieve this connection, tense the muscles around the abdomen and the lower back. If the muscles are loose, only a part of the potential power will be created (Nakayama, 1966:63) (Figures 4 thru 9).

The punch is the very essence of karate (Tsuruoka, personal communication, 2 November 2002). The fore-fist is the most frequently used striking point in karate. It consists of the first knuckle of the forefinger and middle finger. An imaginary straight line can be drawn from the center of the forearm to the point between the knuckles of the forefinger and middle finger. The forearm and the knuckles form a straight line (Nishayama, 1959: 47).

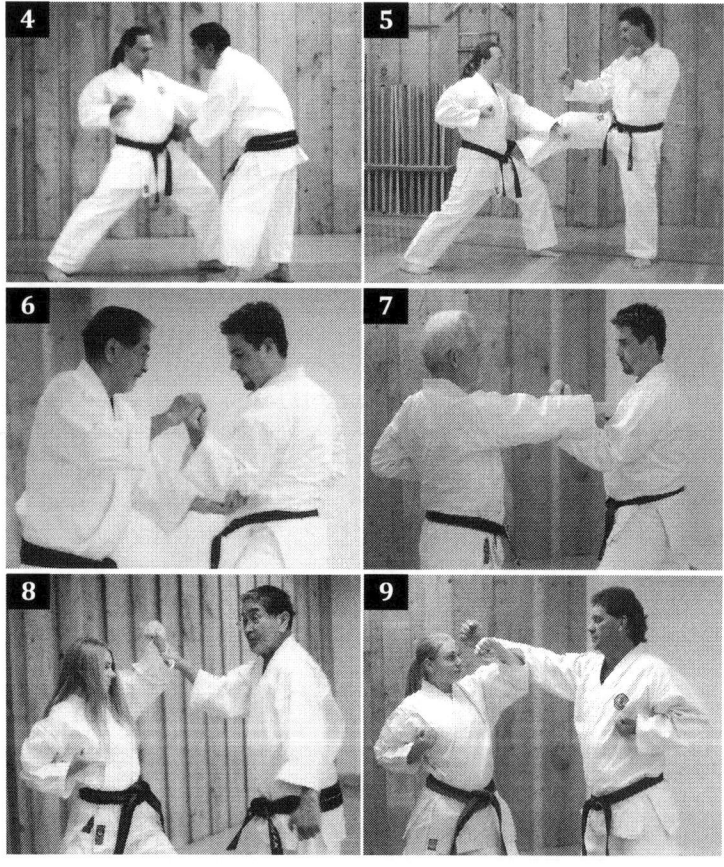

Left column, Tsuruoka Masami making corrections. Right column, applying the principles in practice. Photos courtesy of Robert Toth.

The starting point of a punch is the chamber position. It doesn't matter where the hand is held in chamber. Each of the different karate styles has its own way. The chamber hand creates the rotation and power necessary for a punch. By twisting the wrist, the shoulder will drop and, as the fist is an extension of the elbow, the elbow will scrape the body when the arm is extended for a punch. The punch, then, will have more power. The more the wrist is twisted, the more power there will be in the punch (Tsuruoka, personal communication, 2 November 2002) (Figures 10 and 11).

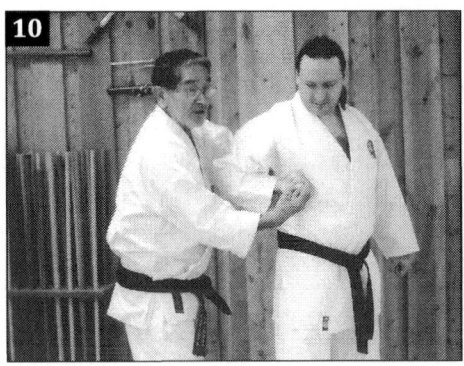 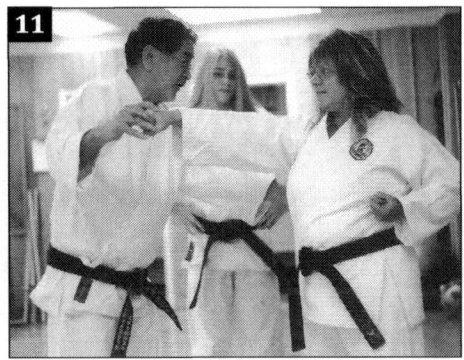

The punch must penetrate. If the punch is jerked out and the fist hits and then stops, it is possible to get tennis elbow (Tsuruoka, personal communication, 2 November 2002). When most people execute a punch, their intent is directed at the surface of the target. The punch is actually meant to extend behind the surface of the target (Bowerbank, 1997: 68).

The arm must extend. Lock the elbow and lock the hip. The shoulders should be square and flat. The shoulder blade disappears as the latissimus dorsi tightens. When punching with penetration, the fist can be felt to go through the opponent's stomach. That is where the injuries should happen. That is why most teachers say to punch though the body (Tsuruoka, personal communication, 2 November 2002) (Figures 12 to 14).

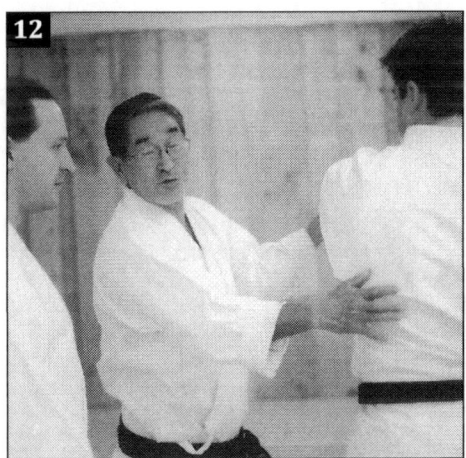 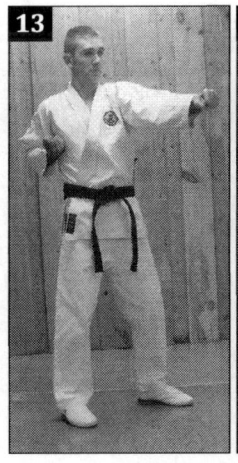 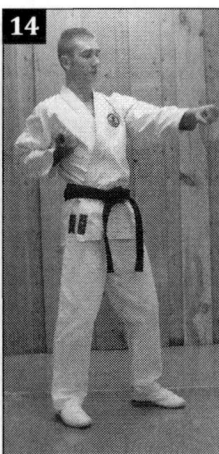

Mr. Tsuruoka points out how back muscles are effected when the arm is chambered and afterward when a punch is delivered. Practicing a basic punch, and letting the hips and shoulders rotate.

Kicking techniques have the most varied methods of application because of the anatomical makeup of the lower trunk and hip area of each person is different. Factors such as flexibility, muscle density, bone length, body fat, and age determine the ability to demonstrate good kicks. Because of these physical differences, karate practitioners subconsciously change the method of kicking rather than follow the ways that were created by past generations.

Contributing factors for maintaining good form for kicking are foot position, hip thrust, retraction, body angle, and balance (Bowerbank, 1997:41, 44). To achieve maximum effect, it is necessary to kick with the whole body and not just the leg (Nakayama, 1959: 136).

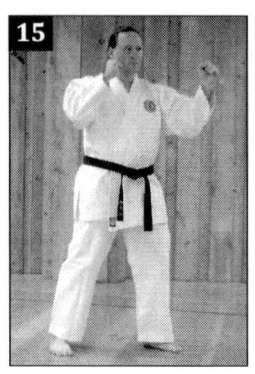 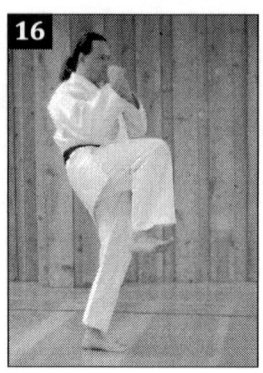 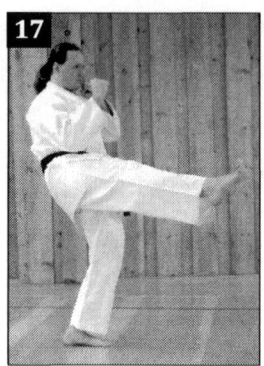 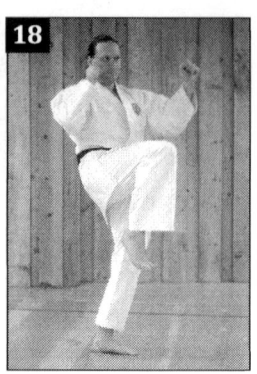

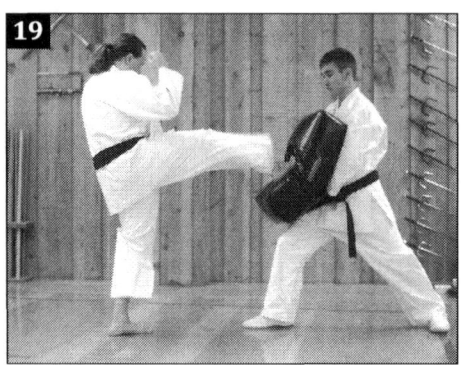 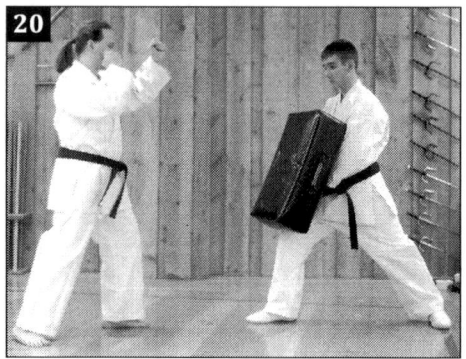

One thing that will enhance kicking performance and give the karate student a better chance to attain technical proficiency is the knee. Too many karate students focus on the end result of a kick. But, the kicking foot only makes contact with the target in the last part of the technique. The knee leads the kick to the target. First, the knee must rise above the belt line before the foot releases. Then, the knee must thrust toward the target. Finally, the knee stays above the waist as the foot retracts after the impact. Finally, the foot is set back down on the floor (Bowerbank, 1997:44–45) (Figures 15 thru 20).

Lifting and bending the knee completely requires the use of the hip and thigh muscles. These muscles are connected to the hip bones. The hips must be stabilized to allow the muscles to operate properly; strong abdominal muscles help this to happen (Nakayama, 1959:138).

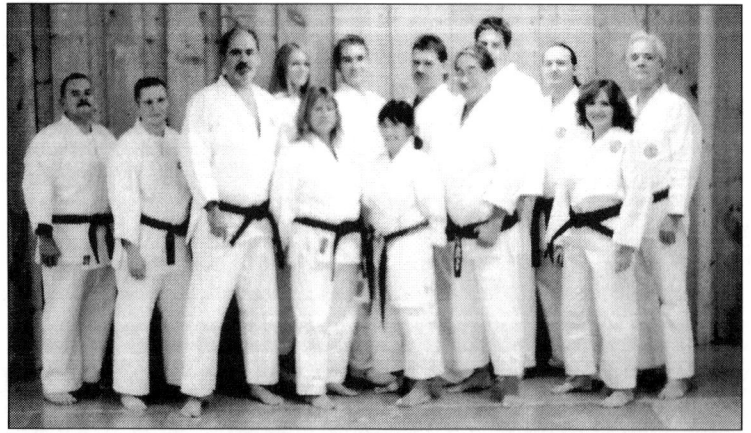

Tsuruoka Masami recently provided instruction for a black belt class hosted by Robert Toth at the St. Catharines Martial Arts Center in Ontario.

Practice of the basic stances, blocks, punches, and kicks should be continuous. It is necessary for karate practitioners to develop a strong foundation of basic techniques because it is only through this method that it is possible to move on to the creative stage of the martial arts. Karate is about creation. It's not about copying. Without creativity, the martial arts will stagnate and die. At the same time, without a foundation of basic techniques, the martial arts will crumble. It is only by practicing and understanding the old techniques that it is possible to create something new.

Most of the old karate masters of the last generation have passed on. Mr. Tsuruoka and his contemporaries were students of the old masters. They learned the old ways. But it was their creativity that brought karate into the 21st century. Hopefully, Tsuruoka Masami's advice will help guide the practitioners of traditional karate far into the next generation.

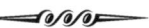

Notes

[1] This interview was conducted with Mr. Tsuruoka at his karate school in Toronto on 22 October 2002.

[2] The Japanese attack on Pearl Harbor on 7 December 1941 brought the problem of resident Japanese in British Columbia into focus. Canada formally declared war with Japan even before the United States did, but it was obvious to Prime Minister Mackenzie King what the war would mean to the resident Japanese.

The Pearl Harbor bombing provided anti-Japanese interests in British Columbia with a propaganda item. Mass evacuation of the resident Japanese was announced late in February 1942 (Adachi, 1991:199, 201).

[3] Chitose Tsuyoshi was born Chinen Gochoku in Okinawa in 1898. He was the grandson of Bushi Matsumura. His martial arts instructors included Kyan Chotoku, Motobu Choyu, Hanashiro Chomo, Higashionna Kanryo, and, most of all, Arakaki Seisho.

Chitose changed his name for personal and political reasons, as was common for Okinawans to do at the time. He attended university in Tokyo studying medicine. While in Japan, he assisted Funakoshi Gichin with instructing karate at one of the first karate schools.

Chito-ryu was not named after him. "Chi" means thousand and "to" refers to China or the Chinese Tang Dynasty. Chitose used the name Chito-ryu to commemorate the thousand years of history behind the art of karate (Sells, 2000:77, 78, 79, 138, 140).

[4] General Douglas MacArthur was the Allied commander of the Japanese occupation in 1945. He effectively, if autocratically, directed the demobilization of Japanese military forces, the expurgation of militarists, the restoration of the economy, and the drafting of a liberal constitution (Encyclopedia Britannica, 2003).

[5] The systematized fighting arts were named after the areas from where they propagated. Shuri-te is found in Shuri and was rooted in Bushi Matsumura Soken's teachings. Naha-te was found in Naha and was the result of a tradition of training originating with Nakaima Kenri and Sakiyama Kitoku. Later tradition says that Naha-te was established by Higashionna Kanryo. Sakiyama and Nakaima brought back essentially the same type of martial art that Higashonna later taught: Southern Chinese gongfu from Fujian Province (Sells, 2000:30, 31, 37).

[6] Kyu are the lower grades of the martial arts below black belt; ikkyu is a first kyu brown belt, the rank right before first-degree black belt; nikyu is a second kyu brown belt (Frederic, 1994:142).

[7] Yamaguchi Gogen (1909–1989) was the head of the Japanese Goju-ryu karate system. He began Goju-ryu karate in 1929 under Okinawan master Miyagi Chojun. In 1935, Yamaguchi organized the All-Japan Goju-Kai Karatedo Association and became its chief instructor.

Ohtsuka Hironori (1892–1982) began martial arts training at six years of age in Shindo Yoshin-ryu jujutsu. Eventually, he was awarded the menkyo kaiden, becoming the successor of this style. A year later, he commenced karate training under Funakoshi Gichin.

In 1939, Ohtsuka founded Wado-ryu karatedo, which became one of the four major styles of Japanese karate. In the same year, he organized the All Japan Karatedo Federation, Wado-Kai, which serves as the worldwide sanctioning body for the Wado-ryu system (Corcoran and Farkas, 1993:363, 396).

Bibliography

Adachi, K. (1991). *The enemy that never was*. Toronto: McClelland and Stewart.
Bowerbank, A. (1997). *The spirit of karate-do: Teaching of Masami Tsuruoka*. Toronto: Morris Marketing.
Corcoran, J., and Farkas, E. (1993). *The original martial arts encyclopedia*. Los Angeles: Pro-Action Publishing.
Encyclopedia Britannica, 1994–2003 ultimate reference suite (2003). CD-ROM.
Frederic, L. (Paul Crompton, Trans. and Ed.) (1994). *A dictionary of the martial arts*. Rutland, VT: Charles E. Tuttle.
Funakoshi, G. (1973). *Karate-do kyohan*. Tokyo: Kodansha International.
Nakayama, M. (1966). *Dynamic karate*. Tokyo: Kodansha International.
Nishiyama, H., and Brown, R. (1959). *Karate: The art of empty hand fighting*. Tokyo: Charles E. Tuttle.

Acknowledgment

The author would like to thank Tsuruoka Masami, Betty Mochizuki, and Monty Guest for the photographs, Adam Kieswetter for proofreading the article, Mike DeMarco for his editorial suggestions, and all of the black belts for their help with the photographs in the technical section.

chapter 42

The Shape of Kata: An Enigma of Pattern

by Giles Hopkins, M.A.

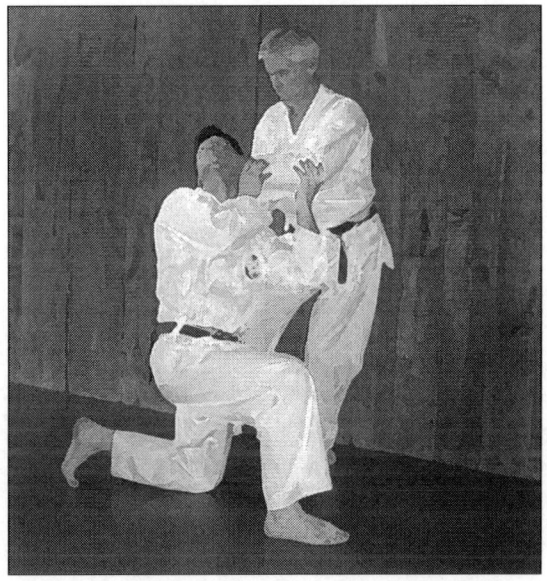

All photos courtesy of Giles Hopkins.

"It should be known that secret principles of Goju-ryu exist in the kata."
– Miyagi Chojun, founder of Goju-ryu

Introduction

Kata has come to characterize karate in the popular imagination much as the *hakama* (skirt-like pant) calls to mind aikido or the slow-motion postures of an old man with raised arms might suggest taijiquan. Certainly there is more to karate than kata—supplementary exercises, strength training, using implements such as the gripping jars (*nigirigame*) or striking post (*makiwara*), prearranged (*yakusoku*) and free-sparring (*jiu kumite*)—but kata is the essence of karate. Katas contain the techniques and the principles of the art. Although in most cases the techniques may seem obvious to anyone watching a kata performance, there is still the question of how one goes about discovering the "secret principles" contained within the kata.

In a short article on karate and Japanese calligraphy, senior Shorin-ryu teacher George Donahue recalled a conversation he had with one of his teachers, Nakamura Seigi, who suggested that there was nothing really hidden within a kata. Everything was there for all to see if they were "willing to use their eyes in an unfettered manner." While this may certainly be true, what, one might still ask, was Miyagi Chojun referring to when he mentioned "secret principles?" Is there more to kata than meets the eye or is this simply a question of semantics? How can something remain a secret if nothing is hidden? Nakamura, Donahue says, "preferred to call the 'hidden' moves 'intermediary' moves, because they occur between the obvious-to-the-eye basic moves" (Donahue, 2003).

Explanations are often quite cryptic in the martial arts, and this would seem to be no exception. There would seem to be nothing between the end of one kata technique to the beginning of the next. The kata is nothing more than a collection of techniques that have been put together in a pattern of movement. But it is this pattern or shape that is distinctive and makes the whole—the collection of individual techniques—greater than the sum of its parts. It is the pattern that contains the "intermediary" moves. So it is through a careful examination of the pattern or shape of a kata that one can discover the "secret principles" of the art.

•••

The classical Goju-ryu katas—what have generally been regarded as those katas brought to Okinawa from China[1]—do not conform to set patterns in the same way that the Gekisai or Fukyu katas, both katas of more modern origin, do. Modern katas like Gekisai I and II, and the Pinan katas of Shorin-ryu, were constructed along specific and easily diagrammatical lines of movement, as if the patterns themselves preceded the techniques, almost like pounding a square peg into a round hole. The shapes of these modern katas have been said to resemble a capital "I" or an "H" or an "X." On the other hand, the classical Goju-ryu katas seem to evidence a more organic kind of growth.[2] One indication of this is that these older katas are never completely balanced between techniques executed on the right and the left sides. This lack of symmetry has led to some interesting speculation about the age and origins of the classical Goju-ryu katas, but much of this research is just that, no more than speculation (Swift, 2002). For practical purposes, it is sufficient to note that all of the classical katas share this quality of asymmetry to some degree.

Consequently, even from the most casual observation of kata performance, one will note that none of the classical subjects begin and end at the same point on the training floor. It would be fair to assume from this that the kata's floor pattern (*embusen*) is an accidental outcome of the techniques that are being demonstrated, and that the kata pattern was never meant to teach balance of movement or symmetry in the application of techniques. While that explanation for kata practice may be at least partially true for the patterns of the more modern katas—what are often referred to as training subjects in Goju-ryu—it is certainly not the case for the classical subjects.

This is not meant to suggest that kata pattern's are completely arbitrary and without meaning. On the contrary, the karate techniques would largely be lost without the patterns. In other words, the kata—and by inference the kata's pattern—must mean more than some have suggested, not simply an elaborate method for training "posture, stance, body geometry, leverage, independent action of the limbs. . . etc." (Johnson, 2000:121). At the very least, without the present shapes of the katas, our understanding of the techniques contained within them would be different, suggesting that the patterns or shapes of the classical katas are not so much related to the solo performance of a kata as they are to the application and meaning of the techniques (*bunkai*). The irony is that though few would debate the importance of kata as an encyclopedic collection of techniques that serve to characterize a martial style, few if any would argue that the kata pattern is just as significant.

Two Views of Pattern

In fact, for most present-day karate practitioners, the pattern has no real significance. If it is discussed at all, it is usually given no more explanation than as a kind of choreography to illustrate what one does when faced with multiple attackers. In this scenario, one begins a kata in the ready position (*yoi*), facing the front or north, using compass directions. If the kata's first move is a turn to the left or west, then the standard explanation has been that one turns to defend against an attack from the side. To continue this scenario, when one turns to the rear (south), the kata is demonstrating how one should respond to an attack from behind. But the absurdity of this explanation of kata—the multiple attacker theory—is shown in any kata where one turns a full 270 degrees (one instance of this occurs in the Goju-ryu kata Sepai). It is obviously ridiculous when one is being attacked from the right side, for example, to turn a full 270 degrees to the left—turning one's back on the opponent in the process—rather than 90 degrees to the right.

Ridiculous or not, if one examines the applications of kata technique practiced in most traditional schools, and even what is shown in any number of authoritative texts, one sees that this multiple-attacker scenario is what informs the way most interpret the techniques of their kata. It is, in fact, reinforced in some schools by the manner in which the kata applications are studied. The student first performs the solo kata. When that is completed, the same student once again begins the kata, but this time with four or five students, each attacking from the prescribed direction indicated by the student performing the kata in their midst. As the student turns to his or her left to execute the first move of the kata, the student standing on the west compass point attacks with the appropriate technique. After the student has dealt with this attacker and begins turning to the right, the corresponding student on the east compass point attacks. The scenario continues in this fashion until the entire kata is completed. But the kata pattern is really insignificant here. In each case, the student has turned to face the attacker, meeting the attack head-on. When the pattern of the kata is used in this manner, it is not teaching movement.

Those who don't subscribe to this theory of multiple attackers, however, still seem to offer no plausible explanation for the many turns and stepping angles or degree of asymmetrical movement shown in the classical katas. Their explanation, based on the direction of attack, argues that the kata pattern sets up an imaginary scenario in which one can learn to respond to an attack from any direction. Certainly there may be some logic to support this view. The "Ha Po"[3]—the classic Chinese poem that seemed to capture the essence of the martial arts for Goju-ryu's founder, Miyagi Chojun—reminds us that "the eyes [should] see in four directions." But one does not need the peculiar patterns of movement evident in the classical katas to teach one how to respond to attacks from different directions. If this were the reason for the kata patterns, one would still be left with the perplexing question of why all kata patterns were not the same. At the very least, one would expect all katas would be balanced to show attacks from complimentary directions if they were meant merely to show the directions of attack. Limiting one's view of the kata patterns to this rather simplistic and not-so-entirely-satisfying explanation seems a bit myopic and, in the long run, misses at least one of the fundamental principles of Goju-ryu: to step off the centerline or, put more colloquially, to get out of the way (Hopkins, 2002).

Indeed, one is left with the impression that whatever key there once may have been to unlock the mystery of kata, it has been lost. Even some of the most knowledgeable karate practitioners and researchers seem to be resigned to accept the mystery and see kata, in the final analysis, as an "enigma" (McCarthy, 2001).

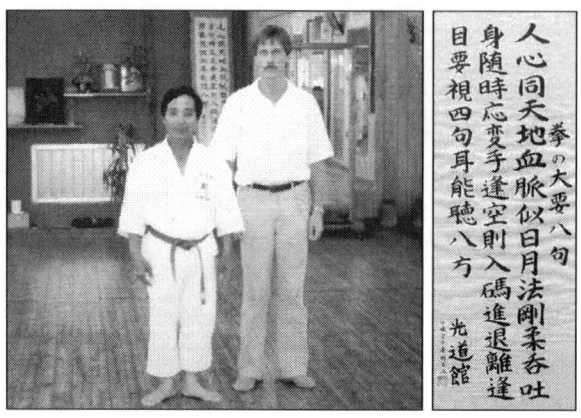

The author with Gibo Seiki. The "Ha Po" scroll is hanging between them in the training hall.

Stepping Off-line

A solution to the kata mystery lies in the kata pattern or shape. The pattern of the classical Goju-ryu katas are meant to illustrate how one should meet or receive (*uke*) the attack. The patterns do show the direction the attack is coming from, but not so that the defender can turn and face the attack, to move either directly into or away from the attack, as is the case in both the "multiple attacker" and the "directional" interpretation of katas. Rather the patterns show one how to step off-line, in most cases, to avoid the attack and then counter.

Consequently, if one's defensive position in relation to the attack is different, the interpretation and application of the techniques will also be different. That is, if the steps and turns in the pattern of a kata are meant to illustrate how a defender steps off-line, out of the line of attack, changing one's angular relationship to the on-coming attack, then how the various blocks and counterattacks are applied against the attacker will also change. This is why one's understanding of a kata's pattern or shape is evidenced in the way one applies the kata techniques; and, conversely, one's misconceptions about the significance of a kata's pattern are also apparent even from the most cursory examination of how one interprets and applies its techniques.

The Lesson of the Eight Directions

The "Ha Po," which one will find in many traditional Okinawan training halls enshrined or displayed somewhere on the walls, also admonishes the student to "hear in eight directions." The eight directions that this refers to are the eight points of the compass: north, south, east, west, northeast, southeast, southwest, and northwest.[4] In a martial sense, the eight directions refer not to the directions of attack but to the directions of defense: that is, how one may move in response to an attack. For example, if one is attacked from the front, one may defend against this attack by moving in any of the eight directions. How one moves in response to the attack is determined by the force, the speed, the commitment of the attacker, whether it is a left or right attack, the balance of the attacker, and one's own balance. One will then respond to the attack by moving to the sides, stepping straight back, moving away at an angle, stepping in at an angle, or stepping directly forward. In martial arts training—and this is certainly true of any of the more traditional martial arts—one trains one's sensitivity or "listening skills," as the Chinese so poetically put it, to "hear" what the opponent is doing to respond appropriately. And there are various exercises that different schools have developed to facilitate this training. The point is that the necessity of developing this sensitivity—how one responds to an opponent's attack—is common to all traditional martial arts, but it has received much less attention in karate.

TECHNICAL SECTION

Since it is the first in the canon of Goju-ryu classical subjects, the Saifa kata is the logical place to begin any study of Goju-ryu movement and the lessons of the eight directions. Saifa illustrates forward angle movement and lateral movement, using the front stance (*zenkutsu dachi*), the parallel stance (*heiko dachi*), the cat stance (*nekoashi dachi*), and what is sometimes described as crane stance (*sagiashi dachi*). The front stance is shown in both forward angle movement—most obviously in the three opening steps—and lateral movement. But while some of these movements may be apparent from any rudimentary performance of the kata or even a basic diagram of the foot positions, other movements—particularly the lateral movements—will remain hidden unless one understands the lessons contained within the shape or pattern of the kata. It should be noted that stepping in kata is dynamic rather than static and the stances do not so easily conform to the rigid classification of names that are necessary for any description in print.

Sequence #1

The first illustration shows the final position of the kata's opening sequence (1a). It is important to begin here if one is to see the transitional move or intermediary technique. Prior to the forward-angle step, there is a shift into a right-foot-forward front stance, with the left hand blocking and the right hand opening at head level (1b). This is followed by a step forward along the northwest angle, the left hand coming up as the right hand is brought down and the knee raised (1c). Most texts that attempt to illustrate or teach kata movement will only include the positions shown in (1a–c). Without showing the transition or intermediary move seen in (1b), however, the application of this sequence is lost. In the application of these moves, one can see how the forward-angle step is used against an attack (1d–e).

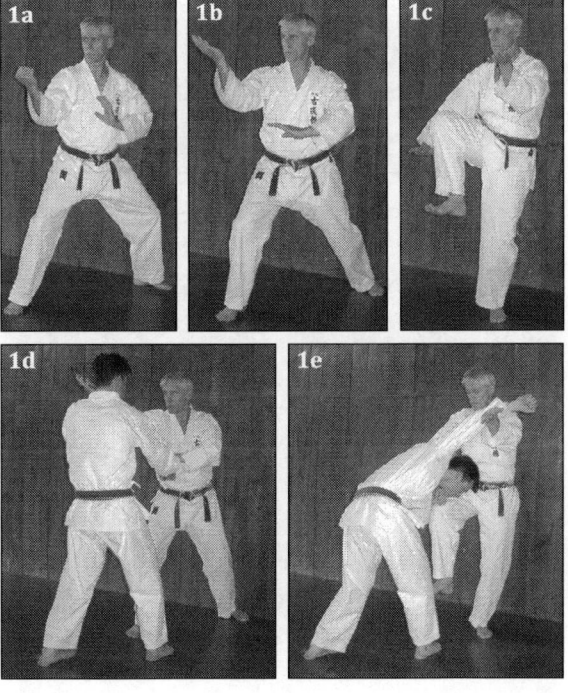

Sequence #2

In this illustration (2a), the final position from the previous kicking sequence is shown: a right-foot-forward front stance and hammer-fist at knee level. Again, it is important to begin here if one is to see the transitional or intermediary technique. In the moves that follow the kicking sequence in the Saifa kata, lateral movement using the front stance is shown (2b–c). This kind of defensive movement is not readily apparent unless one examines the question of why the kata turns a full 180 degrees, from a north facing technique in a right-foot-forward front stance to a south facing technique in a left-foot-forward front stance. Again, the "multiple attacker" or "directional" explanation of kata is less than satisfying here. If one accepts either of these explanations, there is really no need to turn at all or illustrate kata in anything other than a straight line, since one has simply turned to face the attack head-on. But if the attacker is stepping in from the west compass direction with a left attack, then the 180-degree turn shows that the defender has side-stepped the attack, using lateral movement in front stance, and, in the process, established a 90-degree relationship to the attacker.

Consequently, this also changes the way one interprets the hand techniques. The right hand—the hand closest to the attacker—blocks the opponent's left attack, while the defender's left hand simultaneously attacks the opponent's head or neck (2d and 2e). In utilizing the movement shown within the kata pattern, the technique is both faster and more powerful since the entire body and the turning of the waist is employed. In the moves that follow, the opponent's head is brought down and attacked with a half-fist or crab-shell fist to the neck or throat. This is followed by a hammer-fist strike.

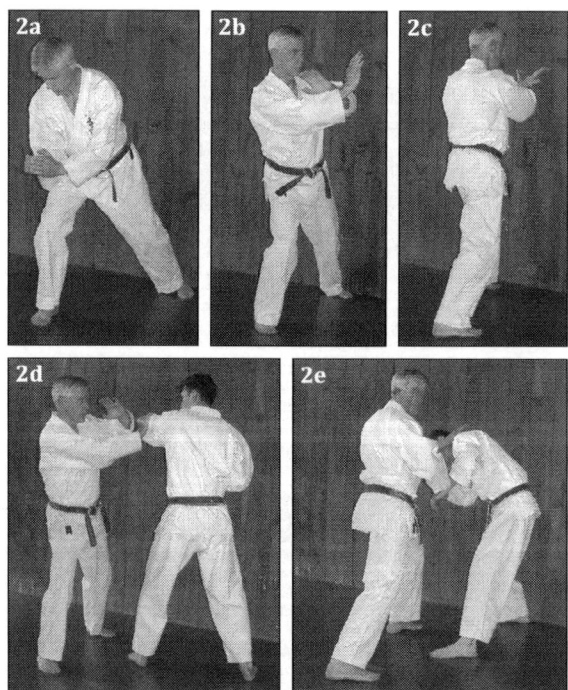

Sequence #3

The first illustration in this sequence shows the final kata position from the previous sequence (3a): a left-foot-forward front stance and hammer-fist attack. In the moves that follow this sequence in the Saifa kata, lateral movement in parallel stance is shown (3b–c). But just as in the previous sequence, the lateral movement is not apparent from the kata movement alone. One must apply the lessons contained within the shape of the kata to see that by drawing the right foot into parallel stance and redirecting one's attention from the rear (or south) to the original front (or north) of the kata, one's centerline has shifted in relationship to the attack from the west. In this move, similar to the opening sequence of the Sepai kata (Hopkins, 2001), the attacker is stepping in from the west compass point with a right attack (3d–e). The left open-hand blocks the opponent's right attack, as the right forearm and hammer-fist is brought down onto the back of the opponent's head or neck. This sequence is duplicated on the other side in response to a left attack, again from the west compass point. The final technique of this sequence—a right-hand grab and left punch, stepping into a right-foot-forward basic stance—I have not illustrated. It should be noted that this "finishing technique" is only shown once, tacked on to the second of these techniques. This is typical of classical katas.

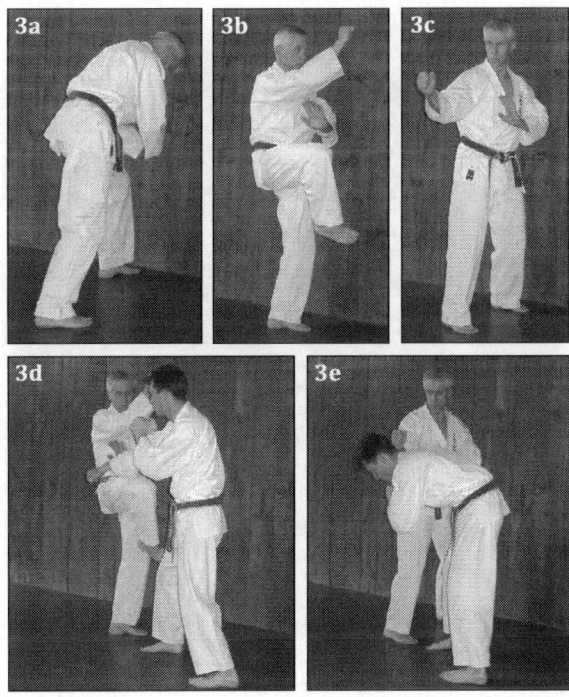

Sequence #4

The first illustration in this sequence shows the final kata position from the previous sequence (4a): a right-foot-forward basic stance with a right hand grab and left punch. In the moves that follow this sequence in the Saifa kata, the final turning block (*mawashi uke*), lateral movement in cat stance is shown. From a rear (south) facing basic stance, the defender steps directly forward with the left foot, pivoting in a clockwise direction to the original front, into a right-foot-forward cat stance (4b–e). Again, though the interpretations of most schools suggest that the attack is from either the south or the north compass point, since one's attention and physical orientation would seem to suggest this, in any practical sense this interpretation isn't very satisfying and by implication suggests that there really is no message contained within the odd shapes and patterns of the kata. If, on the other hand, the attacker is stepping in from the west compass point with a right attack, this last move in the Saifa kata is demonstrating lateral movement, shifting into a cat stance. The left hand is blocking the opponent's right attack (4f), while the right hand is simultaneously brought around to attack the head (4g). Once the head is controlled, the defender pivots back towards the front (north), twisting the opponent's head and neck with the mawashi technique (4h–i). It will be noted that the kata finishes in a cat stance to imply that the knee (*hiza geri*) may be used in the final technique.

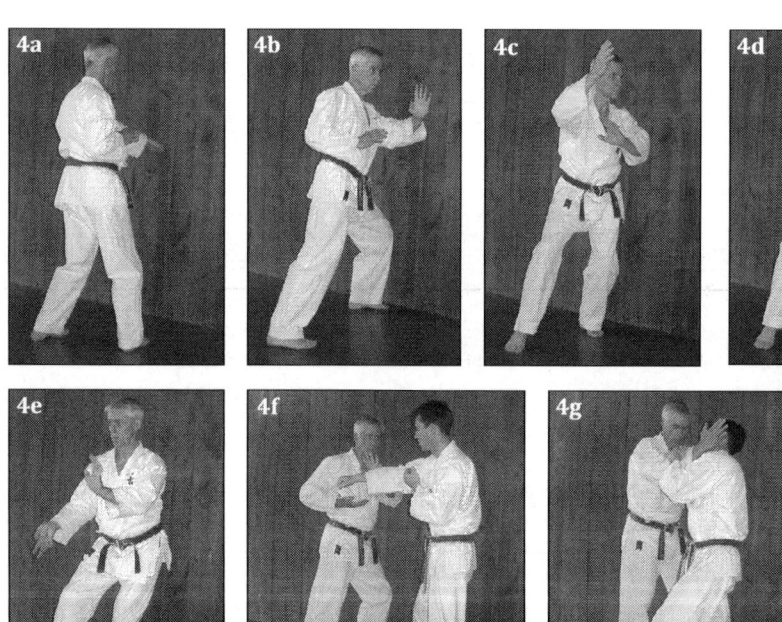

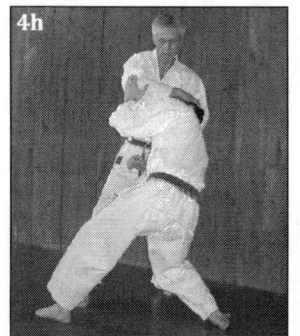

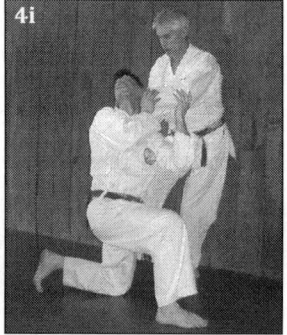

Acknowledgment

Special thanks to Brian Conz, friend and training partner, for his assistance in demonstrating applications for this article. And, of course, a very special thanks to my teachers, Matayoshi Shinpo, Gibo Seki, and Kimo Wall.

Conclusion

This is the lesson contained in the pattern or shape of kata. The classical Goju-ryu katas illustrate how to utilize the various Goju-ryu stances—front stance, basic stance, parallel stance, natural stance, horse stance, cat stance, cross-footed stance—to move in any of the eight directions in response to an attack. Ironically, in learning how to apply the lessons contained within the kata patterns, applying the lessons of the eight directions, we also learn how to apply the hand techniques. If we don't understand the lessons of the eight directions, then we will not understand how the hand techniques are meant to be applied. The key, then, to the understanding and practice of karate, it will be seen, is in the shape of the katas, in the stepping patterns. If one begins to understand what the feet are doing, then, as that old Chinese scholar has said, a journey of a thousand miles truly does begin with the first step.

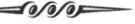

Notes

[1] The open-hand (*kaishu*) katas: Saifa, Seiunchin, Shisochin, Sepai, Sanseiru, Sesan, Kururunfa, and Suparinpei.

[2] I will limit my discussion to the classical Goju-ryu katas, though I believe these points are true of the classical katas of all Okinawan arts.

[3] The "Ha Po" (sometimes called the "Kenpo Hakku") is a poem from the *Bubishi*, a famous martial text reputedly from China and passed down to a number of early Okinawan karate masters. There are many translations and much has been written about its history, its significance in the development of Okinawan karate, and the cryptic nature of some of its contents.

[4] Dr. Yang Jwing-Ming (1996:95) also mentions these eight directions—forward, backward, two sideways, and four diagonal—in discussing movements in White Crane gongfu and martial styles related to White Crane.

Bibliography

Alexander, G., and Penland, K. (Trans. and Eds.) (1993). *Bubishi: Martial art spirit*. Lake Worth, FL: Yamazato Publications.

Donahue, G. (2003, April 1). "Kata, bunkai and calligraphy." http://www.fightingarts.com/ reading/article.php?id=154

Hopkins, G. (2002). The lost secrets of Goju-ryu: What the kata shows. *Journal of Asian Martial Arts, 11*(4), 54–77.

Johnson, N. (2000). *Barefoot Zen: The Shaolin roots of kung fu and karate*. York Beach, ME: Samuel Weiser, Inc.

McCarthy, P. (2001, August 26). "Kata: The enigma of Uchinadi." http://www.fightingarts.com/forums/ubb/Forum10/HTML/000008.html

McCarthy, P. (Trans.) (1995). *The bible of karate: Bubishi*. Rutland, VT: Charles E. Tuttle Co.

McCarthy, P., and McCarthy, Y. (1999). *Ancient Okinawan martial arts: Koryu Uchinadi, Vol. 2*. Boston: Tuttle.

Swift, C. (2002). The kenpo of Kume village: Speculation on the original Nafadi. *Dragon Times*, 23.

Yang, J. (1996). *The essence of Shaolin white crane*. Boston: YMAA Publication Center.

chapter 43

Yagi Meitatsu Discusses the Not-So-Secret Techniques of Okinawan Goju-ryu Karate

by Robert Toth

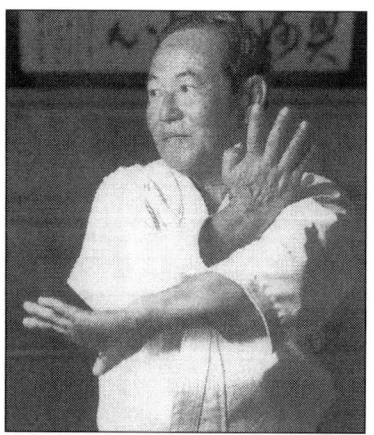

Yagi Meitoku in classic Goju-ryu movement.
All photos courtesy of Robert Toth.

Introduction

A famous man once said, "If you never forget where you come from, you can see more clearly where you're going." Lineage is the credentials that many people use in their search for a good karate instructor. Who did the teacher train with and who did his teacher train with? If possible, the history will be traced back to the absolute beginning. The need to track down the most direct descendent of the originator of a style is a result of the student wanting to learn whatever secrets the originator possessed. If the lineage is direct, it is more probable the secrets of the style will be passed on.

Yagi Meitatsu's lineage is very clear. His father was his only karate teacher. The elder Yagi was also a senior student of Goju-ryu karate founder Miyagi Chojun.

Background of Goju-ryu and Yagi Meitatsu

Miyagi Chojun was born on April 25, 1888 in Naha, Okinawa. The Miyagi family was wealthy as a result of importing medicinal products from China. When Miyagi was five years old, the successor to the main family passed away. As was the custom, Miyagi was adopted as the heir. Miyagi's mother was convinced that her son had to be both mentally and physically strong to face the world as the head of a family. When Miyagi was eleven years old, his mother arranged for him to start martial arts training with Arakaki Ryuko (1875–1961) of Naha (Sells, 2000:81). Arakaki then introduced Miyagi to Higashionna Kanryo when Miyagi was fourteen years old (Higaonna, 1985:25).

Higashonna had established a style of martial arts which was later called Naha-te, a combination of Chinese gongfu and Okinawan techniques (Porta and McCabe, 1994: 64). He had become interested in the martial arts when he was fourteen or fifteen years old. He first trained with Arakaki Seisho, one of the king's warriors. When the Ryukyu Government sent Arakaki to China, he recommended that the young Kanryo study with Kojo Taite of Kumemura village. After two years, Higashionna arranged passage on a ship to Fujian Province, China, to continue his martial arts training. In Fujian, Higashonna became a student of Ko Ryuryu (Sells, 2000:45, 47). Ryuryu, which means "to proceed," was a nickname. Ko is a suffix that means "big brother" (McCarthy, 1995:38). It is not known how long Higashonna stayed in China. But on his return to Okinawa, his fame spread and he taught the martial arts in his courtyard.

Miyagi Chojun trained with his teacher until Higashionna's death in 1915. After this, Miyagi made at least two trips to China to further his knowledge of the martial arts. He then set about perfecting the Naha-te he had inherited from Higashionna Kanryo (Sells, 2000:45, 47, 82).

In 1929, Miyagi Chojun sent his senior student, Shinzato Jinan, to a meeting of various martial artists in Kyoto, Japan. When Shinzato was asked the name of his style, he replied *Hanko-ryu* (half-hard style) rather than admit that the style didn't have a name. After returning to Okinawa, he mentioned the story to his teacher. Miyagi decided a better name would be Goju-ryu. He borrowed the name from a poem in the *Bubishi*, an ancient Chinese martial arts book. The poem explains eight martial arts concepts. One is the idea of hardness and softness (Alexander, 1998:53, 54). The line in the *Bubishi* reads: "The way of inhaling and exhaling is both hardness and softness" (Yagi, Wheeler and Vickerson, 1998:65). Miyagi thought it was important to name his art for the future (Yagi, 2004, e-mail).

Although Miyagi called his style Goju-ryu, he never had a sign with the name written on it at his school. In 1933, Miyagi Chojun's art was formally registered as "Goju-ryu" with the Association for the Martial Virtues of Great Japan (*Dai Nippon Butokukai*) (Higaonna, 1985:28).

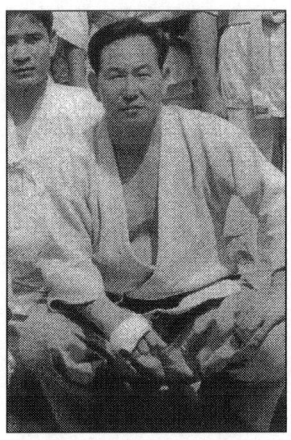 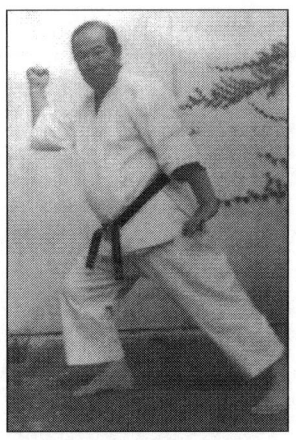 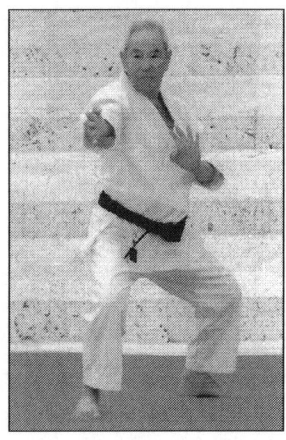

Left: Yagi Meitoku in 1960. Note the bandage on the right hand over his knuckles. The story is that after many years of training with a punching post (*makiwara*), he carved the callouses off his knuckles with a knife and started over again. Middle: Yang Meitoki in his garden dojo. Right: During a demonstration at the Shuri Castle in 1992.

Yagi Meitatsu's father, Yagi Meitoku, was born on March 6, 1912 in Naha, Okinawa (Yagi, Wheeler, and Vickerson, 1998:50). His grandfather took him to Miyagi Chojun when he was thirteen years old. Yagi explained to Miyagi that Meitoku's ancestor, Jana Teido, had been a great man in politics and a great martial artist as well. He hoped that in the future Meitoku would also become a great martial artist (Yagi, e-mail 2004).

Miyagi Chojun was very disciplined and strict. One time a student came to the training hall whistling; Miyagi told him not to return. Another wore a towel around his neck and was also told not to come back (Yagi, 2004, interview). There were only two or three other students training at the time. Later, there would be four or five. During his classes, Miyagi would teach warm-ups, basics, and forms (*kata*) (Yagi, Wheeler, and Vickerson, 1998:56–57).

Many people came to train with Miyagi. He worked them very hard and many students left. If they stayed, Miyagi would teach them the basic Sanchin kata. This would go on for two or three years. It was hard training. Miyagi would leave black and blue marks on his students from checking their stances in Sanchin. The demanding training weeded out all but the most dedicated.

Originally, Miyagi taught only four katas: Sanchin, Seisan, Seiunchin, and Tensho. But later, he taught Yagi Meitoku all the Goju-ryu forms. Yagi, who was only in high school at the time, was the first of Miyagi's students to learn the complete Goju-ryu system (Babladelis, 1992:41–42). This was pre-World War II.

The Second World War was a devastating time for Okinawa and its people. In 1942, the Imperial Japanese forces swept through Southeast Asia. The Japanese felt they were driving the wicked Europeans and Americans out. But by 1943, the tide had decisively turned. Allied forces were pouring into the Pacific and Japan was in retreat. Okinawa formed an outer defense line for mainland Japan and lay in the Allies' path. Naha came under attack for the first time in October 1944. Ninety percent of the city was burned. The city of Shuri was bombed again and again. Okinawan civil defense measures were hopelessly inadequate. Tokyo gave little thought to Okinawa and did virtually nothing to prepare it for invasion. By the end of the Battle for Okinawa it is estimated that 62,489 civilians perished. One in eight of the civilian population was dead. No family remained untouched (Kerr, 2000:463, 465–467, 472).

Miyagi Chojun suffered personal tragedy with the deaths of two of his daughters and a son (Toguchi, 2001:20). As well, Shinzato Jinan, Miyagi's senior student, was killed during the early fighting of the Battle of Okinawa in 1945. There was no karate training during the war. Afterwards, Miyagi taught outside in his yard.

On October 8, 1953, at the age of sixty-five, Miyagi Chojun suddenly died (Porta and McCabe, 1994:69). The Miyagi family held a meeting to decide which of his students their father would have wanted to carry on his system. They awarded Miyagi's belt and uniform to Yagi Meitoku, who was one of his first students (Babladelis, 1992:40).

Yagi named his school "Meibukan" or "house of the pure warrior" to distinguish it from the schools that were opened by other students of Miyagi Chojun (Yagi, Wheeler, and Vickerson, 1998:49).

Yagi's oldest son, Meitatsu, was born in Kume, Naha City, Okinawa, Japan on July 7, 1944. At the age of five, Meitatsu started karate training with his father. They trained in their backyard six days a week for two hours a day (Yagi, interview 2004). Yagi Meitatsu has never read a book about karate or watched a karate video. All of his knowledge about Goju-ryu karate comes from his father and master (Trebilcock, 2004).

Yagi Meitatsu attended university and worked in the United States from 1964 to 1970. He has also worked in Guam, Saipan, and the Philippines.

Yagi Meitoku chose his eldest son to be the first to learn all facets of Meibukan Goju-ryu. Yagi Meitoku gave Meitatsu the title of *hanshi* (IMGKA, 2004) or a respected master and 10th-degree black belt (Farkis and Corcoran, 1983:103, 129). This is the only time Yagi Meitoku gave this title.

On February 7, 2003, Yagi Meitoku died at the age of 92 (IMGKA, 2004). Just five months before his death he gave a demonstration at the Budokan in Naha (Trebilcock, 2004).

Yagi Meitatsu carries on the teaching and traditions of his father. Now at the age of sixty, Mr. Yagi has retired from his profession and devotes all of his time to propagating Goju-ryu karate all over the world. He has said, "This is my responsibility. This is my life."

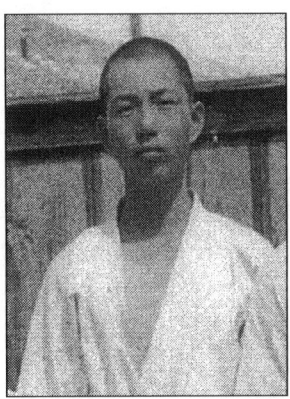 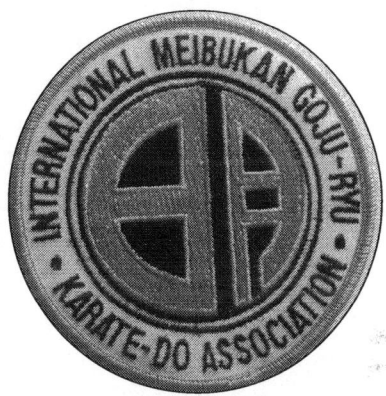

Left: Yagi Meitatsu as a sixteen-year-old black belt. Right: The Yagi family crest was created by Yagi Meitoku. Side by side are the characters for "sun and moon." The sun is bigger than the moon. As the sun and moon traverse the sky, so one must complete the study of each technique. The horizontal line in the "sun" character on the left is thick, while to two for "moon" are thin to symbolize the outside and the inside of the body. The character on the left has no exit, but the one on the right does. This stands for inhaling and exhaling.

INTERVIEW WITH YAGI MEITATUSU

■ COULD YOU EXPLAIN THE THEORY OF GOJU-RYU KARATE?

Go means hard and ju means soft. Physically, both hard and soft techniques are used. Mentally, it is to be soft to other people and hard on yourself. Go or hard is Sanchin kata and ju or soft is Tensho. Sanchin is practiced to create a strong body and to develop internal energy (*ki*) techniques. Tensho is the closing kata. I was told that Tensho was made by the founder of Goju-ryu, Miyagi Chojun. It comes from the Chinese kenpo exercise called *rokkishu*.[1] Sanchin and Tensho have to do with breath control. Sanchin is mostly closed hand and Tensho is mostly open hand.

Philosophically, when you achieve something for yourself, when you've learned something, you have to share it with others. This is inhale and exhale—*go ju*. But I must explain that in my day, we were not supposed to ask questions like this. We just waited until the teacher told us.

■ LET ME UNDERSTAND THIS. ONE OF YOUR GOALS IS TO SPREAD GOJU-RYU KARATE, THE WAY YOUR FATHER TAUGHT IT, ALL OVER THE WORLD. BUT PART OF THAT TRADITIONAL KARATE TRAINING IS THAT THE STUDENT SHOULDN'T ASK QUESTIONS?

Yes (laughs). Sometimes I see white belts or green belts asking, "What does this mean?" "What does that mean?" But I know it's too early for them. Sometimes I'll explain and sometimes I won't.

To take an educational view, when a child is in elementary school and has a homework assignment and the parent does it for him. The child may get 100%, but he didn't learn anything. First let him try. He must labor by himself. If he cannot do it, then you try to help.

I watched my father for fifty years. I waited until he explained or until I could figure it out for myself without being told.

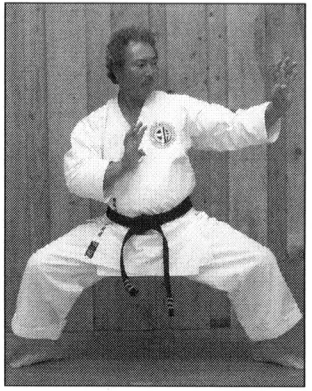 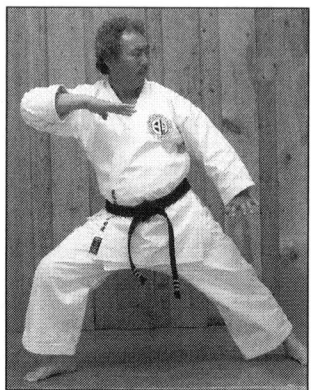

Movements from the katas Seisan (left) and Seipai (right).

■ DO YOU THINK THAT'S WHAT THE STUDENT SHOULD DO TODAY? WATCH YOU FOR FIFTY YEARS?
Yes. That is my desire (laughs).

■ THE IDEA OF DOING AN ARTICLE IN A MAGAZINE WOULD BE TOTALLY FOREIGN TO YOUR FATHER OR TO MIYAGI CHOJUN. THEY'D NEVER CONSIDER IT. BUT IN NORTH AMERICA, THE KARATE STUDENT WANTS TO BUY A MAGAZINE SO THEY CAN SEE PICTURES OF THE MASTER AND LEARN SOME SECRET ABOUT THE MARTIAL ART THEY'RE TRAINING IN. IT'S RATHER DIFFERENT. DON'T YOU THINK?
Many people asked my father to write a karate book. You know what he said?—"My teacher, Miyagi Chojun, didn't write a book so, how can I?"

When somebody studies from a karate book or a video, it's different. You must study physically. If you have videos and books, there's no need to practice. But without videos and books, you automatically practice at least twice a week so as not to forget.

To perfect a kata, it has to be practiced 10,000 times. So if a kata is practiced once a day for a year, it will take thirty years to perfect it.

Some schools have one whole wall of mirrors. But a mirror will not correct your kata. It can only be corrected by the teacher.

In the old days, there was only a small hand mirror in the dojo. My father told me the reason. He said that when you come into the school, you have a mild face before you start. After you've practiced for two hours, you have a hard face. So, when you finish class and are ready to go home, you look in the small mirror until you return to a mild face.

When I tell a story at a seminar, how it is understood depends on how far each person is into their training. Maybe the white belt will understand 30% of the story, a green belt 50%, a brown belt 75%, and a black belt 100%. But some students will understand 120%. They can read between the lines. They can see what I'm trying to say behind the story. This is important. My point is 100% is not enough. There is no short cut. My father, my teacher, didn't teach secret techniques. I had to achieve them myself (laughs).

■ SECRET TECHNIQUES?
Sometimes in the movies they show secret techniques being written onto a scroll

and kept locked in a room. The ninja breaks in, steals the scroll, and studies it. That is not secret techniques. Secret techniques are open to the public but nobody can imitate. Like Bruce Lee, Jet Li, and Jackie Chan. They show everything but other people cannot imitate them. Open to everyone but nobody can imitate. This is the secret technique.

Techniques are different for each person because they depend on physical structure. When my father taught techniques, I could not imitate him 100% because there was different physical ability and we had a different way of practicing. I watched him for fifty years but couldn't do what he did. We had different body structures. Secret techniques depend on the person. You have to be close to the teacher as often as you can because he can't show them in a short time.

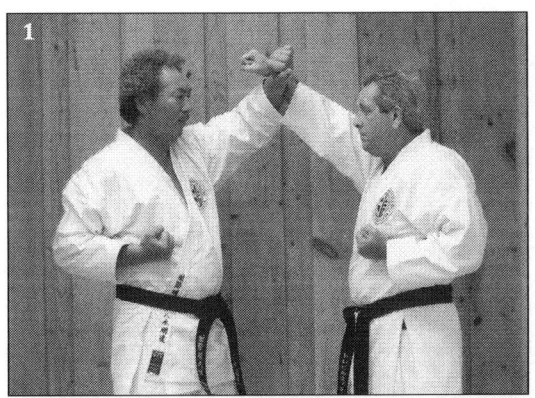
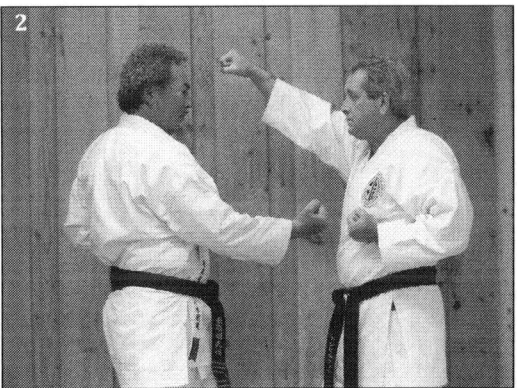
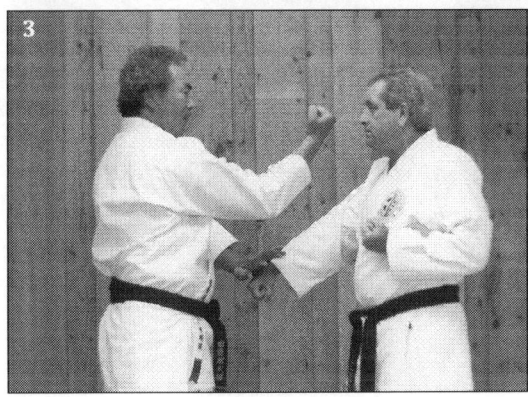
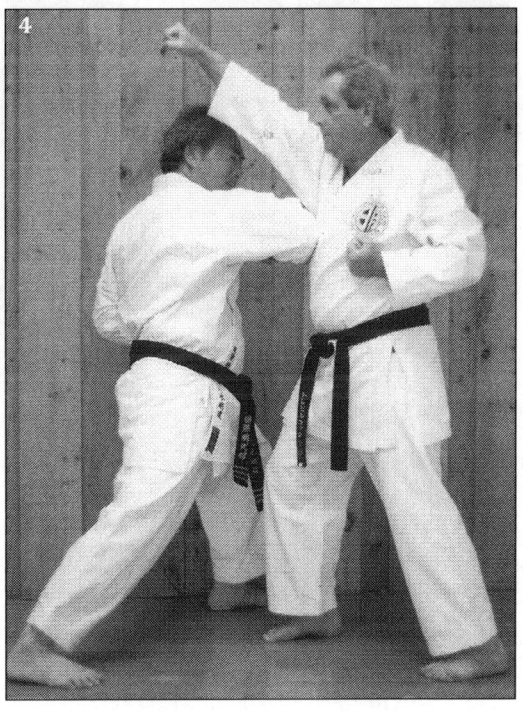

1-4) Mr. Yagi Meitatsu demonstrating several of the conventional techniques as taught by Miyagi Chojun.

■ How do you think karate has changed in Okinawa?

When I was small, we didn't show other people our martial art. We had a high fence around our yard. When we practiced, people would come and try to watch. That was the old days. Today, it's open to everyone.

Even five or ten years ago, I would only teach Meibukan members. Now I have a rounded corner. (Mr. Yagi made as if to cut the corner off of the table we were sitting at with his finger.) I will teach anyone if they are willing to study.

Another change occurred when Okinawa was returned to Japan in 1975.[2] That was the time sport karate or competition karate started in Okinawa. The [All] Japan Karate Association wanted Okinawa to take part in their domestic competitions. A delegation came to discuss the direction the competition would take. We agreed that the free sparring should follow their rules because they started that. But the kata had to be as we did them. But the Japan Karate Association decided that everyone, including Okinawa, had to follow the Japanese standards. Each traditional kata has its own characteristics. But the JKA changed them to make it easy to score for tournaments. And for tournaments they don't practice the katas in the correct order. There is no time for them to study the basic katas of Gekisai Itchi, Gekisai Ni or Sanchin. They skip them. They only know how to win at a tournament.

But we have no intention to argue with the Japan Karate Association. We don't say that they are bad and we are good. It is just different.[3]

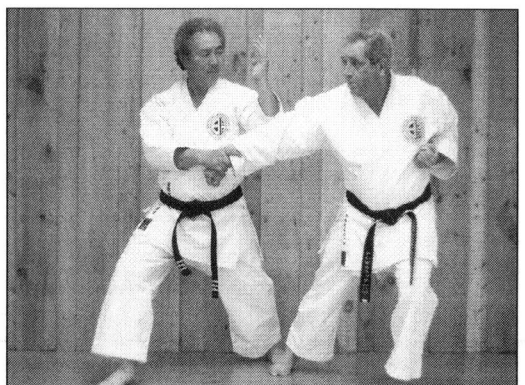 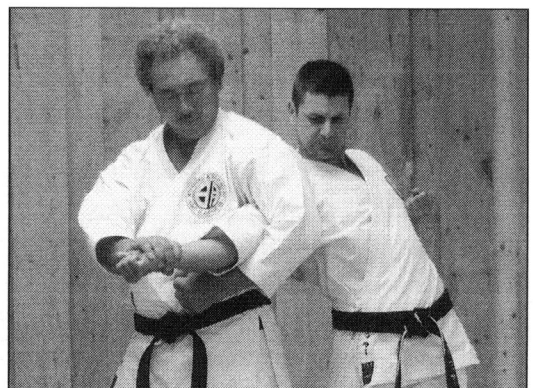

Left, application of a technique from Shishochin kata; right, from Sempai kata.

■ COULD YOU TELL US THE DIFFERENCE BETWEEN TRADITIONAL KARATE AND SPORT KARATE?

The difference between sport karate and traditional karate is sport karate is age-limited. When you are young, you can do sport karate; but traditional karate can be done up until your last breath. Most of the sport karate in Japan is done by university students. But when they leave school and go to work, they stop competing because you cannot go to the company with a bruised eye or broken teeth. Sport karate teaches mostly physical techniques and how to win. Traditional karate teaches how not to lose.

But sport karate is not real fighting. Even the Kyokushin[4] style is not real fighting because they are not supposed to attack the weak points of the body like the eyes. In an actual fight, the opponent will kill you like in a war. So, traditional karate teaches to attack the opponent's weak points.

It's the same with judo and jujutsu. Jujutsu had many very good techniques. But they were fatal techniques. So, Kano Jigoro, the founder of judo, took all the dangerous techniques out and made it safer. Even ladies can compete in judo.

That's why the Gracies are so strong. They kept the traditional ways. In Brazil in the old days, a Japanese jujutsu man taught the Gracie grandfather. He passed it on to his sons and grandsons. Now nobody can win against them. Even the Japanese cannot win because the Gracies know the old techniques.[5]

In the old days, there were many dangerous techniques in karate, as well. I've shown you some. This is real traditional karate. When you make a fist, it's short and dull. If you open the hand, it's long and sharp.

We try to spread traditional karate as we have studied with Master Yagi Meitoku. Our main purpose is not to produce many champions but to produce a fine person. Our teacher always said that, when you study karate, don't put your main purpose to study technique itself, but to study the way of life through karate. Everybody has twenty-four hours in a day. Karate training is only two hours a day. The mental part is the other twenty-two hours. You have to train the spiritual first in order to be a good karate man. Spiritual and physical training have to develop together. We are not perfect. Everybody has good and bad points. It's important to train your heart first.

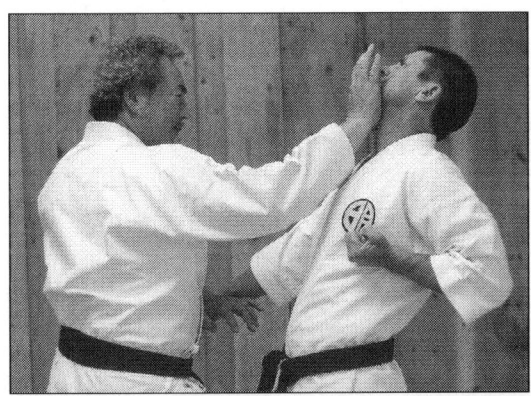
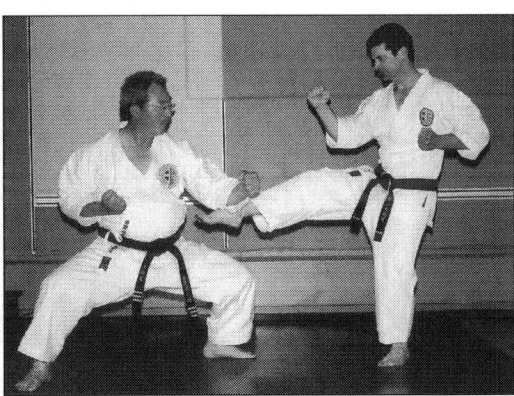
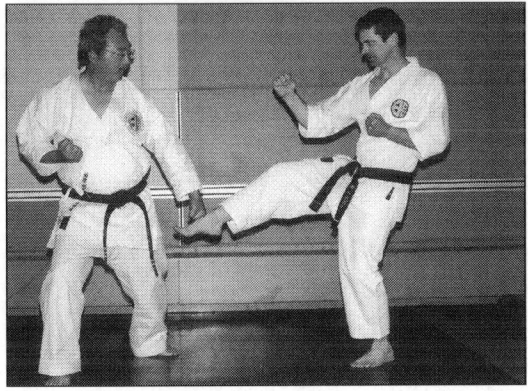
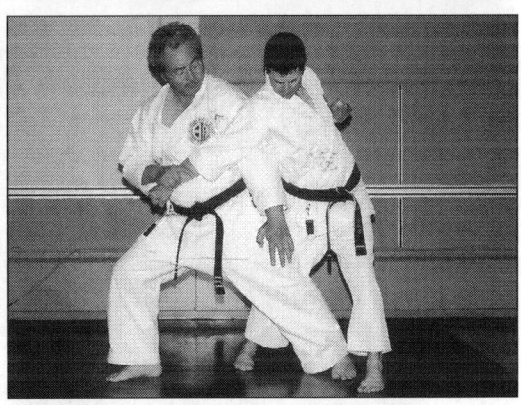

Above: Yagi Meitatsu demonstrating techniques.

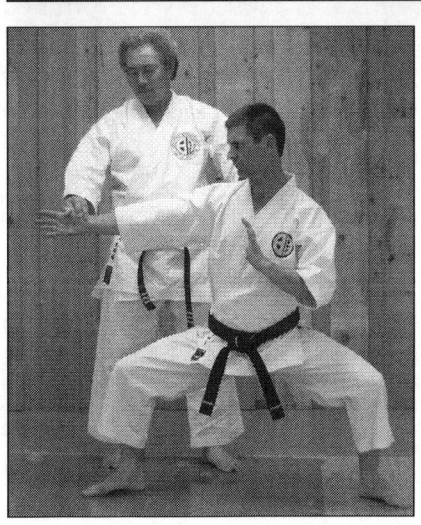

Right: Yagi Meitatsu correcting a technique found in Sempai kata.

People are coming back to traditional karate to study history, applications of movement in katas, and details in technique. Today with the internet and everything, people are learning about Goju-ryu karate and the successor of the style. People from many countries are contacting us for training. At the moment, there are Meibukan Goju-ryu schools in the USA, Canada, England, Italy, Australia, Israel, India, Bermuda, Sri Lanka, and the Philippines.

■ THANK YOU MR. YAGI. I REALLY APPRECIATE HOW MUCH YOU'VE HELPED ME BY ALLOWING ME TO TRAIN WITH YOU.

It's my pleasure.

Conclusion

Martial arts training is like having a puzzle face down on your dining room table. Every time you train, you get to turn one of the pieces over. In time, some of the pieces fit together and the student is able to see what appears to be a picture. Over many years of training, more of the puzzle pieces fit and the picture becomes larger and more detailed.

Sometimes, the student thinks they've found the perfect piece, the one that will make the picture almost complete. But it doesn't turn out that way because our understanding of what the pieces are changes. The martial arts are a puzzle that must be worked on for a lifetime.

Notes

1. *Rokkishu* or "the six wind hands" refers to six types of spear-hand or penetration techniques used in gongfu (Alexander, 1992:52).
2. The American occupation of Okinawa ended on May 15, 1972, having lasted for twenty-seven years. Okinawa regarded the reversion to Japan as the cure for all the real or imagined ills and evils reportedly caused by the Americans (Kerr, 2000:554).
3. The All-Okinawa Karate Federation (AOKF) resisted because many of its members felt that Okinawa, the birthplace of karate, would be dominated by Japanese interests. A split occurred within the AOKF, pitting those who felt that Okinawa should take part in what some saw as the future of karate, against those who pressed for independence and a resurgence of pride in things Okinawan (Sells, 2000:200).
4. Kyokushinkai is a karate style founded by Korean-born Oyama Masutatsu. It was influenced by circular Chinese techniques and the powerful karate of Funakoshi Gichin and Goju-ryu karate. Kyokushinkai advocates body contact to help students overcome fear (Corcoran, Farkas, and Sobel, 1993:67).
5. In 1914, Maeda Esai, also known as Count Koma, came to Brazil. He was a former world champion of jujutsu. He became a friend of Gastao Gracie. As a show of friendship, Maeda taught the son of Gastao, Carlos Gracie, jujutsu. In 1925, Carlos and his four brothers opened the first jujutsu academy in Brazil (Gracie, video 1988).

Bibliography

Alexander, G., and Penland, K. (1999). *Bubishi: Martial arts spirit.* Second edition. Reliance, TN: Yamazato Publications.

Alexander, G. (1998). *Okinawa: Island of karate.* Reliance, TN: Yamazato International.

Babladelis, P. (1992, December). The sensei who received Chojun Miyagi's belt. *Black Belt,* 40–44.

Corcoran, J., Farkas, E., and Sobel S. (1993). *The original martial arts encyclopedia*. Los Angeles: Pro-Action Publishing.

Farkas, E., and Corcoran, J. (1983). *The Overlook martial arts dictionary*. Woodstock, NY: The Overlook Press.

Gracie Jiu-jitsu in Action, video, (1988). Torrance, CA: Brajitsu.

Higaonna, M. (1985). *Traditional karate do Okinawa Goju-ryu, Volume 1*. Tokyo: Minato.

IMGKA (2004). International Meibukan Gojyu-ryu Karate Association website www.imgka.com.

Kerr, G. (2000). *Okinawa: The history of an island people*. Revised edition. Boston: Tuttle Publishing.

McCarthy, P. (1995). *The bible of karate: Bubishi*. Boston: Tuttle Publishing.

Porta, J., and McCabe, J. (1994). The karate of Chojun Miyagi. *Journal of Asian Martial Arts, 3*(3), 63-70.

Sells, J. (2000). *Unante: The secrets of karate*. Hollywood: W.M. Hawley.

Toguchi, S. (2001). *Okinawan Goju-ryu II*. Santo Clarita, CA: Ohara Publications.

Trebilcock, K. (2004, May 14). Interview in St. Catharines, Ontario, Canada.

Yagi, M. (2004, April 16). E-mail communication.

Yagi, M. (2004, May 14). Interview held in St. Catharines, Ontario, Canada.

Yagi, M., Wheeler, C., and Vickerson, B. (1998). *Okinawa karate-do Goju-ryu Meibukan*. Dundas, Ontario, Canada: Action.

Acknowledgment

The author would like to thank Mr. Yagi Meitatsu for providing pictures of his father for this chapter. Also, thank you to Carl Wheeler and Ken Trebilcock for appearing in the photos and their help with the chapter.

chapter 44

Steve Arneil and the British Kyokushinkai: An Interview

by Graham Noble

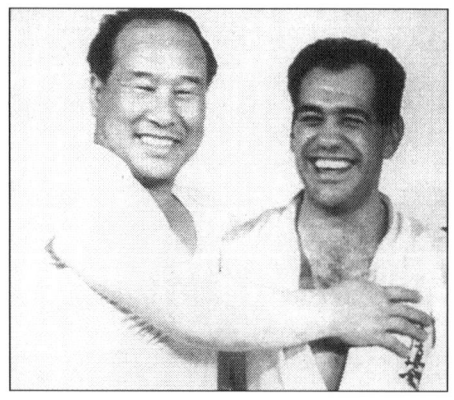 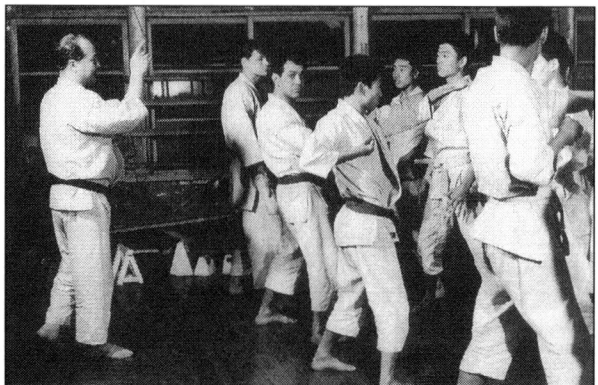

Left: Mas Oyama and Steve Arneil.
Right: Oyama at left instructing at his dojo in Japan. Steve Arneil is second from the left (facing the camera) among the group of students in paired practice.
All photos courtesy of Graham Noble except where noted.

Introduction

This interview with Steve Arneil (8th-dan) was conducted on the eve of the 21st British Kyokushinkai Championships at Crystal Palace, London. Although this occurred in 1996, publishing this interview in the Journal of Asian Martial Arts now makes it available to all interested in learning about a man who is, and has been, a very important figure both in British, and Kyokushinkai karate history. As well as being the leading figure in British Kyokushinkai since 1965, he was the coach of the British Karate Team in a golden era which saw it win the World Championship and become a major force in tournament karate.

His life has been "a life in Kyokushin." He started training at the famous Oyama Dojo when the style itself was only a few years old, lived through its development into a real power in the karate world, and saw at first hand the problems which later set in. These problems led eventually to his break with the headquarters, but his emotional links with Oyama Masutatsu [Mas], and his roots in Kyokushinkai continue to run deep. After the interview, when we talked about the passing of Mas Oyama, and the circumstances which followed, he was close to tears several times.

I really enjoyed my short time with Steve Arneil and his group. The tournament, which I attended, has a deserved reputation for hard fighting, respect, and sportsmanship. My thanks to Liam Keaveney for his hospitality and help in arranging the interview; to Pete Rippin for making the initial contacts and for ferrying me about; and to Steve Arneil himself, for his friendliness, honesty, and straightforwardness.

MEETING MAS OYAMA

■ STEVE, WHEN YOU FIRST ARRIVED IN JAPAN IN LATE 1960, DID YOU GO THERE SPECIFICALLY TO LEARN KARATE?

Hmmm, not really. Coming to Kyokushinkai seemed one of those things in your life which is fated. I never planned it. Actually I had trained before in Africa in Shorin Kempo with a Chinese teacher. I liked that very much. At that time I was also involved in judo, and I liked boxing, but because of the problems in boxing, I concentrated on judo, then kempo.

This was in Northern Rhodesia. I also used to travel down to South Africa. At that time, there was rather a lot of emigration from Japan to Brazil, and when they stopped over in South Africa, we'd meet them and if any had martial arts experience we'd take them to the dojos in Durban. So I was learning karate from this one, from that one, from all kinds of people. I just wanted to learn, and I seemed to be very much attracted to the Eastern forms.

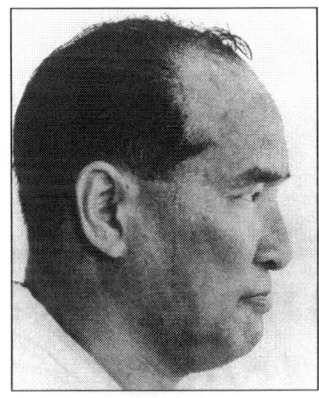

Mas Oyama.
Photo courtesy of the International Karate Organization.

Finally, I decided I wanted to go to the East. My ambition was to go to China, and I did go there and studied in China for a while but we had problems there and had to get out. So I went back to Kowloon, but I wasn't too happy with the teaching there. It wasn't what I'd had in the beginning. Then I was told that I would be suited to a strong form of karate taught by a man called Mas Oyama in Japan.

■ SO HE WAS WELL KNOWN EVEN THEN?

He was heard of. So then I worked my way to Japan and arrived in Yokohama. I didn't speak any Japanese. The only Japanese I knew was "Kodokan" [the headquarters of judo], so I went there and did some judo, and that is where I met my friend, Bob Bolton. I also met Donn Draeger, a great budoman, and we became friends.

I tried some karate dojos. I went to the Shotokan dojo, the JKA, which was just below the Kodokan, and I met people like Kase and so on. It was great, and they were very nice, but—It's difficult to explain, but it wasn't my cup of tea.

I also trained with Yamaguchi, "The Cat." I didn't know it at that time but Yamaguchi had been closely linked to Mr. Oyama. And I thought it was quite good. I liked it.

■ WHAT WAS GOGEN YAMAGUCHI LIKE? DID HE ACTUALLY TEACH AT THE DOJO?

Oh, a very nice man. When I knew him, he was an excellent karate man. And yes, he taught the classes.

■ WAS THE KUMITE HARD?

In those years, yes. With both Yamaguchi and Kyokushin, it was budo. It wasn't classified as a sport. And so the dojo fighting was fairly realistic. The object was to develop high level character, as well as how to fight, how to protect yourself.

Anyway, I spoke to Donn, and he said he knew Mr. Oyama! So he took me up to the first dojo of Kyokushin. That was behind Rikkyo University. When I arrived there—it was just a small place, but you could feel the atmosphere. Donn introduced me to my first contact with Kyokushin, Mr. Kurosaki, a brilliant karate man.

■ Could you tell us something about Kurosaki Kenji. He was known for his strong spirit, wasn't he?

Oh, tremendously strong spirit! He never asked from anybody anything unless he did it himself. He was that type of man. And he was a tremendous motivator, very disciplined, a fine character. Donn introduced me to him and then I sat down to watch the training.

After the training had finished, Donn said to Mr. Kurosaki that I wanted to meet Mr. Oyama and train in Kyokushin. Mr. Kurosaki replied saying that Mr. Oyama wasn't there—he was away teaching in America. But if I wanted, I could come and watch. To me, this was a bit of a shock, as I'd traveled all this way looking for this, and now I was told I could just sit and watch. The other clubs wanted me to join straight-away. I thought it was strange.

■ What struck you about the Kyokushinkai dojo? Why did you feel it was different from the others?

Discipline. Discipline on a very high level, and respect. And friendliness. They would talk to me. I felt they weren't trying to impress me. They were just strong karate practitioners.

Anyway, I said OK. But Donn said, "You have to come every day to watch." I asked when Mr. Oyama was coming back, but they said they didn't know. So I continued to watch, and what I saw I liked. The training was strong. It had rhythm, it was "punch-punch-punch." The teacher was never quite satisfied. Then the fighting started, and I was impressed by that. I wondered why they didn't get hurt, but their bodies were conditioned. And never, ever, did they abuse their position. They knew how far to take it.

■ We sometimes hear stories about bullying in Japanese dojos.

I have heard stories like this, but I can put my hand on my heart and say that I never saw that in the Kyokushinkai dojo of that time. I was treated absolutely fairly as a *kohai* [junior student]. It didn't matter about color or religion or anything. I was a kohai, and I had to do my duties as a kohai. I was treated exactly the same as everyone else. Nobody ever tried to take advantage. What the Japanese white belt got, I got. I've heard stories later on which sadden me, but when I was in Japan everyone was treated fairly.

■ So how long did you sit watching the classes?

About a month. I went up there regularly and sat and watched. Then finally this man walked through the door and I knew immediately it was him. It was just his aura, his personality.

And then Donn Draeger was called because Mas Oyama didn't speak English very much. Donn explained my situation and Mr. Oyama said, "Fine, but you know, if you train with me, you train for life. Think about it. A lot of things can go wrong in life, but you must train in what I teach you." And I said, "Yes, I'll take it on." Then he said, "You start as a kohai, and you must train regularly. If you stop training, we'll kick you out." I said I understood, then he said that as a mark of appreciation, he would give me my first karate gi. And that's where it started.

As a kohai, I had to go in and clean the dojo. It was an old dojo, but man it was spotless. The *sempai* [senior students] would just put their gis on the floor and the kohais would pick them up and it was their responsibility to wash and iron the gis and hang them up on a peg the next day. And if all the gis weren't well cleaned all the kohais would get it in the neck.

And then there was cleaning the toilets out. The first time I had to clean the toilets out, I got the shock of my life. You know Ashihara, the founder of Ashihara Karate? We were kohais together in the dojo. We had to go and clean the toilets, and they weren't flush ones. The toilet then was just a big bucket, and we had to take these buckets out, walk down the road, and throw them in a special area where the truck would come and take it away. And then we had to wash the buckets out with our hands before we put them back. Even to this day, I still shudder when I think about it [laughing].

But then as time went on we trained hard! It was hard training. But it was beneficial training, because we didn't do anything without a reason. It was said to me, and I say this today to my students—"I can teach you, I can help you, but there are two things I can't do: think for you and do it for you. That's your job, and if you can't do it, get out of the dojo."

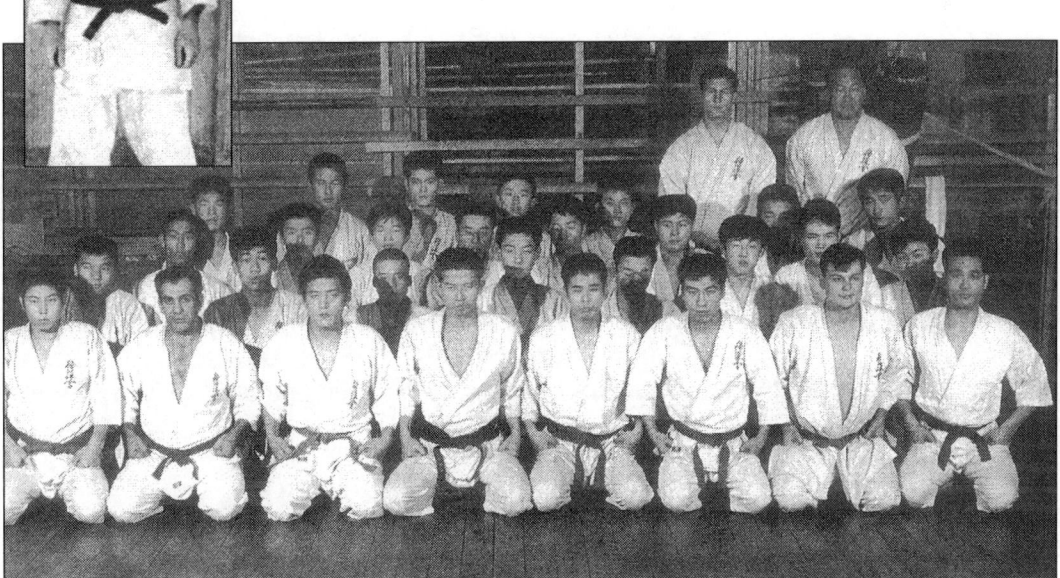

Left: Donn F. Draeger.
Photo courtesy of Robert W. Smith.

Mas Oyama's dojo. He is standing in the back, far right.
Steve Arneil kneels in the front row, second from the left.

■ COULD YOU TELL US A LITTLE MORE ABOUT MAS OYAMA. FOR EXAMPLE, HOW BIG WAS HE—FIVE FOOT SEVEN, FIVE FOOT EIGHT?

Yes, around that. He was a little bigger than me. But at that time he was just a very powerfully built man. He really was.

■ HE DID QUITE A BIT OF WEIGHT TRAINING AT ONE TIME?

He did weight training to supplement his karate, by himself. You know, we'd be doing our punching training, and he'd be lying at the back of the dojo pushing a weight "Uss! Uss! Uss!," while we'd be punching.

■ He'd be bench pressing while shouting the commands for punching?

Yes, while shouting and encouraging us to train harder. That's the way training was with him. Then he'd do squats, and so on.

■ WHAT KIND OF WEIGHTS DID HE USE? HEAVY? LIGHT?

The weights were fairly heavy. He always said that the body itself is very strong, but you should train with weights which supplement your training. You know, he wasn't talking about being a muscle man, posing, or getting cut up. He built his body for power in karate.

■ I SPOKE TO BOBBY LOWE ON THE PHONE ONCE AND HE TOLD ME THAT HE'D SEEN MAS OYAMA BEND A COIN.

I have seen Oyama bend a Japanese coin with his fingers, although I can't vouch for the strength of Japanese coins then.... Still a terrific feat.

■ BOBBY LOWE ALSO TOLD ME THAT MAS OYAMA WAS THE STRONGEST MAN HE HAD EVER MET, NOT ONLY PHYSICALLY BUT MENTALLY.

There's no doubt that Mas Oyama was a very powerful man, physically and mentally, but I wouldn't say he was the only man in the world with these qualities. I also met some people in China who impressed me tremendously with their willpower and their strength, and I've seen others in my travels. But yes, I would say Oyama was one of the exceptional people.

■ I'VE BEEN TOLD THAT AROUND THE LATE 1950S, EARLY 1960S, MAS OYAMA CHALLENGED ALL THE OTHER SCHOOLS TO TAKE PART IN A NATIONAL CONTEST TO DECIDE WHICH WAS THE STRONGEST STYLE. DO YOU KNOW ANYTHING ABOUT THAT?

I've heard of that, but I wasn't aware of any challenge when I was in Japan. The only time when we were part of a challenge, that I know of, was when we were challenged by the Thai boxers. That took place when I was in Japan.

■ SO TO YOUR KNOWLEDGE, HE NEVER BADMOUTHED THE OTHER KARATE STYLES?

No, he never badmouthed any style. All he said was, "We are the best!" He said that "We are budo," and even at that time, the art was changing into a sport. He said that in time to come, a sports-only karate man would find it difficult to deal with a street situation. And his prediction came true. A boy may be excellent at the sport, but not able to deliver in a street situation. Although of course it will help them to some degree.

TRAINING AT THE KYOSHINKAI

■ COULD YOU TAKE US THROUGH A TRAINING SESSION AT THE KYOKUSHINKAI DOJO AT THAT TIME?

OK, I'll take you through an evening session when I was there. Firstly, you had to be there at 7:30. At 7:15, the drums began to beat, and you could hear those drums quite a distance away. When that drum stopped, you didn't bother going into the dojo late, because you just weren't going to train. No excuses.

You began the training by going through the procedures of bowing, meditation, and loosening up and stretching exercises—and the stretching in those days was hard! They would pull your legs apart to work on the splits and I had a hard time with that. I used to play rugby and my legs were quite stiff at that time, but they did get my legs apart! Then you did a lot of physical training like push-ups, and a lot of breathing exercises, because he was very strict on breathing. He said that if a person doesn't breathe, he's dead. So we did a lot of rapid breathing [*nogare*] and a lot of sonorous, abdominal breathing [*ibuki*].

Then we would do our classical warm-up. We would go into Sanchin stance, he would stand in the front, then we would go through the various techniques—fore-fist thrust, back-fist strike, knife hand strike—it would average about seventeen techniques.

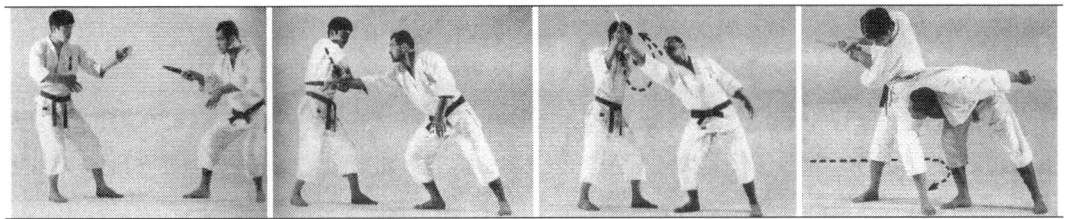

Steve Arneil playing the attacker in the knife-defense
section of Oyama's book, *What is Karate* (1963).
Photo courtesy of the publisher.
Below: More knife-defense technique from *What is Karate* (1963).
Photo courtesy of the publisher.

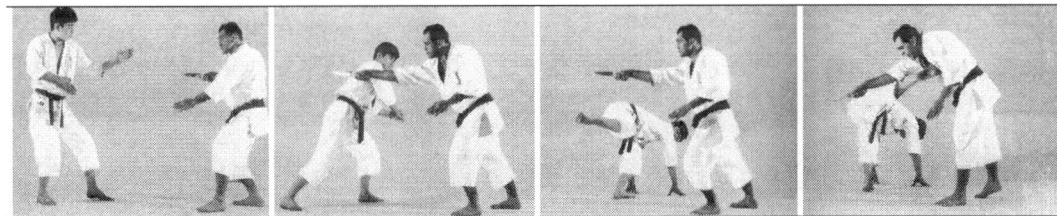

- How many repetitions did you do of each?

Oh Christ—he would start with a count of ten from the highest grade, then the next highest ten, then the next ten, ten, ten—and it would go up to how many black belts there were.

- So Oyama himself would do all this with you?

Oh yes, he trained every time.

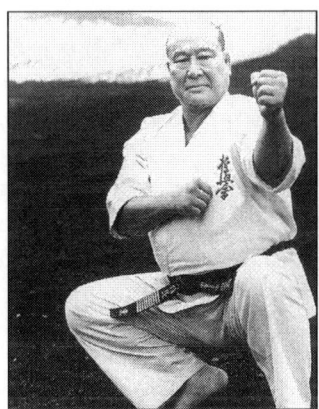

Mas Oyama. Photo courtesy of the International Karate Organization.

- That must have impressed you.

Of course. This is what I liked about him. He did it with us. This is why to this day, I will do my damnedest to train as much as my students as possible. Following on from the hand techniques we would then do the kicks the same way. Then when that was finished, we would go through kihon, the basics, moving through the techniques in forward stance, horse stance, back stance, middle section thrust, upper section thrust, blocks, combinations. He was very, very strict on basics. He wanted the forward stance right, he wanted the back stance, right. Actually he was a bit of a perfectionist and it was very difficult to please him. And until he was happy with it he wouldn't move on to the next technique.

Then we would do free-sparring and that was when you put the little bandages on your fists. That was when the kohais like myself got a little apprehensive. All the black belts would line up, then you had to get up and start from the top of the line, working your way to the bottom. Each black belt had his own ways, and some were heavier handed than others, but they were fair. There were never really any injuries because we were all fairly well trained. The only thing was, we used to hit to the face.

■ THIS WAS WITH THE HANDS WRAPPED?

All we used to do was take some bandages and wrap them round the knuckles so that we wouldn't cut the skin. And you really had to learn to block. If you didn't block, you got smacked. The only thing we weren't allowed to do at that time, was kick to the groin. And we weren't kicking to the legs when I was there. Kicking to the legs only came in after the boys came back from Thailand. Otherwise, it was anything goes.

■ HOW LONG DID THE FREE-STYLE SPARRING [JYU-KUMITE] LAST?

Well, there was no set time. The thing was, at that dojo you started at 7:30, and if he fancied it, you would go on to 12:00. Or if he wanted a short session, you'd finish at 10:00. When you went to the dojo, you went to train and there was no time schedule. If the training ran late, it was your problem how you got home. These were the things you had to accept.

■ DID YOU DO ANY PREARRANGED FORMS BEFORE THE FREE-SPARRING?

Not really. Before free-sparring, we'd do the combinations—moving forward, moving back, front kicks, round kicks, spinning back kicks. We didn't do the things that you saw in Shotokan, for example, the prearranged techniques.

■ SO YOU DIDN'T DO THREE-STEP KUMITE FOR EXAMPLE?

Mas Oyama believed you learned to fight by fighting. Three-step wasn't going to help you with that. For form, you did kata, and believe it or not Mas Oyama stressed kata a lot. He said your kata was there to train you to think. Teaching three-step kumite isn't going to help you in the street. When you did free-sparring, you'd bow, then the guy would throw anything at you he could and you'd have to block it. You didn't say "he's going to throw a roundhouse kick and I'm going to step to the side and then do this or that." He didn't really go for that because he said it was based on a misconception. On the street, no-one would let you know, "OK, I'm coming in with a big round kick."

■ SO HE THOUGHT THAT TYPE OF TRAINING WAS TOO STIFF, NOT NATURAL?

Yes, our fighting was very strong, very disciplined, very accurate, but we weren't like Shotokan, Shukokai, Wado-ryu—you know, block, "bang" counter and then step out—which of course was very good, and I still say is an excellent exercise for karate practitioners. I do it myself now with my students because I think it has a place in a karate practitioner's overall development.

■ DO YOU THINK THIS KYOKUSHINKAI STYLE OF FIGHTING CAME OUT OF MAS OYAMA'S OWN EXPERIENCE?

HE SAID HE HAD FOUGHT BOXERS, WRESTLERS AND SO ON, WHEN HE WAS IN AMERICA FOR EXAMPLE.
I think so, because you know he had to get in the ring and fight under any rules.

■ DID HE SPAR AT THE DOJO WITH YOU?
Oh yes, but very seldom. I am one of the very few people privileged to have sparred with him quite a few times; me and a few other black belts.

■ WHAT WAS HE LIKE TO SPAR WITH?
Phenomenal. You just couldn't hit him. If you kicked him, his hand was there, if you punched to his face, his arm was there. If you moved this way, he was out of the way, if you moved that way, he was in on you. I'm talking of his heyday, when I was around.

I've got a film, which I'm very privileged to have, of me actually fighting him. It was taken in Jordan when I was private tutor to the Royal Family and he came out to see us.

■ WHAT TECHNIQUES DID HE USE IN FREE-SPARRING?
At that time, when I was doing free-sparring with him, he didn't really have the flexibility in his legs that he used to have with the round kicks, but his hands were absolutely brilliant. You know, we'd do the circular blocking movement, and it was like a windmill. Your hand is like a windmill, or a fan. When a fan is going slowly, you can put your finger in and out, but when the fan speeds up, you can't put your finger in. So your reactions and hand speed work in that manner, and that made him almost untouchable.

■ WAS HE QUICK AS WELL, BECAUSE YOU SOMETIME WONDER WHETHER A PERSON WITH A POWERFUL BUILD LIKE THAT MIGHT LOSE SOMETHING IN SPEED?
He was very fast. He was muscular, but he built his body up for the purpose of doing what he wanted to do in karate. He didn't build himself up to pose. His body was big, strong, but it was ready to move like lightning, and powerful enough to do any type of block or defense.

■ COULD YOU TELL US ABOUT SOME OF THE PEOPLE WHO WERE AT THE DOJO THEN. KUROSAKI YOU'VE ALREADY MENTIONED.
Kurosaki was my favorite motivator for fighting. He had the gift of pushing you to the limit, and then he would ask for more.

■ BUT HE WOULD DO IT HIMSELF?
He would be with you, yes. At that time, he was in charge of keeping the high level of fighting up.

■ HE MUST HAVE BEEN WITH THE KYOKUSHIN FROM THE VERY START.
Yes, he was one of the first. Of course, if you were to go back in history, most of the original Kyokushin men came from other styles.

■ I'VE HEARD THAT, LIKE OYAMA, HE WAS WITH YAMAGUCHI OF GOJU AND THEY STARTED KYOKUSHIN AT THE SAME TIME.
I don't really know about that.

■ WHAT ABOUT YASUDA EIJI, WHO DOES THE KATA IN *WHAT IS KARATE* (1959)?
Yasuda Eiji was a good karate man. He was tall, slim...a different character from Kurosaki. Kurosaki would be pushing, pushing, but Yasuda was more easy going. But in

kumite he was like a snake—he would strike so fast you wouldn't know what hit you. He was the type of person who never showed any emotion, so you never knew when he was going to hit you or kick you. He would just look at you, then "bang!" and that would be it. A wonderful gentleman.

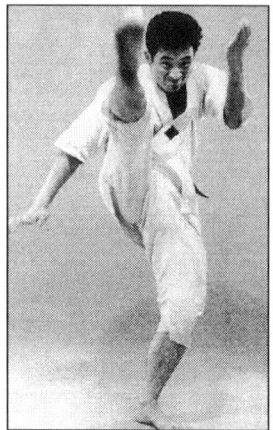 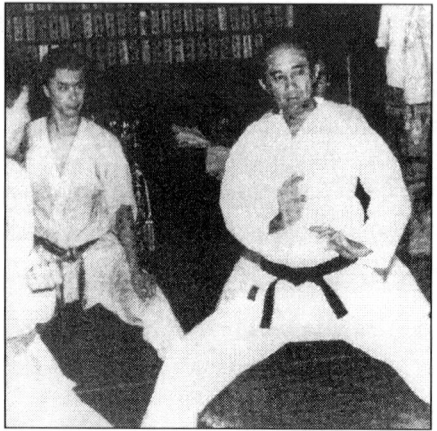 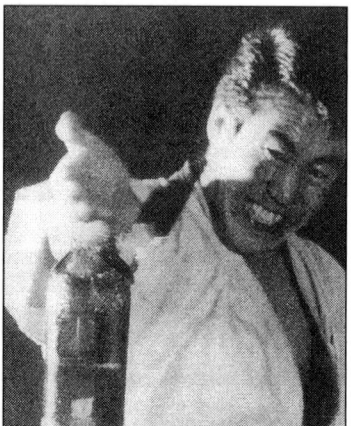

Left: Yasuda Eiji demonstrating Saifa Kata.
Center: Ishibashi Masami teaching.
Right: Okada Hirofumi breaking to top off a bottle.
Photo from *This is Karate* (1965).

■ ISHIBASHI MASAMI?

You don't hear much about him. He kept in the background, but he was a very important person. He was an absolute perfectionist, especially in kata. He really got me into kata, and pushed me in kata. For example, in Saifa Kata, he could put a coin on the floor and start the kata from there. He would do the kata so perfectly that he would finish back on that coin.

He also had a tremendous way of explaining kata in a practical way, not a mystical way. Very down to earth. How you did it, and why you did it that way.

And he also explained that many of the things in the kata may not represent what you see straight-away. In other words, sometimes a move is a link brought into the kata so that it flows, but it has no real fighting meaning. It has purpose in keeping the movement going.

■ AND IT WILL ADJUST THE SHAPE AND RHYTHM OF THE KATA?

That's right. And you know, a lot of people try to create a meaning or application for every movement in the kata. Ishibashi would often say this is just a position, or a linking movement within the kata. Ishibashi was the one who was really in charge of kata at that time, along with Okada Hirofumi.

■ OKADA POSED FOR MOST OF THE PHOTOGRAPHS IN OYAMA'S *THIS IS KARATE* (1965).

Yes, he's in the old books. He was not only a brilliant fighter, but a brilliant kata man also.

■ WHAT GRADES DID THESE INSTRUCTORS HAVE AT THAT TIME?

In those days, I just knew them as "sensei," and a sensei at that time was a 3rd dan. When Mas Oyama came in, I called him sensei too.

- THEY DIDN'T PLACE A LOT OF EMPHASIS ON THE NUMBER OF DAN?

No. You were a sensei. As Oyama said in those years, it's not the grade that makes the person, it's the person that makes the grade. At that time I think Oyama was 6th dan, although I wouldn't put my life on it. I didn't really bother about that. All I knew was he was the Sensei. [Note: In his 1959 book, *What is Karate?*, Mas Oyama's grade is given as 8th dan]. Okada, Kurosaki, and Ishibashi were, I think, 3rd dan.

- THEY WOULD HAVE BEEN THE FIRST GENERATION OF KYOKUSHIN SENSEI?

Yes, they were the first generation of top sensei.

- AFTER THAT CAME THE GENERATION OF NAKAMURA TADASHI, SHIGERU OYAMA?

Nakamura Tadashi, Shigeru Oyama, and myself.

- AND HIDEYUKI ASHIHARA WAS AROUND THEN?

Ashihara was with me. We grew up in Kyokushin and got our grades together. We got our brown belts together. I failed my 1st dan test, but he passed. Then later I passed him and got my 2nd dan before him.

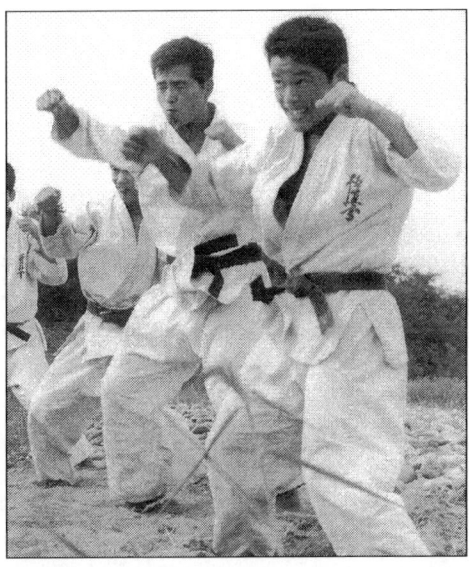

Nakamura Tadashi (left) with Akio Fujihira.

- COULD YOU TELL US ABOUT NAKAMURA?

Nakamura Tadashi was brilliant. He tended to take over, or take responsibility, along with Oyama Shigeru. If it had all worked out as it was meant to, and there were none of the difficulties that happened later. Nakamura Tadashi was groomed to be the next head of Kyokushin.

- HE MENTIONS THAT IN HIS BOOK, *THE HUMAN FACE OF KARATE*.

Yes, he was groomed. We knew it, it was made quite clear, and we accepted he would be the next one to take over. It was intended that, as Mas Oyama got older, he would gradually take control. Shigeru Oyama would be following, and I was following in their footsteps. I was being groomed also—there was no restriction because I was a *gaijin* [non-Japanese]. I was a karate practitioner. I was a 2nd dan when Nakamura and Oyama were 3rd dans.

Then things started to develop. In 1965, I came to Europe and had a lot of hard work, because in those years you had Sensei Enoeda and Kanazawa and Suzuki here. Then I came along and, of course, in those years people thought that only a Japanese could teach karate.

■ BUT MAS OYAMA NEVER BELIEVED THAT?
No. I begged him like hell, "Please send me a Japanese instructor!" He said, "If you're not good enough, you don't deserve to be there. I taught you to be a karate man. Teach you own students, let them learn among themselves." Which I did.

■ HIS TRUST IN YOU MUST HAVE GIVEN YOU A LOT OF CONFIDENCE.
Yes, because you know it was hard work. Let's face it, Enoeda, Kanazawa, Suzuki—they were fantastic instructors.

■ TO GO BACK TO NAKAMURA TADASHI, WHAT WAS SPECIAL ABOUT HIM?
Nakamura was a very powerful, but also a very deep thinking, karate practitioner. There was a lot of philosophy there, and even today with his own group, his philosophy is beautiful and deep. He was a brilliant karate man.

If I can put it this way—Nakamura Tadashi was a good strong karate man with a deep philosophy. He was good all round but his distinctive feature was this deepness. Shigeru was a fighter, and today his own organization will show you that: a fighting style. I was groomed to be in between these two in terms of character. Because I was fanatical on technique, I was also very prominent in kata, and I loved fighting. And even today, in my organization, I try to keep these qualities. I like the basics, the fighting, the kata, and I also like the respect and courtesy of karate as it should be.

The three of us were well matched. Nakamura Tadashi then went to America and did a wonderful job. Shigeru followed him, but before that, Bob Boulton, who was a 2nd dan, came back to Britain. I was going to leave Japan and Oyama asked if I would like to go to Europe to help Bob for a while, because he knew that eventually I wanted to go back to Africa. I said, OK I'll do that. So we came to Britain, but due to the problems in Africa at that time, and with my wife being Japanese, I then made the decision to stay in Europe.

■ IF I CAN JUST ADD ONE MORE NAME FROM THOSE EARLY DAYS — JON BLUMING.
I knew Jon Bluming very well. He was a very robust, very strong fighting man. That's all he ever wanted to do.

■ IS IT TRUE THAT HE HAD A STANDING $10,000 OR, IN SOME VERSIONS, $100,000 CHALLENGE TO FIGHT ANYONE?
I don't know about that.

■ WAS HE TRAINING AT THE DOJO WHEN YOU WERE THERE?
No, Jon had just left. He had left the memory of . . .

■ A LEGEND?
Not a legend, but . . . a madman [laughing]! But, when I say "madman," I say in the best possible way, with a lot of respect. He was just so strong. He was like that at the Kodokan.

■ HIS ABILITY IN BOTH JUDO AND KARATE MADE HIM A FORMIDABLE OPPONENT?
I would say Jon could have got into the Olympics in judo, but because of certain things,

he wasn't chosen to represent Holland. I don't want to go into the politics, but I would say Bluming was better than Geesink. [Anton Geesink won the gold in judo at the 1964 Olympics held in Tokyo]. That's just my own opinion. But he was a brilliant judo man, and as a karate man, he was very good as well.

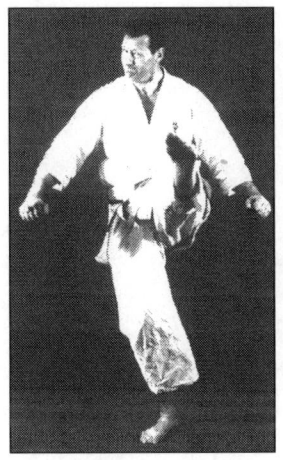 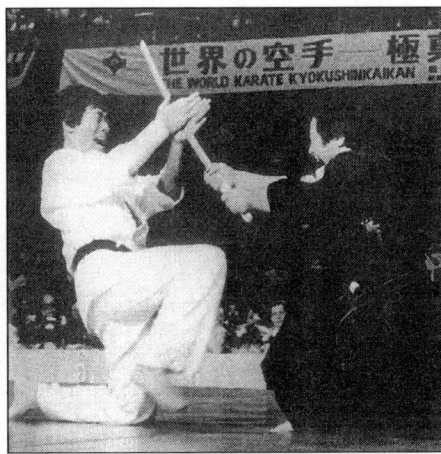

Left: Jon Bluming (photo courtesy of Jon Bluming). Right: Oyama Shigeru (left) in a sword-catching demonstration with Nakamura Tadashi.

THE 100 MAN FIGHT

■ CAN WE MOVE ON NOW TO YOUR 100-MAN FIGHT. YOU WERE THE FIRST PERSON TO COMPLETE THIS TEST?

So I believe.

■ MAS OYAMA MUST HAVE HAD CONFIDENCE IN YOU TO PICK YOU FOR THAT.

I was surprised when he chose me, because people had tried before and been unsuccessful. When he spoke to me about it, I said, "You're crazy!" He said, "I think you can do it." I said, "I don't know," but again he stated that he thought I could do it. "So, would you like to have a go?", he asked, and I replied, "Well, if you think so!"

■ MAS OYAMA SEEMED VERY GOOD AT ENCOURAGING PEOPLE TO TEST THEIR LIMITS.

Yes, but he also formed a judgment of my character. He knew that in my training, I would give nothing but my best. And he knew that if he gave me something to do I would work at it. In any case, he asked me and I said yes. I spoke to my wife about it and she said, "You're crazy!" I told her it would take a lot of training. At that time, my wife was working in a bank and she supported me. Without her, I would never have been able to do it.

So I started to train and it became quite a lonely life. I made my own program up with the help of Oyama. I was up very early in the morning, running up and down hills, a lot of physical training, and working out in the park. Weekends I would go down to the beach and run like hell in the sand.

■ AND THIS WAS ON TOP OF YOUR NORMAL DOJO TRAINING?

On top of my normal dojo training. You know, Mas Oyama didn't say, "Have a break!" But he would monitor me all the time. Then I asked, "When am I going to do it?" He replied, "I'll tell you when. You just work. Don't worry about when you'll do it. Maybe you won't do it." So I kept training, training, and he kept monitoring me, checking my condition, watching me in the dojo, and this went on for six months until I was extraordinarily fit. I breathed, eat, and slept karate. Nothing else.

Then one Sunday morning when I went training as normal, I walked in, and I sensed something different. I opened the dojo doors and they were all sitting there. Oyama Sensei said, "You fight today." I didn't have any time to think about it. And then he said, "Do you accept the 100-man kumite?" I said, "Hai! Yes, I accept the challenge!" So then they phoned my wife to tell her and ask her to pick me up later. Then the fighting started, approximately a minute and a half each fight.

■ THIS WAS CONTACT?

Yes, contact. The only thing was, my opponents couldn't kick me in the legs, but I could kick them in the legs. And no face punches were allowed. If you could knock a man down and he couldn't get up, then the fight would finish and that would help you by cutting down your fighting time. Otherwise, you did the full minute and a half. And then it was "yame" and the next one would get up, then the next one, and the next one. I was able to knock quite a few people down, but it would be ridiculous to say I beat everybody. The object is not to win every fight.

The object is to have the character and condition to stand and fight, to go on. If I'm in charge and you reach a point where you don't know if you are coming or going, I will stop the fighting, and I have done this in many countries. But if you are in the condition to fight, you are allowed to keep on fighting.

So, I survived the 100-man fight. I fought from green belts, brown belts and upwards, and you couldn't say I was treated kindly, because if Mas Oyama had thought one of the fighters was going easy on me he would have said to cancel the fight, so it wouldn't have counted. For them to have been easy on me would have been terrible, so I said to them to come at me strongly, for my sake. And they all played ball and they all fought hard. I was treated fairly all the way through.

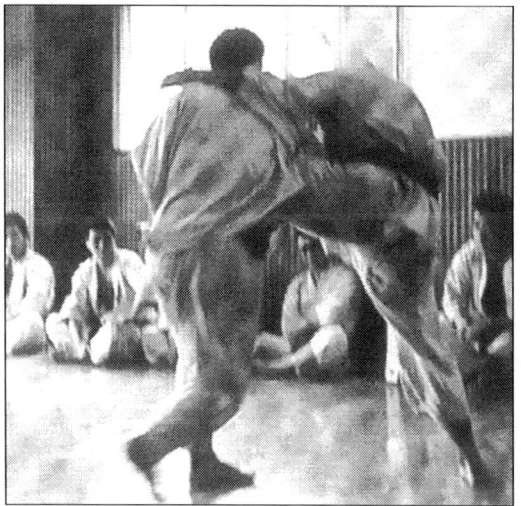 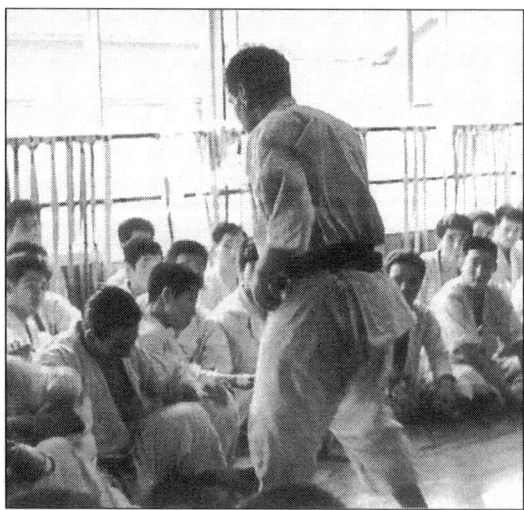

Left: Steve Arneil (right) during the 100-man kumite.
Right: Arneil drives his attacker into the sitting crowd.

You lose count of the fights. You get to a point where you feel your body's going to break up, and then it's purely your mind. So I just fought and fought and fought, and then when Okada came in, and then Shigeru, and then Nakamura Tadashi, I realized it must be getting close to the hundred. When I fought Tadashi he went hard, because he is that kind of man. He's not there to please you, he's there to give you credibility. And after that Oyama gave the order to finish and he said, "You have completed the 100-man kumite." And I shouted, "Yaaagh!" and then, "Uss!" I just stood there, and they all got up and gave me a big clap. It's an inner family affair.

Oyama said, "Take him down and wash him." They took me away, I was covered in blood, and my body was so sore. They washed me clean, and I could see the bruising all over my body. By the time I came back, I saw my wife was sitting there. She looked at me and her expression told me everything. Then they had a bit of a speech, we had some sake. They told me I'd done a wonderful job and they were all proud of me. Oyama put his arm around me and said, "I said you could do it. I'm glad my judgment was good." I said that I was glad I'd accomplished what he wanted me to do. He said, "I think you must now go home with your wife." I said, "I think so too," and that was it.

I walked out with my wife and I walked off as if nothing was wrong, but once I got away from the vicinity of the dojo, I almost collapsed! My wife helped me, she must have carried me back to the station and then our place. And when I got home and undressed, my God, I looked at myself and I looked like a leopard with all the bruising. My wife helped me with the bath and got me ready and I just lay there. And on the Tuesday, I was expected to train again, which I did. I trained very slow, very easy; it was quite painful, but I did it.

That was the 100-man kumite, and it was kept quiet for a long time. I just did something that Oyama wanted me to do. And then it suddenly came out at one of the World Tournaments. It was in the magazine that I was the first man to have accomplished it.

■ YOU MUST FEEL PROUD OF THAT.

I was very proud. But you know, I hear stories about it, and I always say if you ever want to hear about it, speak to me. I'm the one who did it.

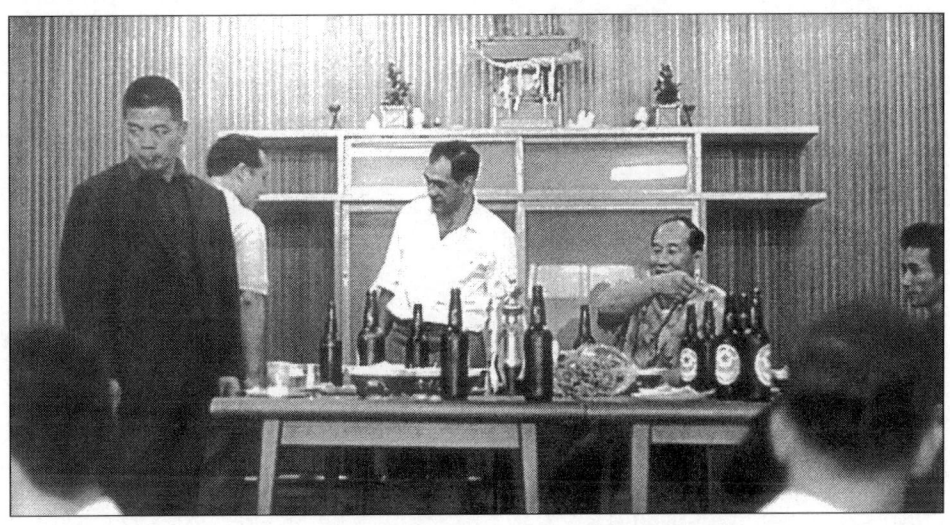

Celebration of Steve Arneil's 100-man fight.
Oyama is seated at the table. Arneil is standing. Kurosaki Kenji is at the left.

■ THERE'S A STORY THAT MAS OYAMA DID A 300-MAN KUMITE.

I've heard that story too, but I can't confirm if it's true or not.

■ DID YOU HEAR ABOUT IT WHEN YOU WERE IN JAPAN?

No, I didn't hear about it then. I knew he'd fought quite a lot of people, but I didn't know anything about numbers or anything. To me the 100-man kumite was just something he wanted me to do, because he said he'd done a lot of fights many years ago.

■ DID THE KYOKUSHINKAI AT THAT TIME HAVE CONTESTS WITH OTHER STYLES?

No. We never had contests with other styles. It was an internal affair between Kyokushin dojos. At that time, the style was growing quite big in Japan, and myself and Nakamura Tadashi were in charge of Tachikawa. It was an American base, and that's how we got into the American scene. We used to go there alternately and teach.

■ WERE YOU THERE WHEN KUROSAKI, NAKAMURA, AND FUJIHIRA WENT TO FIGHT IN THAILAND?

I was training. I was part of that squad. Myself and Oyama Shigeru's brother Yasuhiko were down to go. It was myself, Fujihira, Nakamura and Yasuhiko. I've got a few photos of when we were training. We went to a hut by the river, and we used to run in the water and train, train, train. And then, as it turned out, the squad was whittled down to Nakamura and Fujihira. I had visa problems, and I had to work, and it was difficult. And at that time, Yasuhiko had to complete his law examinations, so it was left to Nakamura and Fujihira.

■ FUJIHIRA BECAME A KICK BOXER LATER.

That's right. After the break with Kurosaki Kenji, he left with Kurosaki and started kick boxing, which he did very successfully.

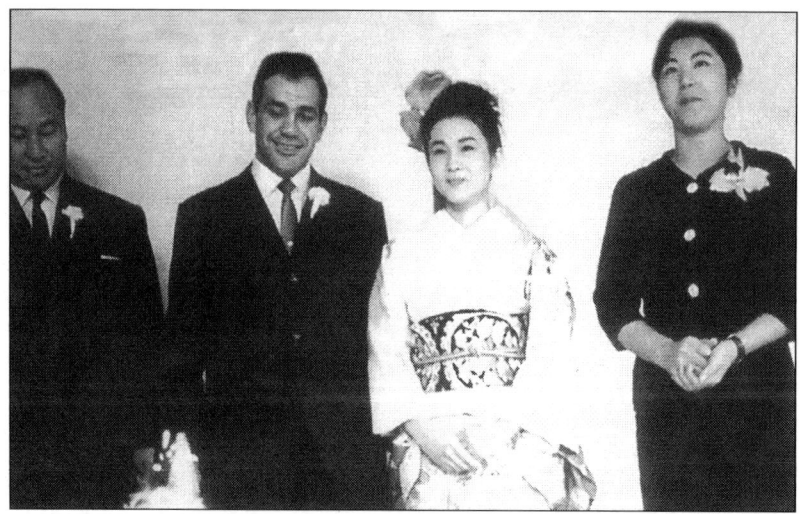

Mas Oyama (left) and his wife (far right) at Steve Arneil's wedding.

■ WHAT WAS HE LIKE? WAS HE A HARD TRAINER?

Fujihira was a small man, shorter than I was, but what a character. What determination! The only way to stop him would be to put a bullet between his eyes [laughing]! That's the only way I can explain it. Oh man, when he was training in the dojo!

■ HE HAD A VERY STRONG PHYSIQUE TOO.

For his size, he was close to perfect. He was really good, and he trained religiously.

You see, the problem with those two was when they were training, we had to do it with them to keep their level up, and we really had to work hard.

How it all happened—the Thai boxers sent out a challenge. They said the Japanese were sissies, they couldn't punch their way out of a paper bag, and so on. They said, "Who will challenge us?" and it was turned down by everyone. Then Mas Oyama said, "I'll challenge you!" So we all went, "Ohhh," because when he said he would challenge the Thais, we knew it would be one of us who would have to go!

In any case, they went to Thailand and they did a very good job. Fujihara won superbly, and so did Nakamura. Kurosaki, as I said, myself and Yasuhiro were suppose to go, but circumstances prevented us. But it was billed for three Japanese fighters, so the Thais said they expected another person to fight. So Kurosaki fought, and you know he should not have fought. But out of courtesy, he fought and he was beaten. He got a broken nose and that type of thing. But as far as we were concerned, our boys had won by taking two out of three. And that's when we got respect from the Thai boxers.

■ WHEN WAS IT THAT KUROSAKI LEFT KYOKUSHINKAI?

It wasn't so long after that. There was some dispute that I don't know about. Kurosaki spoke to me and said, "Look, I have to leave, and Fujihira will be leaving with me. It is up to you to make your own decision." I said, "Thank you." He then said, "Whatever decision you make it will not harm our friendship in any way." And of course he did go, and I stayed along with Nakamura and all the others.

■ THAT MUST HAVE BEEN A BIG LOSS FOR THE DOJO.

Oh yes, it was a big loss. It was a sad time. But life must continue, and I'm sure Mas Oyama felt it as badly as we did. He never showed it, but I'm sure he felt it. Kurosaki was the first of the top men to leave. Why he left, I don't know, but there's something within Kyokushinkai that when you reached a top level like that, something—I don't know, I can't explain. It's happened to me, it's happened to Nakamura Tadashi, it's happened to Oyama Shigeru. Possibly it was politics [with Kurosaki], but at that time, I didn't know.

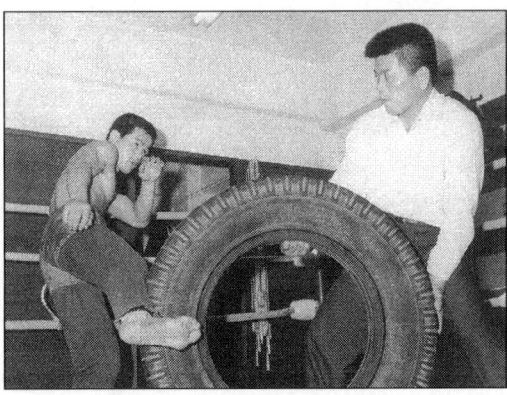

Kurosaki Kenji (left) shown training Fujihira Akio.

KYOKUSHINKAI IN ENGLAND

■ OKAY, SO YOU CAME TO ENGLAND IN 1965?

Yes, in 1965, at Mas Oyama's request, as I said earlier. I met up with Bob Boulton, and we opened up the first dojo at the London Judo Society, which became the London Karatekai.

■ THAT WAS IN THE EARLY DAYS OF KARATE IN GREAT BRITAIN?

That's right, it was very early. That was the time Suzuki and Enoeda had just arrived. Those years were just spent building up the organization.

■ WAS IT HARD?

It was hard, but in a way, it was good too, because the training I was doing was fantastic. People liked it, but if I did that same training today, I'd have no one in the dojo.

■ HAS KARATE CHANGED A LOT SINCE THEN?

Oh yes, things have changed. But, many people ask me how would my students of those years do now. And I have to be honest and say I think they'd get slaughtered, because of the new techniques and training methods that have come in. Where they would win, though, would be in pure determination, spirit. But the technical ability has improved so much with different training methods, and new ways of doing things. I myself was always keen to learn as much as I could from everybody else, and adapt it if I felt it would work for us. And this is the way Kyokushin in Britain developed, but never, ever did I break away from the traditions: the basics, the katas, and the strict discipline of fighting. If you fought somebody and you didn't have the decency to shake his hand afterwards, then don't bloody well fight. And this is the way I still look at my people. And this is why at our championships, if I hear one boo, I am on the microphone immediately to the crowd. It is the worst discourtesy to show to two fighters. If a fighter has made an infringement, then the referees are there to handle it, not people standing up in the crowd and booing.

■ IN THOSE DAYS, THE 1960S AND EARLY 1970S, BRITISH KARATE SEEMED TO BE MORE TOGETHER. IN NATIONAL CHAMPIONSHIPS, ALL THE MAJOR STYLES TOOK PART.

Yes, the good old BKCC (British Karate Control Commission) Championships.

■ SOME OF YOUR STUDENTS FOUGHT IN THEM, BRIAN FITKIN FOR EXAMPLE.

Ah, Brian Fitkin was a brilliant Kyokushinkai man. A good student, and even to this day, I still think very fondly of Brian. But at that time we weren't doing what we are doing now, knock-down fighting, or let's call it the Kyokushinkai way of fighting. We were doing ... and this was very difficult for me ... point fighting or you could say WUKO (World Union of Karate Organizations) type fighting. I wasn't too happy with the idea, but I knew that if I was to survive in this country and promote Kyokushin, I would have to fall into line. I was taught by my teacher to be adaptable, which I was. So I continued to train the way we'd always trained, but I added also the WUKO form of fighting and we became very successful at it. And I was very, very honored when I was approached and asked if I would become the manager of the British karate team. I thought that was fantastic and I said yes, I would like to be, because I also thought it would be a very good opportunity to also get Kyokushinkai known, because I'm a Kyokushinkai man. And it happened at that time that I had in the team—not because they were from my organization—good Kyokushinkai men like Brian Fitkin, Ticky Donovan (because he was Kyokushinkai then), Howard Collins, and various other boys who showed tremendous effort as Kyokushinkai students.

Brian, I would have to say, was the best as far as our WUKO representatives were concerned. He once fought knockdown in Japan, but not thereafter. He concentrated mainly on WUKO. And to me, he was the prize. He was like a stalking tiger. He was brilliant. If he had put his heart into knockdown, he would have been the same in that.

■ HOWARD COLLINS FOUGHT KNOCKDOWN IN JAPAN, DIDN'T HE?

Oh, Howard Collins was brilliant as a Kyokushinkai fighter. He did very well. A tremendous fighter.

■ THE BRITISH KARATE SQUAD WAS VERY STRONG AT THAT TIME.

After a lot of hard work, and by having an open mind, we built up a very powerful squad from all styles, and that was a tremendous experience for me as they also helped me improve my knowledge in all styles.

■ YOU HAD SOME GOOD FIGHTERS.

I'll put my head on the block. I would say my team that won the World Championships, if I could get them today, at the same age, the same level, they would beat the teams now. They were brilliant: Bob Poynton, Terry O'Neill, Stan Knighton, Ticky Donovan, Hamish Adams, Billy Higgins, Brian Fitkin! I'm sorry if I've forgotten some names, but they were great, and they came from all styles. I managed to get them into believing we were one team. It didn't matter what style they came form, we were a British team, and I bred that into them all the time.

And, of course, we beat the Japanese in Paris [1972], which they weren't too happy about, and I told Kanazawa at the time—because he was their manager—"When we meet you again, we'll become the World Champions." He said, "Never!", and I replied, "You watch us!" And then in Long Beach we pulled it off, and I was very happy that I could give my services to my country in this way, and help the fighters for the future. It's turned out excellently too. So far Ticky Donovan [Arneil's successor as British coach] has done a tremendous job and we are still up there, and I hope Vic Charles, who is taking over from Ticky, will continue the tradition of producing strong British teams, because I think at the moment Britain has the highest level of martial art in Europe. I'm talking of the general level. Of course, we have cowboys like everyone else, but if you take the serious practitioners, I think we are a very strong martial arts country.

KYOKUSHINKAI TOURNAMENTS

■ AROUND 1969, THE KYOKUSHINKAI IN JAPAN HELD THEIR FIRST NATIONAL CHAMPIONSHIPS UNDER KNOCKDOWN RULES.

Yes, and soon after that we had our own tournament in this country. In 1975 there was the first World Tournament, and those years were just brilliant.

■ CAN WE TALK ABOUT SOME OF THE FIGHTERS FROM THAT PERIOD, LIKE SATO KATSUKO, THE FIRST WORLD CHAMPION?

Big Sato!—very strong, very dedicated, definitely a world champion.

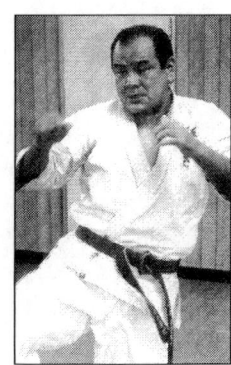

Sato Katsuaki, the first
World Kyokushinkai Champion.

■ Royama [Hatsuo]?

Oh Royama. Royama and I grew up in the dojo. He was my kohai. So were people like Soeno Yoshiji, who's now head of Shidokan karate. So I was giving them a hard time. But these were all good fighters, and gentlemen, and when I say gentlemen, I mean that on a high level. Soeno was one of the best gentlemen I've ever met. Even to this day I have tremendous respect for him, his character, the way he does things.

But people like Azuma, Sato, Sampei, Ninomiya, they were all tremendous fighters. I don't think there was any fighter who didn't deserve the honors he won. Because at that time they were the kingpins; the world around them was still learning the game. And then slowly but surely Europe got stronger and stronger and the threat [to the Japanese] was there. Then the rest of the world developed and it became quite difficult for the Japanese to dominate like before, and the tournaments were no longer one-sided affairs.

■ There was a lot of dissent from the foreign countries about the way some of these tournaments were run, especially the 1991 tournament.

This is one of the reasons I got into hot water, because for one thing I didn't like the way the draw was done. Then I didn't like the way the Japanese could overturn decisions so they went in their favor. I didn't like the conniving that went on. There were times definitely when the non-Japanese fighters were done in. They could have become World Champions.

■ What was wrong with the draw?

Well, how can you do the draw six months ahead then put in a bye for someone? And when the day of the fighting comes, the whole thing is changed. I objected to it and I always made it clear I objected. OK, we fought open weight, so you had to take what came your way. But it was so neatly arranged that the Japanese—and this is no disrespect to the Japanese fighters themselves, they were very good—the Japanese were given an edge, because they fought smaller opponents while our fighters were getting hammered by the big opponents. By the time any of our men got through, they were so beaten up, they would lose.

■ It was also said that the strongest Western fighters were matched against each other in the early rounds.

Of course. It was obvious. I don't have to tell you that. Just look at the tapes. And all this, of course, made me sad, because I never expected this to happen in Kyokushinkai. But then again, politics, sponsorships, all those kind of things were Japanese. I got into a lot of hot water because I was told personally to change a decision and I refused point blank. And I made it clear to my teacher, who I loved very much, that I would grab the microphone and I would tell the whole audience what was happening and then I would walk out. And he said, "I know you will do it, so we won't change the decision." And he smiled at me, and afterwards he said, "You still haven't changed." He respected me for that.

But I can understand his point, because he was under pressure too from many things I don't know about. But I would never be persuaded to change a decision, and I did object strongly. And so did Nakamura, and so did Oyama Shigeru. It seemed like we were just going there as puppets, for their entertainment. We didn't have a hope in hell of winning.

I always said, why don't you do the draw a week before the tournament and do it as it should be done, like we do it here? Our draw hasn't been done yet; it'll be done tonight, the evening before the tournament. But to do it six months before—they gave us all kinds of excuses, but it was just a con.

So the Western fighter would fight against the Japanese, who would be good, but the Western fighter would be better. And then the Japanese would swing the decision on weight, but before they did that, they would look at all the aspects to the thing. So if the foreigner weighed more, they would go on weight. But if it was the other way round they would decide on boards broken, if the Japanese had broken more boards. There was no consistency. They didn't follow the system, which is weights, then boards, then decision. And I was against all this, I argued and protested about it until... Well, things happened. Certain people in my own group took advantage of it, and I got put in the hot seat.

But even at that point I would not change, because Mas Oyama himself taught me to be a man, to keep to my principles, and I know that even to his last day, he would respect me for that because he said to me—obviously I can't prove it—people will have to believe me or not. He told me, "If there's anyone ever who will continue the true spirit of Kyokushinkai, it will be you." And this is my job; I will do it to the end, maybe not under the Japanese flag, but I will do it under my own flag.

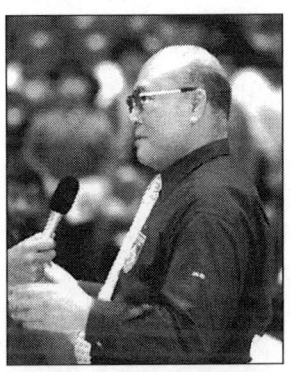

Oyama being interviewed during the All-Japan Championships. Photo courtesy of the International Karate Organization.

LEAVING MAS OYAMA

■ YOU LEFT THE KYOKUSHINKAI ORGANIZATION EVENTUALLY. THAT MUST HAVE BEEN A VERY HARD DECISION FOR YOU.

Oh, it was a hard decision. You know it was my life. I understand Mr. Oyama had no option. He was under a lot of pressure. But there were a lot of false reasons given as to why I left. Supposedly I wanted to take over, I wanted to play God, all kinds of things were said against me. But that's life. If you're in the hot seat, you have to take what comes. But I disputed everything they said. My object was not to override Japan. My object was to give credibility to my teacher, which he wanted. I was always excited when we did well because I was thinking, "Sosai's [the style's founder] going to be very happy." I was for him. I didn't want to be the world controller or the world president.

But some people didn't like the rules I made and they took advantage of it and finally the day came when the old man kensoku'd me. That meant I wasn't put out of Kyokushinkai, but I had to stay in my own dojo. I couldn't go out of my own dojo [to teach or train] and I thought that was ridiculous. When I was kensoku'd, I wrote to my teacher. I said, "You know, we've been around so many years. I grew up in front of you"—because, indirectly, he was like my father—"and you can't tell your son to stay in his room when he's thirty years old. I have done nothing at all to injure you or hurt you. All I've tried to do is give you credibility, and to compliment you on all the things you have done. I've done the best I can, and I cannot accept this." And he replied saying I had to accept it. But when I get someone who I taught from white belt phoning me up and telling me to stay in my dojo—that's enough.

Then the BKK (British Karate Kyokushinkai) made a decision, that if Japan wasn't going to change, then we weren't going to change, because we didn't feel any necessity to. We also didn't like the politics that were going on within our own committee, where members would sit on the committee and then report back to Japan without our knowledge.

Then they said they wanted branch chiefs, and we disagreed as an organization because we didn't see the necessity for branch chiefs. "Branch chiefs" I will say openly, is a gimmick for making money. You know, give me x amount of money and I'll give you a certificate and you're a branch chief. But they broke the rules, because at that time, to be a branch chief you had to have 3,000 members. Some people who became branch chiefs didn't even have five members. I don't like working that way, and the BKK and Europe had functioned very well without branch chiefs. It was country representatives, and they were responsible, with a committee, and the committee made the decisions. But, looking back at it, I can understand why branch chiefs were introduced. It's the domino effect: if one doesn't do it, the next one will. And this is really where Mr. Oyama and myself came to the end of the line. I knew he felt very sad about it, but he was in a position where he had made a decision, and if it looked as if he had gone back on that decision—which I knew he wanted to do very badly—he would have lost face. To me "face" doesn't mean anything, but that is the Japanese way.

Then, finally, I went to Switzerland, where he was supposed to be going. I thought this would be our last consultation, but he didn't turn up. I wanted to meet openly, in front of everybody, so no one would be making up stories. And I feel I was treated badly, after all I had done, because the mandate that the other groups had given me to take to Japan about the fighting and all that—they had all signed it, yet when it came for them to support me, they didn't do it. I never ended up going to Japan. I resigned as European President, and I resigned from Kyokushinkai Headquarters.

And that is when the IFK was created, because I was inundated by people who had the same kind of thinking as I had, who had the same type of problems. They were all ex-Kyokushinkai. I thought, this is crazy, to take this all on at my time of life. But then I thought, why not. Oyama said I must always follow the Kyokushinkai principles, and so I decided I'd do it.

■ How big is the IFK now?

It's big. We've got over twenty countries and we've only been in existence four or five years. We're doing our first world tournament in Moscow next year. It's a healthy organization, but what will take place in the future, nobody knows. My ambition is to create some happiness and the proper spirit of budo.

■ There are now a lot of Kyokushin or Kyokushin-offshoot groups in the world, like Oyama Shigeru's, Nakamura's, and so on.

Yes, but often they have done what I haven't done. When people ask me what style I do, I say "Kyokushin." I haven't changed the style. Oyama Shigeru has the World Oyama style, and he has changed it in line with his ideas. Nakmura Tadashi has his Seido style, and he has changed certain things, although obviously there's a lot of Kyokushin in it. Soeno of Shidokan, he has changed some things. I haven't. I keep Kyokushin techniques and I am a Kyokushin man. The old man made me a Kyokushin man. I took it very seriously when he said I would be a Kyokushinkai man all my life.

What I do know is that if Oyama were alive today, he would be a very, very sad man. He didn't want it to be like this. He wanted a healthy family. He wanted something with credibility. He wanted people to say, "Hey, they're Kyokushinkai. They're a strong group." It was never his intention that things would turn out the way they did, but in a way, he should take some of the blame. He didn't listen to people who loved him very much. I want to keep that spirit of Kyokushin. To me it was beautiful. I was a wild boy when I was young, and I don't know where I'd have been without Kyokushin. So I want to give something back. But no way will I be untrue to my principle—otherwise, what was it all for?

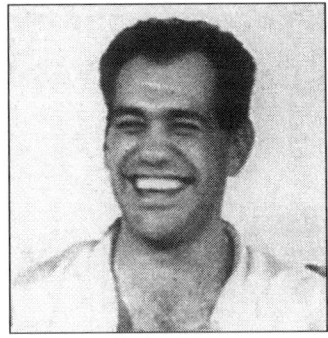

Steve Arneil.

And I want to say, if it wasn't for my good students and a lot of good people around me, I couldn't have accomplished it. So I thank all my students, all my executives and all my coaches for what we've achieved.

References

Nakamura, T. (1989). The human face of karate. New York: World Seido Karate Organization.

Oyama, M. (1966, 1973). *This is karate.* Tokyo: Japan Publications Inc.

Oyama, M. (1973). *This is karate.* NY: Wehman Brothers.

Oyama, M. (1958). *What is karate?* Tokyo: Japan Publications Trading.

Oyama, M. (1966). *What is karate?* NY: HarperCollins.

chapter 45

The Teaching of Goju-ryu Kata: A Brief Look at Methodology and Practice

by Giles Hopkins, M.A.

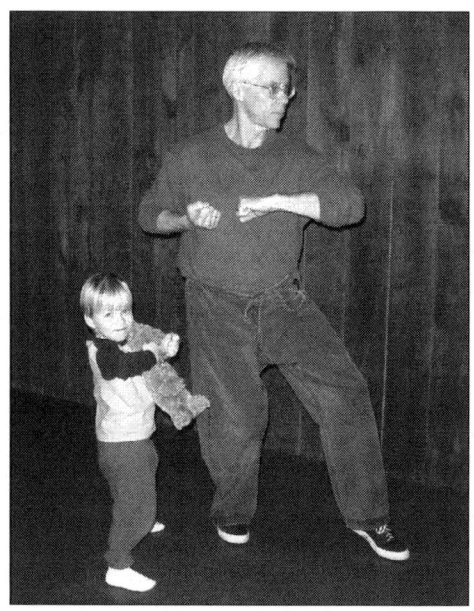

As the author practices a Goju-ryu technique from the Seiunchin kata, his son Noah finds it a natural position to hold his teddy bear.
All photos courtesy of Giles Hopkins.

Introduction

Kata (solo routine) training has become a kind of modern-day Gordian knot; no one seems to have the key to untangle its mysteries. Few seem able to agree on what it means or what it was originally meant to teach. And there are a host of credible explanations that seem to have fueled the debate.

From a historical standpoint, a number of researchers have pointed out that even the origins of various Goju-ryu kata are open to question—some arguing that certain movements are clearly reminiscent of Five Ancestor Fist, others suggesting a link to White Crane, and still others arguing that some form of karate may have been practiced in Okinawa since the 14th century, for all intents and purposes an indigenous Okinawan martial art. This last theory suggests that a blending took place in the early 20th century when a number of Okinawan teachers independently journeyed to China in order to continue their training (Co, 1998; McCarthy, 1995; Swift, 2002).

The question of lineage only further compounds the problem: whose lineage might provide definitive answers about kata? Again, we run into awkward historical questions and a lack of documentation.[1]

Interestingly, some have tried to reconcile these differences of interpretation, side stepping the whole question of historical precedent or lineage, by suggesting that katas contain an almost infinite variety of techniques or different levels of meaning—beginner, intermediate, and advanced levels of kata applications (Heilman, 1997; Higaonna, 2004: 7). Marvin Labbate tries to make this point in discussing what he refers to as "advanced Goju-ryu techniques" (Labbate, 2000). Still others, armed with an arsenal of Japanese terms, describe kata as if it were an onion and the different applications of its techniques merely layers of hidden meaning (Craig and Anderson, 2002). There are even those who see kata as a transcendent and magical experience—as if katas were more shamanistic ritual than practical self-defense; that is, one merely uses them to achieve, through ritualized movement, a kind of trance-like warrior state, similar to what one might find in aboriginal tribal gatherings, the movements conveying a kind of mystical understanding on a subconscious level. Given such diverse views on the matter, it's no wonder that some have even suggested that katas were made to be intentionally ambiguous.[2]

It is my contention, however, that the fundamental problem—what has really fed this seemingly endless debate over the solo kata and its applications—may have more to do with how karate has been traditionally taught than where it comes from or who our teacher's teacher happened to be. It is a question of method, not lineage or historical antecedent, and the method has changed very little over the years. In fact, the methodology of teaching karate has become ritualized as much as anything else in martial arts, to the point where principles have been replaced by repetition. It is the method of instruction that gets passed on in this case, not the knowledge. In the process, the kata becomes something else, no longer a repository of specific self-defense combinations and movement principles. When this happens, the lessons of the teaching aids or mnemonics contained within the katas are largely ignored or forgotten, affecting how we see the applications of each movement.

Pedigree and Pedagogy

The practice of kata has become an almost sacrosanct tradition in karate schools. Over the course of endless hours of kata practice students are told, "Every inch of movement has meaning." With this encouragement, the teacher only hopes that the student will bring life to the kata. The difficulty comes with the student's understanding of this advice and how one learns karate, for the most part through imitation and creative invention.

Most movement, particularly kata movement, is taught through imitation: "monkey see, monkey do." There is little discussion or verbal instruction of kata in traditional schools and perhaps even less in non-traditional schools. Toguchi Seikichi, the head of Shoreikan Goju-ryu until his death in 1998, makes this clear in his description of training in the old days on Okinawa: "Both Higa and Miyagi were very strict and questions were not permitted during training" (Toguchi, 2001:16).

Yagi Meitoku, the senior student to have trained under both Miyagi and Higa, said that training in those days involved long hours of conditioning drills, and only after a number of years would Miyagi even begin to teach kata to a student. Few of Miyagi's students, Yagi says, learned anything more than the "beginner's way, with no understanding of what they were learning." Yagi goes on to say that Master Miyagi "would very rarely give insights or meaning to the kata that he taught until the student showed mastery of the form through hard and consistent training," and few, according to Yagi, stayed long enough to learn anything beyond the rudiments of kata (Babladelis, 1989).

This is still true in most traditional Okinawan schools today. The beginning student simply stands in the back of the room and does his or her best to follow the other students. What little verbal instruction there may be is usually simple and rudimentary: posture, breathing, and stance, for example. Beyond this, of course, the beginning student needs a great deal of repetition. Anything more than this—a philosophical discussion of martial principles, for instance—would be lost on the beginner; he or she has no basis for understanding it. Additionally, one might also argue that this traditional model fits the teacher's natural wariness of beginners, who, for the most part, are not likely to stay long enough to learn what the teacher may really have to teach, to learn anything more than beginner's karate. In the process, the teacher does not give away the "secrets" (the applications, in this case) of the kata to students who are not ready for them. A further rationale is that the movements must be thoroughly ingrained before one learns how to apply them or the movements themselves will be compromised in an attempt to force their application. The teaching method provides a natural safeguard against either of these scenarios. At the same time, however, students are left with the impression that the kata is intentionally cryptic in order to foster the creative interpretation of martial techniques—that is, the applications.

Since the kata is learned through imitation and explanations are rarely given, one is left in most cases to discover meaning for oneself. Anthony Mirakian, a well-known Goju-ryu teacher and early pioneer in bringing Meibukan Goju-ryu to America, supports Toguchi's observation that "there was very little talking" in the traditional Okinawan dojo. Mirakian goes on to say that, "Generally, once a student was shown the kata, he was expected to correct the movements himself . . . the applications were left to the student's imagination and inquisitiveness" (Schoene, 2004).

The trouble is that this discovery method, while rich and imaginative—perhaps even personally rewarding—gives the impression that any interpretation of kata movement that seems to work is okay. In fact, this line of argument suggests there is no wrong or right, just different points of view. However, if there is not strict adherence to both the movements of the kata and the principles of the kata, then one is not exploring the methods of a particular art but rather assigning arbitrary explanations to one's own, sometimes idiosyncratic, movements.

And this is the problem. When students learn kata solely through imitation—rather than in conjunction with a thorough discussion of the martial principles involved and illustrated in the kata—then the movements may be preserved but their applications will be misunderstood. For example, the rhythm and pauses used to teach a kata become habitual in the student, obscuring application combinations and the natural flow of sequences. When the kata is taught, it is slowed down and the techniques are fragmented in order to see the movements more clearly. This fragmentation, however, affects how one sees the applications as well. This is one instance where the teaching methodology—necessary perhaps to instruct a beginner in the rudiments of a particular kata—interferes with a more realistic understanding of the kata's applications.

In his last book, on the "advanced techniques" of Goju-ryu karate, Toguchi, in effect, suggests that he developed his modern training katas to bridge this gap between kata and its applications. (These are the modern Shoreikan katas: Fukyu, Gekisai, Gekiha, and Kakuho). Traditional methods of instruction—that is, imitation without asking any questions—did not satisfy the inquisitive nature of American GIs, and so Toguchi developed a series of basic katas and corresponding two-person drills (*bunkai kumite*) to show applications. He did this, he says, because he "could not speak English" and he believed "a two-person sequence of the kata would give clear answers to the questions posed by the Americans" (Toguchi, 2001:32).

However, these modern training katas do not provide the keys to understand the movement and principles of the original classical katas of Chinese origin.[3] This is particularly true of the two-person sequences that Toguchi developed—their techniques being elementary and the principles of Toguchi's two-person application drills misleading with their straight-line movement. So, even though this did introduce a different methodology into the instruction of karate, it did nothing to explain the movement or techniques of the Goju-ryu classical subjects. The techniques and patterns are fundamentally different.

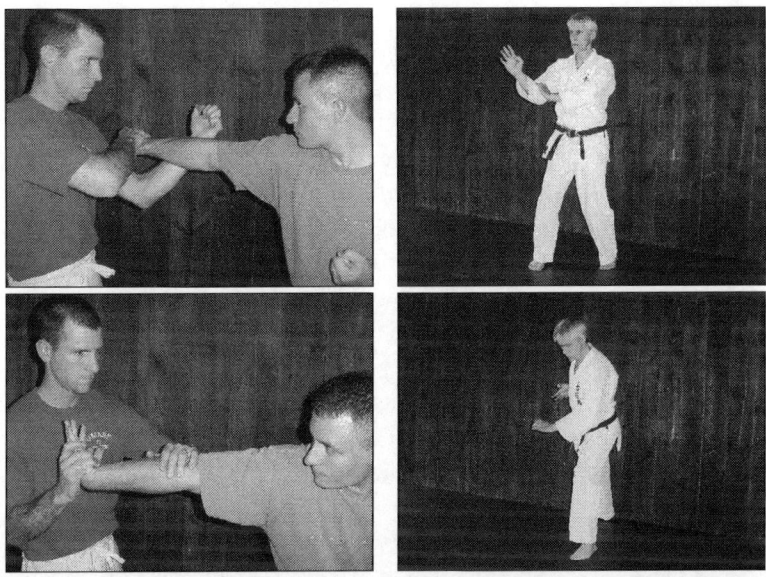

This hand position from Sanseiru kata illustrates another of the mnemonic teaching aids contained within the Goju-ryu katas. The left hand is placed at the elbow to show where the defender would be holding the attacker in this arm-bar technique.

The problem, as McCarthy sees it, is that "the formula once used to interpret its [kata] application principles has all but vanished" (26 August 2001). But it is not the formula that is the problem. The formula is fairly clear once one knows how to look at the kata. It is the methods we use to teach karate that have obscured the message, and the methods have been passed on from teacher to student, maintaining a venerable tradition that in some quasi-religious sense is meant to test the character of the student through long hours of unquestioning repetition. The teacher's methods are not questioned; the teacher has attained his or her own exalted rank through the very means that he or she is using to guide the student. The same understanding will somehow be conveyed to the dedicated student—like a flash of Zen enlightenment—only after years of training. The kata becomes a kind of koan for the karate student; he tests his understanding of the kata as he delves into more and more creative explanations for the applications of the individual moves.

This is the traditional approach to the study of kata. The checks and balances that a thorough understanding of martial principles would provide no longer seem to exist.[4] They have been eviscerated by rationalizations of multiple interpretations or the mystique of advanced levels of understanding. Or they have merely sunk under the burdensome weight and authority of different lineages. Certainly the discovery method is not without its benefits. It forces the student, Anthony Mirakian says, to become "highly observant, one of the most important factors in mastering karate" (Schoene, 2004).

Some Principles Useful in the Analysis of Kata

- Move off the centerline. The stepping pattern of kata teaches this principle. Directional changes in kata show where the attack is coming from and how to step off the centerline in applying the technique. The step and entry technique should be executed in such a way that the attacker cannot attack a second time. This is shown in the kata.
- Katas are composed of combinations or sequences of techniques. Each sequence or series of techniques begins with a "block" and ends with the opponent on the ground or finished. To understand kata, look for the beginnings and the endings.
- Basic techniques that are not shown in specific application sequences are generally put at the beginning of kata and performed in a series of three techniques, as in Shisochin and Sesan, for example. If a technique is performed in response to both a left and a right attack, then the finishing technique of the sequence is often only tacked onto the second technique.
- The legs and arms are connected. Body rotation and stepping that naturally accompanies each technique generates power. There is no chambering of the attacking hand, as it has traditionally been understood.
- Stepping forward with a blocking move in kata implies that one already has control of the opponent. Look for the initial "block".
- Block the arms, but attack the head. Remember that the Japanese word "uke" means "receiving." Using the word "block" creates a rather restrictive and unnecessarily rigid view of these techniques in kata.
- Don't look at final positions to explain techniques. A kata is not static, but always in motion. The real explanation is in the movement—the weight shifting, stances, arm and leg motions—that leads from the previous posture to the final position of the technique one is attempting to explain.
- Movement within sequences should be continuous and uninterrupted. No gaps.

The question is whether this benefit outweighs the drawbacks, considerable as they are, that have led to a general disagreement about kata and its applications.

The way we teach affects our understanding. This is particularly true of those mnemonic teaching aids contained in the classical katas. To illustrate, I will try to show how a few of the techniques of the Goju-ryu kata Seiunchin demonstrate the sort of confusion traditional teaching methods have inspired and led to the very misunderstandings they were meant to avoid—in some cases, obscuring aspects of the kata that would lead to a better understanding of the system as a whole.

The position of the hands in this technique from the Saifa kata illustrates one of the mnemonic teaching aids contained in kata. The left hand is held around the right fist to show where the defender would be holding the attacker in this grab release technique.

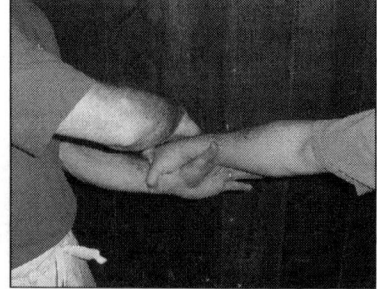
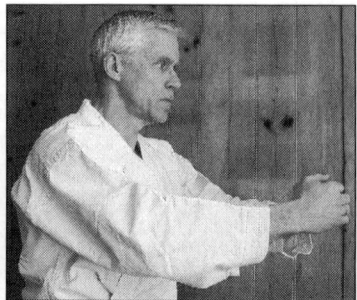

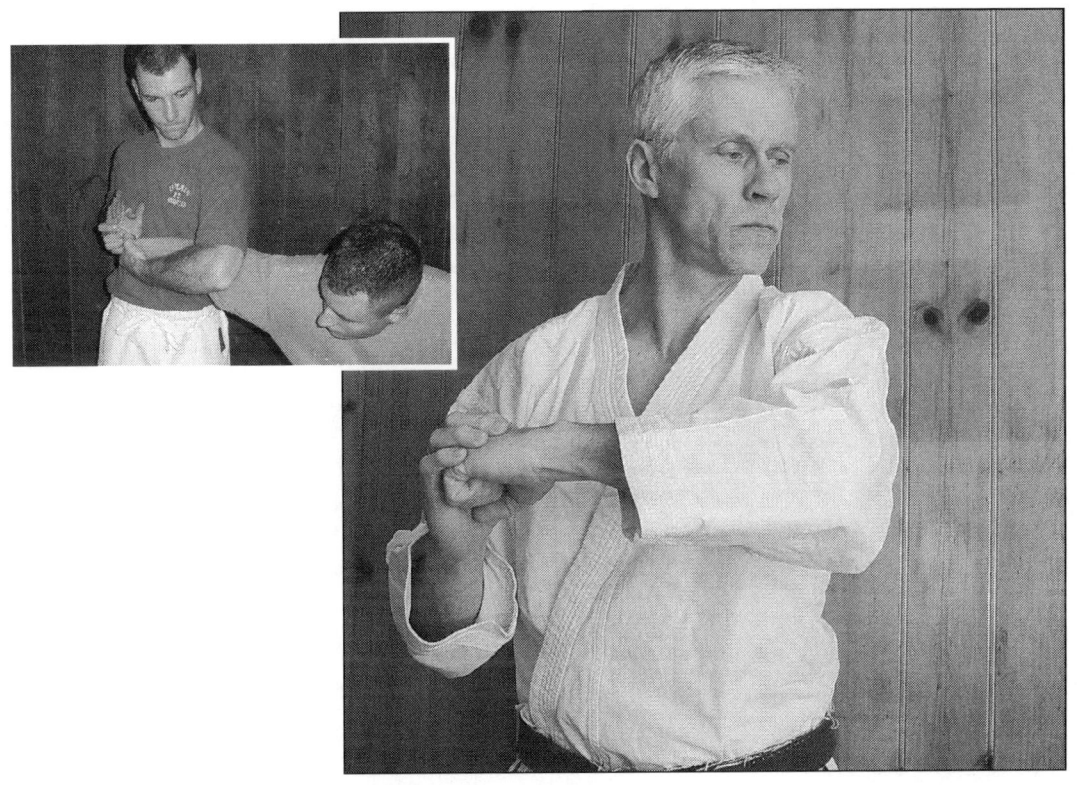

TECHNICAL SECTION

Seiunchin is generally regarded as the second kata in the classical canon of Goju-ryu subjects.[5] Each of the combinations within the kata deals with responses against an opponent's grab or push and shows the defender controlling the opponent as he counter-attacks. Seiunchin contains six of these combinations, not counting repetition: four against wrist grabs and two against pushes or double-hand grabs. The variations—why there are two different responses to a push or double-hand grab and two responses against a cross-hand wrist grab, for example—counter differences in the attacker's strength and commitment to the attack.

It will be apparent almost immediately in some Goju-ryu circles that it is highly contentious to describe the kata categorically as consisting of six combinations of techniques against very specific attacks. To suggest this is somehow blasphemous to those who see kata as a seemingly endless repository of technique.

The way we teach kata, in fact, seems to promote this encyclopedic view of kata. We teach a move at a time, not principles or applications. We dissect the movements so completely that the speed or rhythm we use in teaching becomes so thoroughly ingrained that it frustrates students who try to apply the techniques of the kata in the same manner that they learned them. This method of learning kata has two rather questionable technique. Second, because the kata has been learned piecemeal, we fail to see that the gaps and pauses in movement inserted in places to facilitate learning are not dictated by the application of the various techniques. We tend to disconnect techniques that were meant to be a part of the same sequence. Erroneously, the rhythm and pauses used simply to teach the kata seem to suggest their own applications, or, since they are not recognized as part of the teaching methodology, they interrupt and obscure the kata's more natural application sequences.

Mistakes in Rhythm

Consider the opening moves of Seiunchin kata. The first move of the kata is a step forward, from the beginning ready stance, to the northeast (all directional references assume that the kata starts facing north) with the right foot, dropping into a right-foot-forward horse-riding stance (*shiko dachi*) (1a). The hands open and are brought in front of the body (1b). In some schools, the hands are open, palms facing, with the arms straight, perpendicular to the ground. In other schools, the arms are brought out towards the knees more, with the backs of the hands facing forward. In either case, however, there is no significance to the position of the arms and hands. But since we teach the kata piecemeal, a move at a time, students look for and assign meaning to "every inch" of kata.[6]

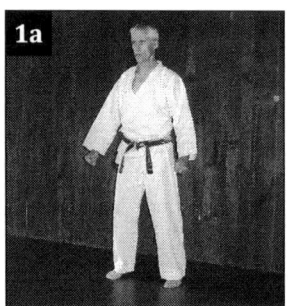
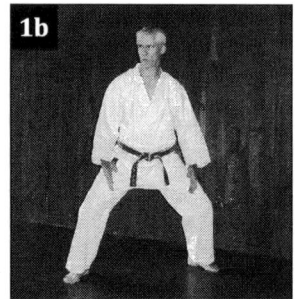

Separating the movement of the feet and hands facilitates learning for the beginner, but this initial rhythm becomes ingrained, repeated by even advanced students, leading to misunderstandings of the applications of the movements. Though it is taught a move at a time, in application the hand techniques that follow are meant to be done at the same time one steps forward into the above horse stance.

Your attacker has grabbed your wrist (1c). As you step to the northeast, on a 45-degree line from the attack and to the outside of the attacking arm, both hands are brought up simultaneously, back to back (1d and f). Your hand then rotates and grabs the opponent's wrist as his other hand, fist closed, is brought down on your attacker's elbow (1e and g). This arm-bar has the effect of bringing your opponent's head forward and down.

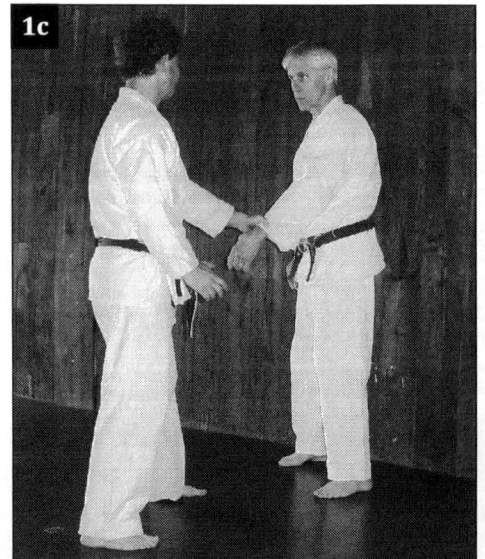
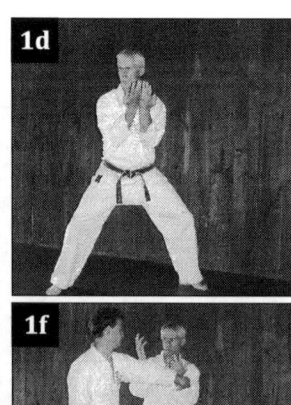
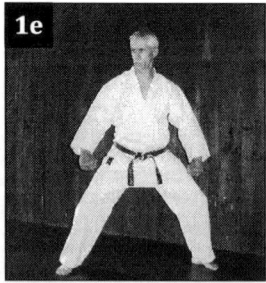
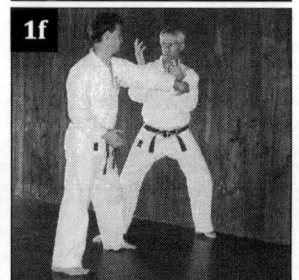
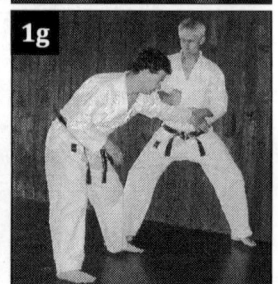

Traditionally, because the application of these kata moves has been left to the imagination and discovery of the student, this technique has generally been explained as a release against a two-handed chokehold or lapel grab. But it makes no practical sense to step forward towards an attacker who is applying a chokehold. However, to the beginning student, who is merely imitating movement when he learns kata, it looks as if both hands are doing the same thing. This is where our methodology—our general reticence in teaching principles—gets us into trouble.

The next hand technique in this sequence of moves has also been fundamentally misunderstood. The katas themselves, as in this hand technique, incorporate mnemonic devices to convey certain principles of movement; that is, certain kata movements are only intended to teach a beginning student how to move and were never meant to be used as applications.

In the hand movements that follow the previous closed-hand grab release and arm-bar (1a–g), both hands are brought up, wrists leading the way, the forward hand at shoulder level and the rear hand to the side of the chest (2a). Since most schools teach kata piecemeal, this palm-up position is seen as having no relationship to the previous technique; however, it is actually part of the same combination. Once the opponent's head has been brought forward and down with the arm-bar, the forward hand comes up to grab the attacker's head (2b and d). As the head is pulled in, the rear open hand is used to attack the opponent's neck or throat (2c and e). The initial palm-up position (2a) is used to remind the student that the elbow should be kept down.

There should be no pause between raising the hand and grabbing the opponent's head. The pause is only used in a teaching sense to check the student's technique, to check that the elbow has indeed been kept down as the hand comes up. This same palm-up movement can be found in a number of places in other Goju-ryu katas, and the same explanation applies. It is not surprising that a Chinese-based system stresses this principle within its pedagogical forms. Classical Chinese martial texts also make a point of mentioning this. Yang Chengfu, the great taijiquan master, reminds us to keep "the elbows folded down," and Wu Yuxiang advises one to "sink the elbows," calling it one of the basic "body principles" (Wile, 1983:6, 27).

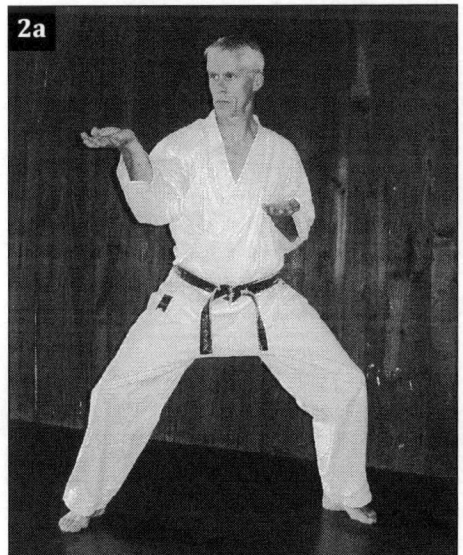
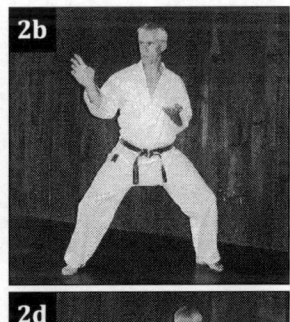
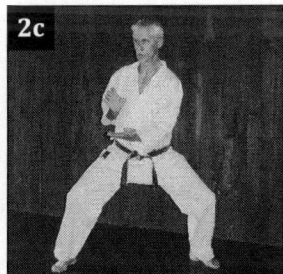
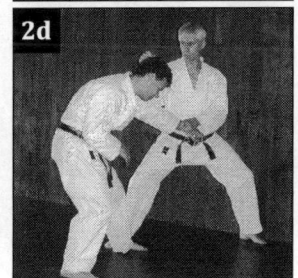
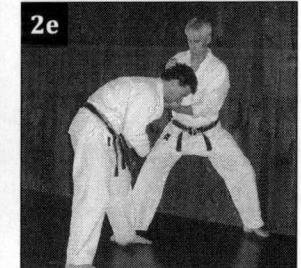

When people fail to realize that the kata itself contains these teaching instructions—whether the teachers themselves have not learned them or students are left to their own devices in how they are to apply the techniques of kata—then each movement is thought to contain application techniques. This movement is often thought to be a chest block followed by a grab (2a–b). But the hand techniques are only separated to facilitate learning proper movement. They are not meant to imply separate applications. One can see, however, that this misconception is a natural outgrowth both of the method by which the movement is taught and the fact that the movement itself contains a mnemonic device that is meant to teach a principle of movement instead of an actual application.

Dissociation of Kata and Applications

While this next sequence of movements in Seiunchin kata (3a–f) may seem to have only a peripheral connection to the problems associated with teaching methodology, the misunderstanding here results from the disconnection we bring to the training hall; we tend to disassociate kata movements from their applications.

In this sequence, after you have grabbed the head and attacked the throat of the opponent (2d–e), you shift to the left into a right-foot-forward cat stance, as the right hand twists and pulls the hair and the left hand grabs the chin (3a–b).[7] Then, shifting forward into a right-foot-forward basic stance, pushing the attacker forward and turning him around, with the right hand pulling the hair and the left hand twisting the chin (3c and e), the defender steps back into a left-foot-forward basic stance, bringing the right elbow up forcefully into the back of the head, neck, or spine (3d and f).

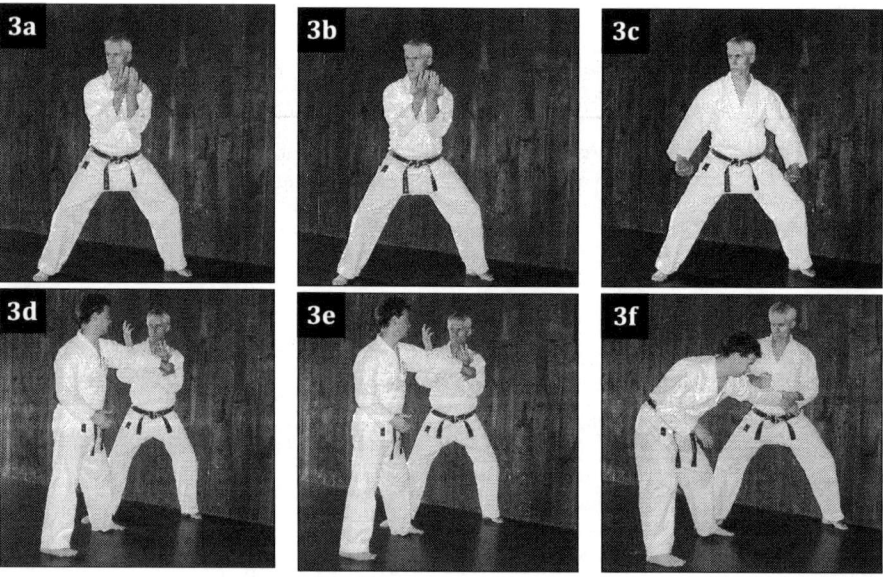

For whatever reason, these applications have not generally been passed on to students. We are dogmatic about preserving the movements of kata, but we tend to see the applications of kata as a creative endeavor, forgetting that the applications (*bunkai*) certainly came before the katas. Perhaps we don't wish to acknowledge the anachronistic nature of an empty hand combat system in modern times, at least the way that it is often studied today. In any case, this sequence of techniques has fed the imagination of students, particularly those raised on the belief that the study of applications is based more on invention than principle.

Failure to Separate Instructional Cues from Application

The next sequence of techniques—the second of the six combinations shown in Seiunchin kata—illustrates the failure to separate the instructional cues within the kata from the application techniques. Like the first sequence, this combination of moves is also a response against a wrist grab. The difference between the two is the strength or commitment of the attacker.

The sequence begins with the right fist being brought into the palm of the left hand in front of the left hip (4a). The hands are then rotated in contact with each other until the right arm is brought across the body to a perpendicular position, elbow down and fist up at shoulder level, with the left palm held along the right wrist, fingers pointing up. At the same time, one steps into a right-foot-forward basic stance to the northeast (4b).

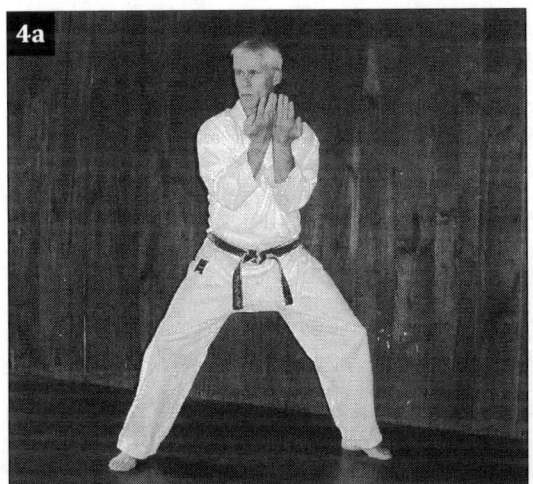

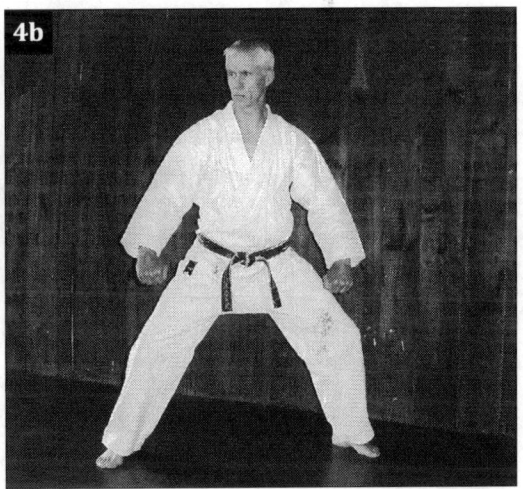

It has always been assumed that this technique demonstrates an assisted block against a very strong attacker who has stepped in with a right punch or has grabbed one's lapel with his right hand. That is, the right arm is blocking and the left palm is pushing against it for support. This is an example of a creative rationalization where there is no foundation of principles or understanding of the mistakes that can arise when one does not fully understand the instructions contained within the kata itself. The confusion comes, in this case, from a too literal interpretation of a movement, one that is ironically meant only to represent an application or to remind the student how the technique should be applied. The left open palm acts as a mnemonic device, reminding the student where on the opponent's body one is applying the technique. One can see the same methodology in Saifa and Sanseiru katas, where again the defender's hand in solo kata is positioned on the body to remind the student of where it will be applied on the attacker [see insets]. In any case, in this technique from Seiunchin kata, it should be clear that the left palm is not simply supporting the right arm, and the right arm is not blocking.

The attacker has grabbed your wrist (4c). Unlike the wrist grab in the first sequence of Seiunchin kata, your attacker here is very strong and locked down on your wrist. As the right hand is brought across to the left hip, the left hand grabs the attacker's wrist (4d). Then, holding onto his wrist, stepping into a right-foot-forward basic stance to the northeast, both hands are brought across the body and up, freeing the right hand (4e). You now continue this sequence by stepping forward, into a left-foot-forward horse stance (*shiko dachi*), along the northeast line, driving your shoulder into your attacker and, breaking his balance, forcing him back and down (4g and h). Holding onto the opponent's wrist and dragging him back, you then step back along the same line, into a right-foot-forward horse stance, using the right forearm—in what is erroneously thought to be a down block—to attack the opponent's head or neck (4g and 4i).

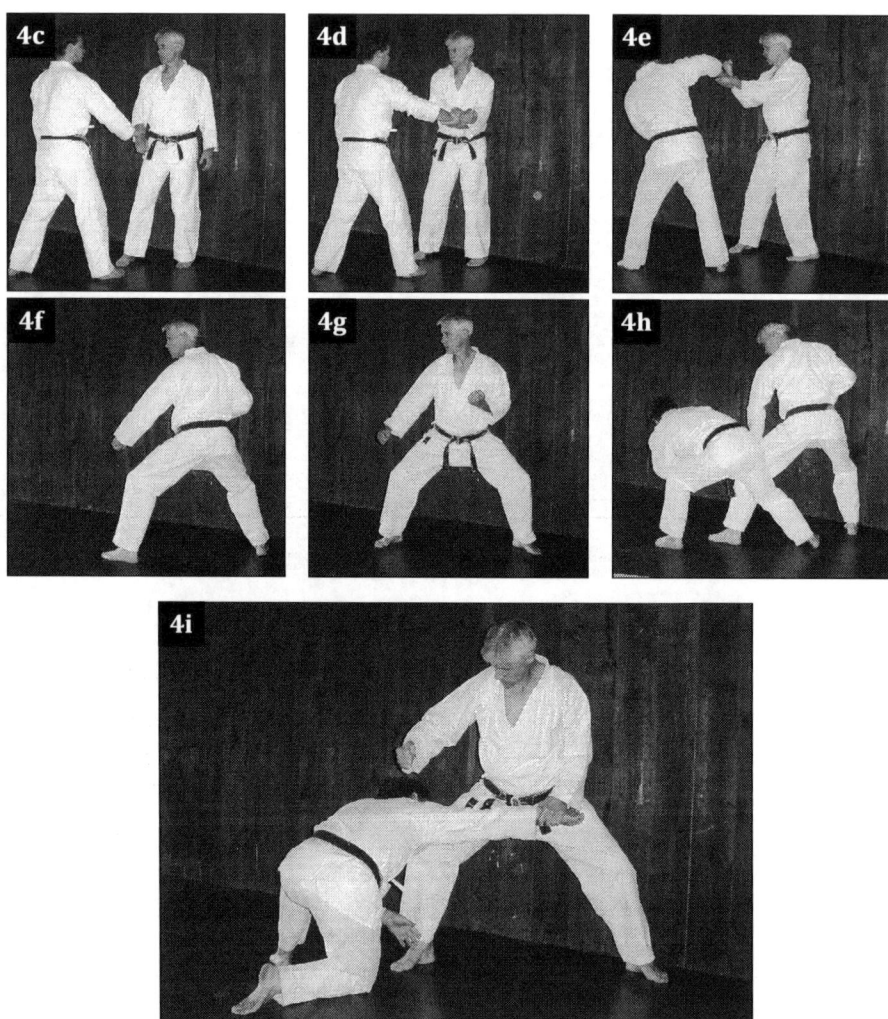

Use of Mnemonic Teaching Devices

Another place where one can see the use of mnemonic teaching devices is the last sequence of Seiunchin kata. Here, you have just completed what are often referred to as two elbow techniques, though the primary function of each of these is a wrist or grab release. After the second of these, in right-foot-forward cat stance (*neko ashi dachi*) (5a–b), you reach over with the left hand to grab the opponent (5c–d). Then, shifting forward, you attack your opponent's collarbone with the right forearm (5e–f).

In the next move of this sequence, you step back into a left-foot-forward cat stance, bringing both open hands into a mountain block (*yama uke*) around the back of your opponent's head (5g–h). Again, because kata is so often taught piecemeal, without any understanding of its structuring principles, this technique has often been explained as a release against a two-handed lapel grab or choke hold. But this series of moves is fairly straightforward if it is executed as a combination of techniques against a single attacker; there should be no gaps in the execution of these techniques.

However, the final technique in this sequence is only implied in the kata. The cat stance acts as a kind of application mnemonic, indicating a knee kick (*hiza geri*). In general, wherever the cat stance occurs in Goju-ryu classical katas, one has hold of the opponent and is counter-attacking from such a close range that the knee, rather than a kick, is the primary technique. In this case, with the forearms and hands of the mountain block being brought around the attacker's head and neck, stepping back and dropping into a left-foot-forward cat stance, the opponent's head is brought forward and down, creating the space to bring the left knee up into the attacker's face (5i). This then, though it is only implied in kata, is the finishing technique in this final sequence of Seiunchin kata.

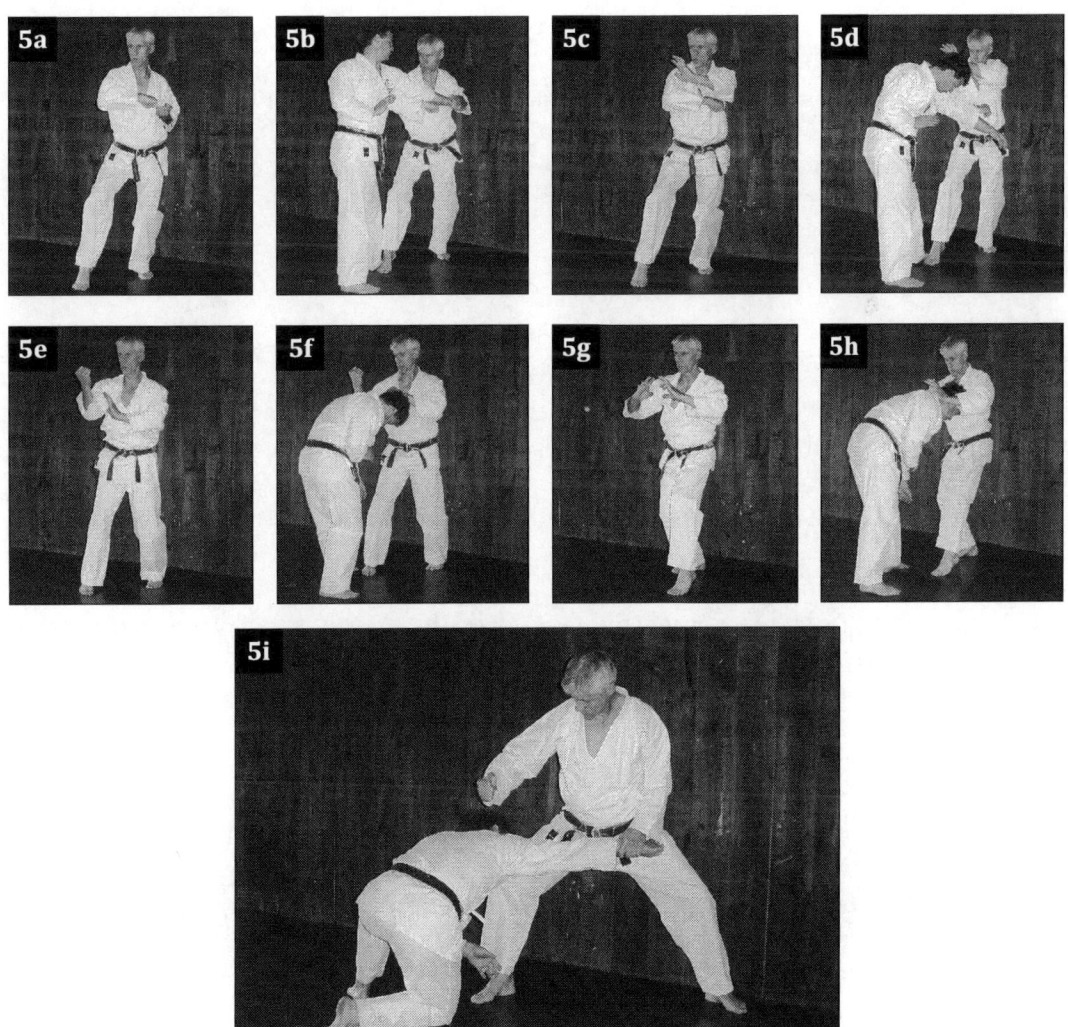

Conclusion

We tend to see mystery where there is only misunderstanding. In the absence of explanation, "secret" or "hidden techniques" (*kakushi-te*) have worked their way into the terminology of kata and the imaginations of students. It is tempting to embrace the mystery of kata as an insoluble conundrum even as we attempt to discover its secrets. After all, we are so often reminded that the journey is more important than the destination. But one should certainly be suspect of anything that purports to offer knowledge wrapped in the cloak of mystery. The Wizard of Oz hides behind a curtain woven of just such whole cloth. Better to unveil the problem, to examine the way we teach and to question what we don't know.

What I have found is that much of the confusion in the way we interpret kata techniques seems to be a natural by-product of the way we teach karate, the way it has always been taught. It has also led, I believe, to a misunderstanding of the patterns and directions of kata (Hopkins, 2004). And, because of the manner in which we dissect kata and train one-point sparring (*ippon kumite*), we have failed to see that katas are composed of combinations or sequences of techniques (Hopkins, 2002).

In certain cases, these differences of opinion or misunderstandings have occurred because some have indeed lost the formula necessary to understand the lessons of kata, but we also need to question our methods. Perhaps it is something rooted in Japanese culture not to question—something inherent in the ethos of martial training that stresses discipline and hard work, built on unquestioning loyalty and devotion to the teacher. On the other hand, there are few teachers, Japanese or American, willing to examine their own methodology, especially when that methodology is part of a long-standing tradition. To question any of this may sound somehow blasphemous. We seem to prefer mysticism to understanding, or at least it would seem so based on the way we teach and the way we study karate.

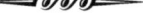

Notes

[1] Upon the death of Miyagi Chojun in 1953, Goju-ryu split into a number of different schools, and over the course of the last half-century, even these schools have broken into different factions. Some researchers have suggested that an analysis of similar kata from different schools might provide valuable clues to the meaning of obscure moves in kata.

[2] This view that katas were used to hide information rather than convey techniques and teach the principles of a martial system seems to have some support in certain quarters. However, it doesn't seem at all logical that the old masters from long ago would hide information from students who had to be accepted by the master, under rigorous character scrutiny, in the first place.

[3] All subsequent references to kata in this chapter refer not to modern training subjects like Gekisai Ichi but to the classical subjects and the teaching of these subjects—Saifa, Seiunchin, Shisochin, Sepai, Sanseiru, Sesan, Kururunfa, and Suparimpei—said to have originated in China, brought to Okinawa by Higaonna Kanryo.

[4] Though it is outside the parameters of this chapter to go into a lengthy discussion of principles of bunkai, it may be useful to mention some in passing. For a more detailed explanation of some of these principles, see author's articles in earlier volumes of the *Journal of Asian Martial Arts*.

⁵ The kanji of Seiunchin is often translated as "control–pull–fight," but the English translation, as well as the kanji itself, has been the subject of some scholarly dispute, which, if nothing else, highlights the difficulties faced by any historical research into the origins of martial traditions. Translations range from "set of pushing and pulling" to "attack distant suppression" to "blue hawk battle." In light of the applications of this kata, however, some kanji and translations would appear to be more appropriate than others.

⁶ There are any number of texts available that will show this first position being used against a bear hug from the rear. There are, however, at least two problems with this interpretation. First, it is not the best or even a very effective technique to use against a bear hug from the rear. And second, the kata doesn't show what one does to the attacker after this; there is no counter-attack if one accepts this explanation of kata technique.

⁷ There is a strong historical component to some of the techniques preserved in the katas that has largely been ignored. As is evident here, these techniques were codified at a time in the past when men generally wore their hair longer or in topknots.

Bibliography

Babladelis, P. (1989). Interview Meitoku Yagi (Goju Ryu). Retrieved on February 1, 2004, from http://www.xs4all.nl/~frits007/history/yagi.htm

Co, A. (1998). *Five ancestor fist kung-fu: The way of Ngo Cho Kun*. Rutland, Vermont: Charles E. Tuttle.

Craig, D. and Anderson, P. (2002). *Shihan-te: The bunkai of karate kata*. Boston, MA: YMAA Publication Center.

Heilman, C. (1997). The dynamics of kata. Retrieved on June 16, 2002, from http://www.ikkf.org/article4Q97.html

Higaonna, M. (February 2004). Suparimpei: Goju Ryu's supreme kata. *Classical Fighting Arts*, (3), 5–10.

Hopkins, G. (2002). The lost secrets of Goju-ryu: What the kata shows. *Journal of Asian Martial Arts, 11*(4), 54–77.

Hopkins, G. (2004). The shape of kata: The "enigma" of pattern. *Journal of Asian Martial Arts, 13*(1), 64–77.

Labbate, M. (2000). Developing advanced Goju-ryu techniques. *Journal of Asian Martial Arts, 9*(1), 56–69.

McCarthy, P. (Trans.) (1995). *The bible of karate: Bubishi*. Rutland, VT: Charles E. Tuttle.

McCarthy, P. Kata: The enigma of Uchinadi. Posted on August 26, 2001, at http://www.fightingarts.com/forums/ubb/Forum10/HTML/000008.html

McCarthy, P. The theory and practice of tradition [sic] karate. Retrieved on January 23, 2002, from http://www.society.webcentral.com.au/Secrets.htm

Schoene, M. (15 Jan. 2004). Interview with Anthony Mirakian Sensei. Retrieved on January 15, 2004, from http://home.achilles.net/~pchan/amintvw.html

Toguchi, S. (2001). *Okinawan Goju-ryu: Advanced techniques of Shorei-kan karate*. Santa Clarita, CA: Ohara Publications.

Wile, D. (1983). *T'ai-chi touchstones: Yang family secret transmissions*. New York: Sweet Ch'i Press.

Acknowledgment

A special thanks to John Jackson, Ole Craig, and Brian Conz for their help in demonstrating applications for this article, and to my teacher, Kimo Wall. Also, a special thanks to my wife, Martha, for her editorial assistance and patience.

chapter 46

The Five Katas of Yagi Meitoku

by Perry Campbell, B.Sc.

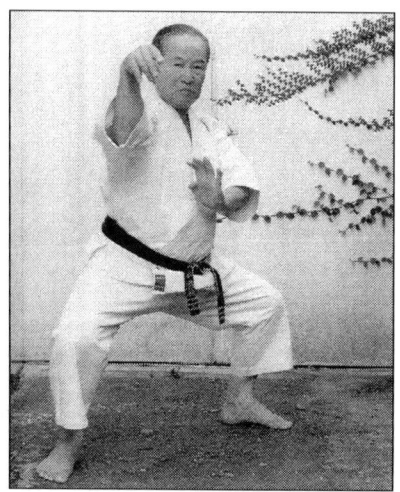

A photograph of Yagi Meitoku in 1985, the year of his 75th birthday.
Master Yagi gave this print to Paul Babladelis in 1989.
All other photographs courtesy of P. Campbell.

Introduction

The passing of Grand Master (*Dai Sensei*) Yagi Meitoku at 91 (February 7, 2003) signified the end of an era in the art of Goju-ryu, leaving a great hole in the Okinawan martial arts community. Mr. Yagi traced his ancestry back to the original thirty-six Chinese families who moved to the Kume district of Naha, Okinawa, more than six hundred years ago, bringing with them, among many things, their martial arts. Yagi Meitoku's love, dedication, and passion for Goju-ryu karate and his teacher, Miyagi Chojun, radiated from him. Mr. Yagi dedicated his life to teaching Goju-ryu's advanced techniques well into his 80's. He left five katas, the Meibuken katas, as his contribution to Goju-ryu karate: Heaven and Earth (*Tenshi*) and the four mythical guardians that protect them: Blue Dragon (*Seiryu*), White Tiger (*Byakko*), Red Sparrow (*Shujakku*), and Black Turtle (*Genbu*). Deceptively simple in format, yet layered with complex theories, the Meibuken katas are Yagi Meitoku's record of the fighting practices, techniques, drills, and innovations he developed over a lifetime of study.

Miyagi's Successor

Upon Miyagi Chojun's passing (October 8, 1953), there were a small group of individuals who felt they were the rightful heirs to the Goju-ryu system: Higa Seko, Miyazato Ei'ichi, Miyagi An'ichi, and Miyagi Chojun's son, Kei. Despite the fact that Miyagi never chose a successor or issued rank to any of his students before his death, very few seniors of the other major Okinawan karate systems disputed Yagi Meitoku's claim as the heir. In the end, the responsibility of choosing a successor fell on the shoulders of Miyagi Chojun's wife and children. According to Miyagi Masu (Tsuru), Miyagi's eldest daughter, choosing Yagi was not difficult. In a letter translated in Ernest Estrada's Interviews, Tsuru said:

> I respect him [Yagi] very much and so does the Miyagi family. Upon my father's death, the family met to discuss who would succeed my father as head of Goju-ryu. The decision was based on who studied the longest, and who was the most dedicated and loyal to my father. It was then that Meitoku Yagi was decided upon to head Goju-ryu. At that time we decided to formally recognize him by giving him my father's karate uniform and belt.

Mr. Yagi's son, Meitetsu, confirmed his father's loyalty to Miyagi. Meitetsu said he could remember each time a typhoon struck Okinawa while Miyagi was alive:

> My father would first go to Miyagi's home to close the shutters and prepare for the storm. Only after Miyagi's home was secure would father return to prepare our home.

To certify the Miyagi family's choice of Yagi Meitoku as the second grandmaster of the Goju-ryu system, they presented him with Miyagi's uniform (*dogi*). Tsuru said:

> It was felt that instructor Yagi was the best person to carry on my father's teachings. So he was asked to continue my father's teachings and also to expand on the teachings so that everyone would know Goju-ryu.

Training with Miyagi Chojun

Yagi Meitoku was twelve years old when his grandfather took him to Miyagi Chojun's school to begin formal training. At that time, there were five or six students senior to Yagi, including Higa Seko, Nakaima Genkai, Azama Kasai (Nanjo Kiju), Toguchi Seikichi, and Sakiyama Tatsutoku.

Instructor Yagi said they did many repetitions of preparatory exercises (*yobi undo*) with each student, counting 100 to 1,000 repetitions of each technique. It was very demanding and most new students went elsewhere to look for easier training. In those early days, Miyagi taught only four katas: Sanchin, Sesan, Seiunchin, and Tensho. These were the open hand (*kaishu*) katas. Of these forms, Seiunchin and Sesan were considered the training katas and had to be studied thoroughly to understand Goju-ryu. Yagi was among the first of Miyagi's students to learn all the katas, including Saifa, Shisochin, Sanseiryu, Sepai, Kururunfa, and Suparimpei, which Miyagi started teaching when Yagi was in his first year of junior high school.

Instructor Yagi said it would take four to five years before they even began learning the kata. Then Miyagi would teach them only one kata for two or more years. He said Sanchin training was particularly severe. Yagi recounted how people would recognize him as a student of Miyagi just from the bruises on his shoulders from Miyagi's severe testing in Sanchin.

In His Later Years

I first met Master Yagi in 1988. I recall wondering what would he be like. Would he be fierce or impatient? I had heard stories of his awesome power. He often broke punching boards (*makiwara*) at will. How he had seemingly little to do with other Goju-ryu styles. So it was a shock that he was nothing like I'd expected him to be. Mr. Yagi was soft spoken, friendly, and tranquil, very much like my grandfather had been. Yet, his eyes were sharp and could change at will into something to be feared, exemplifying his killing stare (*koroshi no mei*). The muscles under the aging skin were amazingly powerful and he moved with graceful fluidity and speed despite his advanced years.

In 1990, when I moved to Okinawa, it was immediately apparent that Yagi's passion had not ebbed. By then he had retired from formal teaching, yet he continued to teach three children's classes each week—a group that he had surprisingly little control over. He would also instruct foreigners in the mornings. The foreigners' visits would generally last two or three weeks. Since I was living there, however, he worked with me each morning and then again in the afternoon, six and seven days a week. Further, he would allow my participation in the children's classes. During this period, despite his occasional bouts with poor health, he would not only come to the dojo to teach two and three times a day, he would practice daily. It was during this period that I began to see how remarkable Yagi Meitoku really was.

At eighty, Yagi was deceptively fluid and quick, and he still possessed great power. Yet there was more to him. He regularly played piano and violin. He was a master calligrapher. In 1988, he was the Japanese champion of Chinese chess (*chunji*). In 1989, he defended his title and became world champion as well. Not surprisingly, his mastery of strategy carried into his martial arts theories, technique, and applications. They are also were embedded within his five Meibuken katas.

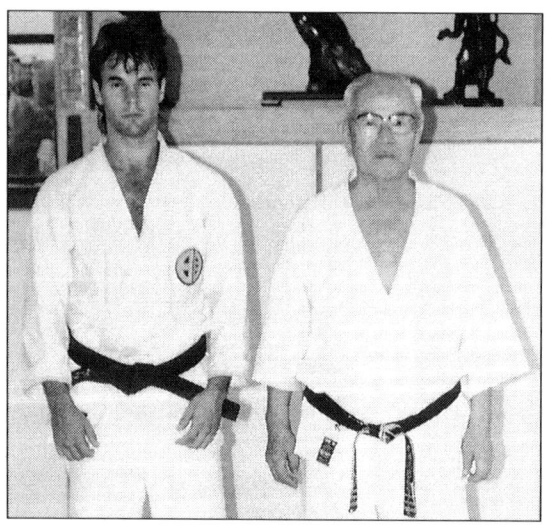

The author with Yagi Meitoku
in Okinawa, 1988.

Influences

Some have said that Mr. Yagi taught the kata "exactly" as Miyagi Chojun taught him, however, this was not the case. As the Miyagi family requested, Yagi Meitoku spent his entire life studying and expanding upon his teacher's teachings. There are several nuances and finer points of the Goju-ryu kata he developed in his later years. Some of these alterations came after even some of his senior students had opened their own schools. Hence, not all of his direct students practice some of his innovations.

In addition to his teacher, Miyagi Chojun, Yagi credited two men who influenced his innovations, although there may have been others. The first was his friend, Ko Shinko—a Chinese martial arts master from Taiwan who is also recognized as having introduced conditioning drills (*kotikitai*) to Okinawan karate. The second was another close friend, Taira Shinken, the weapons master and president of the Ryukyu Kobudo Hozoin Shinkokai. Although each innovation Yagi incorporated was subtle, each notably increased the technique's strength and effectiveness. Not only do the Meibuken katas expand upon Goju-ryu's techniques, they also include the influences of these two men.

The Chinese influence in the Meibuken katas is immediately apparent from the first movement. Yagi Meitoku incorporated the Chinese style of bow and opening—feet are shoulder width apart, hands form a triangle in front of the body at chin level, with the right hand a fist and the left open (a representation of the Chinese character for the Ming Dynasty). The most significant import from the Chinese system, however, is the idea of putting two solo forms together to create a two-man set with almost no alterations to the original forms. At a basic level, these sets contain striking, kicking, and grappling techniques, all executed in continuous motion from beginning to end. At deeper levels, the applications are brutally efficient.

Deceptive Brilliance

I think the two most remarkable aspects of Mr. Yagi's katas is the secret way they pair—Seiryu/Byakko, Shujakku/Genbu, and Tenshi)—fitting together to be practiced as two-man sets. The second is that he developed these kata in his head (bearing in mind that the second kata of each set must be performed reversed—in the mirror image—to make them work together). He did this without the benefit of a partner to ensure that they would be synchronized. These are clear indicators of Yagi's advanced understanding of strategy.

THE FIVE MEIBUKEN KATAS

Heaven and Earth

Originally called Fukyo Kata I and II, Heaven and Earth (*Tenshi*) was Yagi's first Meibuken kata. In the book *Okinawan Karate-do Goju-ryu Meibukan* by Yagi Meitetsu, Carl Wheeler, and Brock Vickerson (1998), Yagi said, "I first got the idea for this kata following a visit to Taiwan." Tenshi is one kata when split into two halves—Heaven and Earth—the halves fit together to form a short two-man set. The kata is characterized by open-hand and finger strikes, double strikes, wrist throws, and scooping the leg. Developed in 1974, Tenshi was an experiment that proved a success and paved the way for the next four Meibuken katas.

Blue Dragon

Blue Dragon (*Seiryu*) is the mythical guardian of the west. The form is characterized by knee kicks, percussion strikes, and powerful waist and hip rotations used in the generation of power in both blocking and striking. Blue Dragon couples with White Dragon to form a two-man set. Thus it contains the attacks and counterattacks for White Dragon.

The rotation of the hips and waist in the wrist block/punch/low block combination is conducted around the body's center axis, with the body upright. Mr. Yagi frequently used a short trident (*sai*) as a model to demonstrate the rotation. Holding the sai perpendicular to the ground, handle upwards, he would rotate the sai clockwise and counterclockwise in his hand. The rotating tangs clearly demonstrate the rotation he wanted.

White Tiger

White Tiger (*Byakko*) is the mythical guardian of the east. The form's techniques are the opposite of those in Blue Dragon. White Tiger is characterized by powerful punching techniques, utilizing upward and downward movement to generate power. This is accomplished by dropping rapidly from a high stance to a low stance, and then springing back to a high stance. The power generated through this dropping and springing proves effective against those of Blue Dragon, which as mentioned utilizes rotation. White Tiger also introduces defending against an attack to the knee.

Red Sparrow

Red Sparrow (*Shujakku*) is Okinawa's mythical guardian of the north. The kata is characterized by open-hand strikes, feinting, rapid hand/foot combinations, and escaping grabbing and locking attacks. When worked as part of the two-man set with its partner, Black Turtle, Red Sparrow is light and quick—like the bird it is named after—and elusive to Black Turtle's grappling holds.

Interestingly, the origin of Red Sparrow's final movement is the same as the second to last movement of Miyagi's original version of Tensho—Heishu Kata Tensho—which Yagi resurrected in early 1991.

Black Turtle

Black Turtle (*Genbu*) is the mythical guardian of the south. This form was completed in late 1990 and is Mr. Yagi's last kata. The mate for Red Sparrow, Black Turtle is characterized by the use of dropping into low, solid stances for blocking and striking. But at times, one springs up to a standing position to deliver a devastating blow. The kata also incorporates grappling. When practiced with Red Sparrow, the grappling and counters flow freely between strikes. This kata's techniques are strong and powerful.

Black Turtle's last movement is also the final movement of Miyagi's Tensho—Heishu Gata Tensho. According to Yagi, the final two movements are actually a Chinese exercise for increasing longevity. Their martial applications, however, are a full Nelson and its counter-technique.

Black Turtle & Red Sparrow
(*Genbu* and *Shujakku*)

The first movements of these two katas with their corresponding partner sequences.

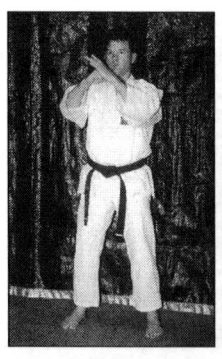 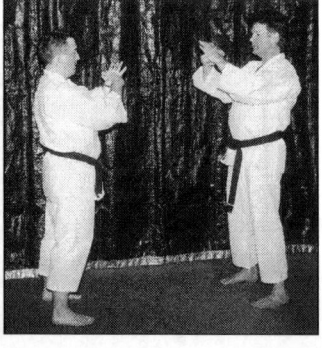

Both the Black Turtle and Red Sparrow katas commence with a formal bow.
Partners pair off in the combined Black Turtle and Red Sparrow katas.

PHOTOGRAPH COLUMN LAYOUT

| Black Turtle | Paired | Red Sparrow |

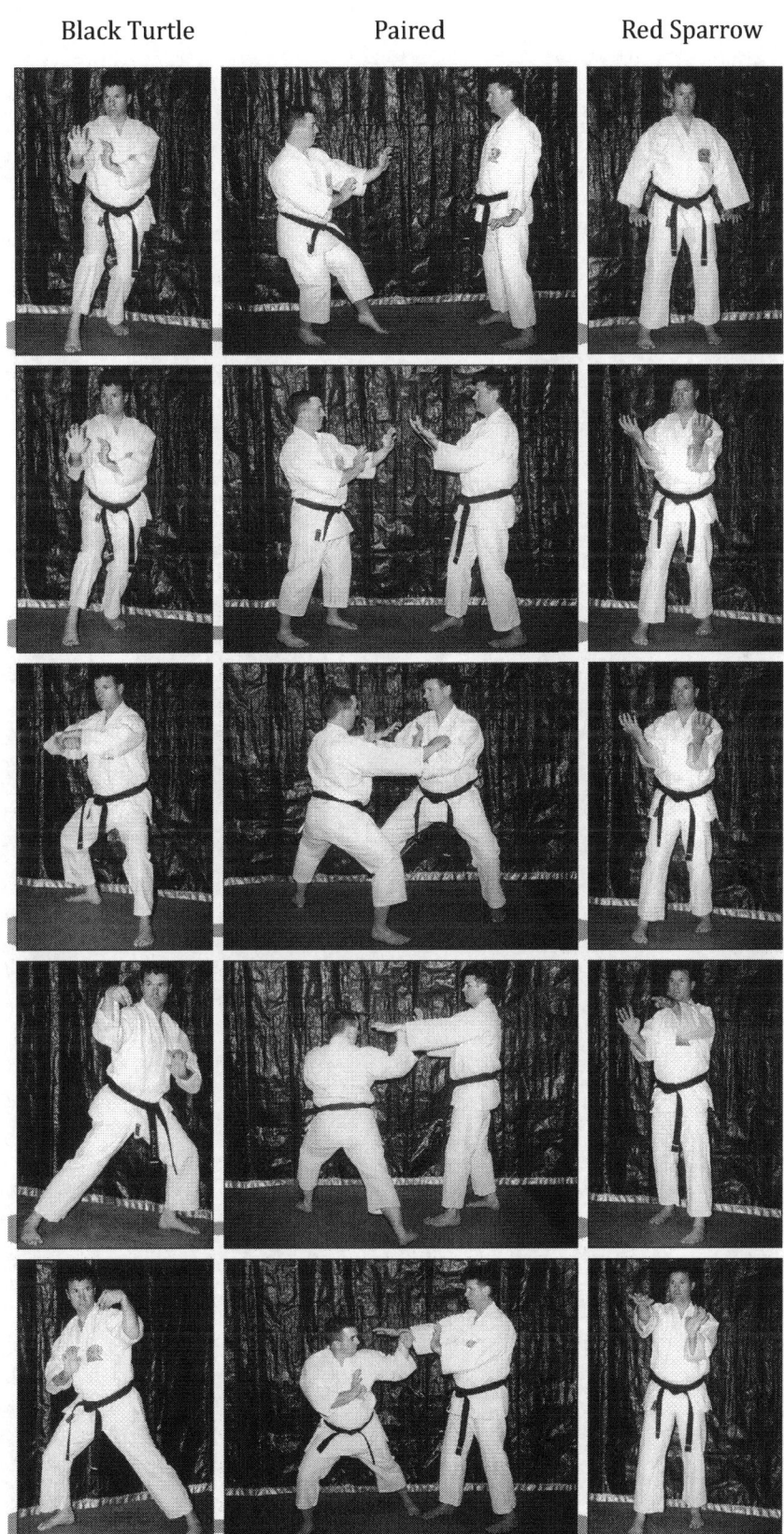

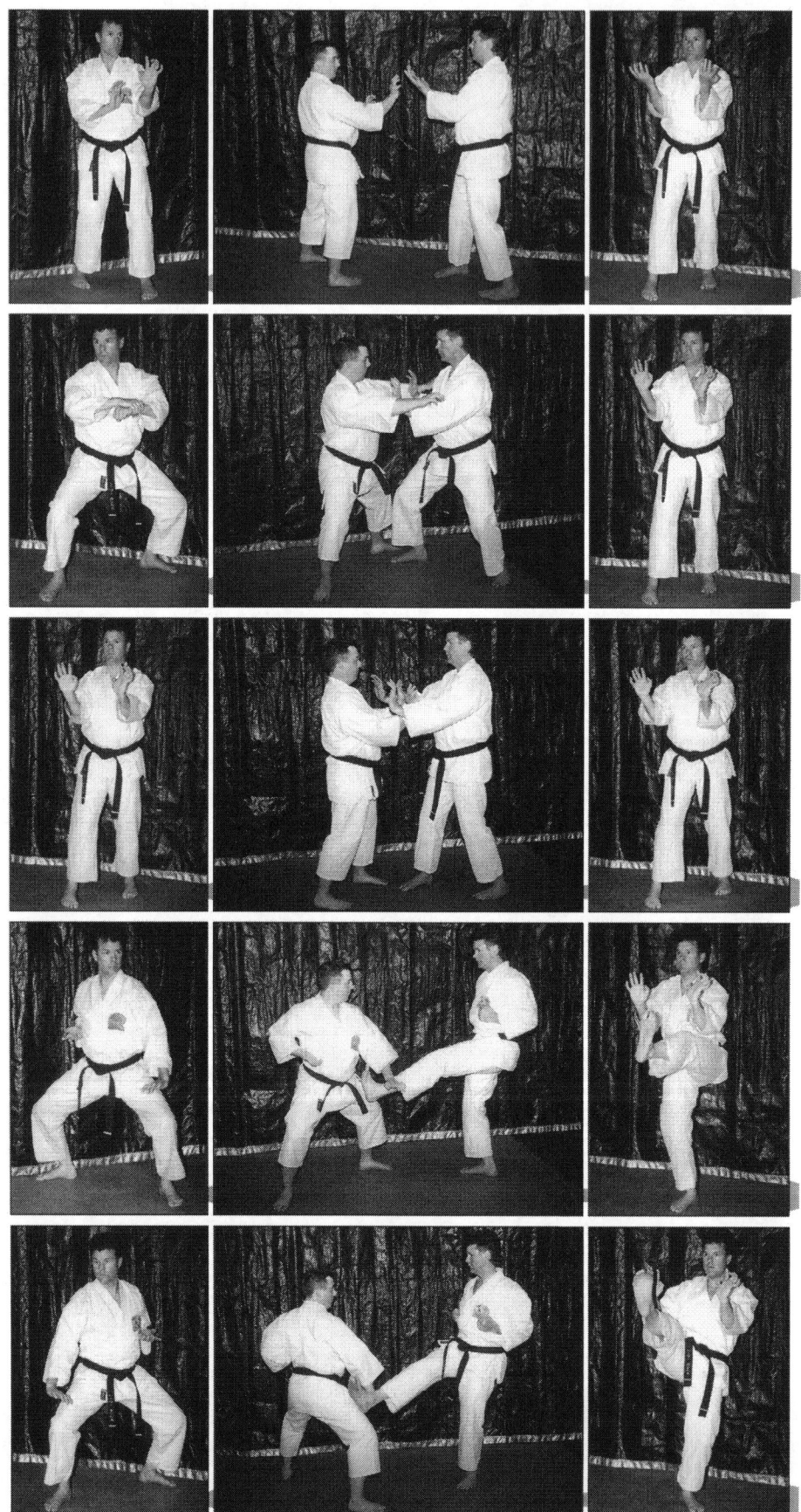

Blue Dragon & White Tiger
(*Seiryu* and *Byakko*)

The first six movements of these two katas with their corresponding partner sequences, beginning with a formal bow.

| White Tiger | Paired | Blue Dragon |

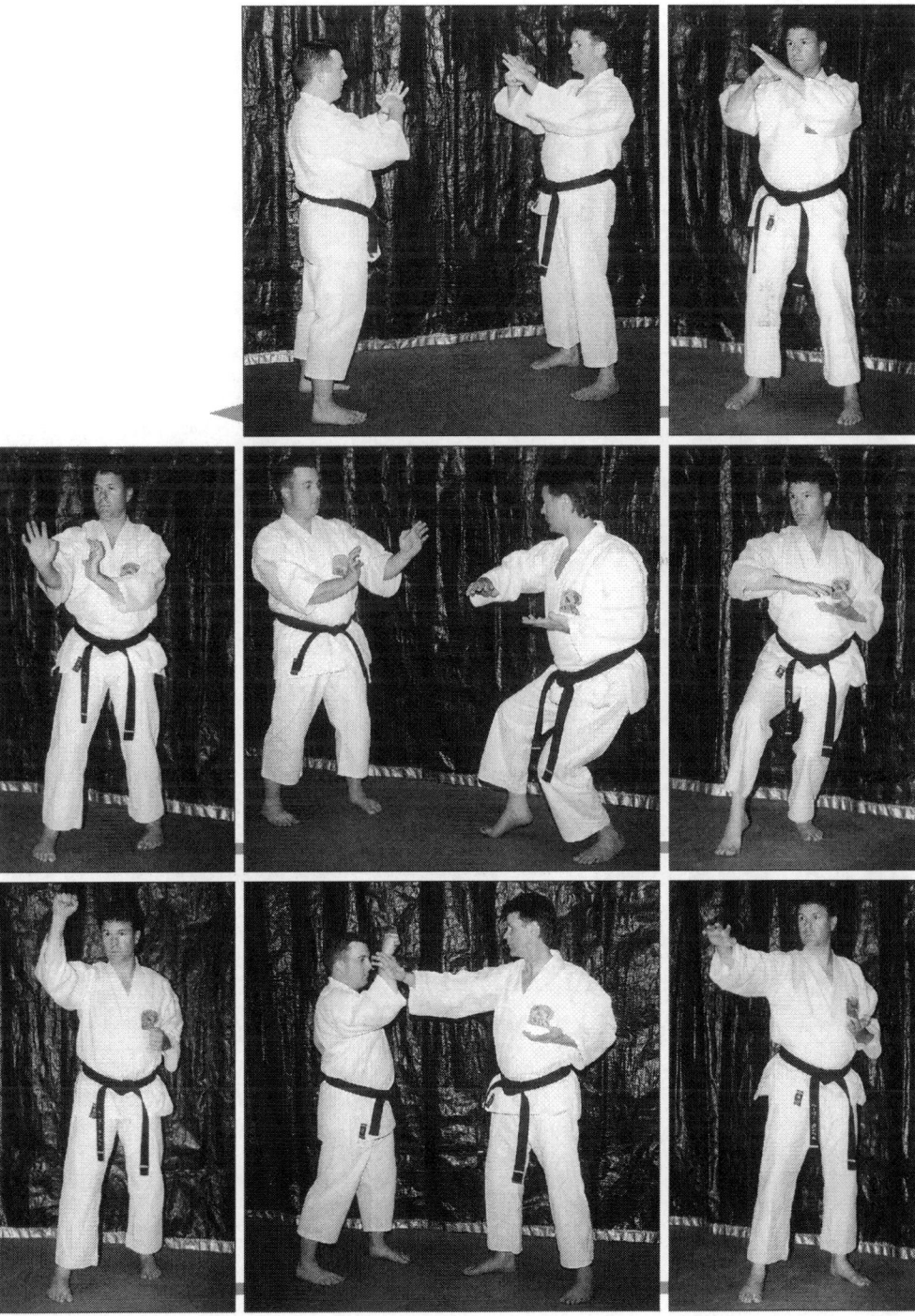

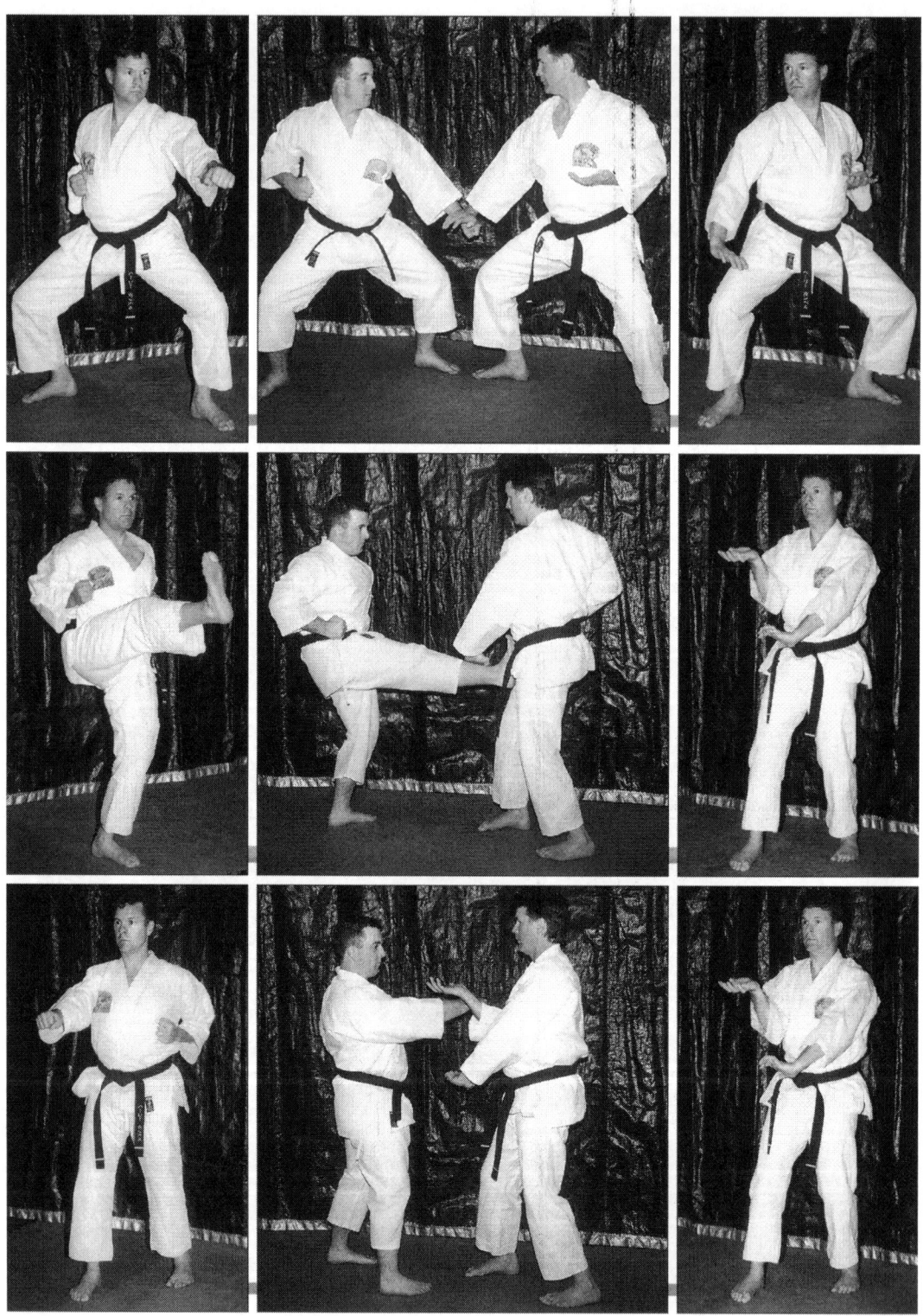

Advanced Applications from Heaven and Earth Kata
(Tenshi)

Tenshi's first movement and application.

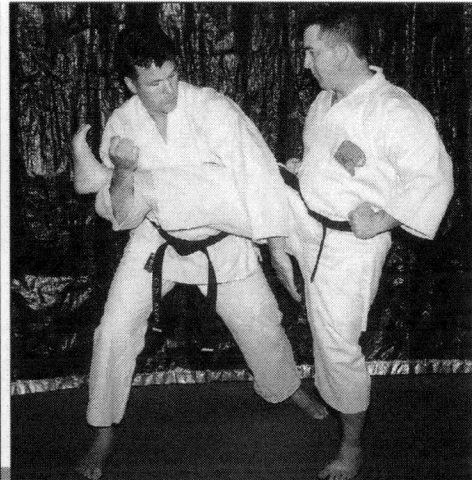

Two later movements found in Tenshi kata and possible applications.

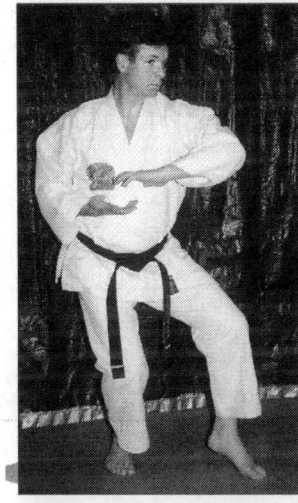
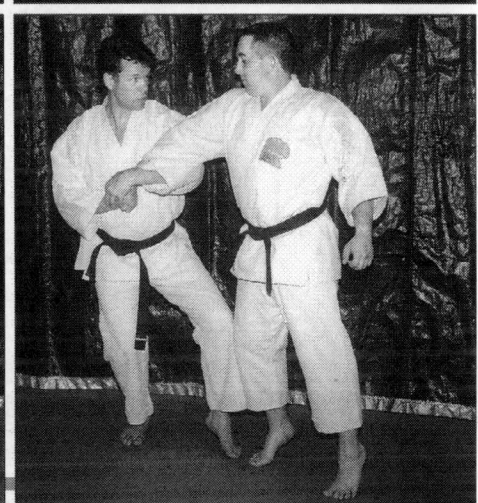
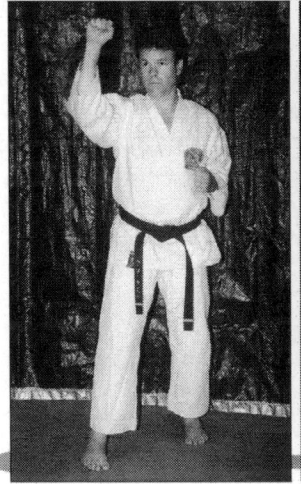
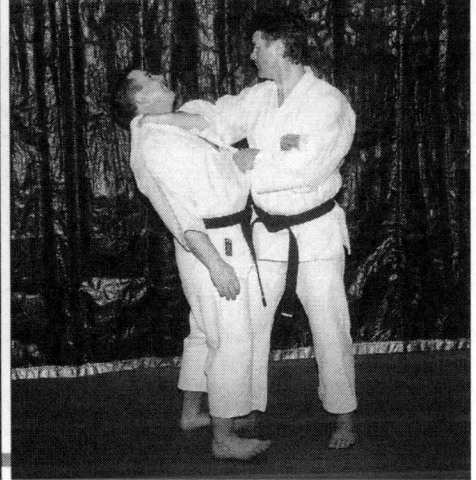

Advanced Application from Red Sparrow Kata

The photograph on the left shows the solo movement in the kata, followed by the series which shows a takedown.

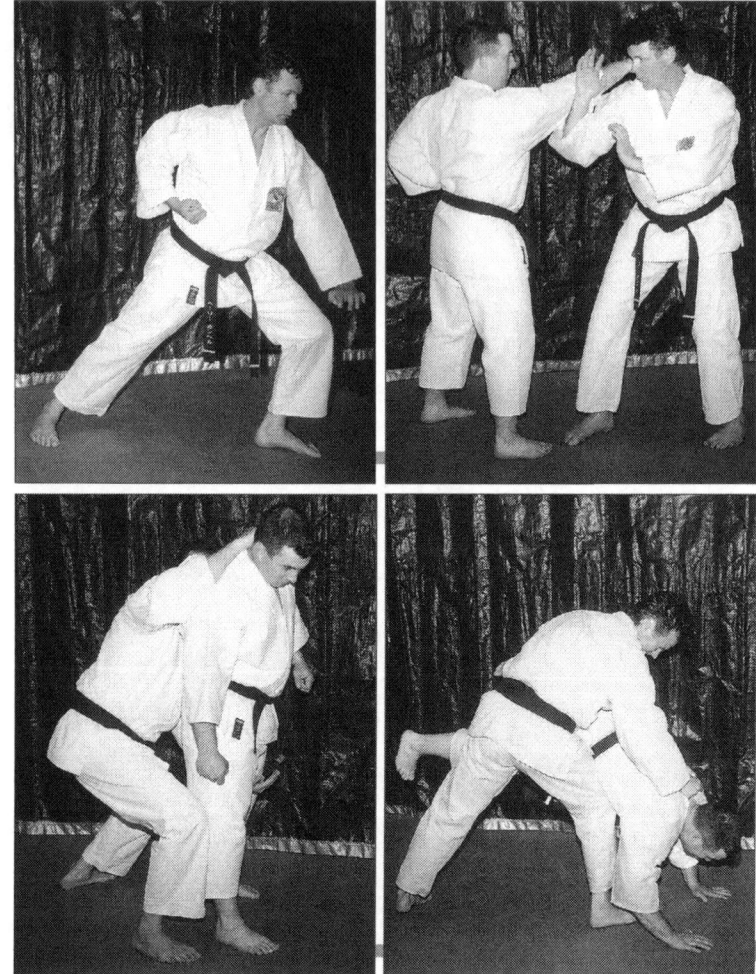

Set-up and finishing take-down.

The Legacy

Yagi Meitoku and his peers are from a period that has been called "the Golden Age of karate." With their passing, the last remnants of their era are disappearing as well. Yet all has not been lost. Along with Yagi Meitoku's direct students who continue his teachings, Yagi Sensei has left a tangible record of some of his knowledge, techniques, theories, and innovations in his Meibuken katas.

chapter 47

The Legacy of Dr. Richard Kim: An Interview with Brian Ricci

by Robert Toth

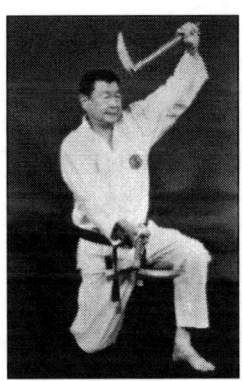 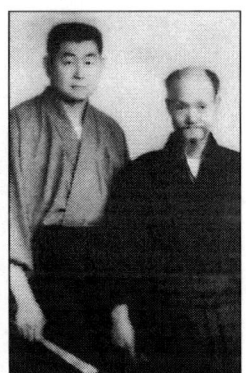

Left: Richard Kim with Yoshida Kotaro.
Right: Dr. Kim demonstrating a technique with sickles.

Introduction

As an artist uses different medium such as clay, paint, or music as a means of artistic expression, a martial artist uses his own life (Kim, 1988). Richard Kim was such an artist. His completed artistic work, his life, went far beyond what most people could ever hope to imagine, let alone accomplish. If the student must surpass the teacher to pay his debt to him, then Richard Kim set the bar very, very high. He was a boxer, soldier, priest (Warrener, n.d.), Ph.D. in oriental philosophy (Warrener, 1982: 65), writer and lecturer, linguist who spoke six languages (Ricci, 2005, May 17), and a martial arts teacher (*sensei*).

Sensei is a term meaning "teacher" or "instructor" used in all Japanese and Okinawan arts. It is written in Japanese with two characters, *sen* (before) and *sei* (life). Within the martial arts context, the sensei is a person with considerable experience of life, some from the normal course of living and some from the martial arts (Castilonia, 1996:143, 144).

Sensei are charged with developing their students to the highest potential and are considered pointers of the Way (*do*) (Sells 2000:369). Sensei are responsible for overseeing the training and personal development of their students. They command absolute respect and authority. The students, in return, accept their sensei's authority and follow his teachings without question (Wingate, 1993:24).

The sensei must constantly exemplify the highest standards of martial art discipline, the whole idea of which is to develop character. The martial Way must be the sensei's way of life, and he must give himself completely to his art in order to pass on the full range of that art's teaching to his students (McCarthy, 1987:10). Dr. Kim was an exemplary sensei.

A Brief Overview of Dr. Kim's Life Story

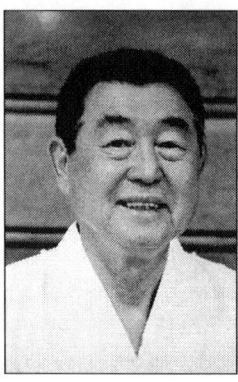

Dr. Richard Kim.

Richard Kim was born in Hawai'i on 17 November 1919 of a Korean father and Japanese mother (Warrener, 1982:91). His father was a landscaper and his mother owned a hotel (Ricci, 2005, May 4). The basement of the hotel was rented to judo instructor Tachibana. When Richard was six years old, his mother enrolled him in judo classes (Warrener, n.d.).

Kim's karate training began in 1927 with Arakaki Ankichi (1899–1927), a disciple of Yabu Kentsu (Kim, 1974:3). Yabu Kentsu had been a student of two great Okinawan karate masters, Matusumura Sokon and Itosu Yasutsune. Yabu was one of the first men to teach martial arts in the Okinawan school system and was known as "The Sergeant" (McCarthy, 1987:32). In 1927, on his way back to Okinawa after a visit to California, Yabu stopped over in Hawai'i. He gave a demonstration at the Nuuanu YMCA on 8 July 1927 (Svinth, 2001:10, 14). After seeing the demonstration, Richard Kim started training in Yabu's Shorinji-ryu style (Warrener, n.d.), which is a synthesis of Okinawan and Japanese karate (Farkas and Corcoran, 1983:242). In the 1930's, Kim met Yabu Kentsu again in Japan and continued training with him (Ricci, 2005, April 21).

"Biggie" Kim, as he was known, spent a great deal of time as a teenager at local boxing clubs, where he acquired boxing skills by acting as a sparring partner for some of the top world contenders (Kim, 1982:6, 7). He later explained what he learned most from boxing was the jab and focus. He also learned the limitations of boxing when he witnessed a Hall of Fame lightweight boxer driven head first into the floor by a Samoan (Ricci, 2005, April 21). Kim had 42 fights in the ring and became the champion of the Orient while living in Shanghai (Warrener, 2001:93).

After graduating from high school, Kim attended the University of Hawai'i. At the university, he joined the Reserve Officers Training Corp (ROTC) and was made a captain. Men who completed the training were given commissions in the US Army Reserve (www.hawaii.edu/armyrotc).

In 1939, Kim arranged to travel to Japan by working on a ship in lieu of payment (Warrener, n.d.). He was able to go to Japan because he had been born prior to the Exclusions Act of 1924 and held dual citizenship (Warrener 2001:93). But upon arrival, he had to "jump ship" because he was underage (Ricci, 2005, April 21). Once in Japan, Kim became a member of the Japanese military (Warrener 2001:92).

In Japan, Kim trained with Yoshida Kotaro in Daito-ryu aikijutsu (Warrener, n.d.). Daito-ryu was one of the most renowned of the old Japanese styles of combat and had been practiced by Minamoto clan warriors for several centuries before the Takeda family inherited it (Ratti and Westbrook, 1973:356). Kotaro had trained with Takeda Sokato (Warrener, n.d.).

Yoshida Kotaro was renowned for his weapon skills (Sells, 2000:135, 137) and was an expert with the spear (*yari*) and the glave (*naginata*) (Corcoran, et al., 1993:396). The training with Yoshida Kotaro was very physical and very harsh. Kotaro taught throwing techniques and also worked with swords and knives. Kim became an apprentice under Kotaro and eventually was given the Daito-ryu *menkyo kaiden* (Warrener, 2001:92). Menkyo kaiden is a certificate that attests to a student's full proficiency and is usually awarded to the advanced student deemed most suited to carry on the art (Farkas and Corcoran, 1983:177).

Richard Kim was then sent to China as an interpreter for a Japanese Imperial Army officer (Ricci Dec. 12, 2005). Here he had the opportunity to study martial arts. Chen Chin-wan taught him a slightly modified version of Yang style taijiquan. He learned baguazhang with Chao Hsu-lie whom he met while in Hong Kong. Kim also trained in Yiquan gongfu with Wang Xiangzhai (1885/6–1963). His first lesson was to stand in a qigong posture known as "embrace the tree" for three hours a day (Warrener, n.d.). While living in Shanghai, Kim also attended St. John's University (Kim, 1982:6–7).

After World War II, Kim owned and operated a bar in Yokohama, Japan. Mas Oyama and Kinjo Hiroshi would come by his house once a week to train. He later met Yamaguchi Gogen through Oyama (Warrener, n.d.). During this period, Kim represented the Seaman's Union in Yokohama (Kim, 1999).

In 1959, Kim moved to San Francisco, California (Kim, 1974:3). He conducted a martial arts program at the Chinese YMCA until his semi-retirement in 1978. Over the years, Dr. Kim traveled all over the world teaching the martial arts. He created a large international organization, the Zen Bei Butokukai, with schools in the US, Canada, and Europe. *Zen Bei* literally translates as "All Rice." Japanese characters, however, can have multiple meanings, depending on the context. The character for "rice" can refer to "people in general." So, Zen Bei can also be translated as "All People" (Foley, 2005, July 3).

In 2000, the Hawai'i Karate Kodanshakai awarded Dr. Kim a tenth-degree black belt (Goodin, 2005). In the same year at a gathering held in a Chinese restaurant in Sacramento, Dr. Kim told the group that he had awarded a seventh-degree ranking to his longtime student, Brian Ricci. That was the only time he had conferred that rank on anyone. It was the highest dan ranking he had ever given (Ricci, 2005, May 22).

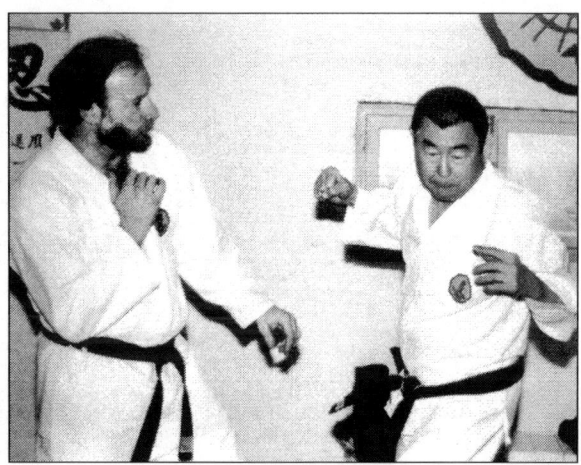

Dr. Kim demonstrating
a boxing technique in Hamilton, Ontario.

Kim Sensei did not attend the annual Zen Bei Butokukai 2001 Summer Camp held at Guelph University in Ontario, Canada, because of poor health. He arranged for Brian Ricci to run the camp in his absence. At a black belt meeting on the first evening of the summer camp, Ricci explained that he had expected that some day Kim Sensei would not be able to teach, but had hoped it would not have been so soon. Ricci made it clear that he had been put in charge of the camp and he intended to fulfill his responsibility to his sensei.

Richard Kim died on 8 November 2001. Brian Ricci has continued his teacher's work in propagating the martial arts. The majority of Kim Sensei's students now train with Ricci Sensei. The Zen Bei Butokukai International Summer Camp at Guelph University continues to be held every year and has grown under Ricci Sensei's care with students attending from all over North America.

BRIAN RICCI INTERVIEW

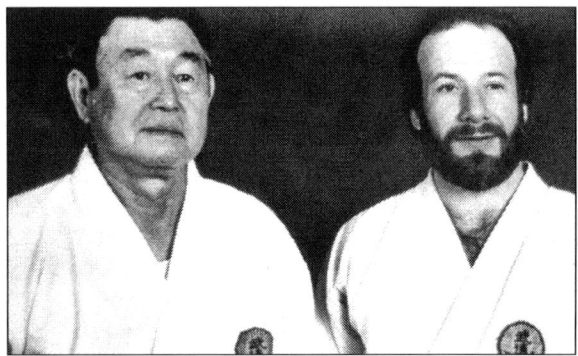

Dr. Kim with Brian Ricci.

The following interview with Brian Ricci Sensei was conducted by Robert Toth on 21 April 2005 in St. Catharines, Ontario.

■ WHEN AND WHERE WERE YOU BORN?

I was born on August 14, 1950 in Everett, Massachusetts, six miles from downtown Boston. Today, I live a half a mile from where I was born.

■ WHEN DID YOU FIRST BECOME INVOLVED WITH THE MARTIAL ARTS AND WHY?

I've always been a movie buff. Watching Jimmy Cagny doing judo in Blood on the Sun or the Mr. Moto movies. Nobody knew what karate was back then, but I knew I wanted to learn how to do those techniques.

It was about 1962 when I went to my mother and said that I'd like to learn jujutsu. She told me to get a book. When I was about 14, I told her that I wanted to learn karate. She said that she didn't want to have anyone in the house who knew how to kill people [laughs]. But in 1965, I had to have a chest operation. When I was leaving the hospital in a cast my dad asked, "Any wish?" I could have anything I wanted. So, I told him I wanted to take karate. From the hospital he took me to a karate school. Then on 15 March, after I healed, I started at a Shotokan karate school.

■ WHO WAS YOUR FIRST INSTRUCTOR? DID YOU GET YOUR BLACK BELT FROM HIM?

Peter Ventresca. Yes, I got my black belt from him in 1972.

■ You don't make your living with martial arts instruction. What all do you do?
I do a number of different things. A lot of things in the movie industry. Stunts and special effects. When I first moved to California, I was living at the YMCA. I heard fire engines and I went out to see what was going on. They were filming the movie Towering Inferno. I met the wardrobe man for the movie and at one point he said to me, "just walk over there." If you look at the Towering Inferno video, near the end of the movie you'll see me walking past behind the actors. Much later I was doing a martial arts demonstration and a fellow came over and asked me if I could coordinate the same kind of thing for special effects in the theater.

If you read the introduction I wrote for Sensei Kim's book, *The Classical Man* [1982], you'll see how I feel about teaching martial arts for a living.

■ When did you first meet Sensei Kim?
I was 23 years old and it was July 1973. I had been training with Luis DeBacario for about two years. I wanted to learn in more depth, so I sent Sensei Kim a letter. He sent word back that I could train and that was it. I decided to quit my job and drove my 1969 Buick from Boston to San Francisco. I arrived at Sensei's dojo and he asked me how I got there. I told him I drove. He said, "You drove?" I said, "Yes. My car's parked out front." He said, "Not anymore." And when I looked they had towed my car [laughs]! I didn't know the law about parking on the street.

■ What was the training like with Sensei Kim then?
There was vigorous repetition. For months there was no katas [forms], just kick, punch, tiger bends, stretching. Then he told me to come to the summer camp in San Diego. He taught five or six katas in one week. In my background, we learned maybe one kata a year. Sensei asked, "How can you learn the advanced kata without knowing the basic kata?"

■ What did Sensei Kim teach at the Chinese YMCA?
Tuesday and Thursday was taiji. Monday, Wednesday, and Saturday was sparring, free style with takedowns, then we'd do mat work from there. And the staff [*bo*]. Just drill and drill.

Sensei Kim always used the words "martial arts." He said karate had limits. You had to become an artist of life.

■ Over the years, you must have seen many people come and go. How did your relationship and your position with Sensei Kim change?
At first I only saw him from across the room. I was invisible. Then in France in 1975, he said to me, "Now I know who to travel with." And I was never excluded. Over time that developed into my being the assistant instructor on the road. He would take me into his confidence and he'd ask, "What should we teach?" I was honored that he'd seek my opinion. Finally, it was, "Brian, run this event."

One of his greatest compliments was when he introduced me to someone in Sacramento. He said, "Rose, meet my friend, Brian Ricci." I was taken back that he'd call me his friend.

■ Why was receiving a dan rank from Sensei Kim so special?
I came from a Shotokan background. Frank Gaviola was from a different background. We felt we were somewhat accomplished martial artists. But to have recognition from Sensei Kim was difficult to earn. The first degree [*shodan*] and second degree [*nidan*]

were working ranks. There were very few third degrees [*sandans*]. Other organizations out there had sixth and seventh degrees that were nowhere near as good as Sensei Kim's black belts. I was a fourth degree for many years. The fourth-dan relationship was different. It meant you were self-sufficient. He wanted to know everything about you. Sensei Kim knew your personality. He knew your moral code in life.

I never asked him for rank. When Sensei Kim sent me the seventh degree, I never told anyone. He announced it at the banquet to celebrate his 80th birthday and his tenth-degree.

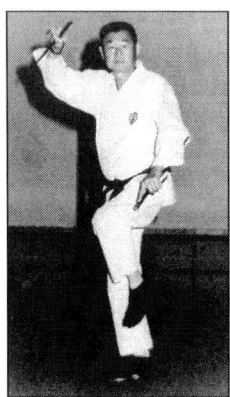 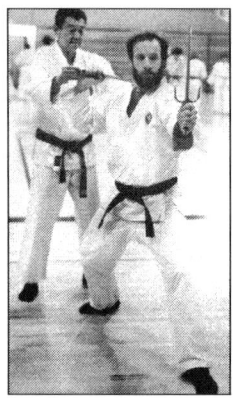

Dr. Kim demonstrates sai techniques.
Brian Ricci adjusting sai technique under his mentor.

■ What is your fondest memory of Sensei Kim?

Sensei's sense of humor. His laugh. We loved to get him going. I remember the summer camp the first time we did a little magic thing called "The Stubby Shapiro Show." It was based on a joke that Sensei had told. But, that day something had ticked off Sensei Kim. He really wasn't in a good mood. But because of the show, Sensei Kim laughed so hard he had tears in his eyes. And I felt so good that we could do something like that to change his mood.

■ What is the most important thing that you learned from Sensei Kim?

Be happy. Enjoy life each day. Live in the moment.

■ The majority of Sensei Kim's students are now training with you. What legacy of Sensei Kim's are you trying to pass on to them?

Tradition. Sensei Kim said that if it comes easy, it doesn't have value. Martial arts tradition has been around for a long time.

■ Can you tell us about the Zen Bei Butokukai International?

Sensei Kim chose the name Zen Bei Butokukai International. As *Zen Bei* means "all people," it reflects his reaching out to everyone. The shape of the crest we use is purely a respect for Sensei Kim.

After Sensei Kim's passing he had left no written instructions as to how things were to continue. But, I like to think it worked out for the best.

■ What do you see for your future in the martial arts?

I enjoy being a vehicle to pass on Sensei Kim's teaching and develop his students to the best of their abilities and to treat all students with fairness and keep his level of teaching.

■ Is there anything else you'd like to say?

We all looked at Sensei Kim as a flawless individual. I got to know him as the man. He made mistakes. But his generosity was to a fault. He always made sure his students got the best.

Dr. Kim was in the true sense a sensei: "One who has gone before" and shares his knowledge with students.

TECHNICAL SECTION

The prototypes of the spear (*yari*) were originally brought to Japan from the Asian continent and enjoyed their greatest popularity after the Mongol invasions of the late 13th century (Draeger, 1973:71, 72). To the Japanese warrior (*samurai*), the spear was second only to the bow and arrow in traditional significance (Ratti and Westbrook, 1973: 241). Even though elaborate spearhead designs took the spear out of the category of piercing weapons and gave it new roles in slashing, hooking, and ripping, the basic mechanics of the spear art continued unchanged and the Japanese samurai trained primarily to be accurate with the thrust (Draeger, 1973:72).

It is interesting to note that the staff (*bo*) was developed at the same time as the art of spear fighting and the boundaries between the two arts have become rather vague. The staff was comparatively less dangerous to practice with than a spear and was often used in the martial art training halls (*dojo*) where spear fighting was taught. In time, the related use of the wooden weapon became so well developed that skilled warriors could be engage in real combat using the staff (Ratti and Westbrook, 1973:305, 308).

Although the Japanese have used wooden weapons since earliest times, the staff was a humble weapon, because the lowliest person could make one. Because of its obvious effectiveness, however, the samurai could not afford to neglect its study (Draeger, 1973:76).

Yoshida Kotaro was known as a spear expert (Corcoran, et al., 1993:396) and Kim often spoke of training with the spear under his teacher (Kim, 1982: 35, 77, 82, 89). Ricci explained many of the kata practiced with the staff that have been passed down from Kim Sensei and taught in the Zen Bei Butokukai are actually spear forms (B. Ricci, 2005, April 21). The kata, Yunigawa no kon, was originally meant to be performed with the spear (B. Ricci, 2005, May 24).

The opening movements of Yunigawa no kon.

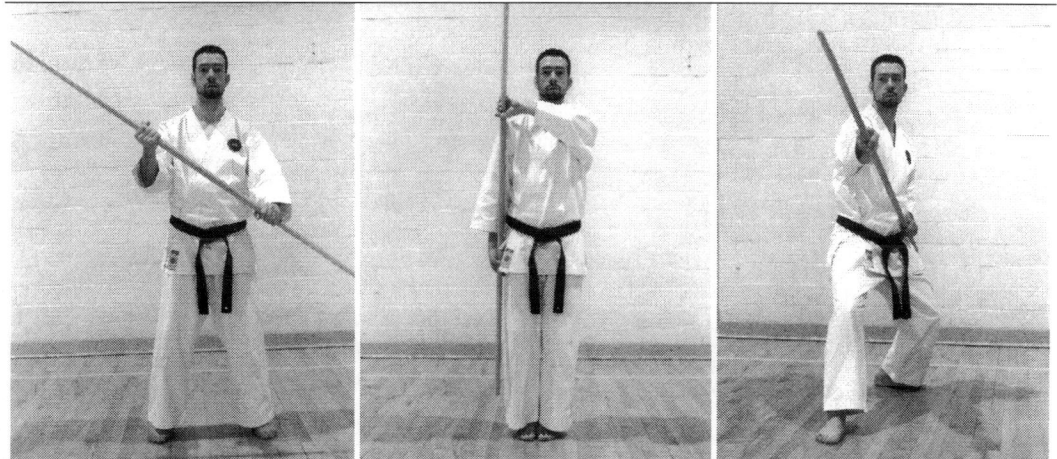

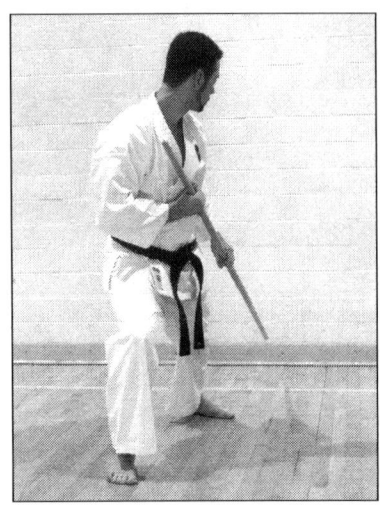
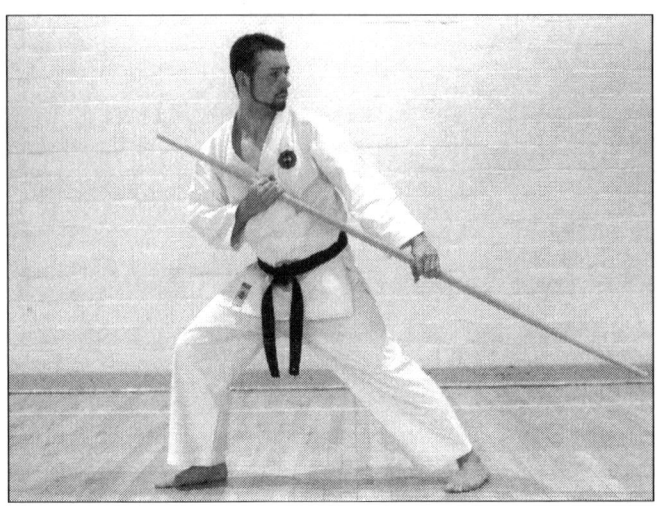
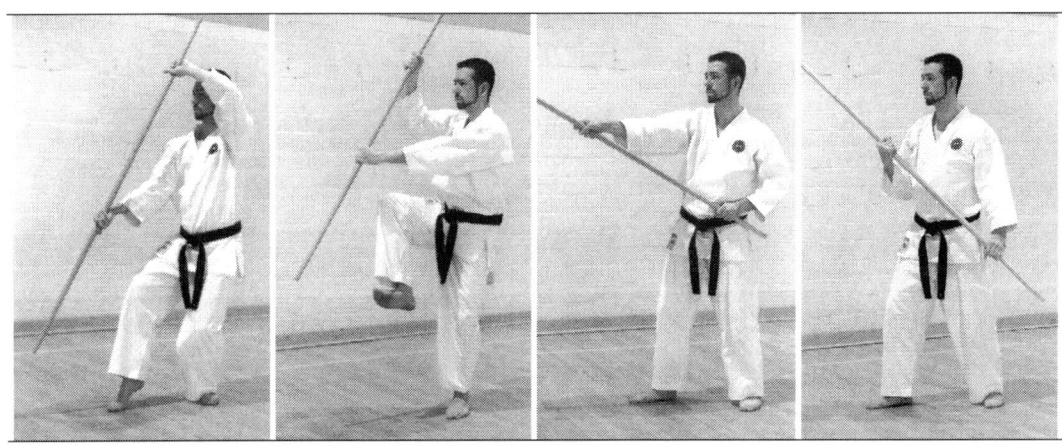
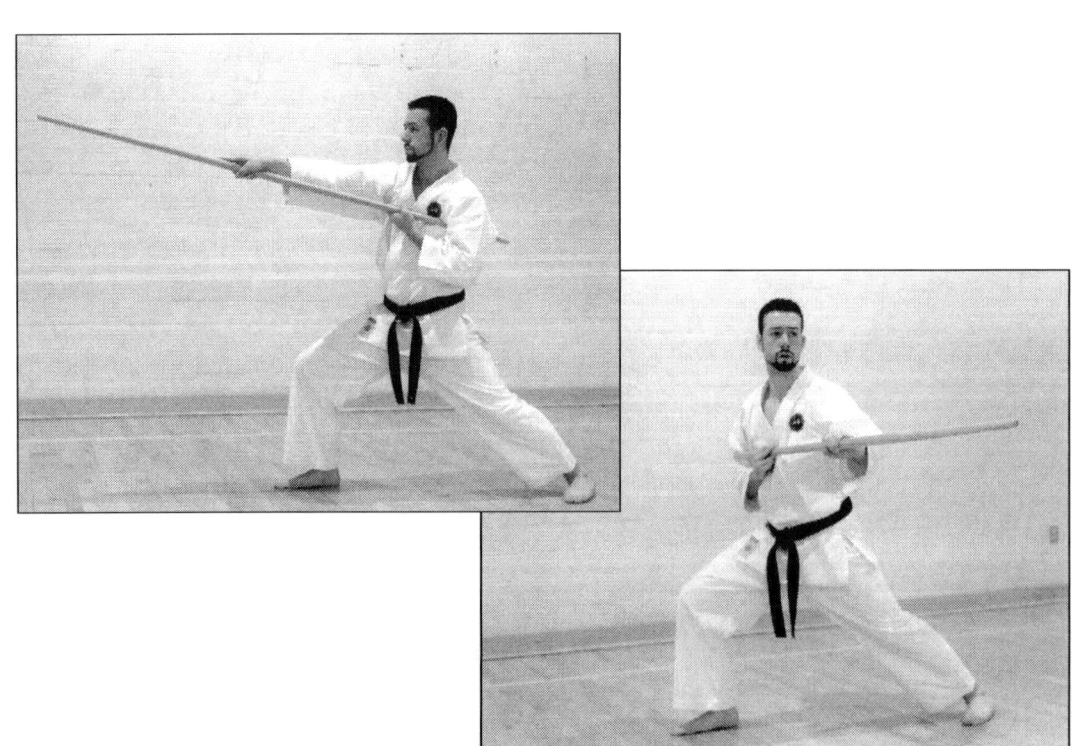

Brian Ricci demonstrates a combination from the Yunigawa no kon. The second move is a retraction of the bo in order to thrust under the opponent's block.

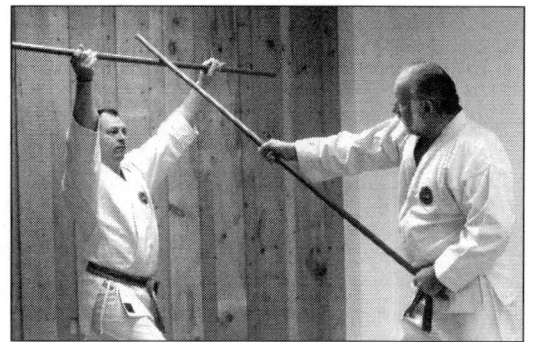

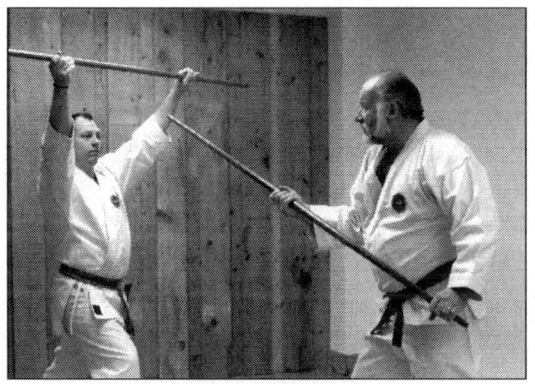

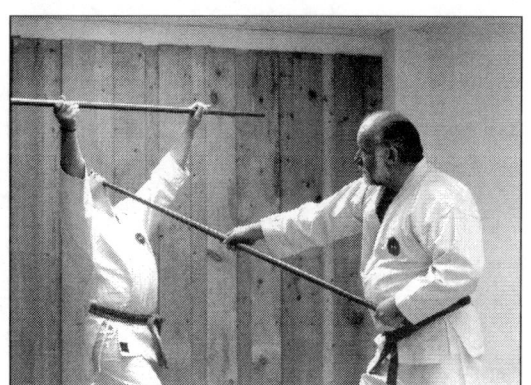

Blocking with the yari or bo is done with the shaft.

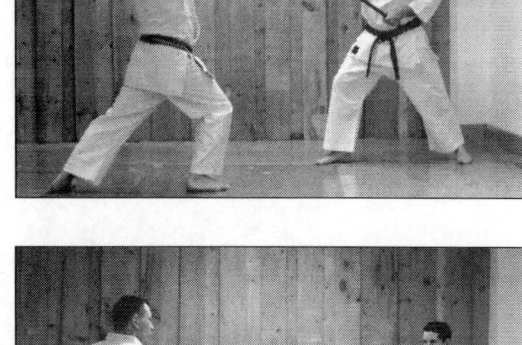

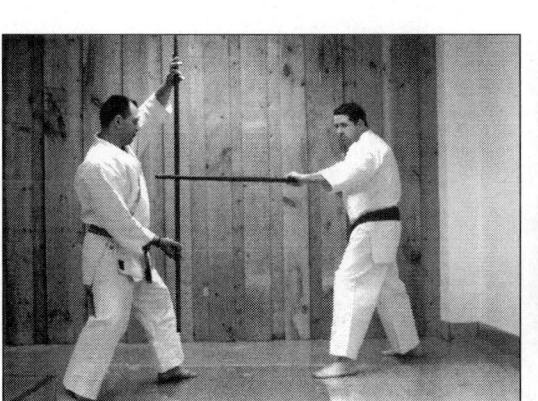

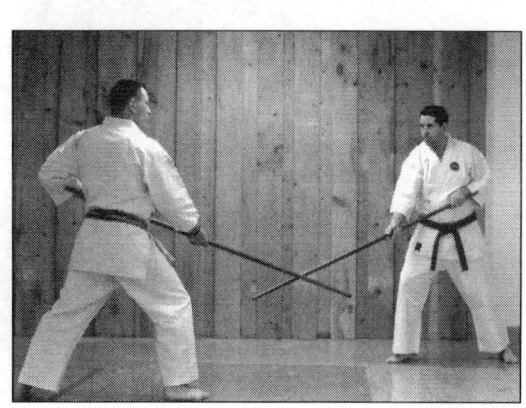

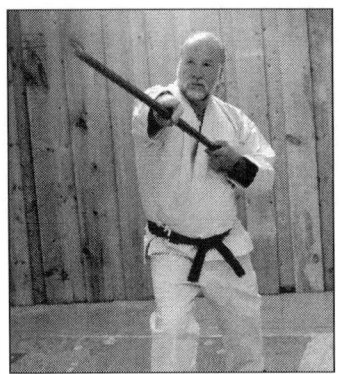 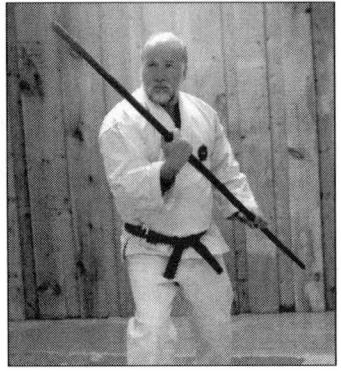

Thrust and retract.

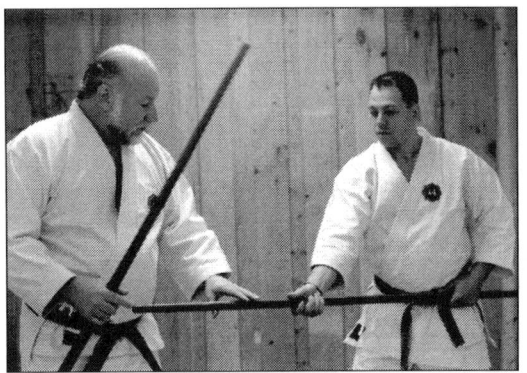 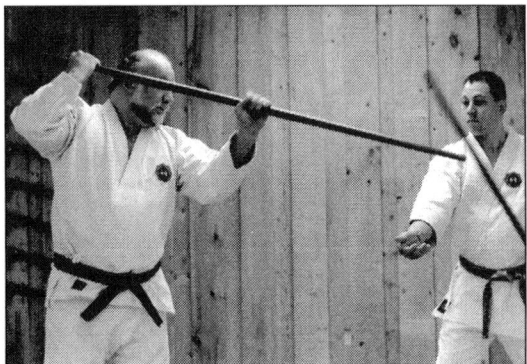

It is important to use a proper grip with the yari/bo.
If the palm is up the weapon can be dislodged with a strike.

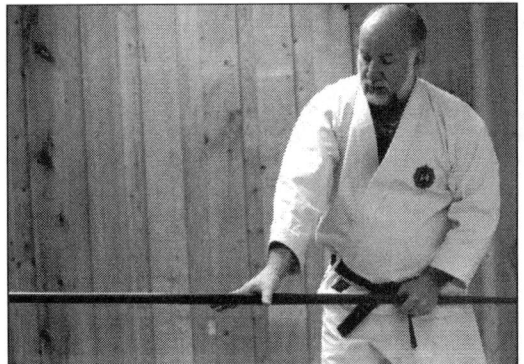 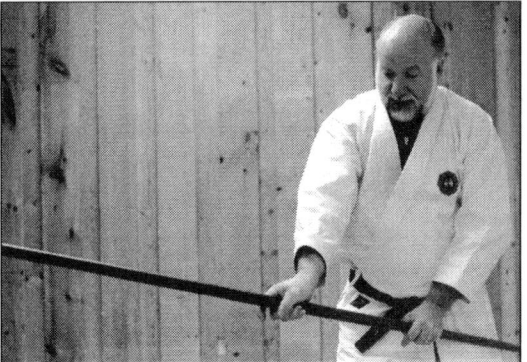

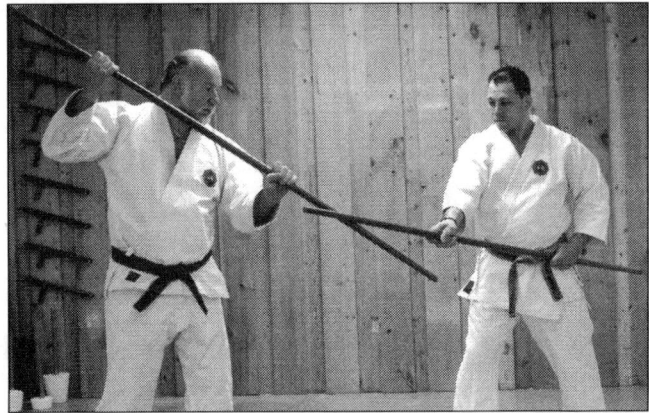

The palm must be down in order to have control of the weapon.

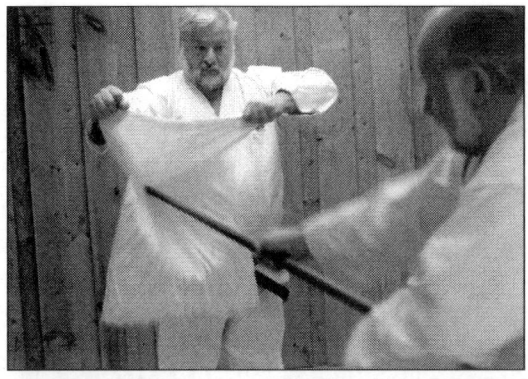 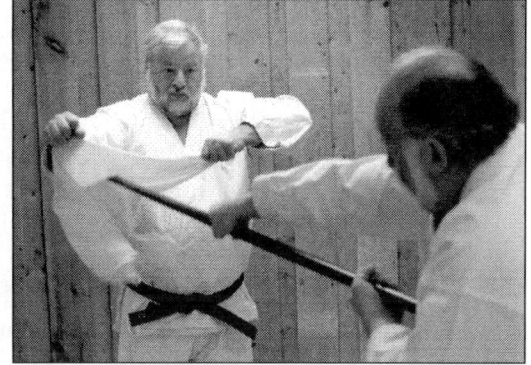
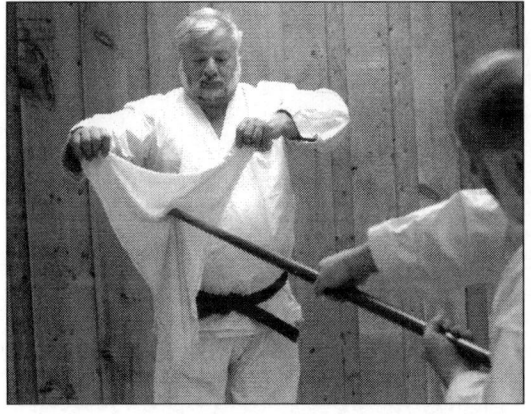 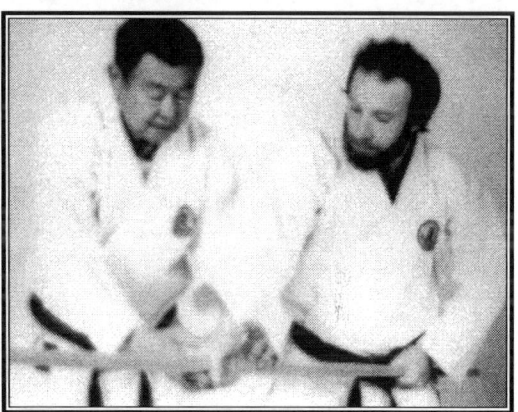

Thrusting with the yari/bo is with a twisting motion. Here Brian Ricci uses a training technique taught by his sensei, Dr. Richard Kim. Dr. Kim had his students use a wet towel to thrust into to show the twisting of the yari/bo.

Conclusion

No one ever will replace Dr. Richard Kim. The circumstances of his life gave him the opportunity to train in a number of martial arts in the countries of their origin during turbulent times. His personal development was a result of his amazing work ethic. Dr. Kim once said, "If you sleep more than four hours a day, you lose."

Today, four years after his death, Dr. Kim's students are faced with the daunting task of passing on their instructor's teachings. Their loyalty and devotion guarantee Dr. Kim's knowledge and wisdom will continue into the next generation. And that generation is sure to view the stories of this great man's life as legend.

―――∞∞∞―――

Acknowledgment

The author would like to thank Brian Ricci Sensei for providing some of the photographs used in this chapter. A special thanks to both Ricci Sensei and Frank Gaviola Sensei for their help and suggestions with the chapter. Great appreciation is expressed as well to Ed Ricci, John Wasilina, Dean and Tony Romanelli, and Kelly Combs for appearing in the photos. The author would especially like to thank Dr. Richard Kim for his guidance.

Notes

[1] Oyama Masutatsu was born Yee Hyung in Kimje, Korea in 1923. In 1937, he was sent to a boy's military academy in Japan. He changed his name and began studying Shotokan

karate. After the war, Oyama studied Goju-ryu karate and eventually created his own style, Kyokushinkai (Corcoran, et al., 1993:365).

[2] Kinjo Hiroshi was born on Valentines Day, 1919. He originally trained in the marital arts with Hanashiro Chomo (1869–1945) and Oshiro Chojo (1888–1935) in Okinawa (McCarthy, 1994:91).

[3] Yamaguchi Gogen was born on 20 January 1909. As a boy, he trained in Japanese fencing (*kendo*) and karate. In 1931, he was introduced to the founder of Goju-ryu karate, Miyagi Chojun (Yamaguchi, n.d.:75–77, 84).

[4] *Butokukai* means "Martial Virtues Association" (Draeger 1974:35).

[5] Frank Gaviola began training with Richard Kim in 1968 at the YMCA in San Francisco's Chinatown. He received his sixth-degree black belt in 2001. He received his associate's degree in architectural engineering from City College of San Francisco. After a 25-year career in engineering, he quit work to teach martial arts full-time in 1992 (Gould, 2002: 22).

Bibliography

Castilonia, R. (1996). *Nuggets in the ground*. LaJolla, CA: International University Line.

Corcoran, J., Farkas, E., and Sobel, S. (1993). *The original martial arts encyclopedia: Tradition-history-pioneers*. Los Angeles: ProAction Publishing.

Draeger, D. (1973). *Classical bujutsu*. Tokyo: Weatherhill Inc.

Draeger, D. (1974). *Modern bujutsu and budo*. Tokyo: Weatherhill Inc.

Farkas, E., and Corcoran, J. (1983). *The Overlook martial arts dictionary*. New York: The Overlook Press.

Foley, S. (2005, July 3). Personal communication with author.

Gould, J. (Ed.). (2002, September). Sensei spotlight: Frank Gaviola. *Martial Virtue*, 22.

Kim, R. (1974). *The weaponless warriors*. Burbank, CA: Ohara Publications.

Kim, R. (1982). *The classical man*. Hamilton, Ontario: Masters Publication.

McCarthy, P. (1987). *Classical kata of Okinawan karate*. Santa Clarita, CA: Ohara Publications.

McCarthy, P. (1994). The world within karate and Kinjo Hiroshi. *Journal of Asian Martial Arts, 3*(2): 90–99.

Ratti, O., and Westbrook, A. (1973). Secrets of the samurai. Rutland, VT: Charles E. Tuttle Company.

Ricci, B. (2005, April 21). Personal communication with author.

Ricci, B. (2005, May 4). Personal communication with author.

Ricci, B. (2005, May 17). Personal communication with author.

Ricci, B. (2005, May 22). Personal communication with author.

Ricci, B. (2005, May 24). Personal communication with author.

Sells, J. (2000). *Unante: The secrets of karate*. Hollywood, CA: W.M. Hawley.

Svinth, J. (2001). Karate pioneer Yabu Kentsu, 1866–1937. *Journal of Asian Martial Arts, 10*(2):8–17.

Werrener, D. (n.d.). Memorial video–Sensei Richard Kim 1917–2001. Private production.

Warrener, D. (1982, May). Richard Kim: The weaponless warrior. *Official Karate*, 65.

Warrener, D. (2001, June). Richard Kim: The classical man. *Masters of Karate*, 93.

Will, J. (n.d.). Gogen "the cat" Yamaguchi: The last interview. *Fighter International*, 24, 26.

Wingate, C. (1993). Exploring our roots: Historical and cultural foundations of the ideology of karate-do. *Journal of Asian Martial Arts, 2*(3):10–35.

Yamaguchi, G. (n.d.). *Karate Goju-ryu by the cat*. Tokyo: International Karate-do Goju-kai.

chapter 48

George Dillman and the Influences in Pressure Point Theory and Practice

Interview by Peter Hobart, J.D.

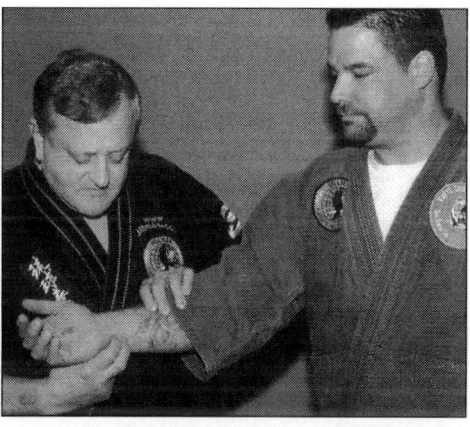

George Dillman indicating pressure points on the arm.
All photographs courtesy of George Dillman.

Almost anyone who has trained in Okinawan or Japanese martial arts over the past three decades will be familiar with the name of George A. Dillman. In 1982, he was described by *Official Karate Magazine* as "one of the winningest competitors karate has ever known" (November, 1982). He was a four-time National Karate Champion between 1969 and 1972, and during this period, he was consistently ranked among the top ten competitors in the nation by many major karate publications. Since that time, his advancement of *kyusho-jitsu* (pressure point theory) has sent shock waves through much of the martial community and turned certain traditional practices on their ear.

Volumes have been written about the technical aspects of his system. What has received somewhat less attention—perhaps eclipsed by the tremendous interest in the practicalities of the art—is an examination of the ideas, principles and beliefs that drive the man. On 21 February 2004, in Freehold, New Jersey, I had the opportunity to present him with a number of questions on such issues as history, tradition, ethics and even philosophy. What follows is a rare insight into another aspect of a man that many people already know, and perhaps others may want to take the time to get to know.

INTERVIEW

■ PETER HOBART: PLEASE DISCUSS THE RELATIONSHIP BETWEEN PRESSURE POINT FIGHTING AND CONVENTIONAL, COMPETITIVE SPARRING.

George A. Dillman: My karate has always been geared at real self-defense —something that will work out on the street—even when I broke down my kata and forms before considering the pressure points, I kept in mind "how would this play out in a real street fight situation?" In the military (police) I was in several encounters where I had to handle some trouble situations and I realized that some of the martial arts techniques that we talked about in the dojo just wouldn't work, and I realized that early on, so I was lucky there. I feel fortunate, though, that I was a sport competitor because had I bypassed that to go into pressure points—which I would have, probably, full-on—if I would have bypassed the sport end of it, I would have lacked a basic ability that I've told people they must have.

We have people that are doing pressure point techniques today that don't compete, they don't spar, they have probably never been in a real self-defense situation and they can't defend themselves. They can learn all the pressure points in the world, but during my sport period, I learned all the things that are actually needed to deliver the pressure points in a real situation, and I developed timing, distance and coordination. If you don't freestyle spar back at your dojo, if you don't pair off and do self-defense, you can't just do pressure point techniques. You could pull one or two off, maybe, for a basic breakaway, but for full-on self-defense you need to develop timing, distance and coordination. That happens—and it happens even more so in a tournament—when the pressure is on, because you have the same pressure, if not a deeper pressure, that you would have in a street situation, because there's thousands of people yelling your name or your opponent's name.

At the same time, that's what made me look for the pressure points, that's what made me find Soken Hohan, that's what made me ask him the question, because I knew we were lacking something. In tournament competition there were several times—and this is the way it was back then, there was no safety gear—when I actually punched some people and wanted to drop them, and they didn't drop. I was told, "One punch kill," "One punch can drop the guy," and I had to be missing something. What is it? Because I just hit this man as hard as I can and they're awarding me a point. Now a point is great, but in a street fight it doesn't mean anything... If I put you in the ring with Mike Tyson and he hits you, he's going to win. You've got to avoid being hit and you've got to be able to get him, and you're going to win.

■ Can you discuss Soken Hohan (b. 1889), Oyata Seiyu, and your first discovery of pressure point theory?

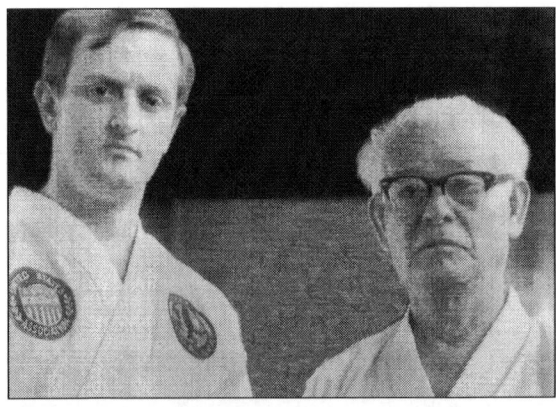

Dillman with Soken Hohan.

I realized I was missing something and I realized that there had to be something in the kata because people were now making up their own katas and forms to music, yet in the Orient they were sticking to those basic Pinan katas, Naihanchi kata, they were sticking to basic katas and teaching them and doing them with a different type of look in their eyes, using *ki* (internal energy), using rooting, using a whole different way of doing forms. I realized that, and I realized that in this country, because we didn't learn the secrets, we were making things up, and I would not fall to that. I asked Soken Hohan, and that's when he gave me the decent answers.

When I got the answers, they were somewhat depressing because I had spent twenty years learning these katas, and now all of a sudden there's no blocks, everything has a serious meaning—every move in every kata—it's just that we didn't know it, and it was right before our eyes. I was actually angry with myself, that I didn't figure it out. The real answers were right in front of my eyes and I didn't see them . . . I needed tournament competition to get me where I'm at today . . . My being good at kata is what led Soken Hohan to work with me. He said to me, "You do such beautiful kata that it hurts me here (indicating his heart) to see that you don't know the answer. You do kata even with spirit. In Okinawa we look that you have spirit to have kata. You have spirit. You just don't know what you are doing with the moves... This what you need to be a master in my country."

In 1983 I ran into Oyata Seiyu. The minute he did his first technique and said, "This is out of a kata," and broke it down, he wasn't on the mat ten seconds and I leaned over—my wife was there—and I whispered in her ear, "That's what Soken Hohan did. This is what Soken Hohan was trying to get across. This is what my notes are about. I have notes on this—on what he's doing right now—now I'm understanding it." Oyata Seiyu gave me the keys to get in the door. I had the door, I had the path, I had the katas, I had the general idea, I knew everything was more serious, I knew there were no blocks, but I didn't know what they were.

■ WHAT WAS IT LIKE TEACHING FOR OVER FIFTEEN YEARS IN COOPERATION WITH WALLY JAY, LEO FONG AND REMY PRESAS?

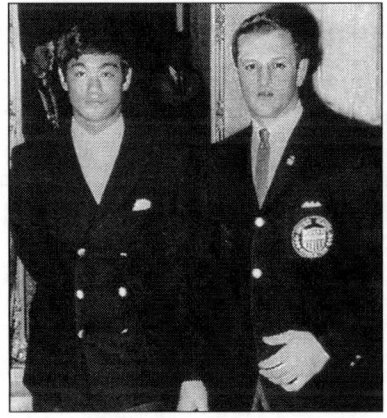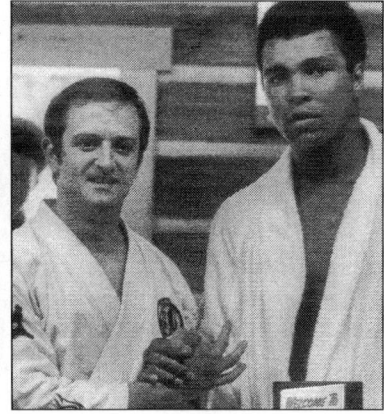

Among Dillman's associates how have influenced his martial art studies have been Bruce Lee and Muhammad Ali.

I attended those people's seminars (Wally Jay, Leo Fong, Remy Presas), I had them in to my school for seminars and we got talking about technique and we wound up sharing. From the minute I saw (Wally Jay) on the mat, I knew that I needed his Small Circle jujutsu for what I was doing. I had an Okinawan master—Oyata Seiyu—who said if you really want to find out the secret, you need a good jujutsu man. Along came Wally Jay, who was the best jujutsu man, and I realized the day he walked in the dojo that it was the Small Circle jujutsu that I was missing. I was able to hit people and hurt them, stun them, but I wasn't able to knock them out as well as I was after studying with Wally Jay. It is that Small Circle theory that he teaches and does that completed my art. He also then found that utilizing pressure points would help him complete his art. He and I used pressure point techniques, but we didn't know how they all fit together in the big package, and now we do.

So we started sharing, which led me over to Remy (Presas). Remy came in, and he started working with me on disarming people, taking weapons away, and I worked with him on pressure point techniques. The three of us had some sessions that I would give anything to have on video. We had some training sessions with the four of us doing and sharing techniques that the average martial artist would find unbelievable. It was fantastic. Remy—I miss him greatly. I always tell people that he was my booking agent. Remy would call me. "You and I will teach a seminar. We will do this in Atlanta, Georgia." I'd ask, "We will?" He'd say, "Yes, yes, you must be there," and then he'd hang up! And he did the same thing with Wally and we put the three of us together, and that became awesome for almost fifteen years.

■ WHAT MAKES A MASTER? HOW WERE YOUR ENCOUNTERS WITH SUCH PEOPLE?

The ability to teach, the ability to get you to do it, there are a lot of people that are good martial artists but they're not good at teaching. Bruce Lee was amazing at getting the concept across. I only worked out with Bruce Lee three times, but he improved my hand speed. He told me right off the bat, "You have to improve your hand and foot speed. You have a lot of power, good techniques, but I can hit you three or four times before you can hit me." Then he did it! But he taught me how to do it too. Then my hand speed picked up.

Daniel K. Pai was one of the unequaled masters in the world. He had so many techniques, but he passed away at an odd time, like Remy Presas, before anyone expected it. Danny Pai was one of the best gongfu teachers at the time. When I had sessions sitting at a dinner table with Bruce Lee and Danny Pai, I just sat and listened. And I was learning more than most people learn in their lifetime in a dojo, over a dinner table. That was amazing—these people could teach by words also, then they could get up and demonstrate.

Robert Trias was one of the first Americans to do the martial arts, and he was a tremendous person and a strong puncher—you wouldn't want to be hit with his punch! I wasn't the size of Robert Trias. Trias was a big, huge strong man, so when he hit, you wouldn't want to be in front of it. But Bruce Lee wasn't, and Bruce Lee made me pay attention to speed and power, because Bruce was a small individual—he was only 5' 7", 125 pounds—so I realized that that was the answer. I just happened to be with the right people at the right time. However, a little credit goes my way because I would seek these people out; they didn't find me.

Ed Parker and I were friends—Ed Parker and Danny Pai were first cousins —and Danny Pai introduced me to Ed Parker, and Ed Parker introduced me to Bruce Lee. Bruce Lee introduced me to Wally Jay and Leo Fong. Bruce Lee sat at my house and said, "Who are some of the toughest fighters on the East Coast—I don't get over here often? Somebody who, if you were going to run into them in a real fight, you'd know you better pay attention and be using both hands." I gave him a couple of names of people I thought of at the time, that I respected and were big, strong fighters. And he took that into his memory bank. I said, "How about on the West Coast?" He said, "There are several," and named them.

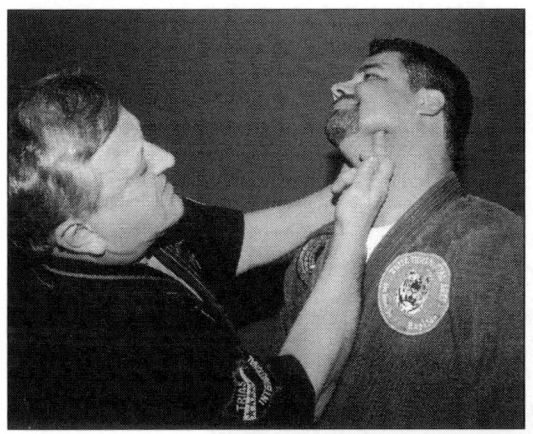
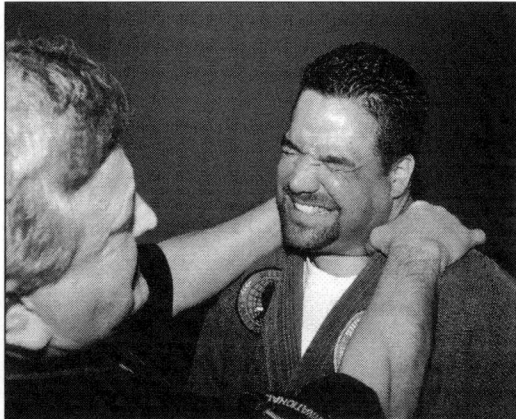
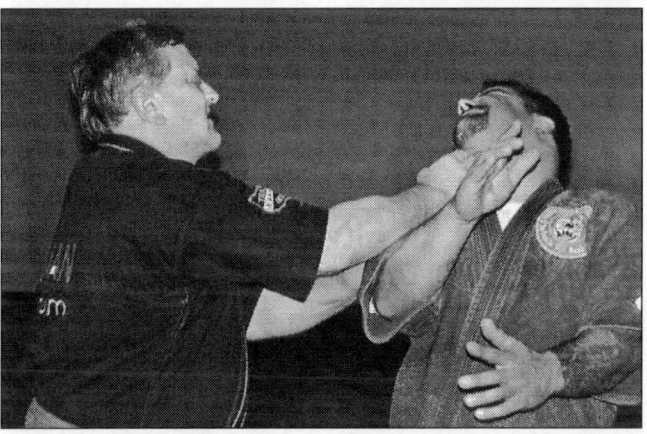
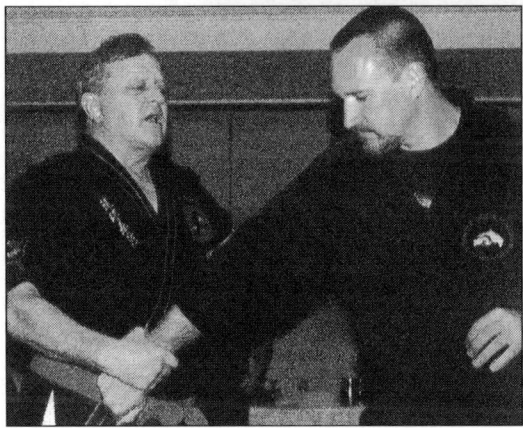
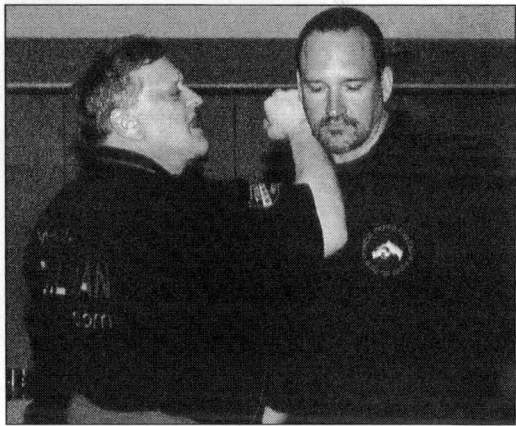

Explaining the locations of pressure points on the jaw, neck and wrist, and how theory is applicable in martial art practice.

Lee said, "there's a guy out there named Wally Jay. You've got to meet and train with Wally Jay at some point. He's a no nonsense person. You ask Wally Jay a question; he does not answer the question verbally. He gets you on the mat and demonstrates it, and you can do nothing about it. I've seen some of the best martial artists in the world get on the mat with Wally Jay, and they get defeated. You've got to train with him. Leo Fong is one of the toughest boxers I've met. You have to slug it out with him, and you have to be ready to take him down, because he will keep coming." After Bruce Lee passed away was when I went to seek out Wally Jay and Leo Fong. I went to Canada to meet with Wally Jay, and took a whole bunch of my students to watch him on the mat, doing his thing, and I approached him about doing a seminar at my school.

■ ON THE IMPORTANCE OF STUDYING AND TEACHING HEALING ARTS IN CONJUNCTION WITH MARTIAL PRACTICES:

Three reasons. The ethical reason, the practical reason... because you as a martial artist have to learn to reverse what you learn how to do. If you hurt somebody, you knock somebody out; you have to learn how to revive them. The third reason is that I, and several other people who are into pressure point theory, are looking for ways to lengthen our lives . . . and I think we're finding it. We're finding better ways to restore our ki energy, we're finding ways to restore after seminars so we're not tired and weak, and that all leads to the healing part of it. We're not only healing, but we're learning the healing within ourselves.

The thing that I found is that most martial artists that are into what I'm into lived into their nineties with complete flexibility. Soken Hohan is on the end of my videotape doing forms. He was 92-years-old. That tape was shot two weeks before he died. Now he didn't know he was going to die in two weeks, but his body was winding down . . . What was amazing was at 92 he could do a kata called Chinto and jump in the air and throw two kicks and he could go to the ground on one knee and get up, and he could do a complete spin, 180 degrees, and not fall over. You go out and take the average man that's 92 and spin him around and he's going to fall over. Well he had complete control of his body, his energy; he knew how the energy spiraled up and down . . . When you spin and move in a kata, you are controlling your energy and sending it up and down through your body. If you know how to do that, it creates health and flexibility.

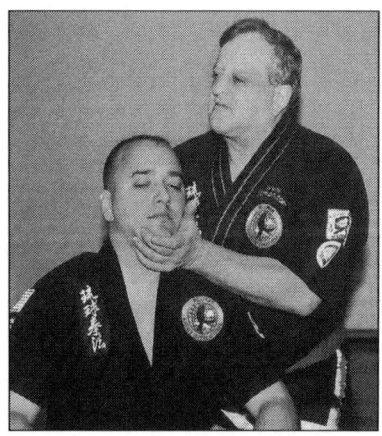 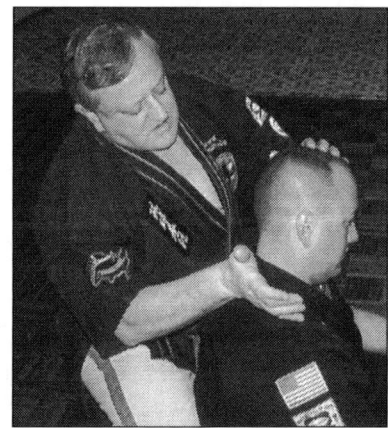

Dillman showing resuscitation techniques.

■ WHAT ARE THE HUMANE ASPECTS OF KYUSHO-JITSU, THE PRESSURE POINT THEORY?

The art that I teach is a lot more humane than punching people in the Adam's apple, poking out his eye, kicking him in the groin—this is what they advise at most karate schools. They're all teaching eye gouges, they're all teaching how to cup hands and hit in both ears. They're all teaching to rip out the Adam's apple or hitting in the throat.

They're all teaching how to kick in the groin. I had to go through that in my mind when I got into pressure points, because I realized how deadly they are, and could be . . . they're just going for what we call "vital points." Vital points like eyes, ears, nose, throat and groin. We have pressure points—there are 361 all over—we have variations to go to because you need them in various self-defense situations. You cannot always get to the eyes, ears, nose, throat and groin—they have a natural defense. There isn't anybody in the world that doesn't flinch at an eye gouge or a groin kick . . . There are pressure points available that give you the exact same result.

■ What importance do emotions play in martial technique?

You read in any martial arts book—any good one—that you should be happy or complacent while fighting. Do not take the anger of your opponent. Anger negates anger. You take two people that are angry, hitting at each other, they cannot do damage to each other. Take one and get him angry, get the other one laughing and he punches the guy that's angry, the guy that's angry will fall down . . . I've been in several self-defense encounters and I didn't realize it, but I was happy and smiling, but I was happy and smiling because I was confident. I knew what I was about to do to this guy, and he's in my face very angry. I didn't understand at that time that it was the happy emotion and mood that I was in that was going to help me drop him.

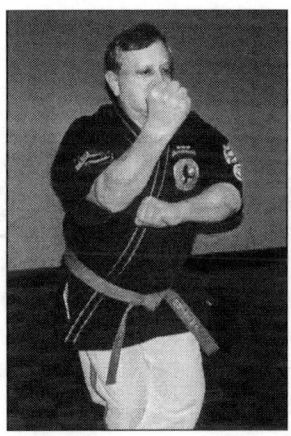 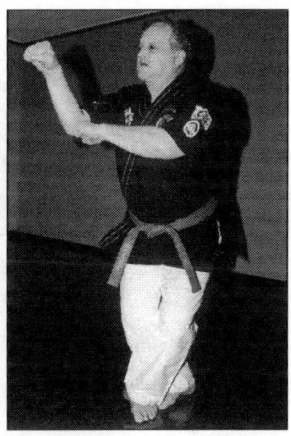

Dillman illustrating how good stances
help the overall techniques.

■ You say that, "The next generation will always be better than the past one. At least that should be the goal of every good teacher. The student should always be better than and surpass the instructor," Does this still holds true?

Oh, yes, they have to, to keep this alive. At one point I was worried about something happening to me. I opened up a secret on the martial arts, and I was worried about something happening to me and no one seeing this. No one knowing about it. So I started teaching it, thinking if I can just get a few people taught to pass this on. Well now there are thousands all over the world. I can name countries around the world that are all doing pressure point techniques . . . We went through a period when people were dropping katas and forms, and that was based on a statement that Bruce Lee made, that I asked Bruce about personally before he died. He didn't mean it the way they were writing it. Bruce Lee said that he did not need katas and forms anymore to fight . . . Everyone looked at that as he didn't need them . . . He said, "Kata and form is you learning how to print the alphabet. You learning how to write. If you want to write somebody a letter right now, you don't print anymore. I think I could stop doing my katas and forms and fight the same, now." He didn't mean don't do them at all.

■ How will your fighting system continue in the future?

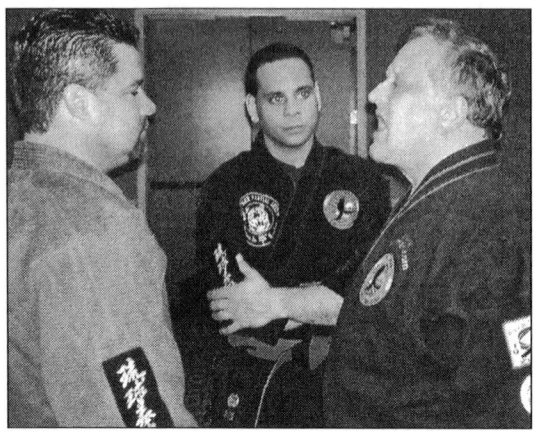 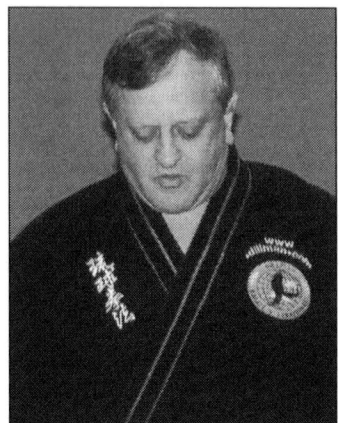

Proper breathing and the use of sound
are part of martial art training.

I want to do a story about that... Remy Presas had a story in *Black Belt* magazine several years ago of who should take over if anything happened to him. We're working with Black Belt now on doing that story, and putting in everyone's picture. But I have a lot of young people that are trained really well, and I know they'll carry the ball, people like Bill Burch, Dr. Chas Terry—he's a medical doctor and an acupuncturist—Ed Lake who went on to acupuncture school, and probably knows more about pressure points than anyone in the system, because he's trained as a doctor and he's trained as a herb person. Dusty Seal is a young man with a tremendous amount of knowledge... the man that helps me write the books, Chris Thomas... I communicate with him daily. He is also a minister... so we communicate on various aspects of self-defense as well as the meaning of all this, tracing it back.

■ What would you want future generations to remember and your influence in the martial arts?

The fact that I made a major change in the martial arts, at least outside of the closed section of the Orient... There are people that are even using my theory that don't understand it well, but they're at least thinking about their forms, their katas, and they're trying to come up with better moves. So I think I've made a major change that I'm happy with, and I think it's going to continue for the rest of time now. If I die tomorrow, I think it's going to continue, because there's too many thousands of people that know and are teaching this theory. There are several things that they're going to have to do and develop and find out on their own, that maybe I didn't teach them if they weren't at the right place at the right time, but they should be able to develop and figure it out. I gave them the pattern to do it. I gave them the roadmap.

chapter 49

Kaho: Cultural Meaning and Educational Method in Kata Training

by John J. Donohue, Ph.D.

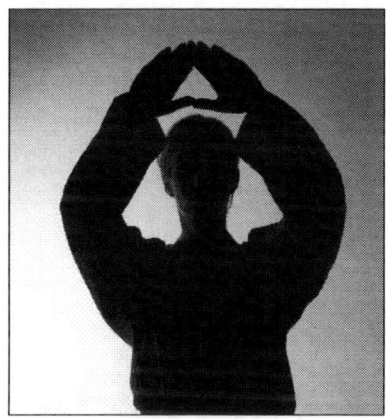

The trainee stands garbed in the robes of a by-gone era, gripping a weapon as deadly as it is archaic. The world tightens down to a small universe built of hard wood, polished steel, cotton cloth, body heat, sweat, and the tidal pulse of heartbeat and respiration. Here, the weapon is wielded in a sequence of moves set down by masters long gone, actions refined and repeated until the performer is lost in the hiss of effort and the focused pursuit of perfection. It is a curious thing, part technical exercise, part performance art, part meditative experience. It is kata.

Introduction

The world of the Asian martial arts is one that has gripped the imagination of Westerners for decades now. Its trappings strike the outside viewer as exotic, its motivations arcane. It is dense with symbolism and occluded meaning. It is rife with opportunity for misunderstanding and romanticization. It is, in short, a social phenomenon that cries out for anthropological analysis.

Students of many modern Japanese martial arts are fond of reminding us, as the Japanese term *budo* implies, that they are really "martial ways." The destination of these ways is varied: they can be understood as systems of physical exercise or spiritual development, as relatively efficient physiological (as opposed to technological) systems, as recreational and competitive sports, or as civilian self-defense methods. In fact, any intense scrutiny of these systems reveals a multifaceted nature in which aspects of all these things can be recognized. The deeper the understanding of budo, the greater their recognized complexity.

This sophistication relates not merely to the techniques and systems themselves, but to the way in which they have been taught within the Japanese martial tradition. This represents another avenue of scientific inquiry for researchers focusing on sociological interpretations of martial arts activity.

I will examine the structure and purpose of the practice patterns known in the Japanese martial tradition as kata. While some Westerners have questioned the necessity for kata training, it continues to form a part of most orthodox martial systems. And the social scientist wonders "why?" This paper examines *kaho* (the use of kata as an instructional tool) from two perspectives: kata training as a cultural activity that has been shaped by the structural characteristics of Japanese culture, and kata training as a highly developed and effective educational mechanism for imparting technical skill in the martial arts.

Kata

Kata forms the backbone of the Japanese traditional martial arts instructional approach (Friday, 1995; 1997). Popularly understood as "forms," kata are a series of movements combined into a performance set. Most traditional Japanese martial arts organizations and systems have a corpus of individual kata that trainees learn at various points in their study. Mastery of individual kata is often linked to promotion. Thus, kata are most immediately thought of as ways to develop student skill.

Kata are more than just performance routines designed to polish technique or showcase ability, however. They are also thought to embody lessons learned by past masters. When we consider that in feudal Japan a warrior's skill was often proven on the battlefield with lethal finality, the role of kata as non-lethal re-enactments of battlefield experience becomes much more understandable. So, too, can we appreciate the reason proponents of the traditional combat-oriented systems (often identified as *bujutsu*, "martial methods") held kata training in such high regard.

The teaching of combat skill, however, does not necessarily mandate such a highly structured, ritualistic approach. Western wrestlers and boxers, for instance, are not schooled through such elaborate patterns. Westerners practicing more modern martial arts systems have abandoned or de-emphasized kata in favor of what they consider more "realistic" and "practical" exercises. For these people, kata practice is a cultural relic, easily jettisoned. It is a contemporary urge for "relevance" that is quite familiar to educators. Yet kata practice persists in many Japanese martial systems practiced today. This persistence argues for a type of functionality that needs to be examined.

Cultural Factors

One source of kaho's continued endurance in the martial arts world may spring from the formative cultural environment of the martial arts. The organization of any human activity reflects its cultural context, and the Japanese martial traditions are no exception. Although the mechanics of fighting are considerably conditioned by human physiology and kinesiology, as well as by the weapons technology being applied, stylistic approaches and organizational patterns are culturally conditioned.

Kata are authoritative things. They are passed on from high-ranking instructors to novices. The criteria used to judge the performance of these sets is one that emphasizes a fidelity to form and movement within the dictates the instructor has established. The student's ability to imitate his teacher in kata performance is considered a key to advancement in rank and status. Kaho's stress of hierarchy, authority, organizational belonging, and conformity all resonate strongly with Japanese cultural patterns.

Indeed, in sociological terms, we can understand Japanese martial arts as corporate entities with a strongly hierarchical organization and an explicit ideological charter. These structural factors condition the process of training to a great degree and so bear some further discussion.

In the first place, Japanese martial arts seem to share a predilection for formal organization that can be contrasted to the approach in other Asian countries. From the Tokugawa Period (1603–1868) onward, we note a marked tendency for martial arts training to be organized in corporate entities (Hurst, 1998). Schools came to have both a physical location, the *dojo* (literally "way place," the training hall) as well as a formal identity. Traditional bujutsu systems were often referred to as *ryu* (literally "streams," which gives some sense of the idea of corporate perpetuation). Usage in more modern martial arts systems known as budo is a bit more varied: some systems maintain the ryu label, others use the more modern designation of *kan* (hall) such as in Kodokan judo or Shotokan karatedo, or *kai* (association) as in Kyokushinkai karatedo.

Whatever their labels, these organizations are hierarchical entities, in which issues of rank (related to skill and seniority) condition behavior. At the pinnacle of the organization is the teacher (*sensei*), who is contrasted with his disciples (*montei*). In addition to this gross distinction, there are finer gradations present as well. Students are enmeshed in a dualistic series of relationships between superiors and subordinates that are modeled on the teacher/student split and that echo general structural principles in Japanese society (Nakane, 1970). Thus, a series of relativistic links between seniors (*sempai*) and juniors (*kyohai*) also shapes behavior in the dojo (Donohue, 1991).

The stratified nature of martial arts organizations is reinforced through their well-known ranking systems. Awareness of rank in these organizations is often buttressed by elaborate symbolic means such as methods of address and ritual bowing. In some systems, elements of training uniforms or their color are used to denote status. The most well-known item of clothing associated with rank is the colored-belt system adopted in many modern budo forms. In this system, trainees are classified according to *kyu* (class) and *dan* (grade). While permutations in hue and numbering are almost as varied as schools themselves, beginners in kyu levels usually wear white belts and, as they progress in rank, are awarded a series of different colored belts, culminating in the black belt, a sign that the trainee has reached dan level.

As they are organized today, budo organizations share a commonality with a widespread organizational type in Japan, the *iemoto* ("household origin," the main house in the traditional arts; Hsu, 1975). Although the Japanese do not formally identify most martial arts organizations as iemoto proper, the arts possess the highly structured hierarchical organization based on personal links between masters and disciples that are central characteristics of iemoto organizations.

As formal organizations, martial arts systems also have an explicit ideological charter—a "mission statement" in the corporate jargon of our times. These charters certainly relate to the philosophical orientation of many Japanese martial arts forms. Broadly speaking, many martial arts, and particularly modern budo systems, are inspired by a mix of Shinto, Confucian, and Buddhist ideas that link training with a type of personal/spiritual development. Much has been made, of course, of the alleged link between Zen and the martial arts (Suzuki, 1960; King, 1993; Leggett, 1978). While it is certainly possible that this connection was important for selected martial artists, it is neither universal nor historically accurate.

In fact, while not for a moment calling into question the sincerity of modern martial artists, an objective assessment of martial arts charters reveal them to be vaguely formulated statements that present these arts as ways to advance the technical practice of the art in question, to celebrate human potential, and to advance causes as diffuse and universally unobjectionable as good sportsmanship and world peace. Charters of this type are useful in that they provide an overarching philosophical rationale (however diffuse) for what would otherwise be merely highly stylized calisthenics. In addition, these charters can be understood as the direct consequence of two things: the need to "rehabilitate" the martial arts after the Second World War and a related attempt to homogenize elements of indigenous Japanese ideology so as to be more easily accepted as these arts spread to the West. It is interesting that this diffuse mysticism has had an unexpected appeal for Westerners seeking alternatives to traditional Western belief systems.

Traditional Asian approaches to learning may also have reinforced an emphasis on kaho. Friday (1995) suggests that the Confucian infatuation with ritual formalism is at least partly the cause. We might also note that the ideographic Chinese writing system demanded a mastery of literally thousands of characters, and a type of fundamental precision was needed to engage in any literary activity. Given the dominant place of Confucianism in Tokugawa Japan, it is not surprising that the rigor of this approach to instruction informed other endeavors as well.

The modern martial arts, the fundamental characteristics of which were shaped by Tokugawa paradigms, are no exception. All trainees, at whatever level, are expected to continue to practice the building blocks of their particular art for a lifetime. These basic elements form the vocabulary of the martial conversation and, as such, need to be continuously polished. These building blocks tend to be embedded in kata. Many a newly minted karate black belt is surprised, on being awarded dan rank, to being reintroduced to the same kata begun as a white belt. Kaho's stress on repetition, rote learning, and stylistic conformity fit very well within the Confucian tradition.

General cultural emphasis on age and seniority also shape kaho. Students tend to learn differing kata in a sequence that is tied to advancement in rank. Their models are "senior" students. And the higher the rank, the more complex the kata and the longer the period of time needed to master it. In the martial arts, there is an explicit belief that the amazing prowess of the master is one that has been forged slowly, over time. It is not a mysterious event. Although it is a supra-rational process, it is the anticipated outcome of practice, refinement, and ruthless self-criticism. The traditional martial arts of Japan reject the "quick and easy" formulations of mass-marketing and run counter to the ostensibly progressive admonitions of Bruce Lee to "absorb what is useful" (1975). The techniques and kata of the art are accepted by trainees as embodying critical martial lessons. The fact that many of these lessons take years to fully grasp does nothing to devalue them. But it once again tends to reinforce a predilection for hierarchy, and kaho fits easily with such an expectation.

KAHO AS TECHNICAL SYSTEM

Certainly the traditional reliance on kaho as a centerpiece of training is not a simple cultural relic. The martial arts are as much focused on product—skills development— as they are on process—the constellation of cultural trappings that surround the arts. As "practical arts," we would expect that the retention of kaho reflects a functional appreciation of the method as a pedagogical tool.

A) Pedagogy

We may posit that kaho must be an extremely flexible instructional tool to survive in the modern dojo. In the first place, we must remind ourselves that martial arts study is voluntary. While school children in Japan are still required to take judo or kendo in school, further training is a result of individual initiative. And in the West, martial arts training halls fall squarely within the category of "voluntary organizations." Participation presupposes a willingness to study, often because of some perceived benefit. But the motivations for training are as varied as the trainees themselves, and so may be the levels of ability. This mandates a flexible technique for teaching that may be one element in ensuring the continuing importance of kaho.

Some students approach the martial arts as exotic forms of exercise. Those of us who have trained in these arts for any length of time, after inventorying the bruises, broken bones, etc. involved may wonder whether there are other activities that create less wear and tear, but it remains that many consider martial arts training a calisthenic activity.

In the West, the allure of fighting skills development often forms a part in martial arts marketing. We might note in passing that this idea is not seriously entertained in Japan. But for Westerners, the hint of Asian mystery and the promise of arcane mastery embodied in every cheap B-grade martial arts movie keeps this questionable self-defense motivation alive. Other students are attracted by the vague yet comfortably exotic ideological trappings of some martial arts systems. They seek a sort of experiential transcendence in their training.

All of which suggests that the student body of a typical martial arts dojo is extremely heterogeneous in terms of personal motivation and athletic ability. This complicates issues relating to "practical" activities such as sparring, where questions of size, strength, endurance, willingness to experience pain, etc. are highly variable. The need for a mechanism for imparting the fundamentals of a particular system, while not introducing unwanted or undue stress on trainees, may well account for an emphasis on kata in training. We note that the more competitive modern forms of the martial arts—that is, those systems that rigidly segregate trainees into classes of higher and lower competencies and are composed of aggressive personalities—are ones that have drifted away from a heavy reliance on kaho as an instructional method.

In addition, we must also remember that the pace of this process of mastery is determined by the individual pupil's aptitude. Martial arts training displays no temporal structure to the training cycle, and entering cohorts are quickly eroded by the notoriously high drop-out rates within dojos. In addition, training may be considered a "spiral" rather than lineal process: trainees continue to refine even the most elemental skills throughout their training careers. Differing physical capacities, levels of emotional maturity, and psychological factors create varying dynamics for each student. Any experienced martial arts instructor knows that there are fairly consistent patterns in aggregate learning, but that each student brings a unique set of strengths and weaknesses to the process. The cyclical nature of training using kata thus permits general progression to take place while at the same time permitting individual focus on specific deficiencies.

Kata practice is also an activity that can be engaged in alone or by groups of students of various age levels or competencies—a key point stressed by modernizers such as Funakoshi Gichin (1868–1957). As such, it is a technique ideally suited to maximizing teachability among heterogeneous populations, an important consideration when we consider the activity's voluntary nature and its existence within a market context.

B) Practicality

There are also basic issues relating to "crowd control" and safety that recommend kaho. It was considered essential in the kobujutsu, the old systems of Japan, which are heavily weapons oriented. In addition to the cultural influences cited earlier, the extreme lethality of edged weapons introduces complications in the teaching method: training must be as realistic as possible, but not induce casualties among the trainees. The mechanics of controlling a class of novices wielding razor sharp or heavy wooden weapons suggests that kaho permitted a replication of successful combat techniques in a choreographed manner.

A room full of students using a slashing weapon like the Japanese sword (*katana*), for instance, provides some real and very serious immediate practical considerations. The wind up and finish embodied in techniques using a three-foot sword create a zone of danger around each swordsman. Trainees need to learn critical issues regarding distance and safe management of the weapon. They need to learn to wield their weapons well and to avoid those of their fellow students. This is not a trivial concern. Note that the sorts of weapons typically used in the martial arts are characteristic of individual, heroic combat styles. The greater the density of fighters in one spot, the higher the likelihood of a literal type of collateral damage. Armies that utilize mass formations tend to emphasize thrusting attacks, since they focus danger to the front and toward the enemy and minimize the possibility of self-inflicted wounds. The techniques developed for the Roman legionnaire's gladius, the Zulu impi's assegai, and the Greek hoplite's spears and swords all support this observation. Japan's weapons systems, forged in a different age, provide unique problems for group practice.

Viewed from this perspective, we can understand kaho's practical aspect as something driven by the need to create a pattern of behavior that protects students from themselves and each other, as well as one that provides an environment in which instructions for complex skills can be communicated, despite the emotional overlay of excitement, fear, and effort.

As mentioned before, kata are also models of success. They are thought to embody lessons learned by past masters. Like all cultural learning, they serve as a type of compacted, highly condensed information stream that holds multiple lessons for practitioners. Thus, kata can be used to teach the rudiments of a system, to refine growing skill, and also to reveal more subtle applications (*bunkai*) to advanced practitioners.

C) Ideas and Emotions

In more modern martial arts forms, the emphasis on kata is also driven by ideological factors that seek to create a mind-set that is not solely focused on combat. In this sense, katas form an integral part of the "moving Zen" experience many people seek in martial arts training—a physically and mentally engaging activity that generates a sense of intrinsic self-satisfaction consistent with the psychological concept of "flow" (see Czikstenmihalyi, 1975, 1990).

The discipline needed to diligently practice and master kata may also serve as a mechanism to test the commitment to an art. Dojos abound with stories of enthusiastic novices whose commitment fades quickly and whose numbers evaporate over time. There may be an element of planning in this phenomenon: martial arts teachers wish to test the commitment and the mettle of potential students—their attitude as much as their aptitude—and kata practice can serve as an excellent vehicle to do so.

There is also an additional ritual and aesthetic quality to kata performance. The stereotyped movements replicated through kata performance may be understood to be doing a number of things: they serve as a public statement of adherence to a particular martial arts style, they are a visible indicator of an individual's acquisition of skill, they provide the opportunity to experience a "flow" experience directly linked to the mystical-religious aspects of the martial arts that attract so many Westerners, and, to the extent that performance is skillful, it draws both observers and performers into an aesthetic community that identifies and reaffirms basic underlying systemic principles.

Conclusion

Westerners tend to view kaho as a cultural relic. Its persistence as a teaching tool in the Japanese martial tradition, however, may suggest that there is a functionality present in the method that is often overlooked. As with most sociological phenomena, there is a complex network of influences at play here.

The tradition of kaho is shaped by two major categories of influences: the cultural and the technical. Cultural patterns inherent in East Asian society during the formative period of martial arts development certainly account for some aspects of these systems: clothing, terminology, etiquette, and even kata practice. This is not, however, the only element at play here.

The fighting systems' overwhelmingly "practical" nature suggests that more mundane factors may be at play. We have identified pedagogical issues that support a continued utilization of kaho, practical considerations that are created by the nature of the human/weapon interface, and more psychological aspects that serve to answer more complex emotional needs of practitioners. It is hoped that the exercise, like the practice of kata itself, assists in revealing the sophisticated and complex nature of these martial systems.

Bibliography

Budden, P. (2000). *Looking at a far mountain: A study of kendo kata*. Rutland, VT: Tuttle Publishing.

Craig, D. (1999). *The heart of kendo*. Boston: Shambhala.

Csikszentmihalyi, M. (1990). *Flow: The psychology of optimal experience*. New York: Harper and Row.

Csikszentmihalyi, M. (1975). *Beyond boredom and anxiety: The experience of play and work in games*. San Francisco, CA: Josey-Bass.

Donohue, J. (1991). The dimensions of discipleship: Organizational paradigm, mystical transmission, and vested interest in the Japanese martial tradition. *Ethnos*, 55, 1–2.

Friday, K., with Humitake, S. (1997). *Legacies of the sword: The Kashima Shin-ryu and samurai martial culture*. Honolulu: University of Hawaii Press.

Friday, K. (1995). Kabala in motion: Kata and pattern practice in traditional bugei. *Journal of Asian Martial Arts*, 4(4), 27–39.

Hanson, V. (1989). *The western way of war: Infantry battle in classical Greece*. Berkeley, CA: University of California Press.

Hsu, F. (1975). *Iemoto: The heart of Japan*. Cambridge: Belknap Press.

Hurst, G. (1998). *Armed martial arts of Japan: Swordsmanship and archery*. New Haven, CT: Yale University Press.

Inoue Y. (2002a). A philosophical look at kata. *Kendo World*, 1(2), 34–38.

Inoue Y. (2002b). The philosophy of kata: Part 2. *Kendo World*, 1(3), 59–69.

Kawaishi, M. (1982). *The complete 7 katas of judo*. Woodstock, NY: Overlook Press.

Kano, J. (1986). *Kodokan judo*. Tokyo: Kodansha International.

King, W. (1993). *Zen and the way of the sword: Arming the samurai psyche*. Oxford: Oxford University Press.

Lee, B. (1975). *The tao of Jeet Kun Do*. Burbank, CA: Ohara Publishing.

Leggett, T. (1978). *Zen and the ways*. Rutland, VT: Charles E. Tuttle Co.

Morris, D. (1965). *The washing of the spears*. New York: Simon and Schuster.

Nakane, C. (1970). Japanese society. Berkeley, CA: University of California Press.

Onuma, H., with De Prospero, D., and De Prospero, J. (1993). *Kyudo: The essence and practice of Japanese archery*. Tokyo: Kodansha International.

Otaki, T., and Draeger, D. (1983). *Judo formal techniques: A complete guide to Kodokan Randori no Kata*. Rutland, VT: Charles E. Tuttle Co.

Suzuki, D. (1959). *Zen and Japanese culture*. Princeton, NJ: Princeton University Press.

Warner, G., and Draeger, D. (1982). *Japanese swordsmanship: Theory and practice*. Tokyo: Weatherhill.

chapter 50

Masaru Shintani:
The Making of a Modern Canadian Karate Master

by Robert Toth

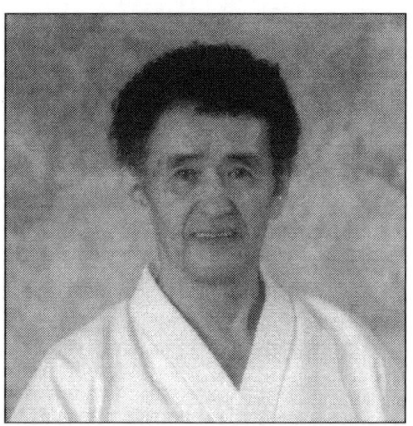

Masaru Shintani, founder of the Shintani Wado Kai karate system.
Photograph dated 1996.

Abstract

This article looks at the life of Japanese/Canadian karate pioneer, Masaru Shintani, from his birth in Vancouver, British Columbia, until his death in Kapuskasing, Ontario. After more than thirty years of teaching, Shintani created one of the largest karate organizations in North America with over 27,000 members. Shintani also invented Shindo, a martial art facilitating the use of an ancient weapon, the short stick, with modern techniques. For this article, many of Shintani's senior students helped to reconstruct his life and explain his complex personality with recollections of their teacher. From the beginning of his karate training in an internment camp, to the eventual achievement of 9th-degree black belt, Masaru Shintani epitomized the modern karate master.

Introduction

This story began twenty years ago when I received a casual introduction to a legend in the Canadian martial arts, Masaru Shintani. I was having a series of treatments for a bad knee at a physio-therapy center in Hamilton, Ontario. After arriving and going through my regular round of ultra-sound on my labored joint, the therapist sat me at a machine for the exercise part of my visit. At a different machine next to me was an older man. How much older than me, I couldn't tell, as he had a full head of curly dark hair and a muscular physique that was apparent even through his shirt. The therapist introduced us by saying, "You two karate guys should get along. This is Shintani" and then walked away.

Of course I had heard of Masaru Shintani, who sometimes went by the name Basil, as he was officially the highest ranked karate black belt in Canada and the head of a large karate organization. Being that I was a lowly new 1st-degree black belt, I was stunned to say the least and mumbled something to him. He looked up at me and asked where I trained and I answered. He politely nodded and said, "That's good karate" and then went back to his exercises. He could have ignored me or he could have slighted my choice of karate schools in favor of his own, but he did neither.

Mr. Shintani told me he was having some physiotherapy done as the result of a car accident in which his back had been injured. He didn't say more and only recently did I learn the complete story. A drunk driver had caused the accident and Mr. Shintani's car had rolled over twice. Despite the injury, he had crawled out of his damaged vehicle and apprehended the other driver (Rempel, 2006 April 17)!

I've never forgotten the simple act of kindness he showed me that day and over the twenty years since then I've always been rather in awe of the Shintani karate organization.

After hearing of his death in the year 2000, I had mentioned to my wife on numerous occasions my idea of writing an article about Masaru Shintani. Finally, after mentioning it yet again she replied, "So, why don't you?" So with that impetus I started the research that led to the following article.

Life in British Columbia

British Columbia is Canada's third largest province. Only one American state, Alaska, is larger in surface. Japan would fit into British Columbia two and a half times (Fodor's, 1991:266).

From the earliest days, settlers on the west coast of Canada were extremely conscious of their British origin and wished to have the colony remain an area populated only by British immigrants. But without increasing its population the province could never become prosperous. The white settlers were constantly concerned over the racial origins of immigrants who came to the area, yet without them there was not an adequate supply of labor. Part of the bargain British Columbia made when they joined the Dominion of Canada was that the Canadian Pacific Railway had to be completed as far as the west coast. In order to do this, the only large supply of labor was the Chinese (Adachi, 1991: 37). When construction of the Canadian Pacific Railway began in 1881, Chinese laborers were imported by the thousands. Employers saw the Chinese as providing cheap and plentiful labor, but white laborers resented the Chinese who were willing to work for a lower wage. So, the political parties in British Columbia adopted an anti-Oriental stand or lose the white labor vote. The Japanese were included with the Chinese in the minds of most of the legislators who attempted to restrict their employment in the province.

Japan's consular representatives in Canada expended a great deal of energy in looking after the welfare of the Japanese immigrants. Much of their efforts were directed against the tendency of non-Orientals to lump Japanese in with Chinese immigrants (Adachi, 1991:38–39, 42).

The attitude of the white population in British Columbia to the Japanese was altered in 1900 when Japanese troops along with British, French, German and Russian, formed an international army that crushed the Boxer Rebellion in China.[1] During the uprising, Russia used this distraction to move a large number of troops south through Manchuria and into Korea. Japan had also coveted Korea, so in response declared war on Russia in February 1904. To Canadians, Japan was now an ally of Great Britain and was fighting a power that had been regarded as one of Britain's most dangerous enemies (Adachi, 1991:44). The war concluded on September 5, 1905 after US president Theodore Roosevelt's peace initiative led to talks between Japan and Russia (Hane, 1992: 176–177). There was worldwide admiration and astonishment over Japan's rise to a position of international power. In the few months following the end of the war only 345 Japanese had entered British Columbia but by 1906 the number had increased to 1,922 (Adachi, 1991:44).

Shintani Family in British Columbia

Until 1909, most of the immigrants from Japan were unattached males and nearly all of them were hoping to make quick fortunes (Adachi, 1991:26). Included were Kanaye Shintani and his brothers. They came from Japan to Canada in the early 1900's and settled on Grouse Mountain (Graham, 2006 April 2) situated just outside of Vancouver on the north shore. Today Grouse Mountain is a popular hiking spot and ski resort (Antonsen, 2006; White, 2006). The Shintanis started a sawmill that became quite profitable. Later, they used their earnings to establish themselves in the cargo ferrying business. At the time there were many ships coming from Japan with cargo that needed to be transferred to the Vancouver ports. Kanaye Shintani found this to be another lucrative business and purchased a ship to transport cargo (Graham, 2006 April 2).

Eventually, the Shintani brothers had accumulated enough wealth that they could marry and they returned to Japan in search of wives. They were intent on *issei*, or first generation Japanese women, rather than those born in Canada because they would be more traditional and more subservient. In Japan, Kanaye Shintani arranged marriage to a young woman from the Matsumoto samurai family (Graham, 2006 March 27). Tsuruye (Canadianized to Thelia) Matsumoto, was brought to Canada in 1918 (Shintani, 1994).

A Japanese wife at that time was simply an adjunct to the husband's needs. She was a person who would look after his wants and relieve his discomforts. Loneliness was the common lot of most of the young wives brought from Japan. Only after having children could they divert their feelings of love to their sons and daughters (Adachi, 1991:90, 91).

The Shintanis were to have six children, four girls and two boys (Shintani, 1994). Masaru Shintani, the eldest son (Elliott, 2000:A8), was born on February 3, 1927 in Vancouver, British Columbia (Shintani and Reid, 1998:6).

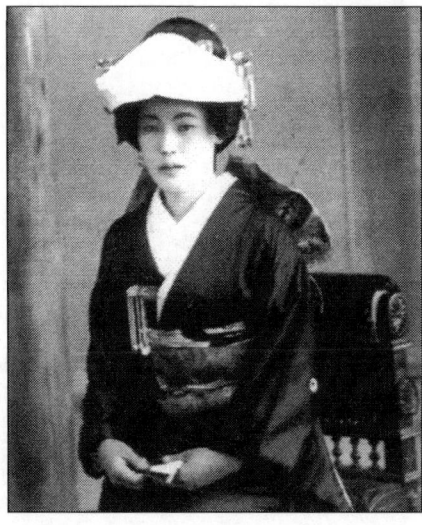

Masaru Shintani's mother, Tsuruye Matsumoto, in 1918.

Masaru Shintani's Childhood

Kanaye was an abusive father (Labbe, 2006 March 27). Masaru explained that his earliest memory of his father was at about three years old. His drunken father picked him up and threw him through a window. His mother came outside to him and they hid in the forest until his father was sober (Shintani, 1994).

When Masaru was seven years old his father was killed in an accident during a drinking party on a boat (Graham, 2006 March 27). Kanaye had climbed onto one of the booms and crawled into a hoisting net. The net was weighted so that it would drop easily when empty. He told the other men at the party to release it and the net dropped to the bottom of the harbor. When the men realized what they had done, they quickly brought the net and Kanaye back to the surface but by doing so he was severed in the boat's propellers (Graham, 2006 April 2).

After his father's death, two ministers by the names of Wilkinson with the Anglican Church of England helped to support the Shintani family (Graham, 2006 April 19). Years later, Tsuruye Shintani would become an Anglican lay minister (Manara, 2006). Masaru attended Japanese school after his regular school hours to learn to read and write the Japanese language. It was at the Japanese school that the young Masaru was first introduced to the martial arts of judo and kendo (Graham, 2006 March 27).

The War in the Pacific began with the Japanese attack on Pearl Harbor on December 7, 1941 (Hane, 1992:310), but Canada declared war on Japan only as a result of the Japanese attack on the British colony of Hong Kong that occurred five hours after Pearl Harbor (Adachi, 1991:199).

By the early months of 1942, the people of Japanese descent living in British Columbia became a problem for the Canadian government. Their removal would greatly simplify the task of defending the coastline against possible invasion and would also remove the source of widespread apprehension among the white population. On February 26, 1942 a formal announcement was made of the mass evacuation of all persons of Japanese origin to a clearing station or assembly center in Vancouver until arrangements could be made for placing them elsewhere (Adachi, 1991:211, 217–218).

In later years, Masaru Shintani spoke of his family being forcibly removed from their home and taken to the camps. He described the situation as "a jumble of terror" (Rempel, 2006 April 17). Shintani's mother, Tsuruye, suffered a physical and mental breakdown over trying to keep her family together. By the time they arrived at the New Denver camp she was quite ill as she would not eat. Masaru fed her like an infant, chewing the food for her and feeding her from his mouth. In time, Tsuruye regained her health (Graham, 2006 March 27).

Karate Class at Relocation Camp

Shintani began his karate training at the age of fourteen in the relocation camp they had been sent to in New Denver, British Columbia. His karate teacher was Akira Kitagawa (Warrener, 1981:6, 8). Masaru first trained in aikido at the camp. He didn't care for it, but Shintani's mother thought the instructor embodied what should be learned in the way of manners and politeness. Akira Kitagawa was just the opposite.

Masaru Shintani and his friends would often see Kitagawa standing in a stream punching and kicking or striking trees with his hands and feet until the bark fell off. The boy's parents told them to stay away from Kitagawa because there was a rumor that Kitagawa had killed two Canadian Mounted Policemen before entering the camp, but that just drew the teenagers right to him (Graham, 2006 March 27).

Shintani admitted that the training with Kitagawa was viscous. It was a grueling self-defense system (Warrener, 1981:6). Akira Kitagawa taught life skills and survival (Lane, 2006). Kitagawa called his karate system Okinawan Te and at the time Shintani didn't know there was any other kind (Graham, 2006 March 27).

August 15, 1945 was the day the people of Japan heard the voice of their emperor for the first time as he broadcast his decision to end the war and on September 2 the day the documents of surrender were signed on board the battleship "Missouri" in Tokyo Bay (Hane, 1992:339). At the end of the war, Kitagawa decided to return to Japan and Shintani stayed in contact with him for years afterwards. Eventually, Masaru was able to visit Kitagawa in Japan before the later died from tuberculoses (Shintani, 1998).

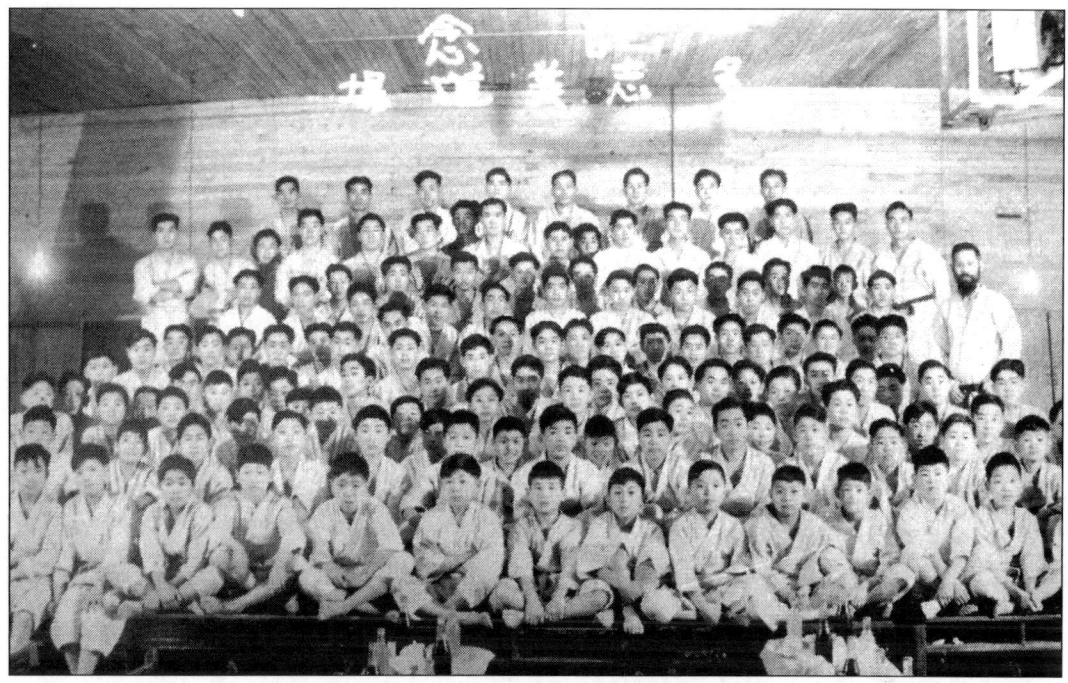

Japanese internment camps in Canada played a significant part in the spread of martial arts throughout North America. By October 1942, the Canadian government had set up eight internment camps in interior British Columbia, including New Denver and Tashme. Over 22,000 people were relocated. This picture shows the 1942 Judo Club, in Tashme, BC. Courtesy of Seichi Tahara. Photograph provided by: Nikkei Internment Memorial Centre Collection, New Denver, BC, Canada. www.newdenver.ca/nikkei/nikkei.php

The Move to Ontario

In 1947, the Shintani family moved east and settled in Beamsville, Ontario where they worked for a local farmer (Elliot, 2000:A8). The area farms wanted the Japanese for fruit pickers and the jobs were brokered by the British Columbia Security Commission (Graham, 2006 April 20). At the time, the Shintanis had thought it would be safer in Ontario than British Columbia, but they were proven wrong. Most people outside of British Columbia had never seen a Japanese person before except as sinister characters in the movies and the evacuation of Japanese in British Columbia was certification by the Canadian government that all Japanese were dangerous (Adachi, 1991:279–280). There were many times that Masaru had to defend himself and he said that he had been lucky to have had Kitagawa as a teacher because the rugged training had saved his life.

In the early 1950s, Shintani started teaching judo and later karate in a shed on the farm. One of his first students was a local police officer who was able to help Shintani avoid prosecution after his frequent skirmishes with local gangs.

Masaru Shintani's first formal karate club was opened at the Hamilton YMCA in 1952 (Graham, 2006 March 27). Later, the club moved to several different locations including a bowling alley and the local Japanese Cultural Centre (Rizzo, 2006). Shintani dreaded professional karate schools and liked to keep a low profile (Lane, 2006).

Meanwhile, the Shintanis purchased a farm in Beamsville and created a successful market gardening business (Elliott, 2000:A8). He also constructed one of the first miniature villages for tourists in the Niagara area (Graham 2006 March 27; Rempel, 2006 April 28). Masaru Shintani loved baseball. He had played in the internment camp in British Columbia during the war (Graham, 2006 March 27) and for a time he was a pitcher (Warrener, 1981: 6, Rempel, 2006 April 29; Rizzo, 2006) for the Cleveland Indians farm team (Elliott, 2000:A8).

Meeting Master Otsuka

Shintani had been taking his mother back to Japan on a regular basis and during one of these trips in the mid-1950s he competed in a karate tournament. At the tournament he met the man that would have a huge effect on his life, Hironori Otsuka (Graham, 2006 March 27).

Hironori Otsuka (1892–1982) began his martial arts training at the age of six in Shindo Yoshin-ryu jujutsu.[2] By 1921, at the age of 29, he was awarded the menkyo-kaiden,[3] designating him a successor and master of the style. A year later he started karate training with the legendary Gichin Funakoshi (Corcoran, Farkas, Sobel, 1993:363).[4]

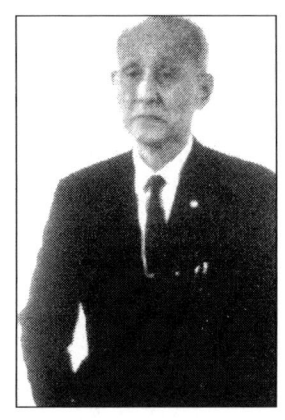

Hironori Otsuka (1892–1982).

Otsuka became known as Funakoshi's best student. He completely immersed himself in karate and assisted Funakoshi in teaching and at demonstrations. But Otsuka was not satisfied with only basics and kata, which was what Funakoshi stressed. Otsuka wanted to develop sparring which Choki Motobu had exposed him to.[5] In 1929 he set up his first independent karate club. Some believe that by 1934 he was given permission by Funakoshi to establish his own group, making him the first Japanese to be so recognized by an Okinawan mentor. Otsuka called his karate system Wado-ryu, the way of peace and harmony. By 1939, Wado-ryu was a popular style fully recognized by the Dai Nippon Butokukai.[6]

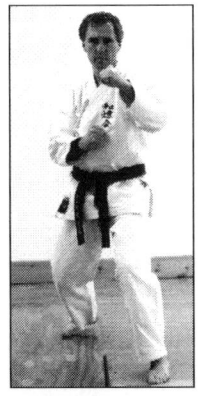 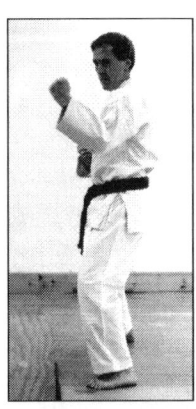 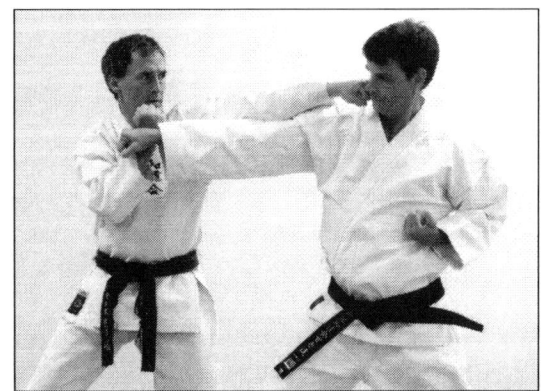

Ron Mattie demonstrates basic *tai sabaki* (body shifting) which is utilized to move off the line of attack. The black line on the floor indicates the line of attack.Ron Mattie and Denis Labbe illustrating tai sabaki with a simultaneous block and counter combination.

The techniques of Wado-ryu emphasized more sparring and practical self-defense training than most karate styles at the time on the Japanese mainland. It also placed less of an emphasis on the number of kata learned. Only nine were required. The basic katas of Wado-ryu, the pinan, were modified from the Funakoshi versions because of Otsuka's association with other karate masters including Kenwa Mabuni.[7] In addition, Otsuka incorporated jujutsu into his karate (Sells, 2000:117–119). Equally emphasized and fundamental to Wado-ryu is *tai sabaki* or body shifting to avoid the full brunt of an attack. Tai sabaki is a technique derived from swordsmanship and blocking movements are often transformed instantly into attacks (Corcoran et al. 1993:80).

For Otsuka, karate-do was primarily a spiritual discipline. In his own words, "Violent action may be understood as the martial arts, but the true meaning of martial arts is to seek and attain the way to peace and harmony" (Corcoran et al. 1993:80).

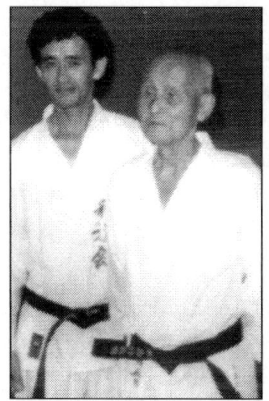
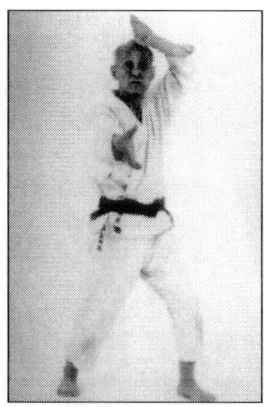
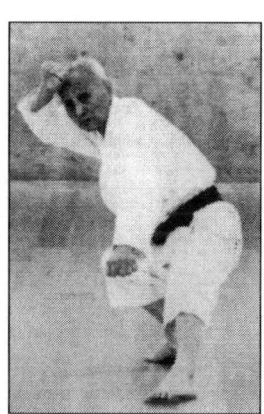

Masaru Shintani with Hironori Otsuka in Lockport, New York, in 1974.
Hironori Otsuka demonstrating movements from the Kushanku kata.

Otsuka developed a very close relationship with Shintani and his mother. Tsuruye Shintani's maiden name was Matsumoto, a very well known samurai family (Shintani and Reid, 1998:6) and that was very important to Otsuka (Graham, 2006 March 27). Masaru Shintani said of Otsuka, "He said 'you come from a fine grain,' and that's why he wanted to talk to my mother. And every time mother would go to Japan, Otsuka Sensei would go to meet her and make sure that she got to my cousin's place and my aunt's place." Shintani said, "I accepted Otsuka Sensei like a father" (Shintani, 1994) and "he treated me like a son" (Shintani, 2005). "He was everything that my mother taught me when I was young" (Shintani, 1994). The thing that existed between Shintani and Otsuka transcended karate. It was as if they followed a particular tradition that no one else did.

Shintani made regular trips to Japan and Otsuka was often in Canada (Graham, 2006 March 27). Otsuka also wrote numerous letters to Masaru and his mother during the 1960s and 1970s. The letters detail Otsuka's travels during the time and offer an interesting insight into the politics of the martial arts in Japan and North America. In the letters, Otsuka tells Shintani to "keep training hard" (Otsuka, 1969 September 17) and "try to master Wado-ryu" (Otsuka, 1972 August 22). Otsuka also suggested that Masaru train with a number of Japanese Wado karate instructors that were visiting Canada on business or attending school (Otsuka, 1972 August 22; 1977, June 17; 1976, April 2).

By 1969 or 1970, Otsuka asked Shintani to officially call his style Wado-ryu and Shintani honored his request (Graham, 2006 March 27). Otsuka wrote in a letter to Masaru Shintani dated July 14, 1974, "Please take care of the Canadian Wado Kai as its representative" (Otsuka, 1974 July 14). In 1979, Hironori Otsuka gave Shintani an 8th-degree black belt plus a 9th-degree black belt certificate for future use. Shintani told Otsuka he would not divulge the 9th-degree certificate until it was needed or until nine years after the 8th-degree rank (Shintani, 1994). Later, Shintani would do the same by postdating ranking certificates for his students (Graham, 2006 March 27; Labbe, 2006 March 27; Manara, 2006; Reid, 2006).

Hironori Otsuka died on January 29, 1982. After his death, the international Wado karate community split into separate organizations. This was triggered by differences in teaching style and leadership (Shintani and Reid, 1998:6). After Otsuka's death, Masaru Shintani became independent of the Japanese organizations, but continued to represent his teacher (Labbe, 2006 March 27). Shintani said, "I've always stuck to sensei's preaching, his philosophy, his humbleness. I copied everything he did. It's just the way a martial artist should really be. I teach with his presence" (Shintani, 2005).

Formation of Shintani Karate

Masaru Shintani broke with the Japanese organizations because he wanted to be in control. His rank was unquestionable. He was senior. He could do what he wanted and what he wanted was to teach in Canada and to bring karate to everyone (Reid, 2006). Shintani believed that anyone could train in his karate (Lane, 2006). His organization was for the most part rurally based in small towns and cities (Rempel, 2006 April 27). He had built up a circuit of schools in Ontario. There were also a number of schools whose instructors only wanted to be affiliated with Shintani without being a part of his organization and that was acceptable to him (Labbe, 2006 March 27).

Shintani was open-minded and he had a very open door policy (Joslin, 2006). He was always willing to teach anyone. He didn't gauge a person by their certificate or their belt, but by who they were. He was very accepting of people (Reid, 2006). Masaru Shintani believed it didn't matter what style of karate a person trained in, it was "all good" because it built spirit and discipline (Elliott, 2000:A8). He had a no-nonsense approach where karate was concerned and he didn't shout like other masters. He spoke softly and the student had to strain to hear (LaPlante, 2006). Learning was highly visual with him (Labbe, 2006 March 27). If he saw someone doing something incorrectly in a class, he'd stop and demonstrate (Graham, 2006 March 27). Masara Shintani had a great knowledge of internal energy (*ki*), body mechanics and tai sabaki. He was like a university professor when he taught (Reid, 2006).

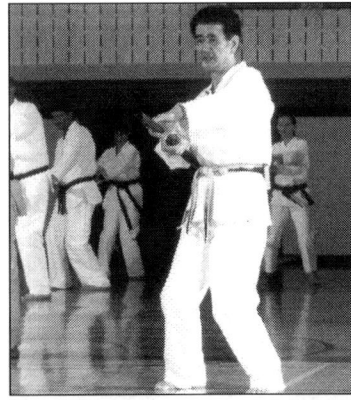 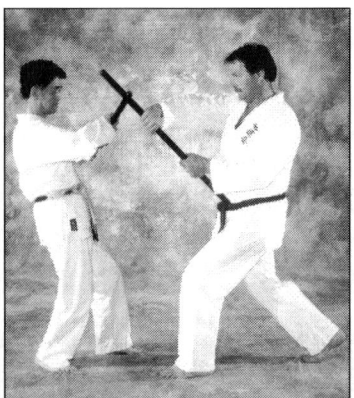 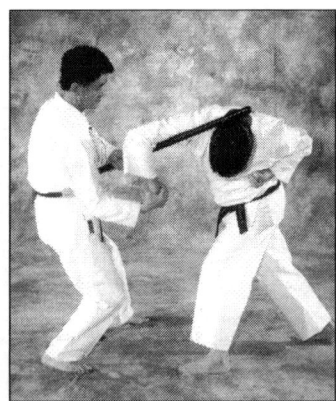

Left: Shintani teaching a Shindo clinic in Delhi, Ontario.
Right: Shintani demonstrating Shindo techniques.

Shintani's Later Years

Joseph Rempel, one of Masaru Shintani's biographers and one of his karate students said, "When sensei Shintani's mother passed away I thought it began the slow death of his own spirit and his own health" (Rempel, 2006 April 21). In fall of 1996, Shintani was teaching clinics in Alberta, Canada and he stayed with Joseph Rempel at the University of Alberta campus hotel. Rempel remembers, "At that point he was suffering more and more from a number of health problems" (Rempel, 2006 April 27).

Dr. Robert Graham, another of Shintani's biographers and also a karate student, was with him the day before Masaru suffered a stroke. Dr. Graham said, "We went out to eat and I noticed when we were walking back that every now and then he would stumble. I had never seen him to not be sure footed" (Graham, 2006 March 27).

After the stroke, which affected his left arm and leg but not his ability to communicate (Labbe, 2006 March 27), Shintani was confined to a wheelchair. But by sheer force of will, he used canes and a walker to continue to teach (Elliott, 2000:A8). Shintani traveled to Kapuskasing in North Eastern Ontario to teach and while there suffered a heart attack. He died during the airlift back to Hamilton's General Hospital (Elliott, 2000: A8). Shintani's ashes along with the ashes of his mother that had been saved after her death were buried at the same time at Woodlawn Cemetary in Hamilton, Ontario. This was done because he was his mother's first-born son (Labbe, 2006 May 13).

Masaru Shintani had lived a simple lifestyle (Rizzo, 2006). He lived in one room with the use of the homeowner's kitchen and bathroom. His room held a chair, a dresser with a small television and a bed (Graham, 2006 March 27). Denis Labbe, the right hand of Masaru Shintani (Lane, 2006) and president of the Shintani Wado Kai Karate Federation, explained, "He had no value of money. He didn't care at all about it. When money came his way he'd help out other people" (Labbe, 2006 March 27). He could have been wealthy, but chose not to be (Reid, 2006). At the time of Masaru Shintani's death, the number of people training in Wado karate in Canada was estimated at more than 27,000 and his organization was one of the largest in North America (Elliott, 2000:A8). The Shintani organization continues to teach the martial arts of Wado-ryu karate and Shindo as taught by its founder, Masaru Shintani.

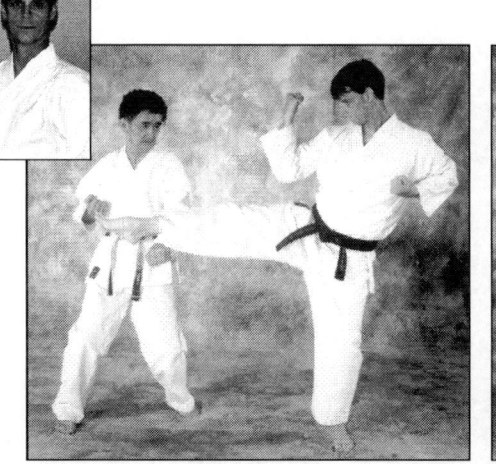
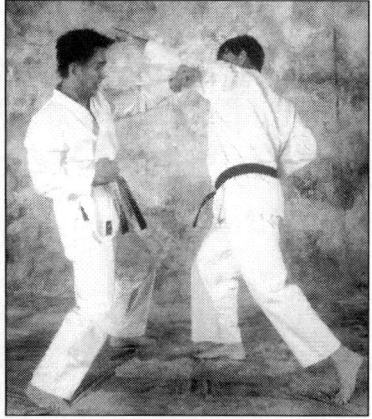

Left: Dr. Robert Graham and Denis Labbe in Welland, Ontario, in 2006.
Middle and right: Denis Labbe helps Shintani demonstrate Wado-ryu techniques in 1996.

SHINTANI WADO KAI TECHNICAL SECTION

Hironori Otsuka (1892–1982) created the Wado style of karate (Corcoran et al. 1993: 363) by combining the Shindo Yoshin-ryu jututsu he had mastered with the Shotokan karate style he learned from Gichin Funakoshi (Sells, 2000:79, 117). Otsuka was also influenced by two other Okinawan masters, Choki Motobu and Kenwa Mabuni. From Choki Motobu he relearned the kata Naihanchi and also received training in sparring or fighting techniques which Motobu specialized in (Sells, 2000:120). Otsuka also trained with Kenwa Mabuni to clarify the pinan katas (Shintani and Reid, 1998: 1). These five simple forms were modified from the method that was used by Funakoshi (Sells, 2000: 119).

Masaru Shintani's version of Hironori Otsuka's Wado karate is also a combination. It is a melding of Otsuka's Wado with the Okinawan Te of Akira Kitagawa.

Like Otsuka, Shintani demonstrated the jujutsu techniques found in the Okinawan forms. Ron Matti shows a combination from the kata Pinan Godan that ends with a jujutsu armbar (A1–A4).

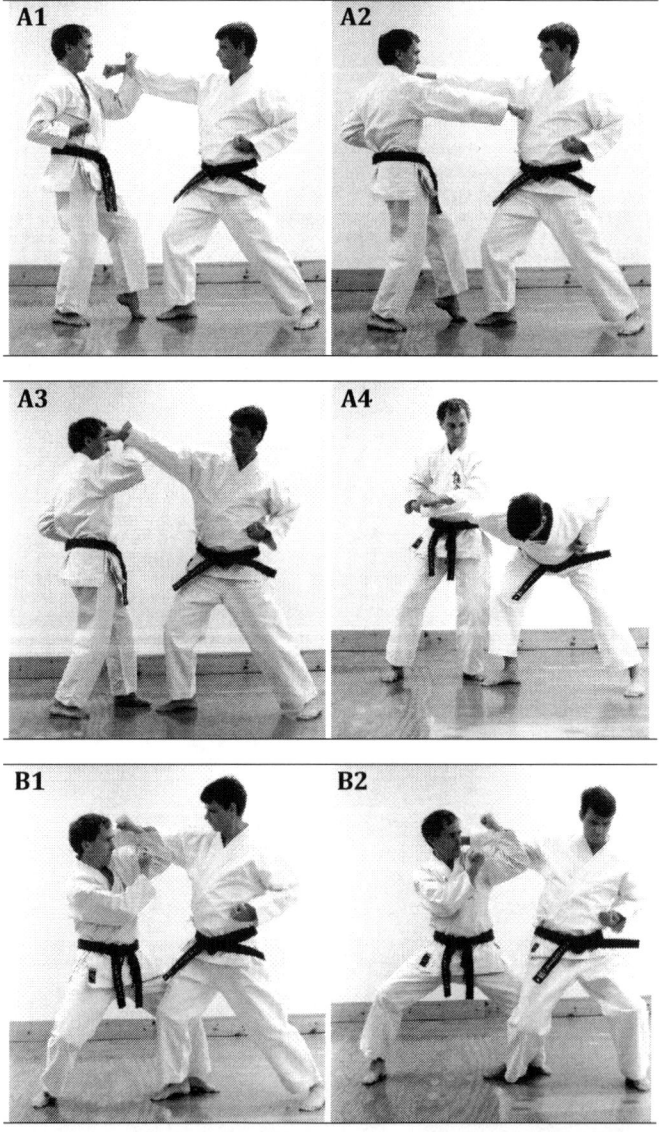

Techniques from the Pinan Godan kata showing an inside block and counter-punch followed by a jujutsu armbar technique. Ron Mattie and Denis Labbe demonstrating.

Ron Mattie and Denis Labbe illustrating one example of the inside fighting style favored by Otsuka and Shintani: blocking on the inside and countering by attacking the opponent's knee.

A basic technique of Wado is *tai sabaki* (body shifting). It is said that the Kitagawa version of tai sabaki is more pronounced. Tai sabaki also allowed a simultaneous block and counter punch response (see photographs). As well, Otsuka and Shintani both favored inside fighting (B1–B1).

The nine katas of Otsuka's Wado-ryu are taught in Shintani's version of the style, but Shintani augmented his syllabus with a number of forms that can be traced back to his first teacher, Kitagawa. Ron Mattie performs the opening moves of the kata Shopai (C1 thru C10).

This sequence of pictures shows the beginning section of the Shopai kata as passed down from Akira Kitagawa. Ron Mattie demonstrating.

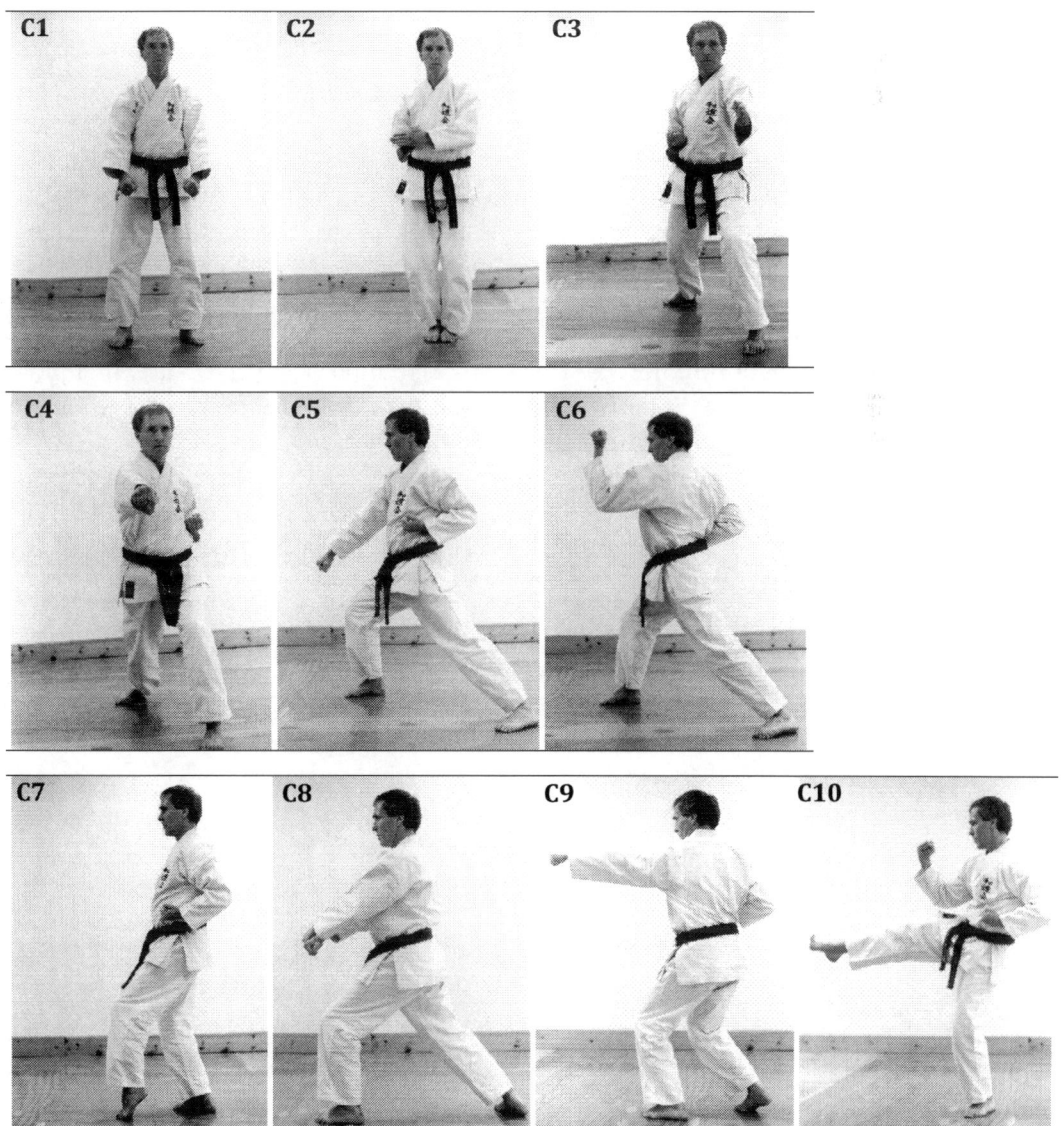

Shindo Technical Section

The techniques of Masaru Shintani's Shindo are different from other stick arts because of the principles of Wado-ryu karate that are used. Masaru Shintani demonstrated Shindo to Hironori Otsuka, the creator of Wado-ryu in 1979 (Perkins, 2006 April 17) and Otsuka gave the system his full endorsement (Reynolds, 2006:5).

Shindo was devised by Shintani in the early 1970s and he started teaching his students the stick art in the late 1980s (Reynolds, 2006:5). At first, it was modelled on a basic kendo movements with added takedowns and locks. Later it changed, becoming modelled more on staff (*bo*) techniques, utilizing a staff with a length slightly shorter than the traditional Japanese half-staff. Initially it was two overhand grips and then it became one over and one under (Rempel, 2006 April 21). The two overhand grips are known as a defensive grip meant for police officers to show a non-threatening posture (D1). The one hand over and one under is an offensive grip that is meant to be more aggressive (Perkins, 2006 May 24) (D2).

One of the core concepts that Shintani taught in Shindo was that it was to be a supplement to karate training incorporating the fundamentals of the Shintani Karate method—sudden explosive action, proper body movement (Reynolds, 2006:6) and sabaki action.

Shindo is the name used to describe the martial art and the stick itself. The same techniques can be done empty handed as with Shindo. It's an extension of your hands (E1, E2, E3). Shintani directed a number of his students to create practice forms using Shindo. Three were to be based on internationally known empty hand katas: Wanshu, Chinto, and Kushanku. They were allowed free reign, but were not to change the distancing and pattern of the existing forms. The students had to interpret the movements in the empty hand form and adapt them to Shindo (Perkins, 2006 April 17) (see G1–7; H1–7). As well, his students in Ontario invented forms called Ciobotie and Shindo Nidan (Perkins, 2006 April 17) (I1–3).

Dr. Robert Graham of Buffalo, New York, put together the form Seishin no Shindo based on the kata Seisho that Shintani learnt from his first karate teacher, Akira Kitagawa (Graham, 2006 March 27). It was one of Masaru Shintani's favorites.

Shintani would have the students show him the forms they were developing for Shindo and he would make alterations to them so as to emphasize what he wanted. For example, he specifically added a rotation movement of the forearms to a part of the Chinto no Shindo form (J1–2).

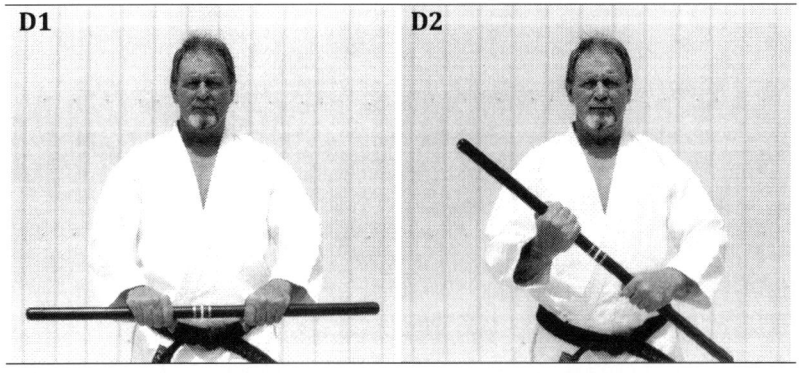

Left: The defensive grip with both hands held on the stick's topside is used to demonstrate a non-aggressive attitude. Right: The offensive grip of one hand over and one hand under is more aggressive. Bruce Perkins demonstrating.

One of Masaru Shintani's goals was to have Shindo taught to law enforcement agencies. He had done a lot of demonstrations to that effect and was on the verge of achieving his goal when he suffered a stroke. Everything in Shindo temporarily stopped. However, before Shintani passed away, he asked Bruce Perkins, one of his students, to put together a training and grading process for Shindo. Perkins and a committee of other Shintani black belts are currently developing the training program (Perkins, 2006 April 17).

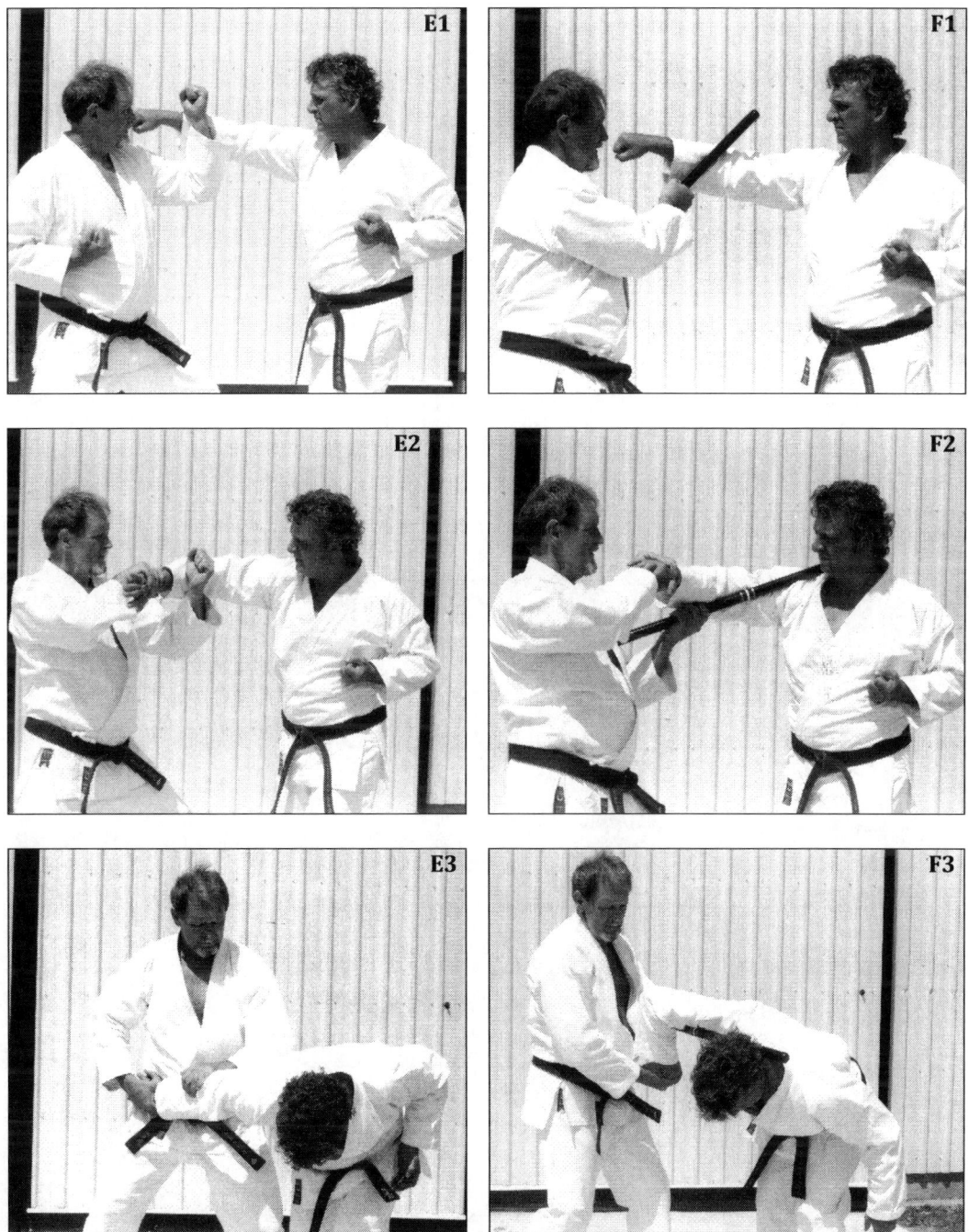

E1-3) Sequences showing a defender blocking a punch, manipulating the wrist, and moving into an armbar with empty hands; and F1-3) the same with a Shindo short stick. Bruce Perkins and James Atkinson demonstrating.

Bruce Perkins, the chairman of the Shindo Federation of North America, demonstrates part of the Chinto kata: G1–7 performed empty handed and then H1–7 with a Shindo short stick.

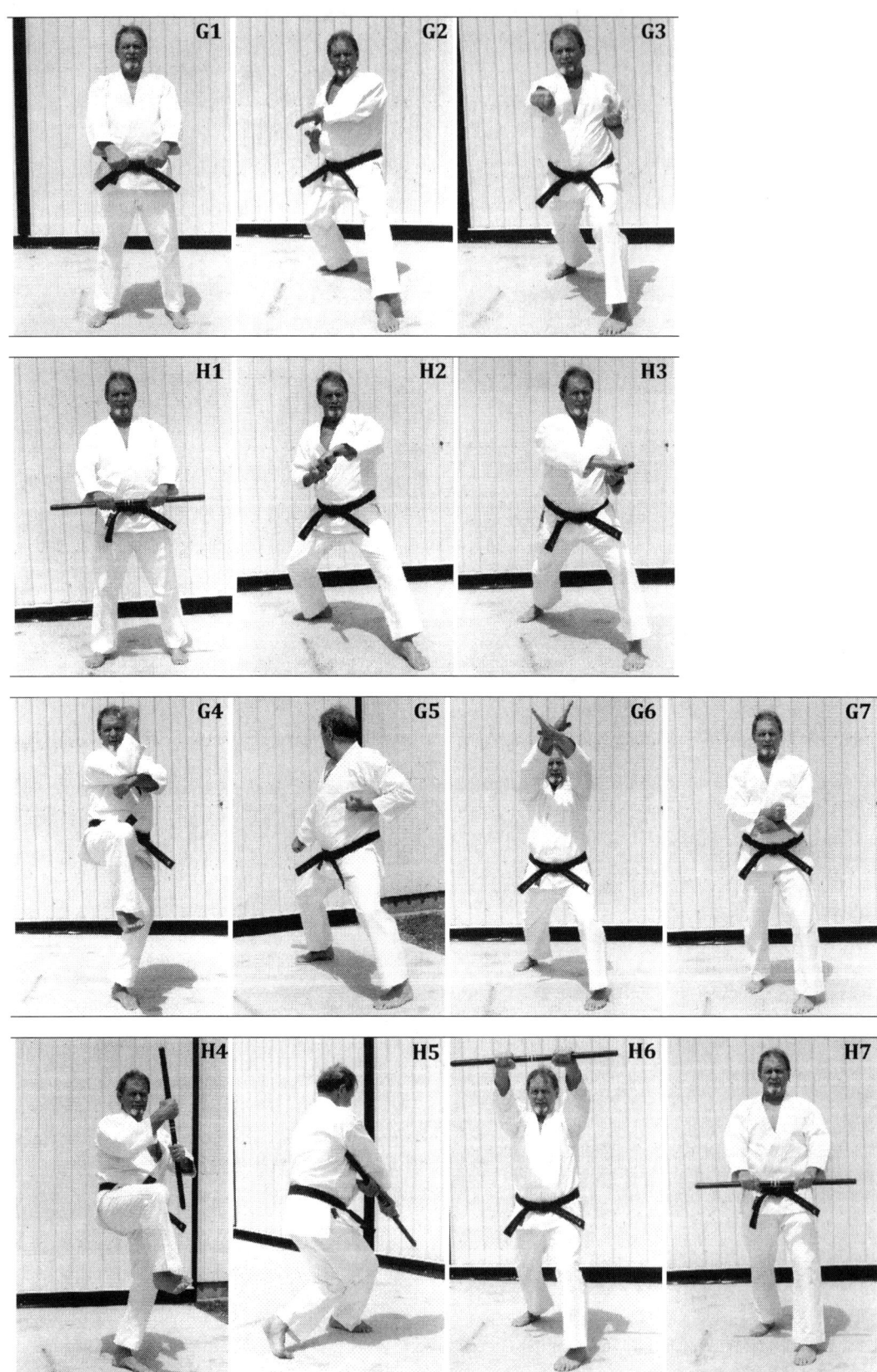

I1-3) Application from the Shindo Nidan kata: scoop block, followed a chokehold, and a takedown. Bruce Perkins and James Atkinson demonstrating.

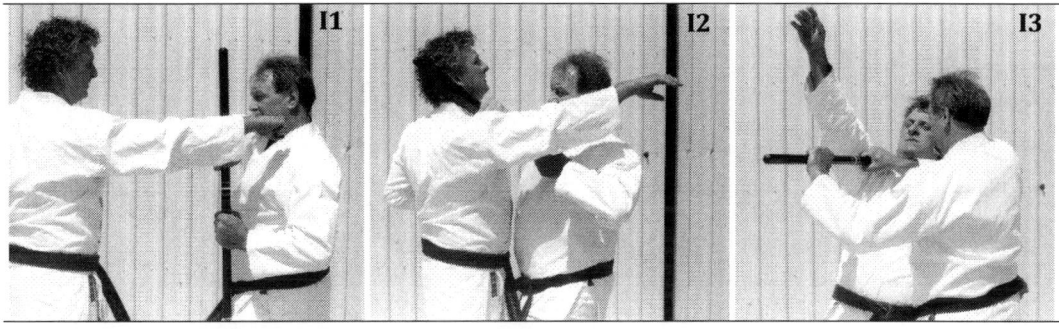

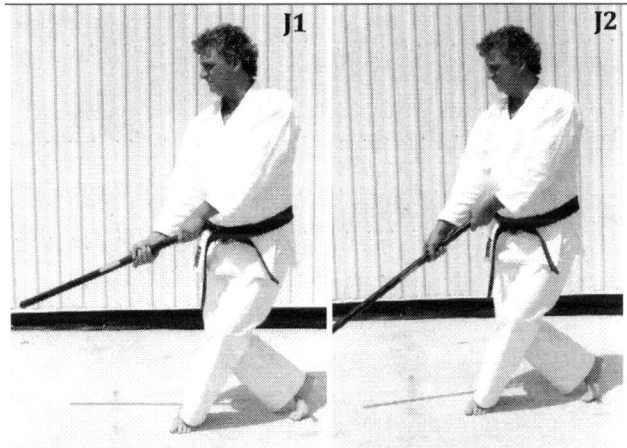

J1-2) One of the details Shintani demanded from his students in the Chinto no Shindo kata was the rotation of the forearm while performing a low block. James Atkinson demonstrating.

Conclusion

A great homage has been paid to Masaru Shintani by his senior students. They received and followed instructions by their teacher as to how they should propagate his martial art. The Wado style of karate as taught by Masaru Shintani has spread all over Canada, the United States, the Caribbean and even India.

Masaru Shintani wrote, "Wado, the way to harmony and peace is the finest quality of the human race with a total goal to peace on earth. We, the Wado students of karate, must be the leaders of unity and happiness throughout the universe and guide our students to the ultimate human alliance with understanding."

The philosophy and karate of Masaru Shintani continues.

Acknowledgment

The author would like to thank all of Masaru Shintani's students who put aside their political differences in order to help with this article. Great appreciation also to Denis Labbe, Ron Mattie, Bruce Perkins and James Atkinson for appearing in the photographs for the technical sections. Pictures of Masaru Shintani are reproduced here courtesy of Denis Labbe and Dr. Robert Graham.

Notes

[1] The Boxers were a secret society in league with the Manchu throne that attempted to drive all foreigners from China (Clubb, 1978:24, 27).

[2] Shindo Yoshin-ryu jujutsu is a Japanese style of armed and unarmed combat (Sells, 2000:117) founded in the nineteenth century (Frederic, 1988:201).

[3] A *menkyo-kaiden* is a certificate of full proficiency in a Japanese martial art usually awarded to an advanced student deemed most suited to carry on transmission of the art (Farkas and Corcoran, 1983:177).

[4] Gichin Funakoshi (1868–1957) was an Okinawan-born karate master regarded by many as the father of modern karate (Corcoran et al. 1993:324–325).

[5] Choki Motobu (1871–1944) was an Okinawan karate master. Born in Shuri, the third son of a ranking lord, as a youth he would often test himself in street fights, but had to train by himself because instructors refused him. Kosaku Matsumora did teach him a few kata because he was impressed with Motobu's ability. Later in life, Motobu received more kata training from Yabu Kentsu (Corcoran et al. 1993:357).

[6] The Dai Nippon Butokukai was founded during Japan's Meiji Period (1868–1912) and set up in the ancient capital of Kyoto in 1895. The organization was built upon the ancient concept of fostering robust strength, indomitable spirit and virtuous character. The Japanese government authorized the Butokukai to research, preserve and promote Japanese martial arts (McCarthy, 1999:73–74).

[5] Okinawan karate master Kenwa Mabuni (1889–1957) founded the Shito-ryu style. He studied Shuri Te from Yasutsune Itosu (1830–1915) and Naha Te from Kanryo Higashionna (1853–1916). Shito-ryu was created by combining the teachings of both (Corcoran et al. 1993:351).

References

Adachi, K. (1991). *The enemy that never was*. Toronto: McClelland and Stewart.

Clubb, E. (1978). *20th century China*. New York: Columbia University Press.

Corcoran, J., Farkas, E. and Sobel, S. (1993). *The original martial arts encyclopedia*. Los Angeles, CA: Pro-Action Publishing.

Eliott, J. (2000, May 12). *Obituary: Karate master's credo of peace and harmony will live on*. Hamilton Spectator.

Farkas, E. and Corcoran, J. (1983). *The Overlook martial art dictionary*. New York: The Overlook Press.

Fodor's (1991). *Canada*. New York: Fodor's Travel Publications.

Frederic, L. (1988). *A dictionary of the martial arts*. Rutland, VT: Charles E. Tuttle.

Hane, M. (1992). *Modern Japan – A historical survey*. Boulder, CO: Westview Press.

McCarthy, P. (1999). *Ancient Okinawan martial arts – Koryu uchinadi, vol.* 2. Rutland, VT: Charles E. Tuttle.

Reynolds, K. (2006, January). Shindo Federation of North America Sept. Grading 2005. In *The Harmonizer, Official Newsletter of the Shintani Wado Kai Karate Federation*, *10*(1).

Sells, J. (2000). *Unante – The secrets of karate*. 2nd edition. Hollywood, CA: W.M. Hawley.

Shintani, M. and Reid, G. (1998). *Wado-kai karate-Kata*. Wado-Kai Karate Association of Canada Victoria, British Columbia.

Shintani, M. (2005). DVD. *Katas – Shintani Wado Kai Karate Federation, Vol. 2*. Omni Media Productions.

Warrener, D. (1981, April-May). Masaru Shintani – Wado Ryu karate master. *Martial Arts World, 4*(2).

Personal Communications

Graham, R. (2006, March 27). Interview in Welland, Ontario.
Graham, R. (2006, April 2). Personal communication.
Graham, R. (2006, April 19). Personal communication.
Graham, R. (2006, April 20). Personal communication.
Joslin, R. (2006, April 26). Personal communication.
Labbe, D. (2006, March 27). Interview in Welland, Ontario.
Labbe, D. (2006, May 13). Personal communication.
Lane, B. (2006, April 26). Personal communication.
LaPlante, G. (2006, May 4). Personal communication.
Manara, D. (2006, April 25). Personal communication.
Otsuka, H. (1969, September 17). Letter to Masaru Shintani.
Otsuka, H. (1972, August 22). Letter to Masaru Shintani.
Otsuka, H. (1974, July 14). Letter to Masaru Shintani.
Otsuka, H. (1976, April 2). Letter to Masaru Shintani.
Otsuka, H. (1977, June 17). Letter to Masaru Shintani.
Perkins, B. (2006, April 17). Personal communication.
Perkins, B. (2006, May 24). Personal communication.
Reid, G. (2006, May 10). Personal communication.
Rempel, J. (2006, April 17). Personal communication.
Rempel, J. (2006, April 27). Personal communication.
Rempel, J. (2006, April 28). Personal communication.
Rempel, J. (2006, April 29). Personal communication.
Rizzo, A. (2006, April 26). Personal communication.
Shintani, M. (1994, September 9). Interview by Bruce Perkins.
Shintani, M. (1998, January 15). Interview by Dr. Robert Graham.

chapter 51

The Stories of Meibukan Gojyu-ryu Karate as Told by Yagi Meitatsu

by Robert Toth

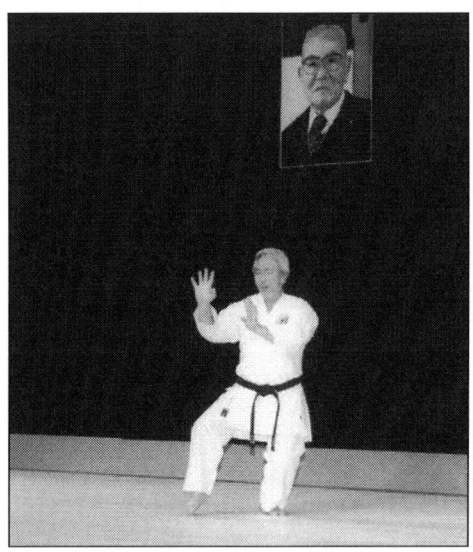

Yagi Meitatsu demonstrating kata in memory of his father. Date: March 2006.

Introduction

The opportunity to spend time with the successor of the Gojyu style of Okinawan karate is not often realized. For this author, the chance has presented itself twice. The first was in May 2004. I had invited Yagi Meitatsu to teach a seminar at our martial arts school in St. Catharines, Ontario. That afternoon, he allowed me to conduct an interview and take some pictures that were published in the *Journal of Asian Martial Arts* (Toth, 2004) as "Yagi Meitatsu discusses the not-so-secret techniques of Okinawan Gojyu-ryu karate."

Sensei Yagi was very pleased with the article. After it was published, when we'd meet for training, he'd introduce me to the attendees and ask if they had read the article. When I approached him with the idea for another article, Sensei Yagi was very much in favor of it.

STORIES

The desire to tell stories and to listen to them is inherent in the human race (Maugham, 1939:xix). Most families have stories that are passed down from generation to generation that help form their history. When Yagi Meitatsu teaches karate, he finds occasions during the class to tell stories about his father or his father's teacher, the originator of Gojyu-ryu, Miyagi Chojun. The stories he tells are all part of his family history and of Gojyu-ryu karate, as well.

On Sundays, Meitatsu's father, Meitoku, would take the family for car trips to look for antiques and visit flea markets. During these excursions, if he was in a good mood, he would regale his wife and children with stories of his teacher, Miyagi Chojun, as well as stories of Miyagi's martial arts instructors, Arakaki Ryuko and Higaonna Kanryo.

At first, Yagi Meitatsu told the stories his father had told him. But the elder Yagi would never tell of his own exploits. So, Yagi Meitatsu also shared stories he knew about his father. These are also part of Gojyu-ryu karate's history.

The stories of the lives of former generations are examples to the people of the modern day (Burton, n.d.:1). In the martial arts, stories are told to educate, instruct, and entertain. Being a part of the martial arts is being involved with a history that stretches back countless millennium. The stories of the past masters help keep us connected to that stream of history that martial artists are all a part of.

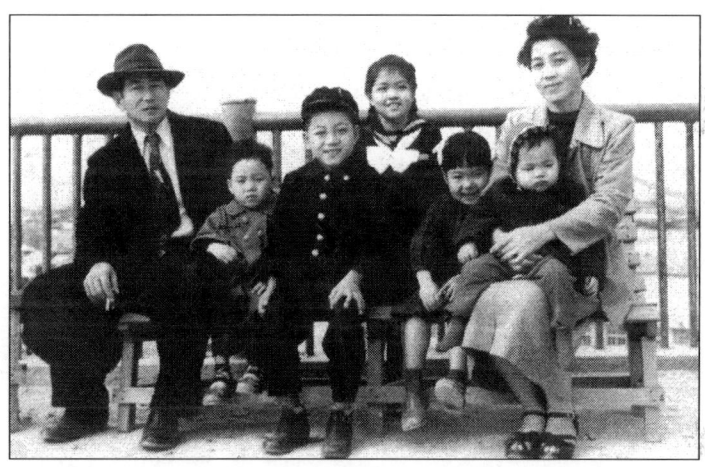

The Yagi family. Meitatsu is the oldest boy sitting next to his sister.

A Short History of Gojyu-ryu Karate

Miyagi Chojun started his martial arts training with Arakaki Ryuko (Sells, 2000:81). Yagi Meitatsu tells the story of Miyagi's first meeting with Arakaki:

> One day, a tough guy was fighting in the street with many people.
> He was so strong that nobody could touch him. The authorities were
> called and two policemen came, but they couldn't control the tough
> either. He was just too strong. The young Miyagi Chojun stood watching.
> Finally, one fellow was able to get the tough guy down and hold him
> easily. Miyagi was amazed and he followed the man to his house and
> asked him to teach him. This was Miyagi's first teacher, Arakaki Ryuko.
> In Arakaki's small house, there was striking post [*makiwara*], stones
> used for weightlifting [*chishi*], earthen training jars [*kami*], and all kinds
> of training items. Arakaki's martial art was about conditioning the body
> first. So, this is how Miyagi Chojun started his martial arts training.
> When Arakaki recognized Miyagi's talent, he introduced him to
> Higaonna Kanryo.

Higaonna is remembered as the man who popularized the Fujian martial arts in late 19th-century Okinawa (Sells, 2000:45, 47). The following story about Higaonna was told to Yagi Meitatsu by his father:

> Higaonna had arranged passage on a ship to Fujian, China, to continue his martial arts training. He knew a man who was captain of a ship and he asked him to take him. Higaonna went to Fujian Province, and started training in the martial arts with Ryoto, a bamboo craftsman. After he studied for about two years, Ryoto found that Higaonna Kanryo had a talent for the marital arts. So, he introduced him to Ryuru Ko. That's the martial arts way. Higaonna trained hard and became the assistant instructor to Ryuru Ko in China. Higaonna Kanryo stayed at Ryuru Ko's house. Higaonna would sleep on the first floor and Ryuru Ko slept on the second floor. Higaonna had a bamboo bed with a thin blanket. That way he wouldn't sleep easily and he'd wake up quickly, like an animal, and when people would come he would hear them. Higaonna stayed at Ryuru Ko's house for seven or eight years.
>
> After eight years, Higaonna Kanryo went back to Okinawa. But before he left China, Ryuru Ko told him, "Don't teach the martial arts too easily." When Higaonna Kanryo returned to Okinawa, he didn't teach for almost twenty years. In that way, he kept his word to his teacher.
>
> People in Naha recognized that Higaonna was a great martial artist and many famous people wanted him to teach. Finally, after twenty years, he began to take students. Among them were master Miyagi Chojun, Juhatsu Kyoda,[2] and Shiroma Masahige.[3]

Miyagi Chojun trained with Higaonna Kanryo until Hiagaonna's death in 1915. Afterwards, Miyagi made at least two trips to China to further his knowledge of the martial arts. He then set about perfecting the Naha-te he had inherited from Higaonna (Sells, 2000:45, 47, 82). As a small boy, Yagi Meitatsu remembers meeting Miyagi Chojun. These are stories about Miyagi Chojun told to Meitatsu by his father:

> There are no fighting stories about Miyagi Chojun. In fact, for most of the masters there are no fighting stories.
>
> One time, Miyagi Chojun was attacked by three toughs. Miyagi curled himself into a ball to protect himself. Although the three men punched at him, they couldn't hurt him because he had developed his body to such a high degree. Miyagi covered his face with his hands, watched and waited for one of the men to kick him. When this happened, Miyagi caught the man's foot and threw him to the ground. The other two ran away.
>
> •••
>
> Miyagi was very strong. When he squeezed raw beef it would come out between his fingers like hamburger. He could crush young bamboo. The technique he used is something that has to be trained. It's all finger power. The thumb is not used.
>
> When Miyagi Chojun was young, about twenty-five years old, a tough guy came from mainland Japan to do demonstrations. The man's manager would offer a bet that would pay back ten times if anyone could knock the tough guy down. There were some martial artists that paid the fee, punched the man but couldn't knock him down.

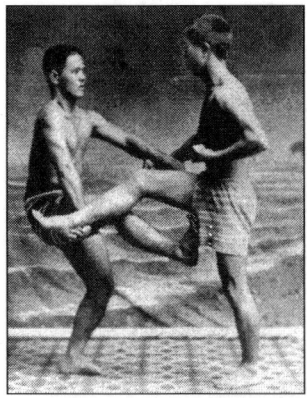
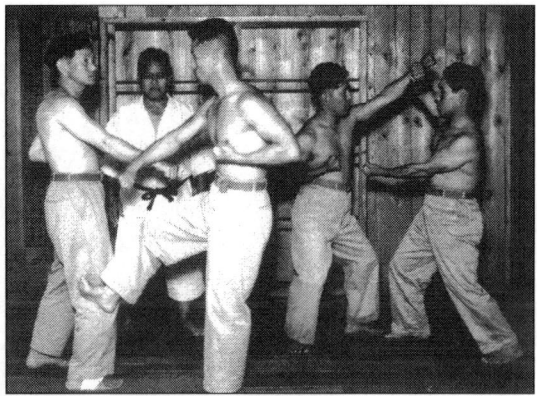
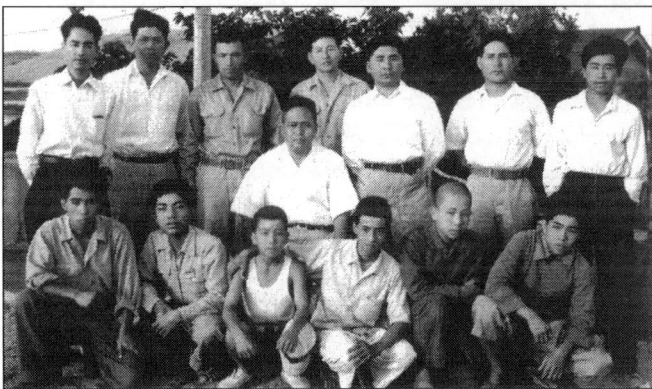

1) Miyagi Chojun with Kyoda Juhatsu.

2) Miyagi Chojun with a group of students. Yagi Meitoku is in the middle of the back row.

3) Miyagi Chojun teaching after World War II. The period can be determined by the U.S. Army issue pants worn by students. Yagi Meitoku is on the left.

When he was younger, Miyagi's name was Machu. Someone asked him, "Machu, can you do it?" Miyagi replied, "Maybe." So, he paid the fee to the tough guy's manager. Miyagi stood in front of the man, punched him and the fellow fell down. The tough guy complained, "Why did you punch? I wasn't prepared." With the other martial artists, they would wait for the tough guy to be ready before they punched him, but Miyagi didn't wait. He punched him before he could prepare. This just shows how smart Miyagi was. He was a very smart young man.

•••

When Miyagi Chojun was teaching he didn't have a dojo. He taught in his backyard. He would tell the students, "Move that stone over there. Relocate that plant over there." After two hours he'd say, "OK. You must be tired. You can go home." The next week he'd have them move the stones and plants again, but to different locations. Some of the students got tired of it. They thought that Miyagi wasn't teaching anything, so they went to another dojo where the teacher taught forms [kata]. After a few months, there were only two or three students left with Miyagi and only then did Miyagi start to teach.

There were two reasons he did this. First, Miyagi was watching the personality of each student. Second, in the Gojyu system, it's important to make the body strong first. Remember, Ryuru Ko didn't want Higaonna to make learning the martial arts too easy and Higaonna had passed that on to Miyagi.

•••

Miyagi Chojun was a very severe instructor. When a student came with a towel wrapped around his neck to the dojo, he was told not to come again.

When another student came to the dojo whistling, he was told not to come back. Miyagi said, "If you'd show disrespect like that to my face, what would you do behind my back?" Miyagi was very severe.

•••

A long time ago the Butokukai[4] invited Miyagi Chojun to demonstrate in Tokyo. Miyagi couldn't go. To be frank, he got sea sick when he traveled by boat. So, he sent his senior student, Shinzato Jinan.[5] At that time, in Japan, they had many different kinds of jujutsu[6] and kenjutsu.[6] After the demonstration in the changing room, some of the Japanese martial artists came to Shinzato and said, "We have names for the different styles of our martial arts. What is the name of your style?"

At that time in Okinawa, the art was just called *te* or *tode* to represent "Chinese Hand." So, when Shinzato returned to Okinawa, he reported this story to Miyagi Chojun. Now, Miyagi's family was rather well off and he knew of the old Chinese martial arts manual called the *Bubishi*.[8] Higaonna Kanryo also used to tell Miyagi about the *Kempo Haiku* ["Fist Way Eight Poems"] that is in the *Bubishi*. The two words Miyagi liked the most from the Kempo Haiku was "gojyu."

•••

Miyagi had two favorite philosophies. The first was: to study the martial arts, you have to train in spiritual training before physical techniques. Even if you have good techniques, if you don't have a good heart, people won't follow you. The second was about how there is no competition for flowing water. It will just naturally go from up to down and someday, it will reach the sea. These are Miyagi Chojun's favorite philosophical concepts.

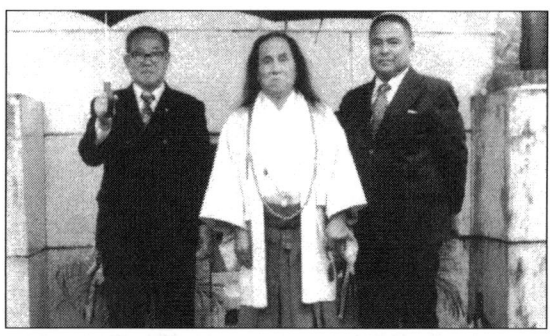

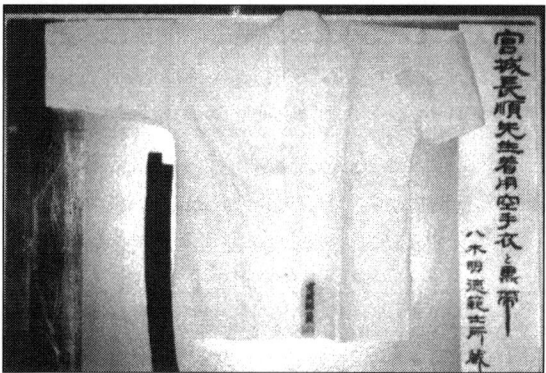

Left: "Fist methods, eight poems" from the *Bubishi*. Top right: Yagi Meitoku, Yamaguchi Gogen, and Ken Miyagi at Miyagi Chojun's grave. Bottom right: Miyagi Chojun's uniform and belt.

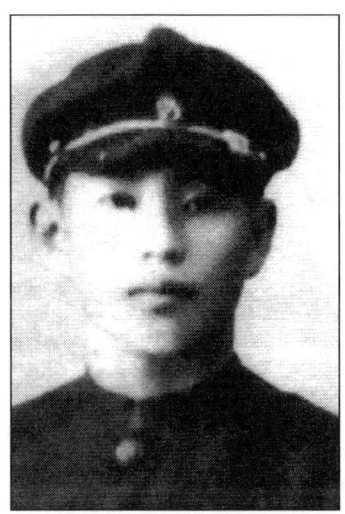 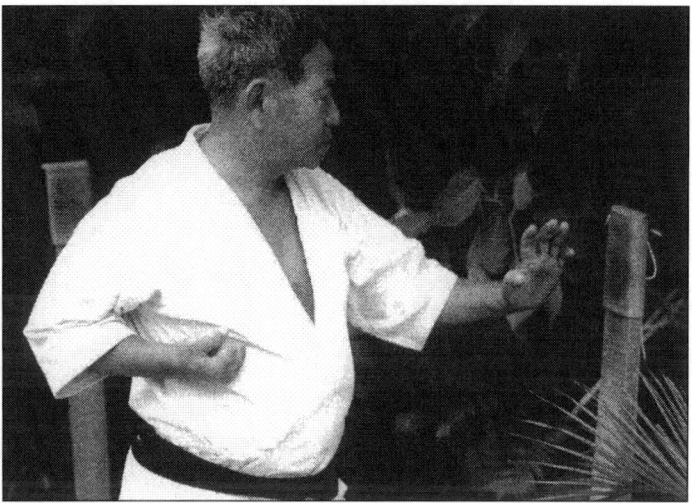

Left: Eighteen year old Yagi Meitoku in uniform. Right: Yagi Meitoku working with a makiwara in the garden dojo in the mid-1980s.

Gojyu-ryu was the first Okinawan karate style to be named (Yagi, 2006). In 1933, Miyagi's style was formally registered as "Gojyu-ryu" with the Butokukai (Higaonna, 1985: 28).

Yagi Meitoku was born on March 6, 1912 in Naha, Okinawa. His grandfather took him to Miyagi Chojun when he was thirteen years old (Yagi e-mail, 2004). In the early days, they taught only three kata: Sanchin, Seiunchin, and Seisan. Only the successor of the style would be taught all of the other kata. Miyagi taught Yagi Meitoku all of the kata (Yagi, 2006).

After Miyagi's death in 1953, the Miyagi family chose Yagi Meitoku to carry on the Gojyu-ryu karate system. At that time, he was given Miyagi Chojun's uniform and belt as symbols of his inheritance (Babladelis, 1992:40). Yagi named his school Meibukan ("House of the Pure Warrior"; Yagi, Wheeler, and Vickerson, 1998:49). Meitatsu started training with his father at the age of five and trained with him for over fifty years (Yagi, interview 2004). These are some of the stories Yagi Meitatsu told about his father:

> Yagi Meitoku had a very strong punch. It was strong enough to break a makiwara. I remember when I was small my father would put a makiwara near a wall with a small string between the makiwara and the wall. My father would punch the makiwara and it would move a little closer to the string. After two or three months the makiwara would touch the string and he'd move the string farther away. He'd move it again and again.
>
> •••
>
> If someone had a new makiwara in Naha, Meitoku would often ask, "Can I try your makiwara?" They'd say, "Sure." But they wouldn't expect Yagi to be able to break it. Yagi Meitoku would punch the makiwara, and boom! He'd break it. So, later on people would say to each other, "If you build a new makiwara, don't tell Meitoku or he'll come and try it out and break it."
>
> Later, when we would test our black belts, we'd have a makiwara test. In our style, we don't have any free fighting; only kata. So, after the student would demonstrate kata, they'd have to punch the makiwara. If they were not strong enough ... well, maybe next time.

When Yagi Meitoku was in the Japanese military, he was in a group that had to take care of the horses. At that time, if a horse would bite, he'd have a red ribbon tied on top of its mane. If a horse kicked with its front legs, he would have a yellow ribbon on its neck. A horse that kicked with its rear legs, he would have a blue ribbon tied to its tail. One time there was a horse that had three ribbons because he bit and kicked with both its front and rear legs. Nobody wanted to look after it. So, the officer in charge said, "Yagi, you take care of it." So, Yagi did. Usually there was no problem.

Then one day, Yagi went to the barn and the horse was uneasy and he tried to push Yagi into a corner so he could bite him. Yagi avoided the horse. A few days later, Yagi went back to the barn. The horse was tied up, so it couldn't escape. Yagi held the horse's rope and hit the side of its face many times with his fist. The side of the horse's face was very smooth like a makiwara, and Yagi could break a makiwara. So, he punched the horse many times. Finally, the horse fell down. Just at that moment, two or three soldiers were walking by and saw what happened. At least they saw Yagi punch the horse and the horse fall. The next day they told everyone, "Don't fight with Yagi. With one punch, he knocked down a horse!

At that time in the Japanese Army when someone made a mistake, the officer in charge would slap everybody in the unit one by one. One day there had been a mistake made in Yagi's group and the officer came to punish them. This was after the horse incident. Yagi was standing third in line. The officer came up to the first man and slapped him, then the second man and slapped him. He skipped Yagi Meitoku, then slapped the fourth man. Maybe he had it in his mind that Yagi would block and hit him back. This story was told by a classmate of Yagi Meitoku's and not by Yagi himself.

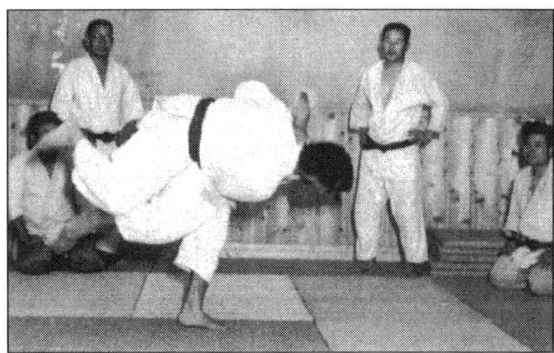

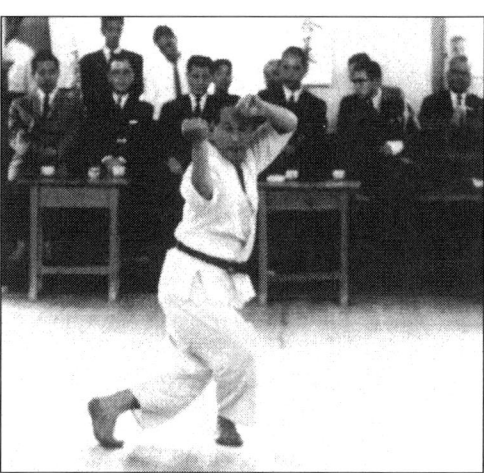

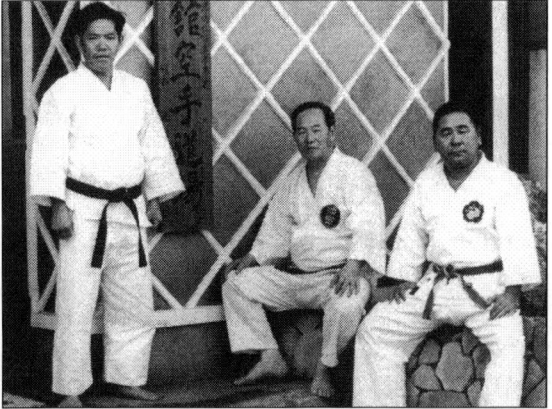

Top left: Yagi Meitoku was ranked in judo while he served as the chief customs officer for Naha City. He is seen here teaching judo.

Top right: Demonstrating the kata Seipai in Tokyo in the early 1970s.

Left: Kobudo master Matayoshi Shimpo (1922–1997), Yagi, and Toguchi Seikichi (1917–1998).

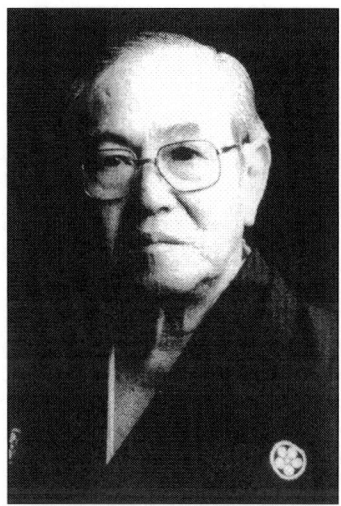 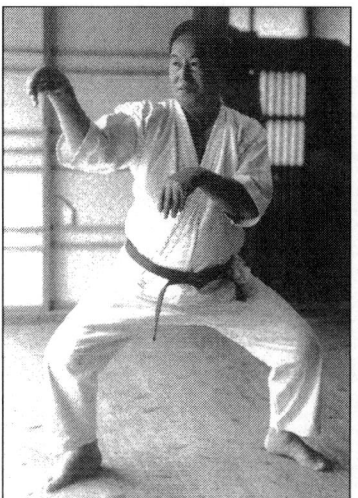 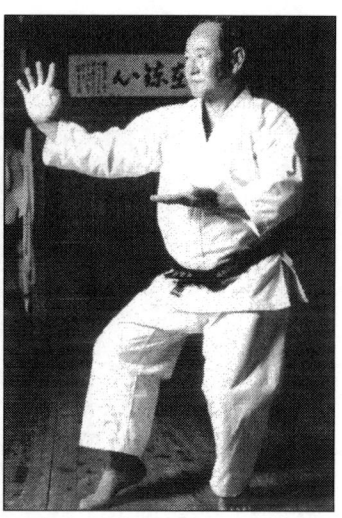

Yagi Meitoku in a formal portrait and in poses from the kata Sanseiru (left) and kata Kururunfa (right).

Yagi Meitoku chose his oldest son, Meitatsu, to be the first to learn all facets of Meibukan Gojyu-ryu (IMGKA, 2004). Yagi Meitatsu was born in Kume, Naha City, on July 7, 1944. At the age of five, Meitatsu started karate training with his father. They trained in their backyard six days a week for two hours a day (Yagi, interview 2004). Meitatsu tells these stories of training with his father:

> We used to practice six days a week, Monday through Saturday. We'd do apparatus training [*hojo undo*], chishi, kame, and forearm training [*kote kitae*]. The kote kitae was not just with one partner. We'd change partners over and over again. Then we'd do Sanchin. Everyday we'd do this and our arms were always bruised with no time to heal. After practice, we'd go and buy ice in a bucket to drink. This kind of training made a strong body, but when I'd go to school my hands would shake so much I had trouble holding a pencil.

•••

Yagi's students were taught to clean up the dojo before class and not afterward. That way the teacher could see the most serious students were the ones that showed up early to do the cleaning. The others would just show up in time for class.

When they were young, Meitatsu and his fellow students would bring water for the teacher during a break. They'd also turn the teacher's sandals at the door to point toward the exit, so it would be easier for the teacher to slip them on and be on his way.

•••

During winter training [*kangeiko*], there was no heater in the school. During the last two weeks of December, we'd practice from 4:00 to 6:00 am. At first, many people came to train, but it was too early and because it was December they were too busy so, after a week, only two showed up. Yagi Meitoku did this as spiritual or mental training.

People have asked if my father trained my brother and I special. We were the same and equal to other people, but we always had to work harder than everyone else. I remember the senior students would chase after me with a stick to make me move faster. Every day we'd run barefoot for about twenty minutes. When I was small, I used to hate my father. Every day we had to practice, six days a week. Every New Year there would be a number of famous performers on television, but I had to miss the show. There was no video then. So, when you missed the show, that's it. But today I appreciate what my father did.

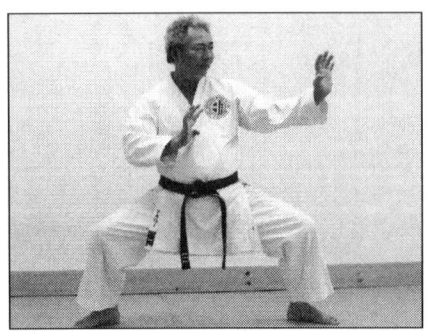

Yagi Meitatsu in a pose from the kata Seisan.

Our "two-years practice" [*ninen geiko*] was 11:00 pm December 31st to 1:00 am January 1st. The last hour of the year and the first hour of the New Year we would practice. So, the last hour of this year and the first hour of the next year you finish with karate and start with karate. You don't see your family or your girlfriend—you see your teacher and your karate group. From 11:55 to 12:05, the last five minutes of this year and the first five minutes of the New Year, we would meditate. The last five minutes of this year, you think back to what happened in the year. The first five minutes of the New Year, you make decisions or goals for the New Year. Those ten minutes are very important. Then, after the one hour training in the New Year, we would all run to the Naminoue Shrine[9] to pray. Judo and kendo students, also in their uniforms [*dogi*] would be there, too. But now it's very crowded, so we don't go anymore.

•••

Sometimes people ask me if I like karate. I still don't know. My father made me practice. I had no choice. I believe that people don't choose a profession. The profession chooses people. The first son has an obligation that must be fulfilled. I was never told this, but I felt the responsibility. I started my sons in karate training when they were three years old. Now they are 28 and 29. They're teaching while I'm away.

When asked if he thought his oldest son would carry on after he retired, Meitatsu answered, "I hope so."

TECHNICAL SECTION — FOREARM TRAINING

Kote kitae means forearm training. In Gojyu-ryu karate, the body must be trained first. Kote kitae conditions the forearms to make them capable of delivering strong blocks and punches. The kote kitae drill was taught by Miyagi Chojun to Yagi Meitoku and passed on to his son Meitatsu when he was a boy. As a boy, Meitatsu would train with his father's much older and larger students. When performing the kote kitae, some of the senior students would be soft with him, but others would hit hard. Partners would be changed over and over again.

There is a hidden technique within the kote kitae drill. As the arm comes up to strike the partner's arm, it simulates poking to the eyes. Eyes cannot be hit with an up to down attack as other strikes are delivered in Gojyu-ryu, but they can be struck from below.

Forearm Training

1-2) Right arm middle block and low block.
3-4) Left arm middle block and low block.
5-6) Both people step forward with the right foot while performing a middle block and low block.
7-8) Both turn and face each other with left foot in front, while performing a middle block and low block.
9-10) Step back with left foot and continue with middle block and low block.
11-12) Left arm middle block and low block.
13-14) Both step forward with the right foot, while performing a middle block and low block.
15-16) Both persons turn and face each other with left foot in front while performing a middle block and low block.
17) Back to the beginning and repeat ad infinitum (same as beginning #1).

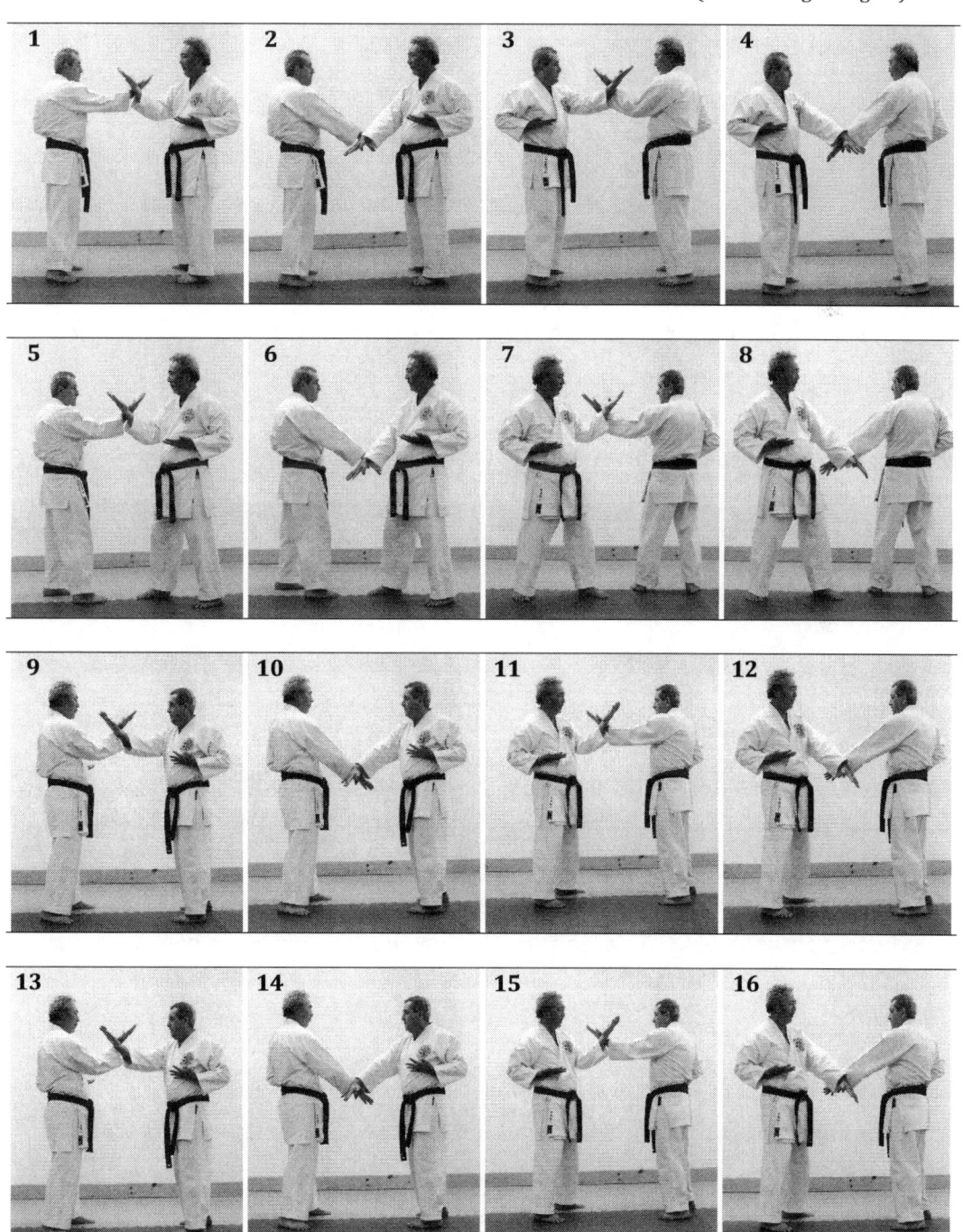

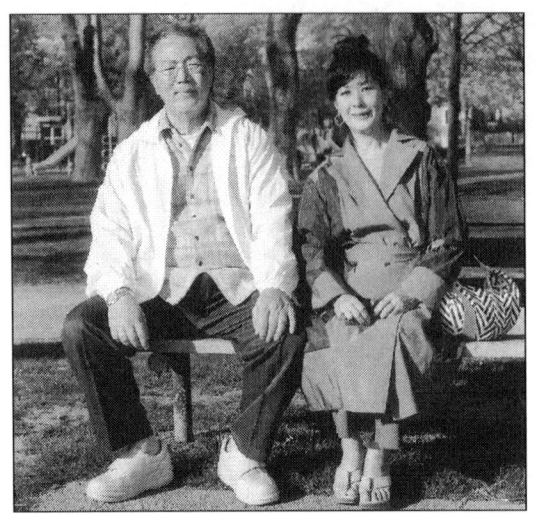
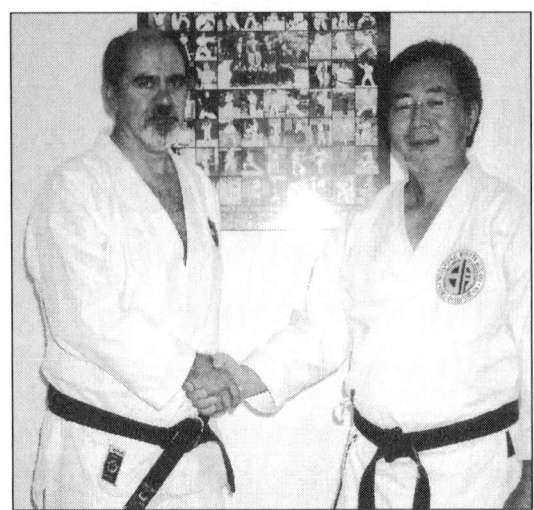

Meitatsu and his wife Noriko at Montebello Park in St. Catharines, Ontario, Canada.
The author with Yagi Meitatsu in Brantford, Ontario, Canada.

Conclusion

The stories of the Yagi family make up the history of Gojyu-ryu karate. Whether they are anecdotes about Miyagi Chojun and his teachers or the reminiscing about Yagi Meitoku by his son, they are all a part of the greater legend of the martial arts. Another volume of stories is in the making as Yagi Meitatsu continues his obligation to his father by spreading Gojyu-ryu karate around the world. The Okinawan karate master meeting new people and teaching his family art in the United States, Canada, Poland, England, and other countries guarantees a new batch of stories that will be passed on to the next generation.

NOTES

[1] *Gojyu* translates as "hard and soft." The normal spelling "goju" leads the non-Japanese speaker to pronounce the term harsher and give it the meaning of "fifty." Yagi Meitoku pointed this out to Ken Trebilcock during a 1995 trip to Okinawa. Yagi Meitatsu likes to use the spelling "gojyu" with the softer sound of "jyu" because it offers a more correct phonetic rendering of the term (Trebilcock, 2006).

[2] Juhatsu Kyoda (1887–1968) founded the style called To'on-ryu (McKenna, 2000: 33).

[3] Masahige Shiroma (1890–1954) was also known as Gusukuma Shimpan. He was one of the most talented karate teachers to outlive the war. His peers considered him a brilliant technician. Unfortunately, he is also one of the least known of the old Okinawan masters. He is most remembered as a Shorin-ryu stylist, but had also trained in Naha-te (Sells, 2000:146, 176).

[4] The *Butokukai* (Martial Virtues Society) was founded during the Meiji period (1868–1912). The Japanese Government authorized it to research, preserve, and promote Japanese martial arts (McCarthy, 1999:73, 74).

[5] Until his death during World War II, Shinzato was Miyagi's senior student (Sells, 2000: 105).

[6] *Jujitsu* ("gentle art") is a Japanese method of unarmed combat that uses the human

body as a weapon.
7. *Kenjutsu* ("sword art") is the traditional, aggressive method of swordsmanship practiced by Japanese feudal warriors.
8. *Bubishi* means "to provide military ambition." It is an anthology of the history, philosophy, and application of Chinese gongfu. It is presumed that the *Bubishi* was brought from Fuzhou, Fujian, China, to Okinawa sometime during the mid-to-late19th century (McCarthy, 1995:12, 13, 14).
9. The Shinto shrine at Naminoue overlooks Naha harbor (Kerr, 2000:415, 452).

Bibliography

Babladelis, P. (1992, December). The sensei who received Chojun Miyagi's belt. *Black Belt*.

Burton, R. (n.d.). *The Arabian nights*. New York: The Book League of America.

Farkas, E., and Corcoran, J. (1983). *The Overlook martial arts dictionary*. New York: Overlook Press.

Higaonna, M. (1985). *Traditional karate do Okinawa Goju ryu, Volume 1*. Tokyo: Minato Research Publications.

Higaonna, M. (1995). *The history of karate*. Thousand Oaks, CA: Dragon Books.

IMGKA (2004). International Meibukan Gojyu-ryu Karate Association website www.imgka.com

Kerr, G. (2000). *Okinawa – The history of an island people*. Boston: Tuttle Publishing.

Maugham, W. (1939). *The teller of tales*. New York: Doubleday, Doran and Company.

McCarthy, P. (1995, summer). The search for the Bubishi. *Budo Dojo Magazine*, 12–14.

McCarthy, P. (1999). *Ancient Okinawan martial arts, Volume 2*. Boston: Tuttle Publishing.

McKenna, M. (2000). To'on-ryu–A glimpse into karate-do's roots. *Journal of Asian Martial Arts*, 9(3):32–43.

Ricci, B. (2006, September 18). Personal communication.

Sells, J. (2000). *Unante: The secrets of karate*. Hollywood, CA: W.M. Hawley.

Toth, R. (2004). Yagi Meitatsu discusses the not-so-secret techniques of Okinawan Gojyu-ryu karate. *Journal of Asian Martial Arts*, 13(4), 60–71.

Trebilcock, K. (2006, December 6). Personal communication.

Yagi, Meitatsu (2004, April 16). E-mail communication.

Yagi, Meitatsu (2004, May 14). Interview held in St. Catharines, Ontario, Canada.

Yagi, Meitatsu (2006, May 1). Interview held in St. Catharines, Ontario, Canada

Yagi, Meitatsu (2006, October 21). Interview held in Brantford, Ontario, Canada

Yagi, M., Wheeler, C. and Vickerson, B. (1998). Okinawan karate-do Goju-ryu Meibukan. Dundas, Ontario, Canada: self published.

ACKNOWLEDGMENT

The author would like to thank Sensei Yagi Meitatsu for providing the pictures of his family and of Miyagi Chojun. All of the other photos were taken by the author. Thank you, as well, to Ken Trebilcock for appearing in the photos in the technical section and for his help.

chapter 52

Politics and Karate:
Historical Influences on the Practice of Goju-ryu

by Giles Hopkins, M.A.

Illustration courtesy of iStock.com
All photographs courtesy of Giles Hopkins, except where noted.

Introduction

A few years ago, I happened on a translation of the minutes of the 1936 meeting of karate masters, government officials, and journalists in Patrick McCarthy's *Ancient Okinawan Martial Arts: Koryu Uchinadi*. The meeting was sponsored by the Ryukyu Newspaper Company, but its primary organizer was Nakasone Genwa (1886–1978). Though Mr. Nakasone went on to publish a number of books on karate (Karate no Kenkyu, 1934; *Karate-do Taikan*, 1938; *Kobo Kenpo Karatedo Nyumon*, 1938, with Mabuni Kenwa), he seemed a curious figure to be so instrumental in this gathering of prominent martial artists. McCarthy notes that after graduating from college, Nakasone moved to Tokyo, became involved in the socialist movement there, and "served as the publisher of its newspaper" (1999:58). It struck me then that this ancient tradition of martial arts—a tradition, it has been suggested, going back to Bodhidharma—was not immune to the pressures of politics and different social agendas. Perhaps I was naïve to think there was anything that could survive the insidious influence of politics.

As I closed the book, I thought about my impressions of Okinawa. I could hear crickets in the distance. Dogs were barking and it was hot and humid.

It was hot there too. In Okinawa, we slept on tatami mats in a small apartment that

Matayoshi Shinpo sensei (1922-1997) had given us for the summer, just above the vegetable market—my teacher, me, and one other student. Trucks from the countryside began their deliveries at three or four in the morning. Awakened by the dogs and the constant jockeying of delivery vans through the small streets, we were tired by mid-day. The soft tar in the road yielded under the weight of each step. Sweat dripped down the center of our backs, soaking our shirts. June bugs screeched like cats held at bay when small boys trapped them with butterfly nets and stowed them safely in cages tied to their belts.

We were usually up soon after sunrise, setting off in search of coffee through the seemingly endless market stalls of Heiwa Dori (Peace Street)—a maze of intersecting covered alleyways, restricted to pedestrian traffic, that began after World War II as a marketplace run by the widows of Okinawan soldiers. In the aftermath of the war, wing sections of downed fighter planes were dismantled and used for shelters, many of them making up the walls and roofs of the original market. Now, of course, it's all very modern; Naha, the capital of Okinawa, is mostly concrete and glass.

But not far from the office buildings and department stores that crowd the center of Naha, one can still see wooden houses with sliding doors and tile roofs that survived the devastation of the war. Walking through the narrow streets, where potters have continued to make the old jars that karate students (*karateka*) call gripping jars (*nigirigame*), one can still experience glimpses of an Okinawa that has all but disappeared. The signs are still there, pointing the way to an old craftsman who still makes the traditional Okinawan weapons or to a small training hall (*dojo*) tucked away at the end of a narrow alley. Most of the young people in Okinawa are playing baseball on hard-packed dirt fields. But a few still find their way to the dojo, their shoes lined up just inside the door. The cadences of training can be heard from the street. Though many things have changed, Okinawa has managed to survive the terrible events of the 20th century. But the gnawing question remained—at what cost?

Sitting in my kitchen that evening, thinking about McCarthy's book, I sensed that Okinawan karate may also have been under attack in the first half of the 20th century—even before the Second World War—and it was an attack that seemed to be far more subtle, and yet, for that very reason, potentially far more significant for the martial arts.

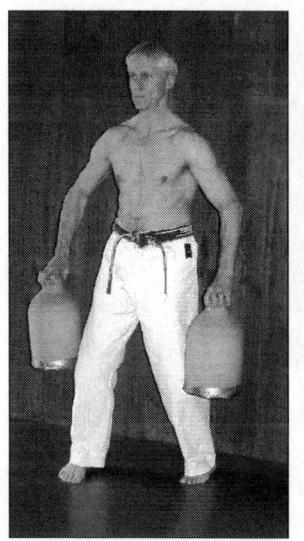 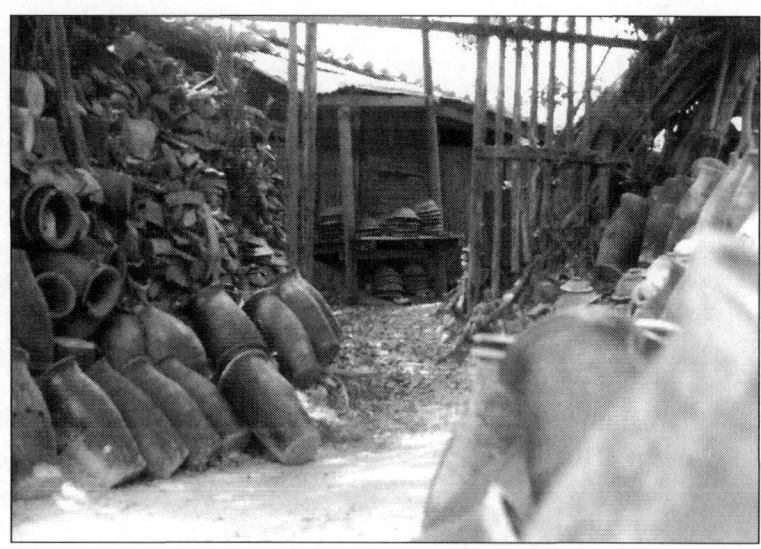

Above: The author with gripping jars (*nigirigame*)
and an old pottery shop where they are made.

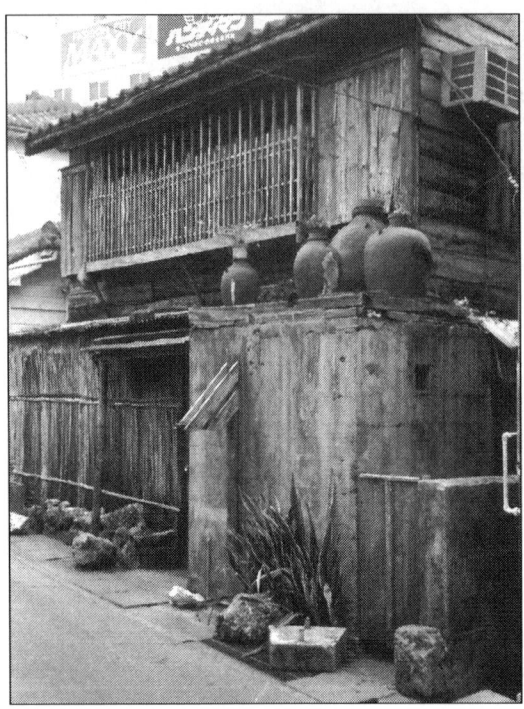
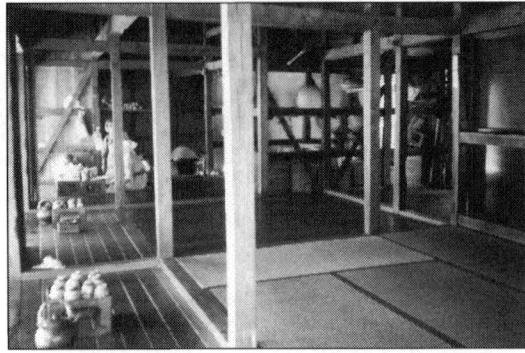
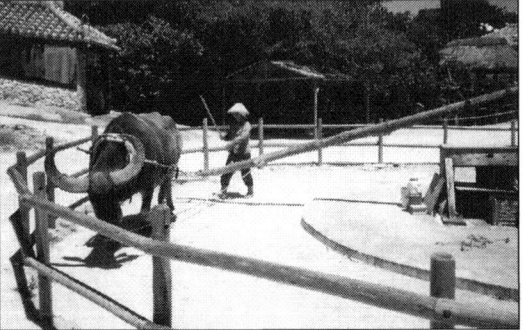

Left: An old style house in the midst of Naha city which managed to survive WW II.
Right: The interior of an old style house. Turning a grindstone with the help of ox power.

The Realities of History

Many of us still naively believe that traditions—or the high-mindedness of certain larger-than-life individuals—may protect a practice from the social or political influences of the world in which it exists. In some circles, there is the rather ingenuous notion that traditional arts are somehow independent of politics. But everything is political in one sense or another.

To suggest that any martial art, traditional or otherwise, can develop in a political vacuum is to say that it exists outside of history. This is the same as arguing that Shakespeare or Mozart or Picasso are somehow independent of the historical events that in fact shaped them. We are tempted to imagine that their work exists outside history because it seems transcendent—that is, it resonates today as much as it did with generations of sympathetic students of the arts in the past—but it is just not the case.

In the martial arts, we have ritual and tradition, both serving to preserve our practice and connect us to the past in a way that would also seem to transcend historical evolution. It is an inescapable irony that in practicing traditional karate—an admittedly anachronistic pastime—we wish to connect with some evanescent past, shrouded in the mists of legend, while at the same time disavowing any connection with modern history, in this case the influences of the 20th century.

As students of history, however, we must try to understand these historical influences in order to understand what we practice today. How can we separate what is truly traditional from what is merely expedient, the essential from what has been grafted on to it out of political necessity?

The underlying agenda of the 1936 Ryukyu Newspaper Company meeting—etched in fine print between the lines of text—was to find ways to popularize karate, make it more acceptable to the public, and give it a less violent image. In the process, there was a not-so-subtle attempt to make karate less Chinese, to Japan-ize karate. Were there underlying political reasons for this push to change and popularize karate?

Japanese Politics in the Early Years of the 20th Century

In 1936, Japan was awash with fear and domestic terrorism. The previous decade in Japanese politics saw a "resurgence of right-wing patriotism, the weakening of democratic forces, domestic terrorist violence (including an assassination attempt on the emperor in 1932), and stepped-up military aggression abroad" (Library of Congress, "The Rise of the Militarists," hereafter, LOC Militarists). Japan had already withdrawn from the League of Nations and military leaders were looking for any excuse to strengthen their hold on Manchuria "as an industrial base, an area for Japanese emigration, and a staging ground for war with the Soviet Union" (LOC Militarists).

Hirohito had taken the throne in 1927 and nationalist groups were calling for a return to traditional Japanese values—"the ideals of . . . self-sacrifice in service of the nation"—to the "exclusion of Western influences" (LOC Militarists). Since the first Sino-Japanese War of 1894-95, Japanese military leaders were embarking on more and more provocative actions in Manchuria and attempting to exert more control in Japanese governmental affairs "aimed at setting up a national socialist state" (LOC Militarists). Even European nations and the United States were seen as a threat since the last decade of the 19th century—and unquestionably in the aftermath of the 1900 Boxer Rebellion—interested in dividing China into various "spheres of interest," a policy they euphemistically referred to as "carving up the Chinese melon" (Hooker, 1996). Though Japan appeared to be as hegemonic as any European power in the decades that followed, one can certainly understand the rise in militaristic nationalism to protect their regional interests. But perhaps the motivation of Japan's military leaders was prompted by nothing more than an age-old animosity between China and Japan. Was this the divine retribution to be visited on China in response to the invasions of Kublai Khan so many centuries before?

In any event, this rekindling of patriotic zeal coupled with an anti-Chinese bias is evident in the minutes of the 1936 meeting, and it had two quite important effects on the martial arts: The first was the push to popularize karate and develop a curriculum that could be safely taught in schools, a sort of quasi-martial training to indoctrinate the youth. In order to do this, the public perception of karate would need to be changed from a brutal form of hand-to-hand combat to one of physical education. In fact, if one could emphasize spiritual as well as physical development, it would be even better. The second effect would be to separate karate from its Chinese roots; change its name; and make new, Japanese forms (*kata*).

The Situation in Okinawa

In his short essay An Outline of Karatedo, which McCarthy dates March 23, 1934, it is evident Miyagi Chojun was already thinking about the nature of karate and its popular perception by the time of the 1936 meeting. In this early essay, Miyagi emphasized that "training in karate-do improves one's health" and that "physical and mental unity develops an indomitable spirit" (McCarthy, 1999:51). Certainly, these were laudable goals and might even convince a wary public that the aim of true karate practice was in keeping with traditional Japanese values and would develop physical as well as spiritual strength in Japan's youth. Though at times in the minutes of the 1936 masters meeting, it would seem that there were disagreements—most notably over the place and importance of classical (of Chinese origin) katas—it is clear that the participants were generally united in their efforts to popularize Okinawan karate.

Some have suggested that the impetus for this move may have had more expedient financial motivations behind it. The post-war depression of the 1920's hit Okinawa perhaps harder than other parts of Japan. Broadening karate's appeal would benefit karate instructors financially at a time when most Okinawans were not very well off. George Kerr sums it up succinctly, if somewhat dryly, when he states that "Okinawa suffered extreme hardship; the prefecture was at the bottom of the list in the distribution of aid on a national scale" (1958:434). On average, the standard of living seemed to be increasing in the first two decades of the 20th century, but Okinawa's economy was still "last and least in comparison with the advances which had been made in other prefectures of Japan" (Kerr, 1958:434). Why the disparity?

Okinawa itself exerted little influence over its own affairs as a young prefecture and certainly less over Japanese national interests, having "only five representatives in a Lower House membership of 381" (Kerr, 1958: 428). As early as the first Sino-Japanese War, "Official [Japanese] policy stiffened and remained hostile thereafter to all local traditions and folkways which marked off Okinawans from other loyal subjects in the empire" (1958:422). Prejudice towards these poor country cousins more often than not seemed to dictate policy. As Kerr points out, the Okinawans had almost no influence in the "matter of appointments to the governorship" (1958:429) and, by 1919, Okinawa "showed increasing export deficits" (1958:432).

The island's economy gradually came under the control of the central government and Japanese industry, yet the Japanese Government seemed to offer little in the way of aid or reform. So much so, Kerr suggests, that it seemed as if "'Economic colonization' had replaced 'political colonization'" (1958:432). To cope with a poor economic outlook and an increasing population, the government encouraged emigration. As callous as this "solution" seems to be, "By 1930, more than 54,000 had left Okinawa for foreign lands" (Kerr, 1958:438), sending money home, aiding development, and adding a source of revenue that was not dependent on the national coffers, exactly what the government had been hoping for.

The second step the central government took to address economic problems had the two-fold benefit of not only defraying the cost of local governmental services, but also ensuring a sort of civic-mindedness in Okinawan citizens. The government encouraged participation in any number of local associations. Membership was supposedly voluntary but, as George Kerr points out, "everyone in a community was expected to belong to one or more of the associations" (1958:429). The associations made "contributions of time, labor, material, or money" to provide for "the costs of fire fighting, road repair, maintenance of shrine grounds and parks, work on public buildings" and the like (Kerr, 1958:429).

In addition to economic difficulties, the first quarter of the 20th century also saw an Okinawan crisis in health and healthcare. This was not surprising given the economic hardships the Okinawans faced, but there was also a shortage of doctors. The Ryukyu Islands were not an attractive location after one had spent years studying to become a doctor—no one was going to get rich in Okinawa. "Okinawa Prefecture had the lowest recorded venereal disease rate" in Japan in 1905, but 25 years later Okinawa "had the highest rates in the country for both venereal disease and tuberculosis" (1958:440). Because Japan was preparing for war in the 1930's, "there was a quickening interest in national health standards and public welfare" (Kerr, 1958:440)—certainly something a number of karate teachers must have been aware of when they noted the health benefits of karate training in their writings.

The Japanization Program

Though Japan may have been reluctant to address economic and political problems —that is, to offer any sound economic solutions or provide any significant political autonomy—in Okinawa, it did not seem slow in recognizing the need to assimilate the erstwhile Kingdom of the Ryukyus. This was the real goal, and "the educational system took the lead in the 'Japanization' program" (Kerr, 1958:447). Where "speech, dress, and food habits set the Okinawans somewhat apart" (Kerr, 1958:454), education was a means to minimize if not completely erase these differences.

The number of schools increased dramatically in the first thirty years of the 20th century and so did the number of matriculating students. Education was at least a long-term means for improving the economic outlook of Okinawa, but it also served the more immediate purpose of indoctrination, creating a sense of national identity.

A growing sense of national pride seemed to accompany the defeat of China in 1895 and no doubt helped to bolster the central government's efforts to assimilate the younger generation of Okinawans. According to Kerr, "the traditions and history of old Ryukyu meant little to them" and "Chinese learning withered away with the older generation" (1958:445). Kerr suggests that it also "quickened a desire to be considered 'up-to-date' at Naha and Shuri, and to abandon old-fashioned customs" (1958:442). The younger generation in particular took up "the changing fashions" and even went so far as to take "distinctly Japanese names" (Kerr, 1958:442).

Sports, particularly the Japanese sports of kendo and judo, were central to this effort to bring the once independent Ryukyu Kingdom under the banner of the Japanese Empire. Exercise and athletics not only satisfied a need to address recent health concerns in Okinawa, but also "played an important part in Japan's assimilation program," Kerr notes (1958:446). Okinawan karate, introduced to the schools in the early years of the 20th century and fully integrated as "a part of the regular school curricula" by 1933 (McCarthy, 1999:49), could only benefit from this association, many must have thought, particularly if it were to introduce "new" katas and terminology that would be seen as Japanese (rather than Okinawan or Chinese). It was the means to keep a tradition alive in the guise of something new. It may also have been the impetus for Okinawan karate teachers to seek recognition and grade from Japan and the Dai Nippon Buto-kukai, which recognized karatedo as an official style/tradition (*ryu*) in 1933 and granted Miyagi Chojun the title of kyoshi (All-ryu Network, "Chronology 1900–1949.").

Certainly one should acknowledge that assimilation is never as easy as it might seem in retrospect. The younger generation aside, there were others in Okinawa, foreigners included, who were very much interested in promoting and preserving Okinawa's history and traditions. A few Okinawan scholars, though trained and educated at Japanese universities, were taking an interest and writing attention-getting articles. Interest in some circles was enough to prompt the formation of an "Association for the Preservation of Historic Sites and Relics of Okinawa" (Kerr, 1958:456). By 1930, Shuri Castle had been declared a "National Treasure" and a four-year program of restoration and repair had begun (Kerr, 1958:456).

But this interest in the past, however small it may have seemed to the general populace, "was not at all to the liking of the military men and extreme nationalist agitators at Tokyo, and led to a minor crisis in Japanese-Okinawan relations on the eve of the Pacific War" [1937–1945] (Kerr, 1958:456)—nor was it to the liking of those in positions of power. After public outcry questioning government tactics "to suppress local peculiarities of speech and custom," according to Kerr, the governor stated "vigorously the official view that every vestige of Okinawa's provincial individuality must be erased" (1958:457).

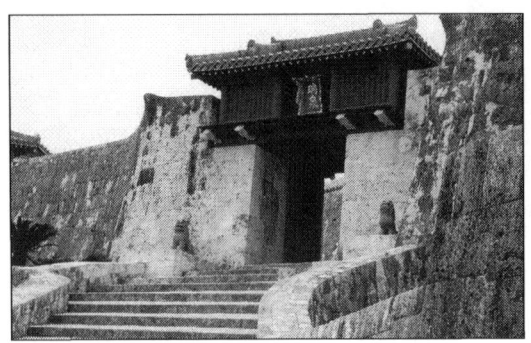 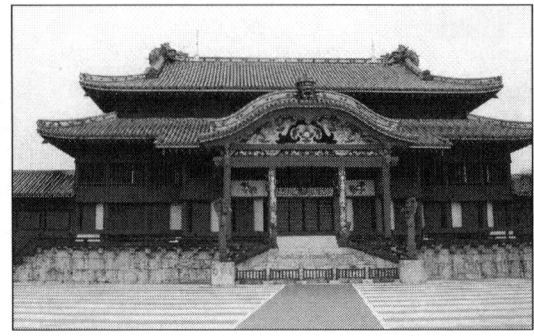

Left: The walls and entry of the reconstructed Shuri Castle.
Right: A reconstructed Shuri Castle — perhaps once the symbol of the Ryukyu Kingdom.

Admittedly, this is a brief outline of the political and economic influences at work in Okinawa in the first decades of the 20th century, but it is enough to raise questions about the direction karate took in the years and decades that followed. Did economic hardship play a significant role in the push to popularize karate? In popularizing karate, was the essence of karate watered down to the point where it was no longer a deadly martial art but merely an athletic endeavor to promote spiritual and physical well-being? Did the rise of the Japanese militarists and an aggressive foreign policy towards China cut the ties of tradition and serve merely to bolster the idea of karate as a sport—to Japan-ize what had long been referred to as "Chinese hand"?

The effort to make karate more appealing to the general public may have come from a need to offer something positive, some cultural palliative, to counter the economic hardships of the times; the island was over-crowded and economically depressed with very little political influence of its own to remedy its ills. But it also may have been politically motivated—part of an attempt to assimilate the Okinawans and remove Chinese influence.

In any event, this push toward physical fitness and an "indomitable spirit" is something that reflected the militant nationalism and aggressive foreign policy of Japan in the 1930's. It had been building steadily in the early years of the 20th century, and played out in Japan's imperialistic incursions into Manchuria and later in China proper. This was the atmosphere that informed and in some sense shrouded the 1936 masters meeting sponsored by the Ryukyu Newspaper Company. Less than a year after this meeting, the Second Sino-Japanese War began.

The 1936 Masters Meeting

The larger question for Okinawan karate, of course, is whether politics and the economic realities of the day had any significant and lasting effect on the development of karate in the 20th century. We know at least that the name changed. According to the minutes of the 1936 meeting, Nakasone Genwa's first order of business was to recommend that the name of Okinawan karate be officially changed, using the Japanese characters for "empty hand" instead of the characters for "Chinese hand," as had been the tradition. Though there seems to be no real objection to this name change, some participants at the meeting pointed out that the general population recognized the term *toudi* (the Okinawan Hogen term for Chinese hand), or more simply *te* (hand). At least in part, it seemed to be a question of familiarity, what was recognizable. Others, however, pointed out that there were those—particularly in the school systems—who "resent[ed] the term *Tou* [China]" (McCarthy, 1999:64).

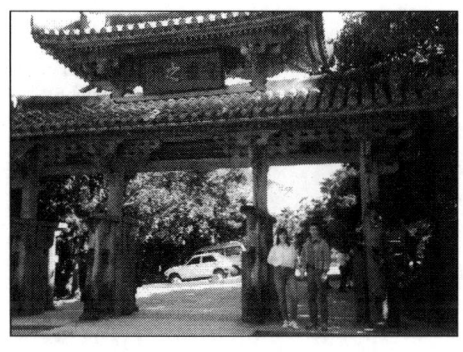

The author and his wife Martha at the old Shuri Castle Gate.

In this case, it seems fairly clear that this is a political issue—a change in tradition driven by the exigencies of contemporary politics. In fact, in view of Japan's overall assimilation program, growing animosity towards China, and disparaging view of Okinawan culture one would certainly expect this move. But, one might ask, what's in a name? As Miyagi sensei suggests: "Names change, like examples do, it depends upon the times" (McCarthy, 1999:61), as if to imply that this would be a change in name only, having little other effect on the practice of karate or how it was taught.

Of course, less cynically, in making karate seem more Japanese, it might also make it more acceptable to the general population. Yet which changes are acceptable because they are inconsequential and which changes are unacceptable because their effect is detrimental? Certainly when we look back on the efforts of the more militant Japanese nationalists to "erase" Okinawan traditions, we are appalled and recognize how destructive such an attitude is. How then should we look at the seemingly innocuous changes suggested by politicians, military leaders, and journalists at this 1936 masters meeting?

The second order of business at the 1936 meeting, forwarded by Vice Commander Fukushima Kitsuma of the regional military headquarters, was to recommend that new katas—Japanese katas with Japanese names—be created. Behind this suggestion, coming as it does from outside the circle of Okinawan karate masters, is the need to eradicate evidence of Chinese influence on Japanese culture. Ostensibly, of course, the discussion is again couched in terms that suggest a need to popularize Okinawan karate, which, as Nakasone Genwa suggests, "is in a slump these days" (McCarthy, 1999:65). However, in no uncertain terms, Miyagi says that "the classical kata must remain" (McCarthy, 1999: 65). In fact, he reiterates this point, underlining the importance of the toudi katas to an understanding of the art, saying, "classical kata must remain intact, otherwise they will be forgotten" (McCarthy, 1999:66). It is easy to understand why he was so insistent when one remembers the first precept of Goju-ryu put forward by Miyagi: secret principles exist in the Goju-ryu katas—and of course the katas he was referring to here are the classical katas of Chinese origin.

Yet even Miyagi, echoing a number of the non-martial artists at the meeting, agreed that new kata, "suitable kata . . . for students from elementary school to university level, should be developed" (McCarthy, 1999:65).[1] The question for Miyagi Chojun was whether one could do both; that is, popularize karate and preserve its traditions without losing the essence of the art.

Preserving a Tradition

Miyagi was adamant about preserving the old katas—the classical subjects. But the bunkai—the analysis of katas or the applications of the techniques—did not need to be taught. Without knowledge of the bunkai, the kata movements merely become dance or at best an agreeable form of exercise. Karate remained intact, but it was fundamentally different—it was safe. It could be used to promote health. One would become stronger and healthier, gain confidence and polish one's spirit, but no one would get seriously hurt. Here was the means to preserve and popularize what was essentially an anachronistic and brutal pugilistic endeavor, in reality meant to kill or maim.

This might explain why Mabuni Kenwa's Kobo Jizai Goshinjutsu Karatedo Kenpo and a number of his other works that included discussions of katas, published in the 1930's, only show very elementary bunkai, not the katas' more deadly applications (See inset comparison). Mabuni was a close friend of Miyagi's, active in the Ryukyu Tou-te Kenkyukai, an association founded in 1918 to preserve the Okinawan martial arts. Mabuni also stressed the health aspect of karate training and one of its primary goals, that of "cultivating a strong, healthy body and mind" (McKenna, 2002:13), echoing many of the same sentiments or repeating many of the same reasons that Miyagi had emphasized in his earlier *Karatedo Gaisetsu*. In fact, Mabuni quotes *Ito Daisho*, saying that karate training would "instill patriotism and train individuals to stand-up in times of crisis for their country . . . an effective form of mental training" (McKenna, 2002:14).

There were other ways to preserve the techniques of kata and bow to the pressure to popularize karate as well, to change the public perception of karate, stressing the idea of physical and spiritual development. The Goju-ryu kata *Tensho* (revolving hands) is a case in point.

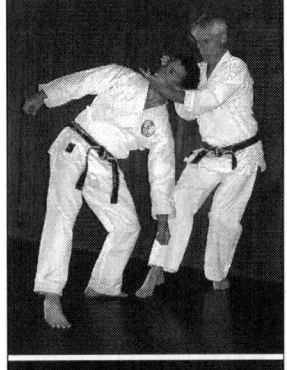
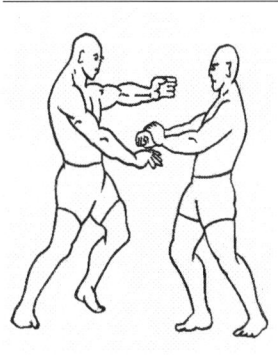

The drawings (adapted from Mabuni, 2002) and photographs show differences in interpreting applications. These attempt to illustrate the point made in the text that Mabuni may have downplayed the deadliness of karate to adapt to a political agenda.

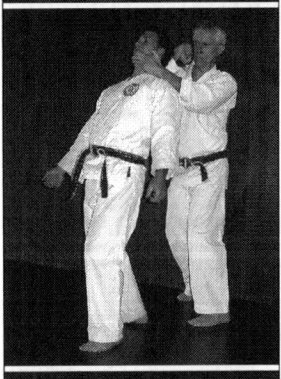
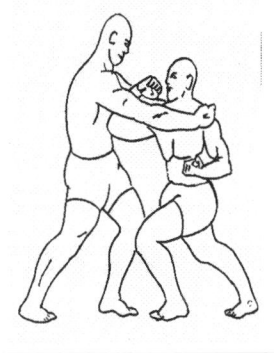

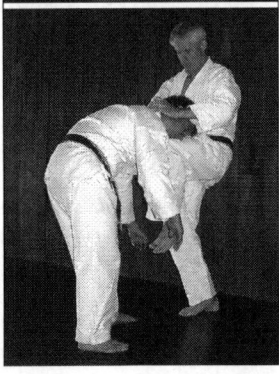
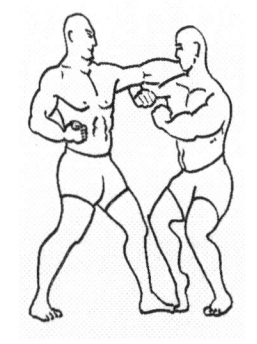

Tensho Kata

In his Karatedo Gaisetsu, Miyagi Chojun refers to Tensho as a fundamental exercise (*kihon kata*), similar to Sanchin kata. With the practice of these exercises, Miyagi says, "students learn to regulate their breath while coordinating it with the use of their power in a correct posture." The purpose of kihon kata, he states, is to develop "a strong physique while encouraging a budo spirit" (Miyagi, 1934/1993:23). The focus here is placed on posture, breath, skeletal alignment, muscular development, and so on—in a word, physical and spiritual development rather than the practice of clearly defined self-defense scenarios.

These katas differ then from the open-hand formal exercises (*kaishu kata*) that contain, as Miyagi says, "both offensive and defensive techniques in various paradigms" (Miyagi, 1934/1993:24). In other words, kaishu kata—Saifa, Seiunchin, Shisochin, Seipai, Sanseiru, Seisan, Kururunfa, and Suparinpei—are composed of combinations that show specific applications, while the kihon kata—though they contain fundamental or basic techniques—are used to condition the body and train posture and breathing. And for anyone familiar with Goju-ryu training, there is a distinct difference in the place of kihon- and kaishu-kata in training.

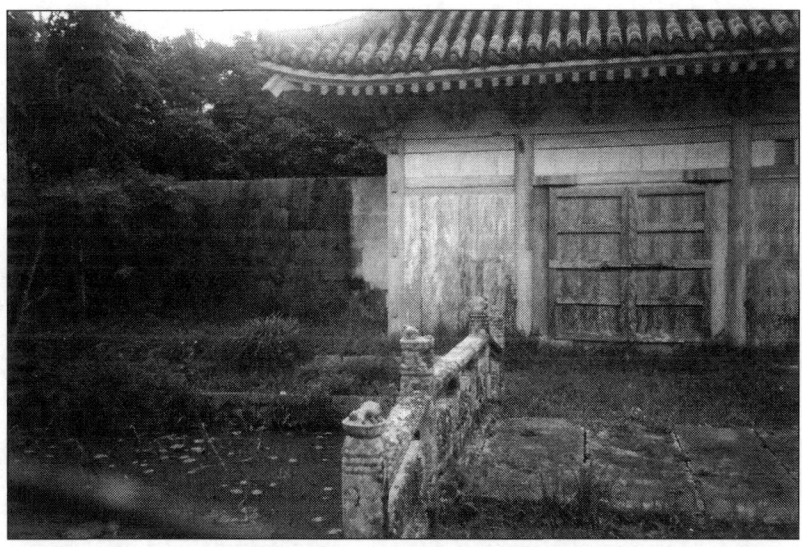

An old style building near the Shuri Castle.

The kihon kata Sanchin is taught very early, at white-belt level, and developed over the course of years of strenuous practice. The breathing is audible and the techniques, basic punches and blocks, are performed slowly with tension in sanchin stance (*dachi*). The teacher usually calls the student through the exercise and does a hands-on check for proper balance, alignment, muscular tension, and the like. It is often said that Sanchin, or "three battles," trains the mind, the body, and the spirit.

On the other hand, the kihon kata Tensho is taught at a higher level, at brown-belt or as an advanced black belt kata. Whereas the practice of Sanchin kata often begins formal class training, Tensho is often used to end training. If Sanchin is used to develop the hard aspect (*go*) of Goju-ryu, Tensho is said to develop the soft side (*ju*). Sanchin is a part of the Goju-ryu curriculum that Miyagi learned from Higashionna Kanryo and presumably one of the katas Higashionna brought from China. The history of Tensho kata, however, is a good bit murkier.

After a decade training with Higashionna, Miyagi Chojun went to China, by most accounts to visit the places his teacher had trained and meet Higashionna's teacher, Ko Ryuru. Miyagi was traveling in the company of Go Kenki (Wu Xiangui), a Chinese tea merchant living in Naha and a friend of Miyagi's, who acted as translator. Go Kenki was also a White Crane gongfu teacher (*shifu*).

There are differing opinions as to the duration of either of Miyagi's research trips to China (he would return in 1936, again in the company of Go Kenki). Were they a matter of weeks, months, or years? Was he there only long enough to observe training methods and techniques, or did he learn katas and study with a Chinese teacher? [See Ravignat, 2004, for some interesting discussion of what Miyagi may have brought back with him from China.] The question is how influential or productive these trips were for Miyagi.

There has been some recent speculation that Miyagi did not find Higashionna's teacher, who may in fact have been Wai Xianxian, not Ko Ryuru (Ravignat, 2004). Without this link, it is difficult to know what Miyagi studied in China or how much of an influence it had. Some researchers suggest that Miyagi may have developed Tensho from his study of rokkishu found in the *Bubishi* or that it is based on a Five Ancestors Fist gongfu form or perhaps a Wing Chun form (McKenna, 2006). Others have suggested that the main influence in Miyagi's development of Tensho kata was really Go Kenki, who was living on Okinawa, and who had been training with and sharing White Crane gongfu techniques with some of the great teachers in Okinawa for some time (Ravignat, 2004, part II).

In any event, what research and tradition both suggest is that Miyagi formalized the movements of Tensho kata and added it to the curriculum he had learned from Higashionna, whether it came from his research in China or his studies with Go Kenki in the Kenkyukai. What is not clear is why Miyagi felt a need to introduce these particular techniques into the Goju-ryu curriculum; that is, since there is no need to introduce something that is already there, what was missing?

The other question—apparent to anyone familiar with the training of Tensho kata in a traditional Goju-ryu dojo—is why Miyagi chose to downplay the applications of the techniques in Tensho, referring to it as a kihon kata. Used in this fashion, the emphasis, as in Sanchin kata, is on developing breathing and, for lack of a better word, internal energy (*ki*). Its soft, flowing hand movements seem more closely related to qigong than karate, and yet this is how it has been preserved in the traditional training regimen of Goju-ryu. Even to use it as a kind of pushing hands or arm conditioning exercise (*kakite*) as Marvin Labatte suggests (Labbate, 2001), merely reinforces the notion of using the kata as a form of physical and spiritual conditioning.

There are, however, very real self-defense applications contained within Tensho's flowing hand movements, yet they are rarely ever trained as such. Historically, the implication is that many teachers, Miyagi included, may have felt a need to de-emphasize karate's brutality in favor of its health benefits. The structure of Tensho kata and the manner in which it is generally performed both tend to hide the martial techniques and their applications. Emphasizing these aspects of Tensho may have satisfied a certain political agenda.

What Was Lost

The structure of Tensho kata raises a number of interesting questions, since it is different from Goju-ryu's other classical kaishu katas. The other katas have clearly designed combinations that show quite specific application sequences, composed of entry and controlling techniques and finishing techniques (Hopkins, 2002); Tensho does not. Appearances suggest that Tensho was constructed over the basic framework of Sanchin—three steps forward and three steps back, in basic stance (*kihon dachi*), finishing with a circular block (*mawashi-uke*)—to preserve a set of basic hand techniques—techniques that showed a similarity to the established canon of Goju-ryu katas, but were different enough that they needed their own kata to preserve them intact.

If the kata techniques are rearranged into blocks and attacks—admittedly an exercise that raises red flags for some purists and certainly some questions of interpretation—one will see five blocks and five attacks covering the upper, middle, and lower target areas. They are done first with the right hand, then with the left hand, and finally with both hands (see illustrations 1a-e and 2a-e).

Tensho Kata   1a-e → blocks   2a-e → attacks

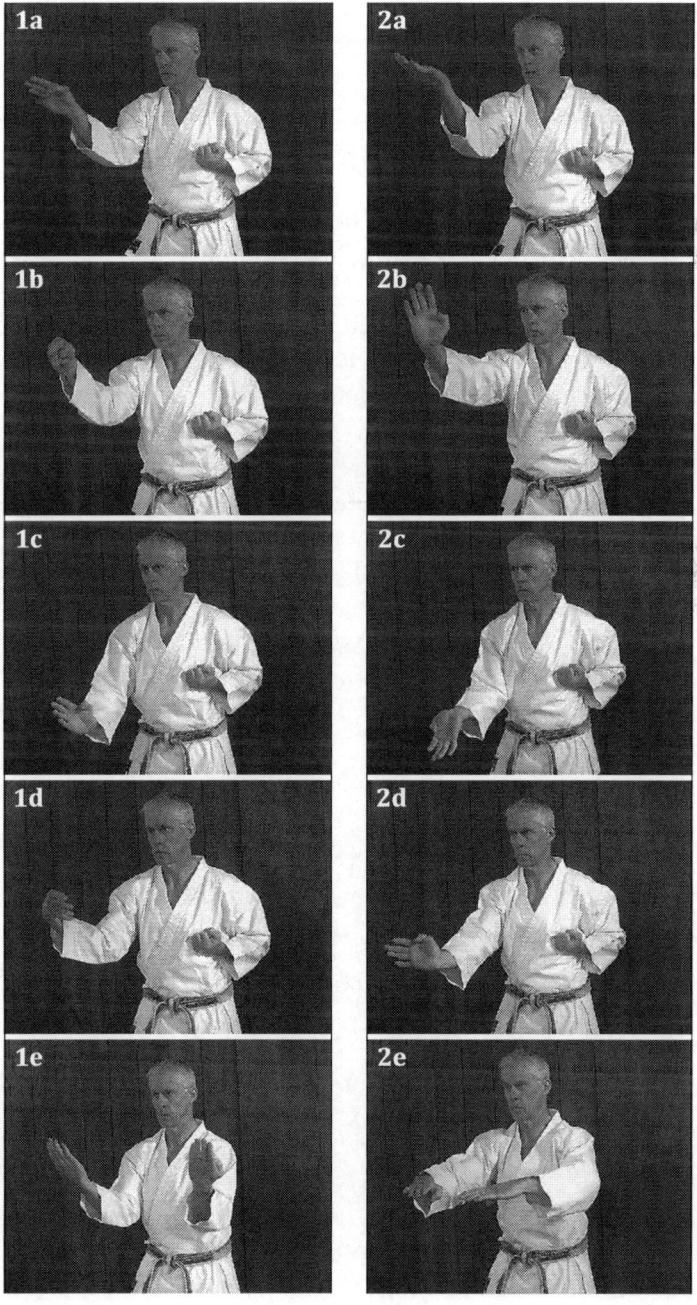

By appearance, they seem to be White Crane in nature, similar to some of the open-hand techniques of other Goju-ryu katas. It is easy to find palm strikes, knife-hand (*shuto*) attacks, and open-hand blocking in other katas. Yet this very similarity raises the question of why Miyagi saw the need to add these particular techniques to the Goju-ryu canon; that is, what is distinctive about Tensho kata?

The first and perhaps most obvious difference is that the hand techniques preserved in Tensho are executed off the front foot, unlike so many of the attacking hands in the other katas. (For example: Sanchin kata executes punches almost exclusively off the rear foot—that is, a left punch, for instance, from a right-foot-forward stance—as do Seisan, Sanseiru, and Suparinpei. See picture 3 of punch from Saifa).

Another noticeable difference is that Tensho lacks any real movement of the feet in relation to the hand techniques—that is, the hands move independent of any stepping or turning of the body. This is very different from what we generally see in the other Goju-ryu classical katas, suggesting two possible explanations: One, Tensho's hand techniques are merely that, hand techniques or basics, if you will, and they are not shown in application the same way techniques are shown in the other classical katas; or two, they are shown from a set stance position because they represent "inside" techniques, quick hand responses when the defender cannot move to the outside of the attack.

One of the fundamental principles found in the kaishu kata would suggest that the defender's first inclination in applying the techniques found in Goju-ryu katas is to move to the outside of the attack or to employ what some Chinese styles refer to as a "changing gate" method of first moving and blocking to the outside and then changing to the inside as one counterattacks. This is illustrated by the patterns and stepping inherently connected to the techniques' applications (Hopkins, 2004).

On the other hand, the techniques of Tensho kata seem to work as inside techniques, suggesting one thing that Miyagi may have thought was missing in Goju-ryu.

The other difference one notices is that the blocks and attacks are executed with the same hand, unlike the kaishu kata where the initial block and attack is generally simultaneous, blocking with one hand while attacking with the other (see picture 4 of Seipai double technique in cat stance). Together these differences suggest techniques that are meant to be used as "inside" counterattacks; that is, the opponent attacks with a left upper-level punch and the defender (using the kata's first technique) blocks with the right wing-like hand and immediately follows it with a right knife-edge (*shuto*) attack to the opponent's neck (see illustrations 5a and 5b). This is the kata's first block-and-attack sequence.

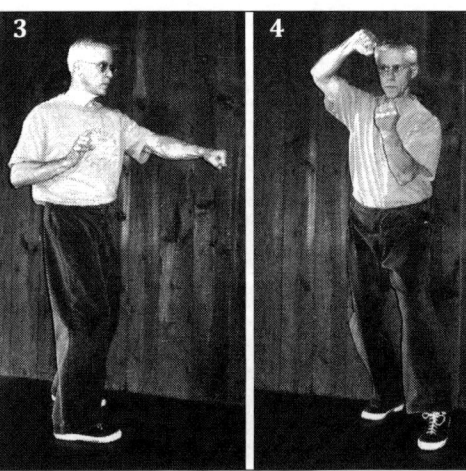
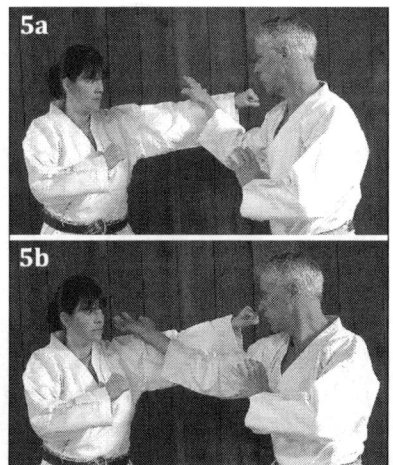

The kata's second sequence is a bit more problematic. The kata's structure obscures the technique's application, and the breathing pattern—underscored by its status as a kihon kata—does not correspond in each case with the technique; that is, inhaling on blocks and exhaling on attacks is not necessarily the rule in Tensho.[2]

As the kata is performed, the first sequence is followed by an upper-level palm strike (see 6a). Then the hand is brought to the side (either to the hip in some schools or to the chamber position by the ribs in others) in a circular motion, followed by a lower-level palm strike, fingers pointing down (see 6b). One can see that in the performance of the kata, Miyagi has chosen to put two attacks together, an upper-level and a lower-level palm strike. He follows these two attacks with the two blocks that are meant to accompany them: a rising wrist block (see 6c) and a dropping wrist block (see 6d). These blocking moves might, in fact, be more easily referred to as "painting the fence," as they are described in the 1984 *Karate Kid* movie.

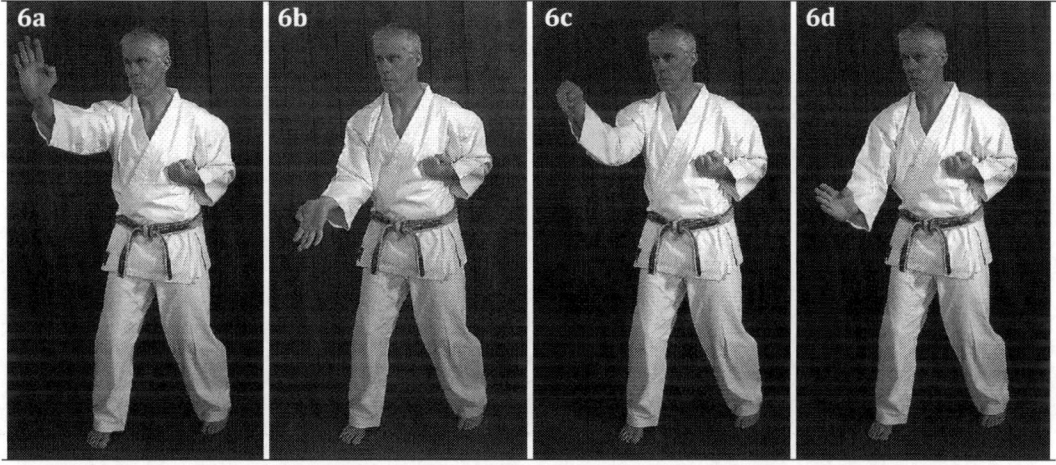

In application, the opponent attacks with a left punch, either to the chest or head. The defender blocks with the rising wrist block, followed immediately with a palm strike to the face (see 7a and 7b). It is important when executing each of Tensho's blocking positions that the elbow be kept in and down.

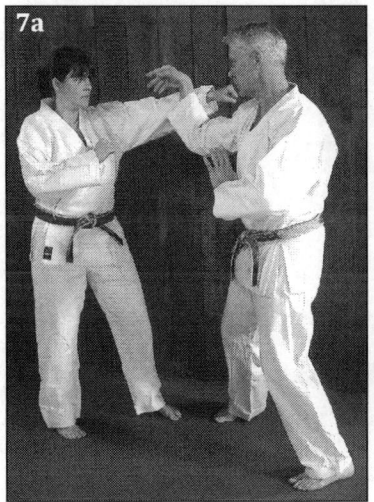
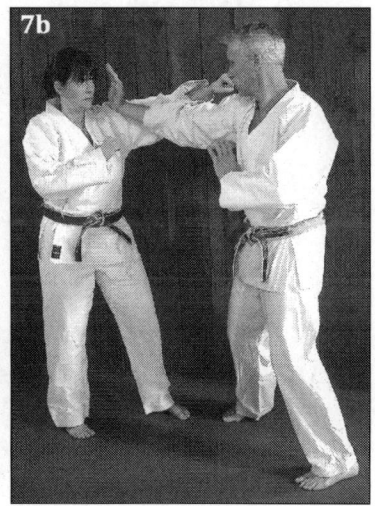

The next application sequence shows the opponent attacking with a left punch, either to the chest or stomach. The defender blocks with the dropping wrist block, followed immediately with a palm strike to the opponent's stomach or groin (see 8a and 8b).

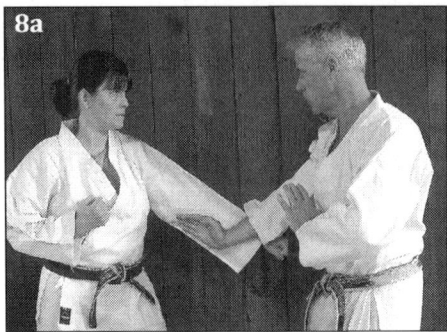 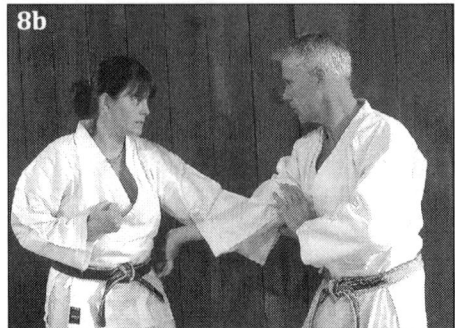

It is easy to see the simple logic and effectiveness of these techniques. But it is also easy to see that by rearranging the sequence of the techniques, the kata's structure effectively obscures any understanding of how to apply them. In addition, by emphasizing deep, rhythmical breathing and slow hand movements the focus is placed on health and conditioning more than self-defense and martial effectiveness.

The next application sequence shows the opponent attacking with a left middle-level punch. The defender blocks with a horizontal or side wrist block, followed immediately with a palm strike to the opponent's ribs (see 9a and 9b). Again, it is important that the elbow be kept in as the forearm is canted out. This series is performed in application the same as it is in kata.

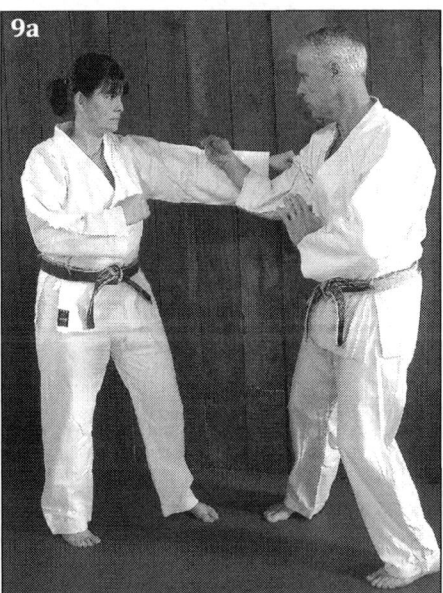 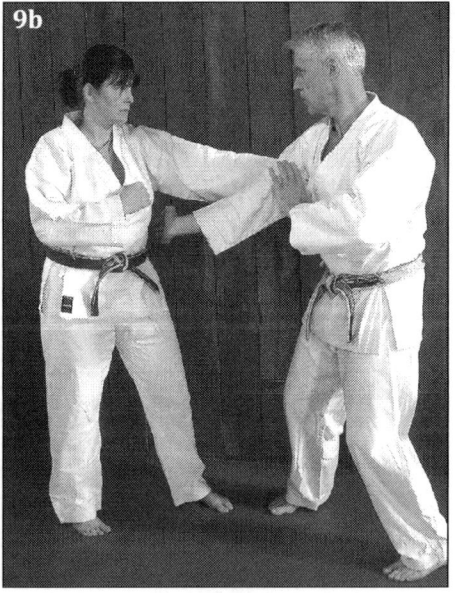

The final block and attack sequence—if one does not include the ending mawashi-uke since it is certainly not unique to Tensho—is only shown in the kata as a double-hand technique stepping back. It is done three times in the kata. It shows an inside forearm block, followed by a spear-hand (*nukite*) attack. If it is executed singly against a punch, it shows the use of the fingertips in striking (see illustrations 10a and 10b).

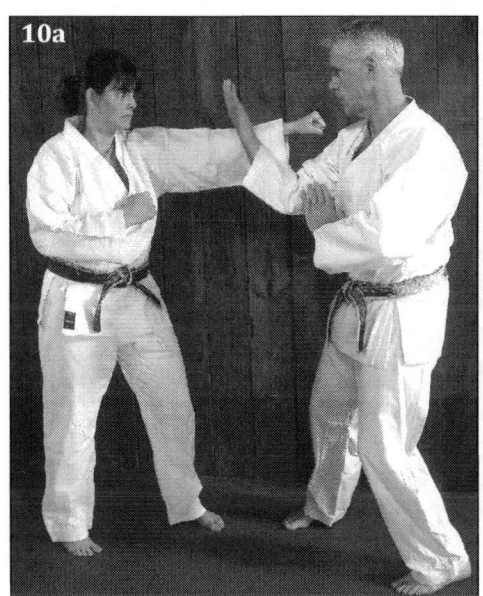 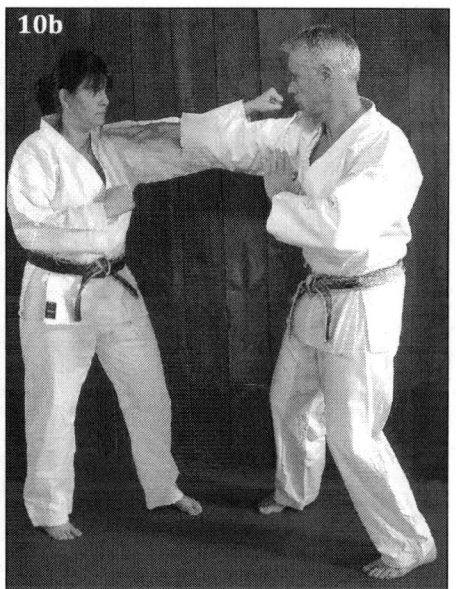

Thus the kata shows methods of striking, from knife-edge to palm to fingertips, and blocking, from the wrist to the forearms in a variety of angles, all from an inside and close-in position, utilizing the same hand for both block and attack. Certainly there are disadvantages to this same-handed block and attack defense. For one, it is slower than blocking with one hand while simultaneously attacking with the other. It also requires more advanced timing. However, there are also advantages. One is that the defender's counterattacking hand is already on the inside of the opponent's guard. As the opponent senses the attack, his flinch response is to pull his own hand in to cover. Doing so, however, merely facilitates the defender's attack, helping to pull the shuto, in the first block and attack sequence for example, into the intended target.

While the techniques of Tensho seem straightforward enough, they are difficult to apply in reality; they require a greater degree of expertise than many of the "outside" blocking and attacking techniques of the other katas. The techniques of Tensho also demand a certain understanding of "short power"—that is, the ability to attack without chambering the hand. What is clear from this analysis, however, is that Tensho kata should also be trained with speed and power—the techniques were meant to be used. In most cases, students engaged in the practice of Tensho look as if they are painting elaborate pictures in the air or blessing the masses as if they were martial monks performing magical rites.

Tensho will no doubt remain a kihon kata in the Goju-ryu classical kata canon, and students will continue to perform it in a slow, rhythmical fashion, focusing on breath and posture, connecting in some spiritual way with the great teachers of the past. We may never know why Miyagi chose to conceal the applications of Tensho. But we should remember that what we take for tradition was itself shaped by the necessities of another day. Like other times, politics and economics are constantly at play, and it is probable that they had a profound effect on the practice of karate and the way it was preserved. Perhaps, if we are careful, we can scrape off some of this veneer of political influence or economic expediency and get at the substance underneath it all—in this case, the essence of the art or what it might have been originally.

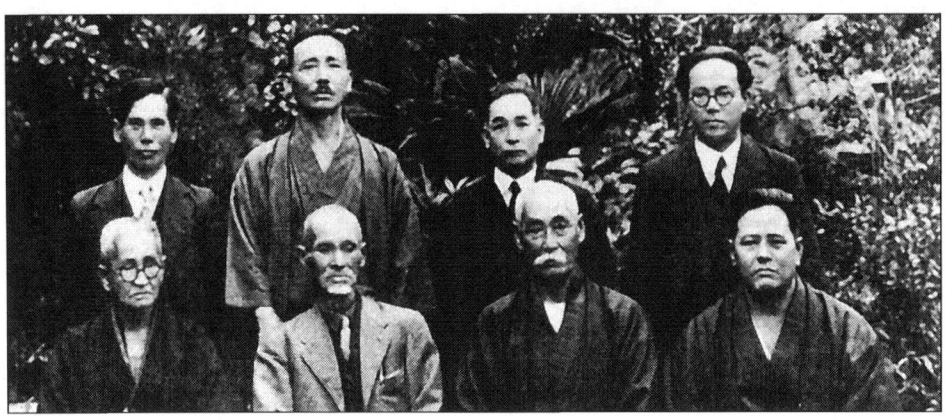

1936 Meeting of Karate Masters. Photograph courtesy of Graham Noble.

Conclusion

It was the end of the summer. The sounds of the market woke us for the last time. We still hadn't gotten used to it. This was not the contemplative silence of a Japan one sees in a Hiroshige print. When we arrived in Okinawa almost two months earlier, we found it to be full of surprises. It had seemed then as if Okinawa had been covered in concrete after the devastation of the Second World War. We had expected something different, but the magic and mystery of Okinawa was still there, just beneath the surface.

We often stopped to visit with Matayoshi's wife, before heading off on our explorations, just as we did this morning, our last. She offered us rice balls and we talked with her as she collected money from the small farmers or gardeners that rented space in the market to sell their produce. Her granddaughter, Nami, played in the back of the office. Some mornings Matayoshi himself would come by and haul us off to visit a famous dance teacher or we would all climb into someone's offered van and head off to see the sights of Okinawa.

But this morning we were waiting for a van to take us to the airport. To pass the time, Kimo Wall[3] was doing magic tricks for Matayoshi's granddaughter. When he held his hands out, palms up, to show her that they were empty, she looked up with surprise.

"*Doku des'ka* (Where is it)?" she asked. The coin had disappeared.

"I don't know," Kimo said, with feigned innocence. "I've forgotten where I put it. Maybe it's lost." Matayoshi laughed too. He had seen these tricks before. In a minute, the coin would appear again from behind Nami's ear or it would fall from the air as if by magic, our attention on other things.

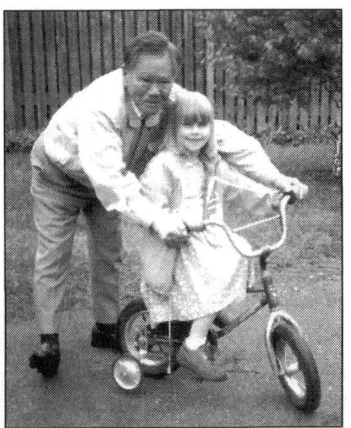

We look to see what is hidden in the hand, but we don't see it. Sometimes I wonder what else is hidden, what else may have been lost with the deaths of so many of the old masters, lost like Nami's coin, or whether we have simply forgotten where and how to look.

Matayoshi Shinpo with
the author's daughter Emily.

Acknowledgment

A special thanks to John Jackson for help in demonstrating applications, along with my wife Martha, and our daughter Phoebe for taking the pictures.

Notes

[1] By 1940, Miyagi sensei, with Nagamine Shoshin of Shorin-ryu, had created Gekisai dai Ichi kata for use in middle schools (All Gojuryu Network, "Chronology 1900–1949").

[2] It is interesting to note that if one adheres strictly to this "rule of breath," as Labbate does in his 2001 article, one must rather awkwardly interpret the more obvious shuto attack of the first sequence as a block.

[3] Kimo Wall, 7th-dan, studied Goju-ryu under Higa Seiko and kobudo (ancient weapons) under Matayoshi Shinpo (1921–1997). In addition to the martial arts, he studied healing arts as well. He lives in Panajachel, Guatemala, where he teaches martial arts and Thai massage (*Nuad bo rarn*).

Bibliography

All Gojuryu Network. Chronology 1900–1949. http://www.gojuryu.net/view page. php?page_id=31

Hooker, R. (1996). Ch'ing China: The boxer rebellion. Accessed on July 10, 2006 from http://www.wsu.edu:8001/~dee/ching/boxer.htm

Hopkins, G. (2002). The lost secrets of Okinawan Goju-ryu: What the kata shows. *Journal of Asian Martial Arts, 11*(4): 54-77.

Hopkins, G. (2004). The shape of kata: The enigma of pattern. *Journal of Asian Martial Arts, 13*(1): 64-77.

Kerr, G. (1958). *Okinawa: The history of an island people*. Rutland, Vermont: Tuttle.

Labbate, M. (2001). Tensho kata: Goju-ryu's secret treasure. *Journal of Asian Martial Arts, 10*(1): 84-99.

Library of Congress. A country study: Japan. "The rise of the militarists. http://lcweb2.loc.gov/frd/cs/jptoc.html.

Library of Congress. A country study: Japan. "Two-party system." http://lcweb2.loc.gov/frd/cs/jptoc.html.

Mabuni, K. (2002). Kobou jizai goshin-jutsu karate kenpo. Translation and commentary by Mario McKenna. Internet publication.

McCarthy, P., and McCarthy, Y. (1999). *Ancient Okinawan martial arts: Koryu Uchinadi, Vol. 2*. Boston: Tuttle.

McKenna, M. (2006). A little more on Tensho and Rokkishu. Accessed on Aug. 4, 2006 from http://okinawakarateblog.blogspot.com

Miyagi, C. (1934/1993). An outline of karate-doh. Translated by Patrick and Yuriko McCarthy. Fujiwara, Japan: International Ryukyu Karate Research Society.

Ravignat, M. (2004). The history of Goju-ryu karate: New ideas on Goju-ryu's direct Chinese ancestors. www.meibukanmagazine.org

chapter 53

A Preliminary Analysis of Goju-ryu Kata Structure

Fernando Portela Câmara, Ph.D. and Mario McKenna, M.Sc.

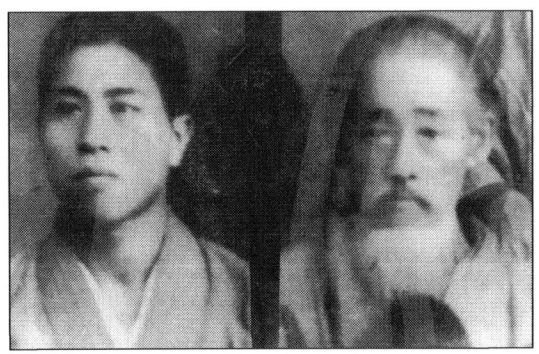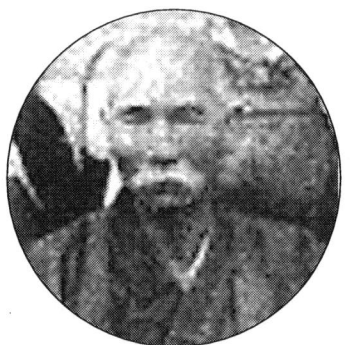

Higaonna Kanryu and his student Kyoda Juhatsu (left).
Right: Itosu Anko – the person most responsible for modernizing karate-do.
All photographs courtesy of Mario McKenna.

Introduction

Goju-ryu is the name of a karate-do style Miyagi Chojun (1888–1953) organized in the 1930's. Miyagi alleged that his system originated from a Chinese *quanfa* (*gongfu*) school established in the city of Naha in 1828 (Miyagi, 1934) and credited Higaonna Kanryo (1853–1917) as the primary source of the system. Yet when we examine modern Goju-ryu we can see several important influences on its development. These include the modern karate method developed by Itosu Ankoh (1830–1916), the indigenous Okinawa Hand (*ti* or *te*) tradition and Miyagi's personal studies.[1] We will discuss each of these briefly below.

Itosu taught the first karate classes publicly as part of elementary school physical education curriculum in 1901 and later on at the junior high school level (Iwai, 1992; Okinawa Prefectural Board of Education, 1994).[2] Itosu's method included a number of key points (Kinjo, 1999; Murakami, 1991):

1) the development of a new series of introductory kata named Pinan,
2) the standardization of existing kata,
3) the emphasis on mental and physical discipline,
4) the cultivation of morality, and
5) the de-emphasis on pure combative technique (Kinjo, 1999; Murakami, 1991).

Itosu's method was continued and improved upon by subsequent students and teachers such as Funakoshi Gichin, Chibana Choshin, and Mabuni Kenwa; and formed the basis for modern Okinawa and Japanese karate.

The influence of Itosu's method on Miyagi was critical to the future development of Goju-ryu. According to Kinjo Hiroshi, Goju-ryu is a modern style in line with Itosu's karate model (Kinjo, 2007). Kinjo argues that both Itosu and Higaonna organized karate in 1905, however only Itosu's model was adopted by the Okinawa Prefecture Education Department. It was rumored that because of Higaonna's focus on Sanchin kata training that it was considered unsuitable for developing adolescents (Kinjo, 2007). That coupled with another rumor that Higaonna drank excessively stopped Higaonna's karate from being introduced into the school system. Miyagi was a student at the first prefecture junior high school during the time that the Itosu model of karate was introduced and would have learned karate from Itosu and his student Chomo Hanashiro.

As an adult, Miyagi organized the karate that he had learned from Higaonna and had it accepted as part of the Okinawa prefecture commercial school. This was Miyagi's karate which he would later call Goju-ryu. It is interesting to speculate if one of Miyagi's motivations for having Goju-ryu introduced into the school system was the memory of his teacher's grief and the early popularity of Itosu's karate.

In contrast to karate-do, Ti is a pre-World War II generic term referring to the non-kata based unarmed combative traditions practiced on Okinawa (Hokama, 1999). It does not refer to a specific method, system, or style of combat. The oral tradition of the older Okinawan karate teachers refers to postures, stances, techniques, etc. with the generic term Ti. Interestingly, according to Morio Higaonna, Miyagi Chojun only referred to what he taught as Ti (Higaonna, 1998).

Lastly, there are several, but under-documented accounts of Miyagi Chojun researching other fighting systems. When investigating Miyagi Chojun's life, we see that he spent most of his life's energies and his family fortune to studying the fighting arts. During his studies he came into contact with such fighting traditions as Fujian White Crane boxing (*baihequan*), Tiger boxing (*huquan*), Monk Fist boxing (*lohanquan*), and possibly Five Ancestor fist boxing (*wuzuquan*) (Kinjo, 1999; Tokashiki, 1991). This raises questions regarding the continuity in the kata passed on by Miyagi Chojun.

Goju-ryu's Kata Catalog

In the late 1930's, Goju-ryu apparently consisted of eight kata: Seiunchiun, Saifa, Shisochin, Sanseru, Seipai, Seisan, Kururunfa, and Suparimpei / Pechurin; and two basic exercises that were adapted into a kata format, Sanchin and Tensho. In the early 1940's, two basic introductory kata were added to the system: Gekisai I and II.

Kanzaki Shigekazu (b. 1928) and Murakami Katsumi (b. 1927) were disciples of Kyoda Juhatsu (1887–1968), a long-time student of Higaonna and Miyagi's senior. Both men claim that Higaonna Kanryo taught only the katas Sanchin, Sesan, Sanseru, and Pechurin. Examining these four forms reveals that each kata has an asymmetric pattern. That is, kicks are done predominantly with the right leg and upper body techniques are frequently done with only one side of the body.

The katas Seiunchin, Saifa, Shisochin, Seipai, and Kururunfa are of note in comparison to the four previously mentioned katas, as they are symmetric forms. Kicks and techniques are frequently done with both sides of the body. Seiunchin, Seipai, and Kururunfa are mentioned in the late 1930's in the written works of Mabuni Kenwa (1889–1951), a karate teacher and friend of Miyagi's. Miyagi's early students also mention Seiunchin as one of the older katas he taught. In contrast, Shisochin and Saifa are not mentioned in any published karate list of the 1920's or 1930's. Interestingly, Miyagi was apparently the only person to pass on these five katas.

Alternate Sources

There appears to be a lack of written documentation on the origin and transmission of Goju-ryu katas. In addition, testimonies from older teachers are filled with contradictions and inconsistencies. Taking this into account, the origins and lineage of Goju-ryu kata remain unclear.

According to noted martial arts historian Hokama Tetsuhiro (Hokama, 1999), there are six ways to analyze Okinawan karate-do katas:

1) methods of walking, hand use, and technique utilization,
   e.g. Sanchin, Shisochin;
2) names of the founder or originator of a particular tradition
   e.g. Kusanku, Wansu, etc.;
3) names of specific areas or districts in which the tradition
   was practiced, e.g. Shuri, Naha, Tomari;
4) the religious or spiritual principles inherent within a tradition,
   e.g. Suaprempei, Seipai;
5) the metaphysical or transcendental aspects of a tradition
   (catharsis / purification / Zen), e.g. Sanchin, Tensho; and
6) the implied movement of animals.

Of these six methods, the analysis of methods of walking, hand use, and technique utilization in Goju-ryu kata may provide an interesting and useful means of investigating their origin and development. In this paper, the structure of the eight Goju-ryu katas will be analyzed by the exploratory statistical technique of cluster analysis to obtain a classification of these katas and formulate ideas about their origins.

Data Mining

Data mining can be defined as the science of extracting useful information from large data sets. In other words, data mining provides a practical means for the classification and distinction of large amounts of data. We can think of data mining by using an analogy of mining for gold. A data miner looks for "gold" (useful knowledge and information) by "striking ore" (mountains of data) by using different kinds of tools (such as a statistical technique). Data mining then is a technique to help us distinguish gold from ore.

In order for us to "mine the data" contained in the Goju-ryu katas, we classified each kata on the basis of repeated patterns or themes found in them. Goju-ryu katas show a recurrence of patterns that can be used as an inventory for classification. For example, the following characteristics can be observed in the original Higaonna katas (Sesan, Sanseru, and Pechurin/Suparimpei) as stated by Kanzaki and Murakami:

1) all begin with three steps forward from the Sanchin exercise,
2) all have a four directional (or cross) performance pattern,
3) two of them (Seisan and Pechurin/Suparimpei) have three steps in Sanchin stance while performing double open-hand blocks (*osae-uke* and *sukui-uke*).

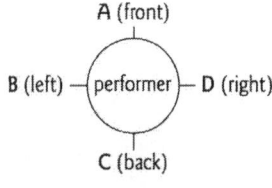

In addition, these katas have associated asymmetries:

1) kicks are performed with the right leg;
2) punches are concluded with the left fist.

In contrast, Saifa, Shisochin, Seipai, Kururunfa, and Seiunchin are symmetrical katas. Shisochin, Saifa, and Seiunchin begin with three advancing steps while repeating the same technique, but do not follow the Sanchin stance or pattern. The majority of techniques from these five katas are performed with both sides of the body, making them symmetrical.

Based on these observations, two senior Goju-ryu instructors identified ten themes among Goju-ryu katas. Each kata was then rated by the instructors for the presence (1) or absence (0) of each theme (Table 1). The predominant theme was symmetry of a kata and was defined as the percentage of repeated techniques with both sides of the body. A kata was considered symmetrical if it had greater than 20% repetition of techniques on both sides of the body.

Only the classical katas were used, as these are the forms that have been thought to have been passed down from Higaonna Kanryo to Miyagi Chojun. Therefore, the katas Sanchin, Tensho, and Gekisai were not included in this analysis. Tensho and Gekisai were excluded as they are modern exercises while Sanchin has almost complete symmetry.

TABLE 1:
OCCURRENCE OF PATTERNS IN THE CLASSICAL GOJU-RYU KATAS

Themes / Kata	Sanseru	Sesan	Suaprempei	Saifa	Seiunchin	Shisochin	Seipai	Kururunfa
1. Sanchin	1	1	1	0	0	1	0	0
2. Sesan	0	1	1	0	0	0	0	1
3. Three-theme	1	1	1	1	1	1	0	0
4. Cross pattern	1	1	1	0	0	1	0	0
5. Maegeri	1	1	1	1	0	1	1	1
6. Kansetsugeri	1	1	0	0	0	0	0	0
7. Nidangeri	1	0	1	0	0	0	0	0
8. Other kicks	1	1	1	0	0	0	0	0
9. Assym. kicks	1	1	1	0	0	0	0	0
10. Symmetry	0	0	0	1	1	1	1	1

NOTE: *Sanchin* = Sanchin Pattern; *Seisan* = Seisan pattern; *Three-theme* = beginning kata with three repetitions; *Cross pattern* = Four directional pattern; *Maegeri* = front kick; *Kansetsugeri* = low side kick; *Nidangeri* = double kick; *Other kicks* = other kicks; *Assym. kicks* = kicks done with only with right leg; *Symmetry* = >20% of repetition for both sides.

A cluster analysis was then performed. Cluster analysis allows for the classification of different things or objects into similar groups (clusters). The analysis separates each kata into a different group so that one kata is more similar with others within its group compared with other katas outside its group. This allows the separation of data into meaningful sets that share common characteristics. Cluster analysis forms a tree-like structure known as a dendogram to visually show the groupings of different things, in this instance kata. The clusters analysis was performed using the statistical program SPSS (V14.0).[3] These techniques allowed for the classfication of Goju-ryu katas to provide insight about their structure.

Results and Discussion

Cluster analysis based on the categorization of themes in Table 1 revealed that the classical katas consisted of two clusters (Figures 1). The first cluster included Sesan, Superimpei/Pechurin, and Sanseru. The second cluster included Saifa, Shisochin, Seipai, Kururunfa, and Seiunchin. The first cluster was labeled the Higaonna cluster (Cluster H). The second cluster was labeled the Miyagi cluster (Cluster M). This raises some important questions in the development of modern Goju-ryu as formulated by Miyagi Chojun.

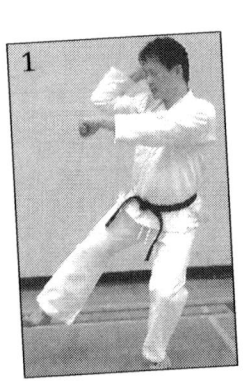
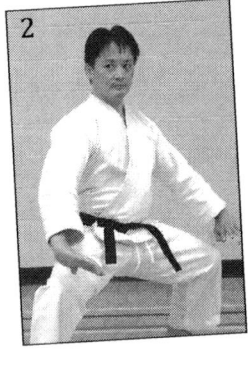
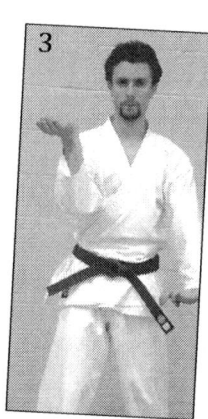
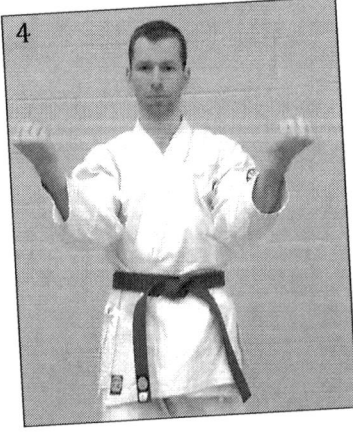
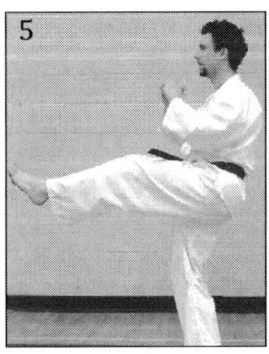

1) Knee kick (*kansetsugeri*).
2) Opening movement from the seiunchin kata.
3) Scooping block (*sukui uke*).
4) Sanchin stance — a fundamental posture found in Goju-ryu and katas from the Naha city area.
5) Front kick (*maegeri*).

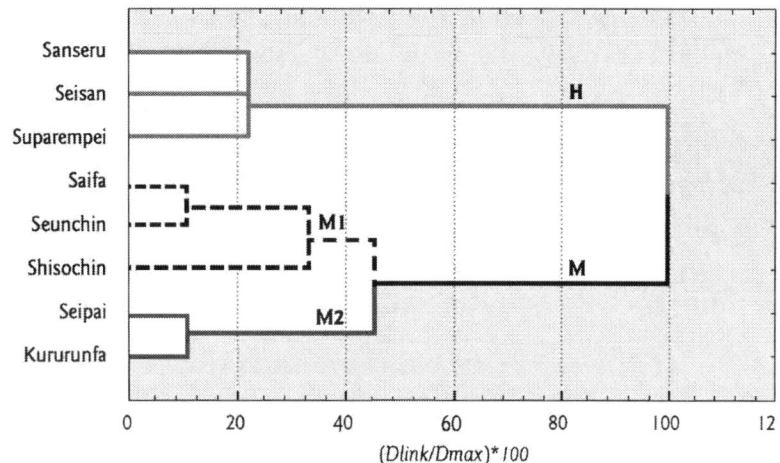

FIGURE 1
Tree Diagram for the Eight Classical Goju-ryu Katas
Complete Linkage, Squared Euclidean Distances

The above chart visually portrays the results of the cluster analysis. It is referred to as a dendrogram or a tree-like diagram. This shows the relationship between the different katas and the groups they form. We can see that the Higaonna or Cluster H (50% black line) consists of Sanseru, Seisan and Suparempei/ Pechurin. In contrast we can see the Miyagi or Cluster M (black line) consists of Saifa, Seiunchin, Shisochin, Seipai and Kururunfa. Looking closer we can see that the analysis broke down the Cluster M further into two smaller groups: Cluster M1 (dash line) which contains Saifa, Seiunchin and Shisochin, and Cluster M2 (70% black line) which contains Seipai and Kururunfa.

First, could Cluster H be considered an indigenous boxing method while Cluster M be considered Chinese boxing? On March 19, 1866, the last group of Chinese envoys visited Okinawa. Documented within the program of this last visit was a demonstration of boxing and weaponry by Aragaki Seisho[4] and others at the Ochayagoten[5] in Shuri Castle. Several kata names were listed including Sesan and Suparempei/Pechurin (McKenna, 2001). Both of these katas are part of Cluster H. Therefore, these two katas were practiced on Okinawa before Higaonna Kanryo reportedly left for China and could be considered indigenous. We can hypothesize that due to the grouping of katas in Cluster H, that Sanchin and Sanseru may also have been practiced during this time, suggesting that Cluster H represents an Okinawan boxing method. Further corroborating evidence can be seen if we examine the curriculum of Kyoda Juhatsu's To'on-ryu which contains only four kata: San Chin, Seisan, Sanseru and Bechurin. Therefore, we can speculate that Cluster H may represent the original Nahate kata (Sanchin, Seisan, Sanseru, and Suparempei/Pechurin) as argued by Kanzaki and Murakami.

Second, these results suggest that Higaonna Kanryo was responsible for the introduction of Cluster H, but there is no clear proof that he was responsible for the introduction of Cluster M. The other kata found in Cluster M seem to be from different system(s) from the original four as found in Cluster H, and seem to be more of an addition to that curriculum rather than an integral part. We can also state that Cluster M appears for the first time as part of Miyagi Chojun's teachings.

It could be argued that the four original kata of Cluster H were beginner forms and only Miyagi Chojun learned the other more advanced forms found in Cluster M. However, as Hirakami (2001) points out, looking at the technical content of the four kata found in Cluster H, it is difficult to maintain this theory. Therefore, it is interesting to theorize that Cluster M represents newer Chinese katas introduced by Miyagi Chojun after Higaonna's death in 1915.

Finally, if Higaonna Kanryo taught the katas that form Cluster M only to Miyagi Chojun, then Higaonna passed on two or more different systems. That is, Higaonna passed on a modified version of what constitutes the original fighting arts of the Naha City area as represented by the katas Sanchin, Sesan, Sanseru, and Suparempei/Pechurin. This then begs the question, where did these additional katas come from? Did they originate from Higaonna's teacher in China, Ru Ru Ko, or did they perhaps come from someone else?

NOTES

[1] The characters used by Itosu to render karate would be pronounced toudi in Okinawan dialect, meaning "Tang/China Hand" showing a Chinese origin or influence.

[2] Although this is contradicted in Morio Higaonna's book, *The History of Karate: Okinawan Goju-ryu* (1998).

[3] In SPSS (V14.0), the cluster analysis uses the average linkage as an algorithm for amalgamation and squared Euclidian distances.

[4] Aragaki Seisho (1840–1920) is considered to be Higaonna Kanryo's first boxing teacher.

[5] The royal tea house located in Shuri Castle.

BIBLIOGRAPHY – ENGLISH

Higaonna, M. (1998). *The history of karate: Okinawan Goju-ryu*. Thousand Oaks, CA:Dragon Books.

McKenna, M. (2001). Exploring goju ryu's past: Myths and facts surrounding Higashionna Kanryo, pt. 1–2. *Dragon Times*, 18-19.

McCarthy, P. (1993). *An outline of karatedo*. International Ryukyu Karate Research Society.

BIBLIOGRAPHY – JAPANESE

Hirakami, N. (2001, May). Secret of Nafadi and Fujian boxing, pt. 1-2. *Gekkan Hiden*, 110–114.

Hokama, T. (1999). *Okinawa karate-do kobudo no shinzui*. Naha: Naha Shuppansha.

Iwai, T. (1992). *The ancient transmission of karate-jutsu*. Tokyo: Aiyudo.

Kinjo, A. (1999). *A true record of the transmission of karate*. Okinawa: Tosho Center.

Kinjo, H. (2007). Seitokukai Homepage. http://skrt.s43.xrea.com/karatejp/modules/xoopsfaq/index.php?cat_id=7

Murakami, K. (1991). *The heart and technique of karate*. Tokyo: Shinjin Butsu Orai Sha Hakko.

Okinawa Prefectural Board of Education. (1994). *A basic investigative report into karatedo and kobudo*. Ginowan: Yojusha.

Tokashiki, I. (1991). *Gohaku-kai yearbook* (Vol. 4). Naha: n.p.

ACKNOWLEDGMENTS

Thanks to Fred Lohse III for proofing and editing the manuscript; and Justin Chin, Maik Hassel, and Oliver Riche for posing for the photographs.

chapter 54

Defending to the Four Direction: Evolving Uechi-ryu's Hojoundo Exercises for Advanced Students

br Ihor Rymaruk

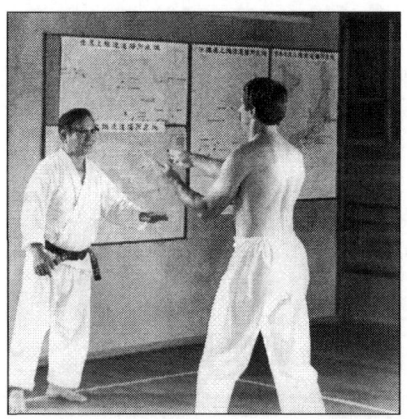

Master Uechi Kanei directing Rymaruk's Sanchin practice, Futenma Dojo, 1982.
All photographs courtesy of Ihor Rymaruk.

Brief Background of Uechi-ryu

Uechi-ryu is one of four major karate styles on the island of Okinawa. It is uniquely different in that it has not lost its resemblance to its southern Chinese roots. At its core are the three katas that Uechi Kanbun (1877–1948), the founder of Uechi-ryu, brought back from China after spending thirteen years on the mainland as a student and then taught at his own school—sanchin, sesan, and sanseru. In 1940, Kanbun's students renamed Uechi's school from Pangainoon-ryu Karatejutsu Kenkyu-jo (Half-hard, Halfsoft Style Empty Hand Technique Study Hall) to Uechi-ryu Karatejutsu (Uechi's Art of Empty Hand).

Uechi Kanei (1911–1991), Kanbun's eldest son, authorized a group of senior practitioners to piece together the fighting techniques that Kanbun taught. Between 1950 and 1960, Uechi-ryu took on, for the most part, its present-day format. Five beginner and intermediate katas were developed based on the original three katas. A series of warmup exercises were added and the hallmarks of uniquely extrapolated techniques from Kanbun's fighting style were used to make up the formal exercises (*hojoundo*). Uechi-ryu's core of kata and techniques has been consistent for over fifty years. During those years, various two-person drills were developed, but there were no universal changes in how students practiced these core exercises. The practice of Uechi-ryu in the main schools on Okinawa is consistent, yet none are carbon copies of each other.

Training on Okinawa is a dream for most karate enthusiasts; however, the difficulties of travel, language, and time prevents most from attaining that dream. A few dedicated individuals were privileged to be a part of Uechi Kanei's dojo. My first certified Uechi-ryu instructor, Frank Gorman, and now my present teacher, James Thompson, both instructed and practiced Uechi-ryu as taught by Uechi Kanei. Thompson trained exclusively at the main dojo in Futenma Airbase under the direct tutelage of Uechi Kanei for almost ten years, a unique accomplishment for a non-Okinawan at that time. Being a part of Uechi Kanei's dojo was a special experience for me as well with the realization of being part of an organization greater than any one school. Today, there are many transplants from other countries that have fallen in love with the island culture and its people, and practice the martial arts on a regular basis. Some have become head teachers in their own Uechi-ryu dojo.

Enhancing the Standard Formal Exercises

Hojoundo practice basically consists of thirteen hand and leg exercise combinations that always begin with a block, and is normally practiced as a group without regard of rank. Traditionally, hojoundo exercises are practiced while standing in place, and the exercises remain the same for the beginner, intermediate, and advanced students. That is, in the Uechi style, there is no progression of difficulty to challenge more advanced students. After executing thousands of repetitions, the training drill is embedded in muscle memory and becomes a natural reflex or habit. Practicing hojoundo is a great workout at any level, and it is a good feeling to be able to execute techniques on autopilot without errors. We believe that martial arts training consists of mind, body, and spirit, Currently, our destination in our training journey is to react with an empty mind. In essence, an empty mind is not necessarily lacking in knowledge, but it is conditioned to respond to any challenge without thought.

As I evolved in my understanding of Uechi-ryu, I began incorporating various stepping sequences into my practice of the formal exercise. The culmination of which is the evolution of old ways done with a new twist, which I call "Defending to the Four Directions." Teaching new students and developing their foundations is still done in the time-tested traditional manner. However, as students progress in rank and understanding, it seemed logical to challenge the student's comfort zone as they moved through the ranks of beginner, intermediate, and advanced levels. After all, I too, still a beginner, also needed to push, explore, and take my own understanding to different levels. Taking students out of their comfort zone by putting hojoundo into motion, builds on what students can already do extremely well in a static position, and helps students to discover, through struggle, that there is a continued need for greater mental as well as physical training challenges. Incremental additions to training drills have the benefit of maintaining a student's thirst for new information, and demonstrate that the level of one's training is only confined by one's own limitations. Evolution is a friend, stimulated and influenced through diligent repetitive training and time.

It is important for all new students to develop and understand the original format of the formal exercises as developed and practiced by Uechi Kanei. Without this original format, there is no style of Uechi-ryu. Once a student can perform the formal basics smoothly and without any hesitation, he or she is ready to add life to the static formal exercise training regime. Once the formal exercises are learned, students are typically taught two-person control fighting drills. These drills (*kyu kumite*) are the real beginnings of developing timing and distancing and simple blocking and striking. However, these drills do not incorporate the formal exercises in a realistic defensive or offensive manner, and actually relegate them as warm-up for kata, without much exploration or practice of real benefits for practical self-defense. Furthermore, the hojoundo exercises assume that all attacks come from the front only. Hojoundo's application may be understood by the masters, but it should not take years for students to make the leap to the practical application stage.

I began searching for ways to help students understand and bridge the gap to the application of hojoundo. Hojoundo are preformed in an hourglass (*sanchin*) stance with a designated foot forward. The first modification I incorporated for intermediate beginners was to alternate arm movements. That is, to practice an exercise that is intended to be executed with a left arm block, for example, by alternating left then right with each repetition. This changes the flow of the original combination, but not the combination itself. If the standard way is to do a certain technique off the lead leg only or off the rear leg only, I practice the upper body combination without regard to which leg is forward. I would keep my stance stationary, but alternate the hand combinations. After all, students should be able to apply combinations that they have learned regardless of which foot is forward. Plus, the added benefit of alternating sides is that your uniform will no longer bind at the shoulders or arms from doing the same repeating motion.

As I became comfortable practicing in this ambidextrous stationary manner, I found that the realism of fighting movements was still missing, and that the traditional format of blocking off a specific foot was not being applied. Realistic fighting is rarely if ever a stationary activity without footwork, and it is important to maintain the style's foundations. So, for my intermediate and advanced students, I took the next step, and put hojoundo into motion with a simple step. This was accomplished by stepping forward and executing a given combination until there was no room to go forward, at which point we would step backward executing the same combinations before moving on to the next. This allowed for the alternation of arms during the practice of the combination without compromising the standard format of hojoundo. While stepping forward or back is not a unique way of practicing basics, as many other styles do so during their basic drills; it is just not how traditional Uechi-ryu hojoundo was practiced. When there were a lot of students in class, and space was very limited, I would have students take one step forward, execute the combination, step back, and execute the combination for six to ten repetitions (A1-3). This method worked out well, and the step forward gave the feeling of being on the offensive, while the step back gave the feeling of defense. Thus, hojoundo took on the motions of an ocean wave, moving forward, closing ground/offense, and moving back, giving up ground/defense.

Maintaining good form will likely be a challenge for intermediate students; however, the more accomplished a student becomes, the easier it will be for him/her to maintain his/her sanchin root. Through the stepping motion, students can better visualize the application of each hojoundo exercise, even though they will still assume that the attack they are fending off is coming from the front.

Sequence of Hojoundo Exercises Used with Defending to the Four Directions

1) circle block, front kick
2) circle block; hook punch
3) high block punch, middle block punch
4) circle block punch, palm block punch
5) circle block chop, back fist, punch
6) circle block, elbow strikes
7) finger strikes
8) four-way wrist blocks
9) fish tail blocks

Stepping to the front and to the back is the fundamental footwork.

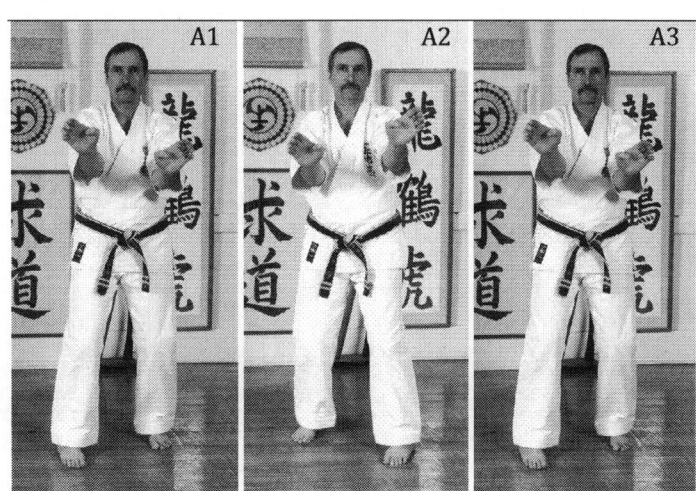

TECHNICAL SECTION

Defending to the Four Directions

The next logical progression for the practice of hojoundo is to appreciate that attacks come from all directions. "Defending to the Four Directions" was conceived about two years ago as I monitored and critiqued students' leadership and teaching skills while continuing my personal development and study in the back row next to my new white belts. This technique was developed as I experimented with ways to give my Uechi-ryu formal exercises a more practical and realistic twist.

This exercise along with the use of strong visualization increases the practicality of Uechi-ryu in a self-defense situation and challenged even the most advanced student. You will have trained to defend in any direction of multiple incoming threats while staying true to the founders and foundations of Uechi-ryu. "Defending to the Four Directions" is not a very complicated drill; it's just not for beginners. This multidimensional addition to hojoundo makes Uechi-ryu a more realistic close-in fighting system.

To execute the "Four Directions" foot work, you will need to understand two basic turns, a 90°pivot turn, and a 180°turn known as a sanchin turn for its execution from the sanchin stance. To make the 90°pivot turn, start in a sanchin stance with your left foot forward. Your big toe of your back foot should be in line with the heel of your front foot, and your feet should be approximately shoulder width apart. Pivot on the balls of your feet to face your right. Your right foot will now be your front foot and your left foot will be your back foot (B1-2). You may also choose to begin with the right foot forward, in which case you will pivot in the same manner to the left. Always pivot to the direction of the rear foot.

To execute a sanchin turn, begin in a sanchin guard position with one foot in front of the other, toe heel on the same line, feet shoulder width apart. Pivot on the ball of your hind foot, turning the heel toward your supporting front leg. As you start turning, to your left if your right leg was forward, or to your right if your left leg was forward, turn your hips and shoulders in the direction of the turn before moving your front leg. Plant the heel of C1 your pivoting leg on the floor and bring your other leg around smartly so that the toe of that foot is in line with the heel of the pivoting leg. Ultimately, your front leg will become your hind leg as you turn your body 180°to face the opposite direction that you started from (B3-4). Once you have mastered these turns, you are ready for the "Four Direction" cycle.

Begin the "Four Directions" cycle by standing in the Sanchin guard position with

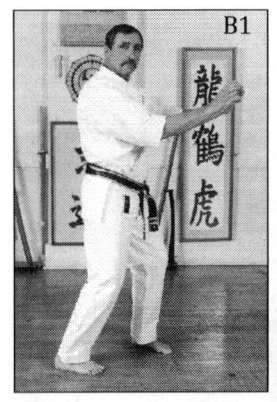
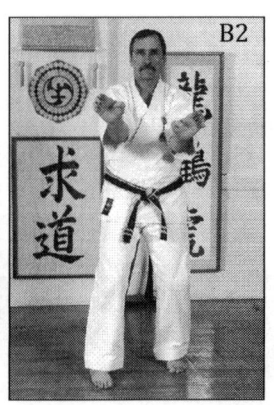
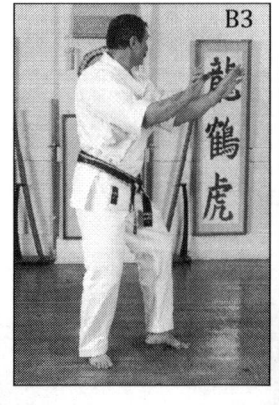
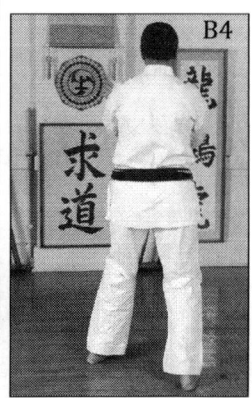

your right foot forward (C1). Step forward with the left foot (C2). Next, pivot 90° to your right (C3). Now execute a sanchin turn, turning 180° toward your left (C4).

Repeat the 90° pivot turn to the right, followed by the 180° Sanchin turn to the left, until you have faced all four cardinal directions, and are facing the direction you began in (C5-17).

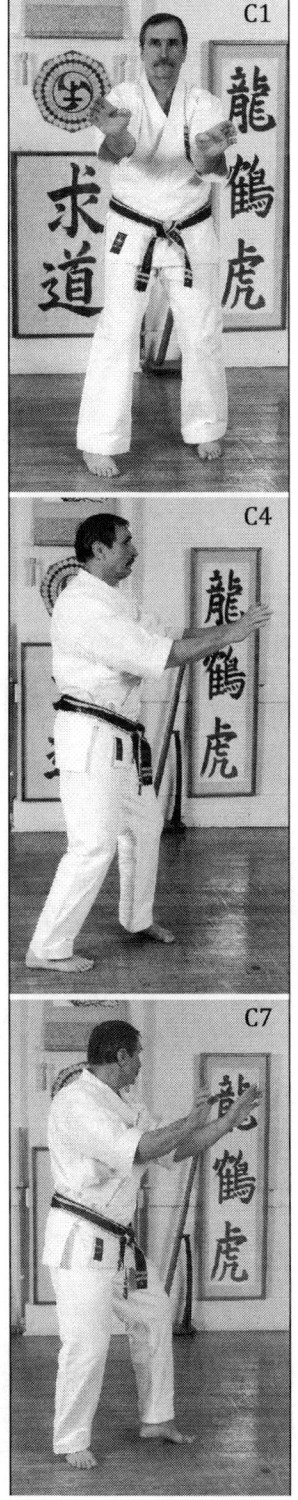
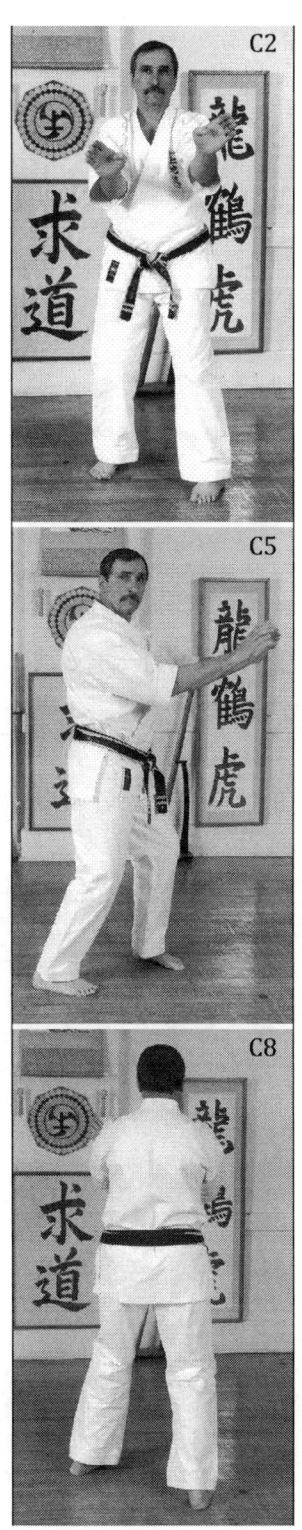
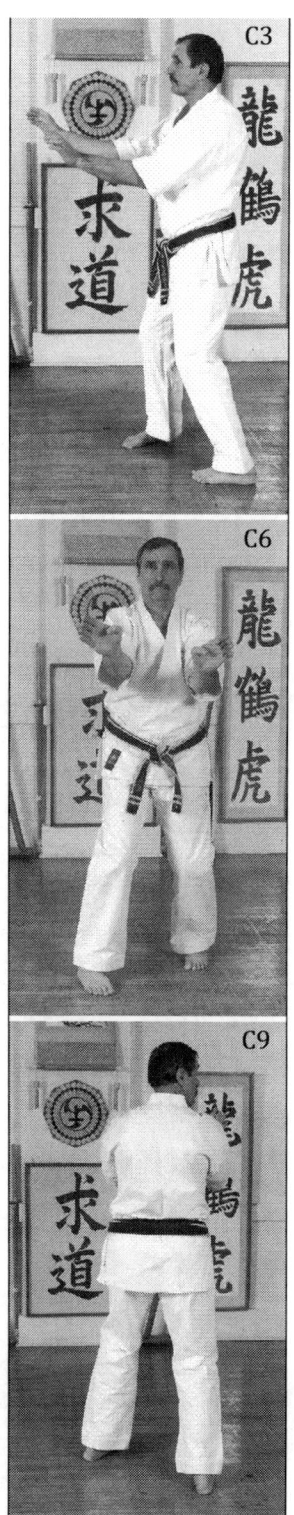

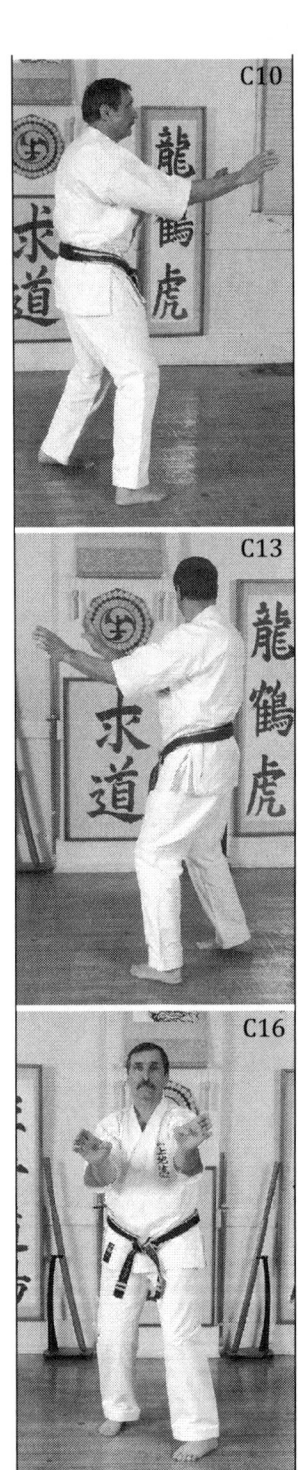

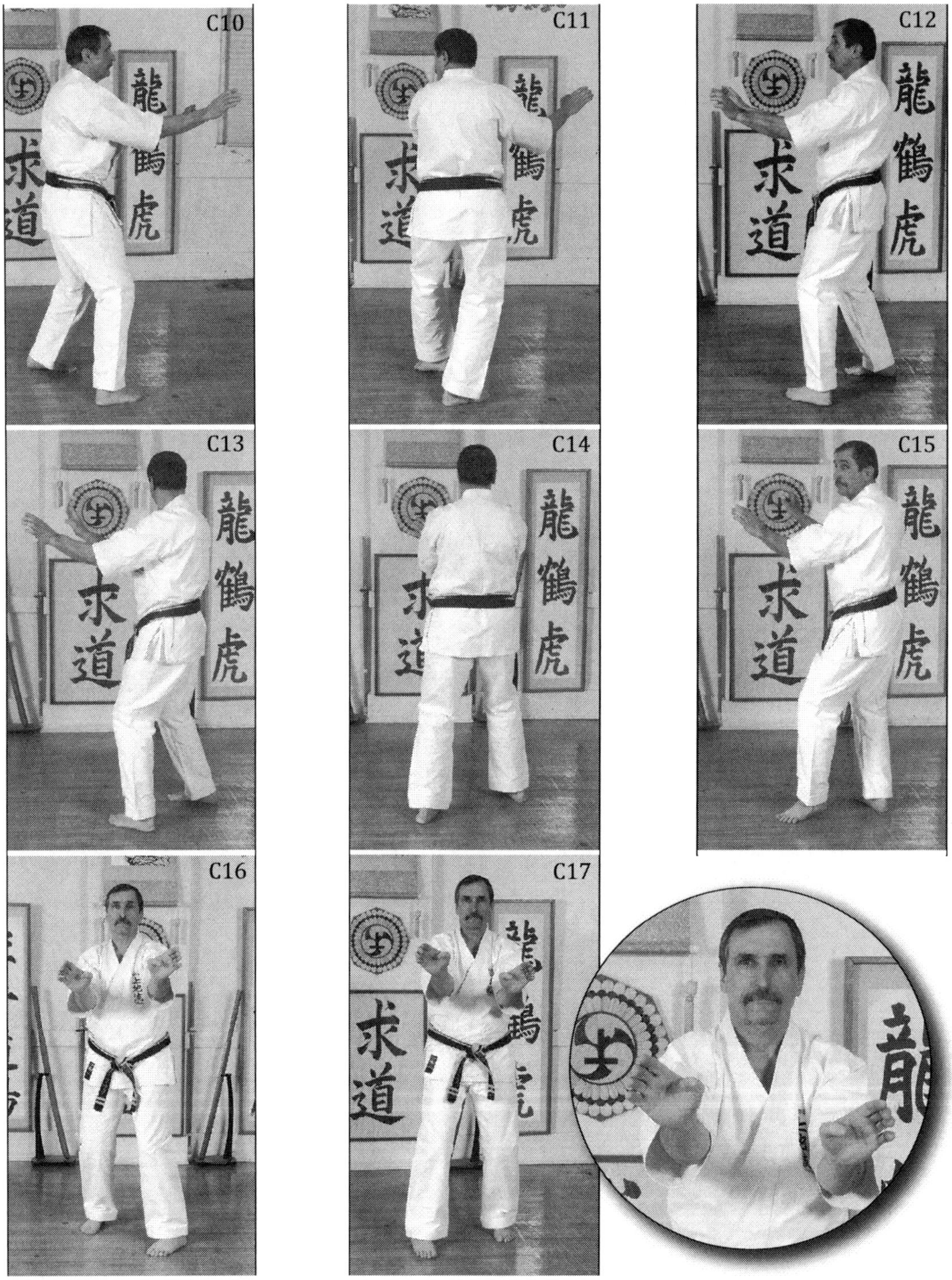

Four Direction Practice

Once you have mastered this pattern of turns, you will be ready to add hojoundo exercises. To do this, simply execute a hojoundo exercise after each turn. You may do the same drill throughout the cycle, or you may do a different drill between each of the turns. A compplete cycle of the "Four Directions" technique applying the circle block hook punch exercise of hojoundo is profided in D1-36. This set begins with a step forward followed by a step back before the cycle begins (D1-7).

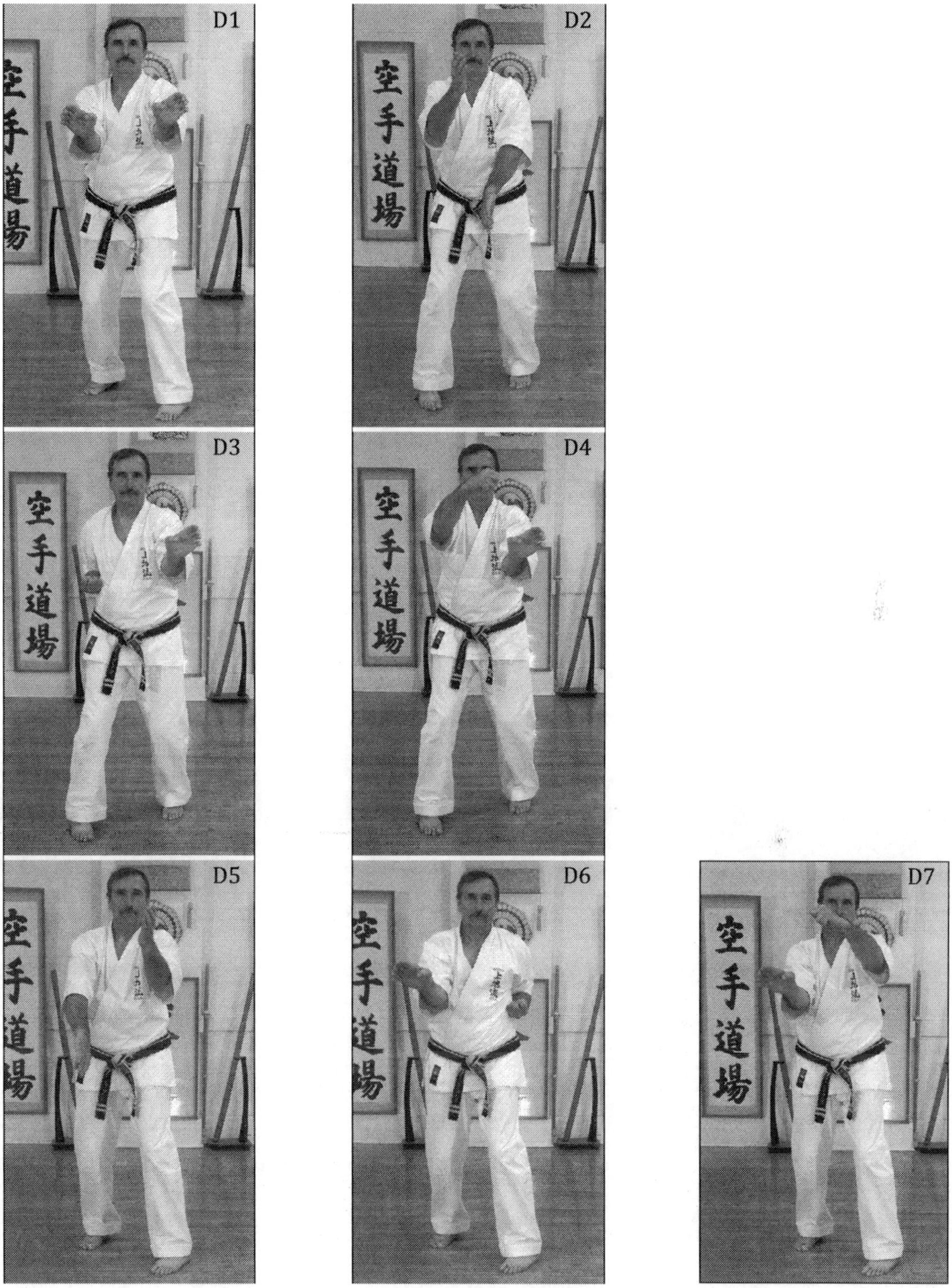

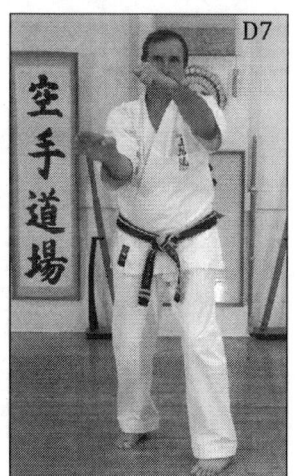

D1-4 From the left guard position, step forward with you right leg. Execute a left circle block off the rear leg and a right hook punch off the front leg. Always come to the guard position after completing each combination.

D5-7 Step back with right leg and execute a right circle block followed by a left hook punch.

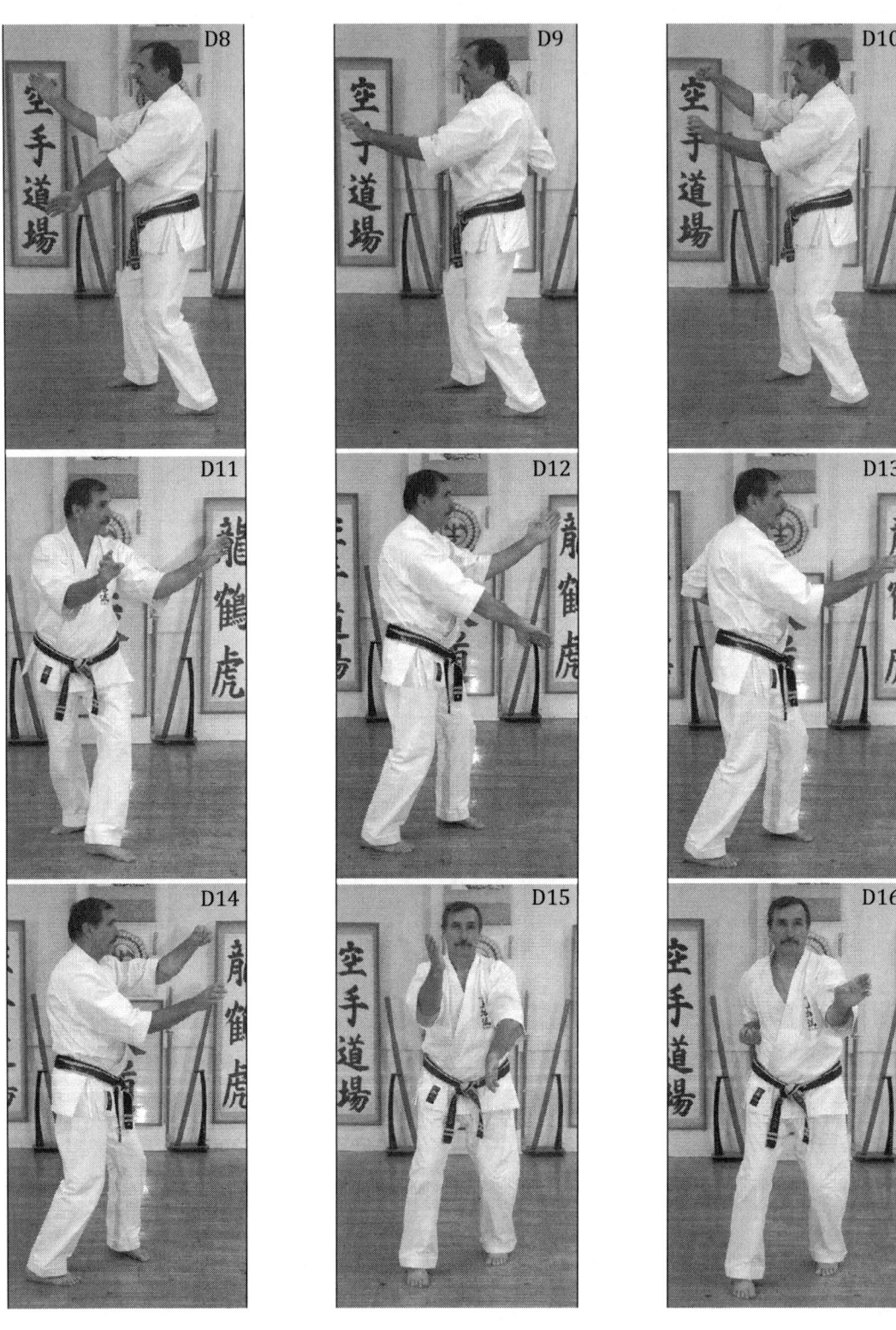

D7-10 After delivering the left hook, return to the guard position. Pivot 90° on the balls of your feet to the right, and execute a left circle block and right hook punch.
D10-14 From the guard, turn 180° and execute a circle block off the rear leg and a hook punch off the front leg. Return to the guard position.

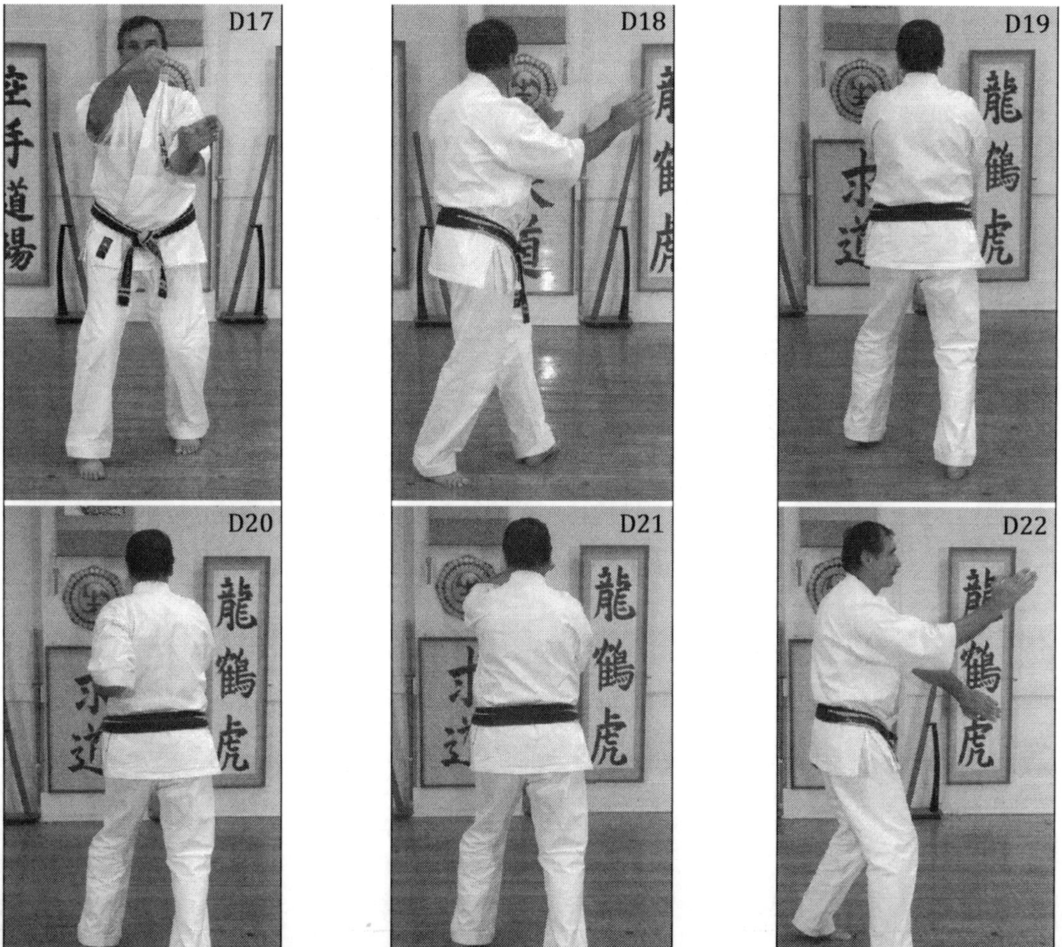

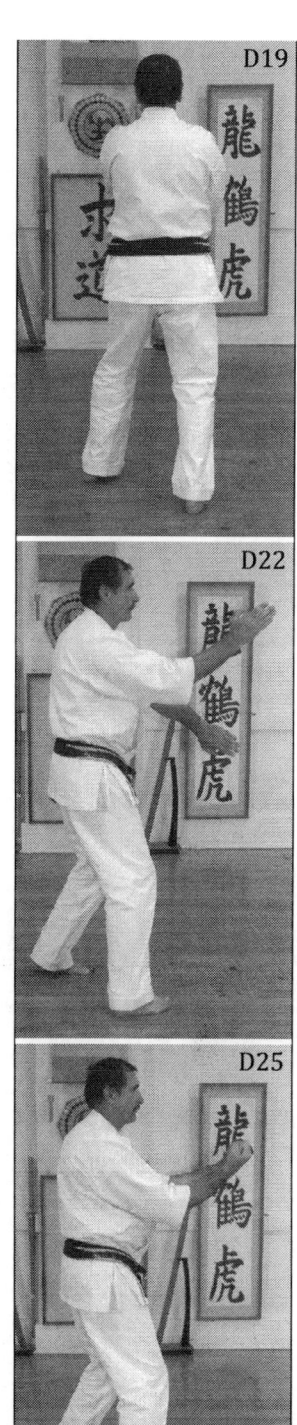

D14-17 Shift you weight slightly onto the balls of your feet and pivot 90° to the right. Perform a circle black and hook punch combination.
D17-21 From the guard position, execute the second 180° turn. Perform a circle block and hook punch combination.
D21-25 From the guard, pivot 90° to the right and execute circle block and hook punch combination.

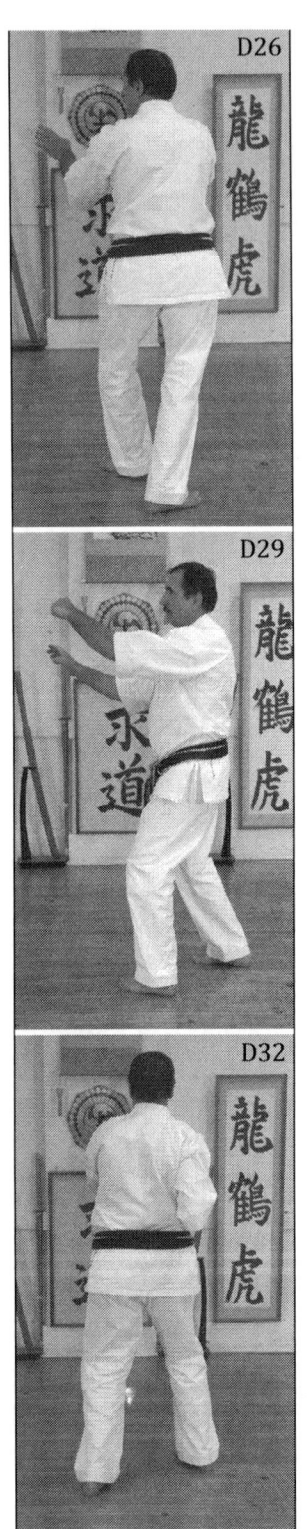
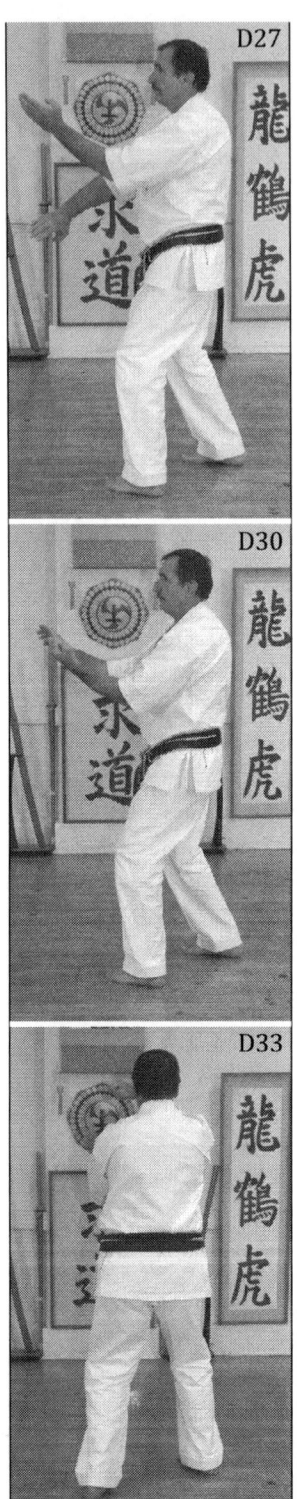
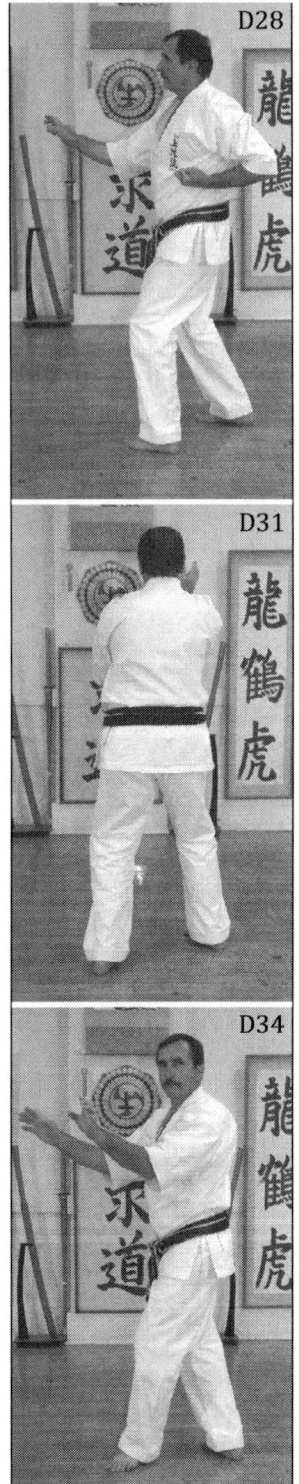

D25-30 Bring your hands to the guard position, execute a 180° turn, and perform a circle block and hook punch combination.

D30-33 After completing the combination, bring your hands to the guard position and pivot 90° to the right. Execute a circle block and hook punch combination.

D33-36 After completing the combination, bring your hands to the guard position, and turn 180°. Perform a circle block and hook punch combination. This is the end of the four direction cycle. At his point, you can continue the same sequence for several more repetitions, or you may move on to the next combination.

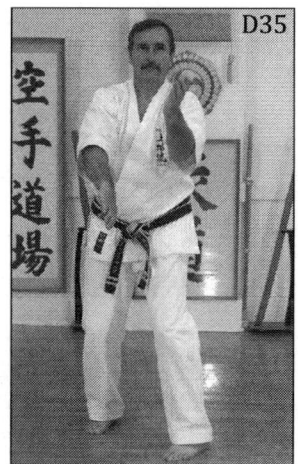 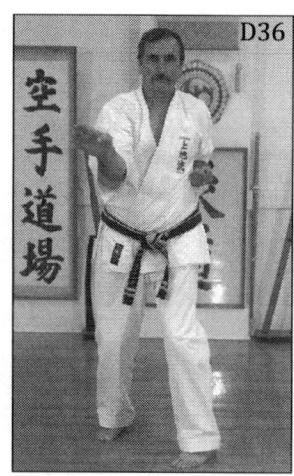

"Defending to the Four Directions" can be applied to most hojoun-do exercises, except for the side snap kick, and the three stepping drills. Keep in mind you can practice the "Four Directions" beginning with either foot forward, as called for by the hojoundo exercise you wish to practice. If you are training solo, you may change the direction of the flow of the exercise at any time by pivoting to the direction of your choice. For example, you may wish to begin with your right foot forward, in which case you would simply pivot to your left instead of the right, then execute sanchin turn as usual. You may also wish to add stepping forward or backward in between turning. For group training, be sure to establish the direction of movement first so as to reduce confusion and collisions.

Four Direction Application

You may find this technique challenging at first, or find that your once solid form may become sloppy. As you continue to practice in the four directions, your mind will become sharper, and your body will create new muscle memory that will make the drill easier to execute. You will be able to further hone your skills, and may even find that you utilize hojoundo techniques more often in self-defense applications. An example of how the "Defending to the Four Directions" technique may be applied is provided using circle block hook punch in E1-25.

E1-3 The defender on the left steps in and performs a circle block to check the attacker's left guard followed by a hook punch.

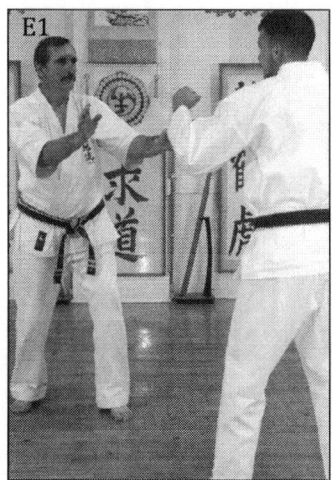 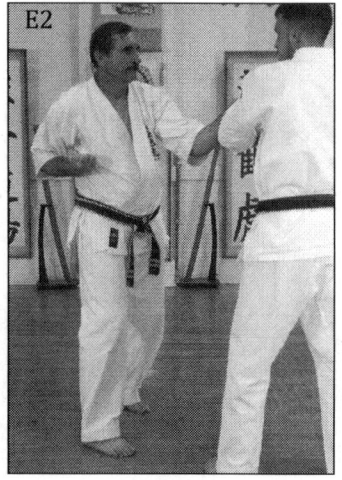 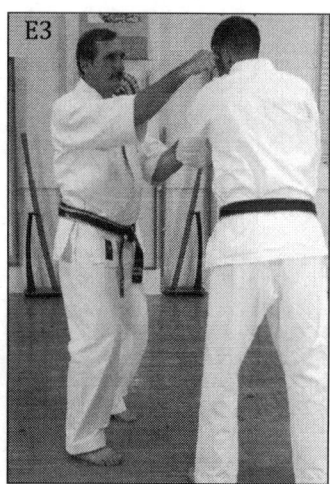

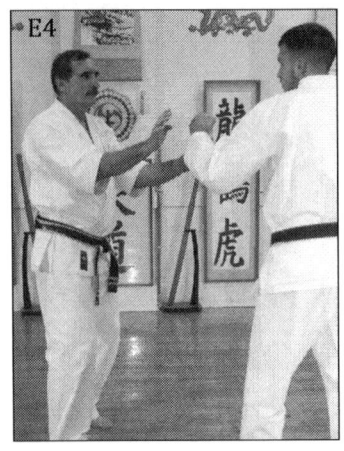
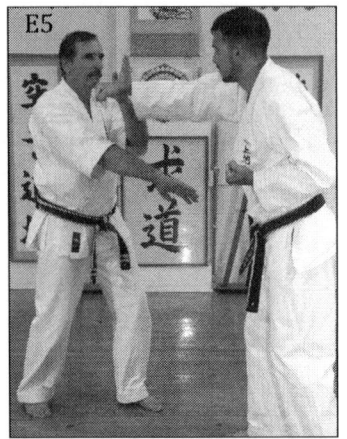
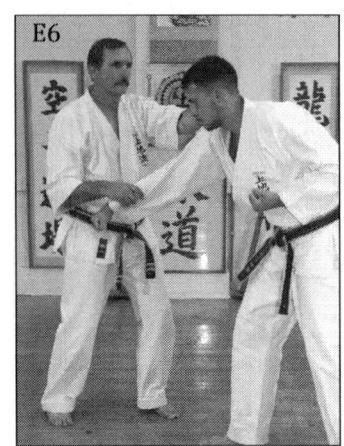
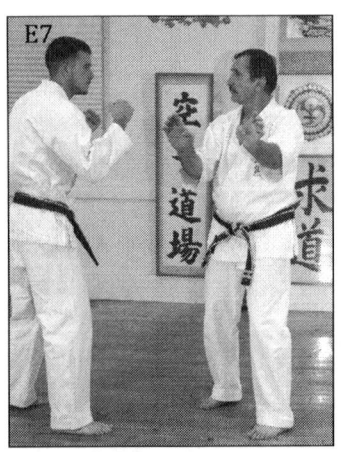
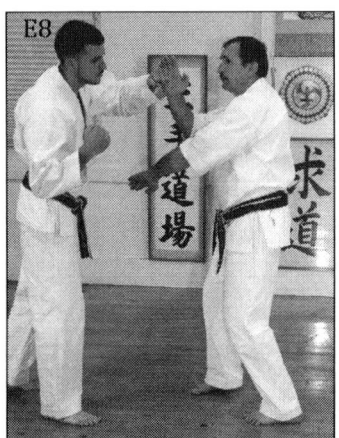
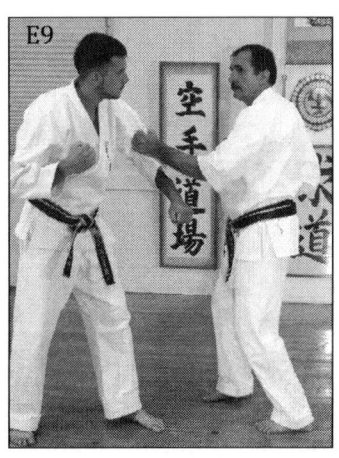
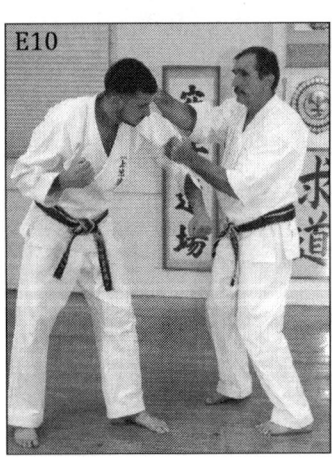
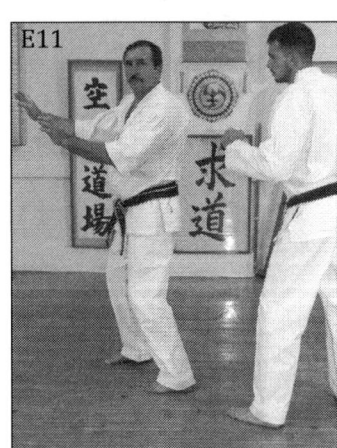
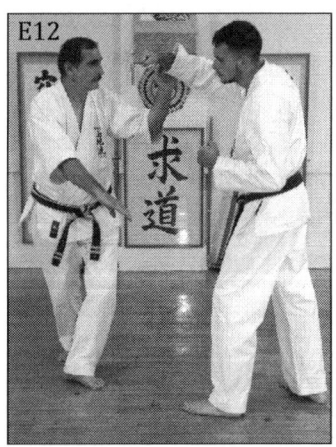

E4-6 From the guard position, the defender steps back against the attacker's punch. He then executes a circle block and finishes with a hook punch.
E7-10 The defender (on the right) is threatened with an attack. He pivots 90° to the right and neutralizes the left punch with a circle block. He then counter-attacks with a hook punch.

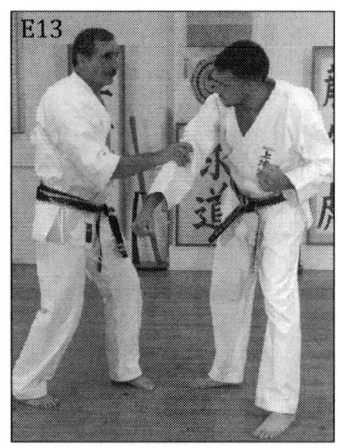
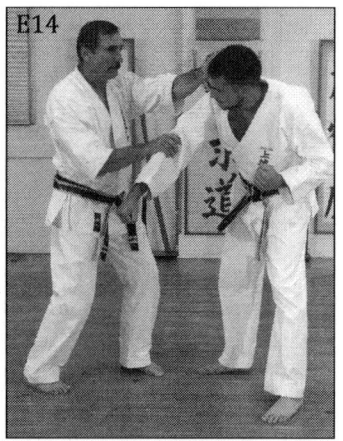
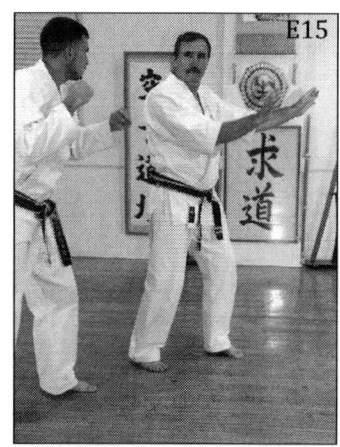
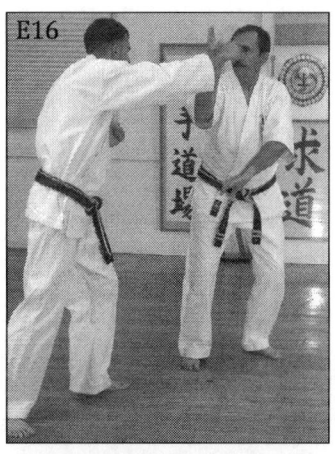
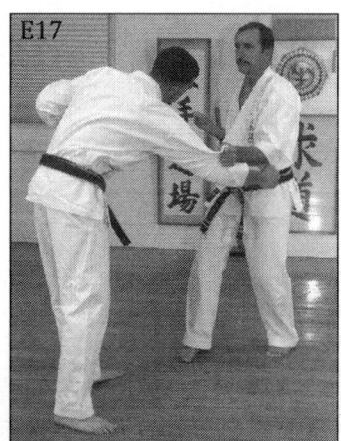
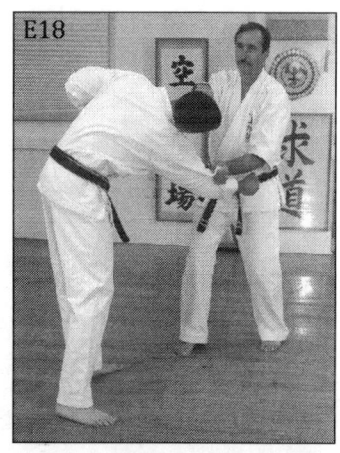
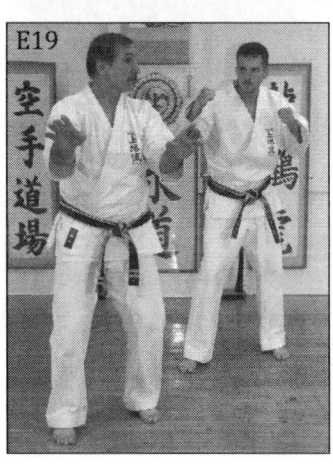
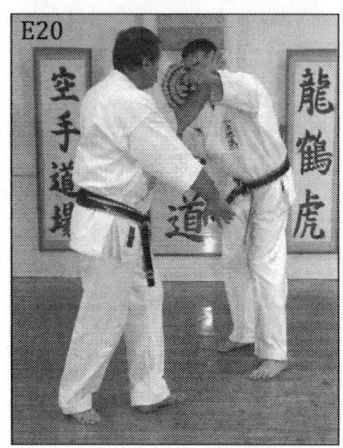
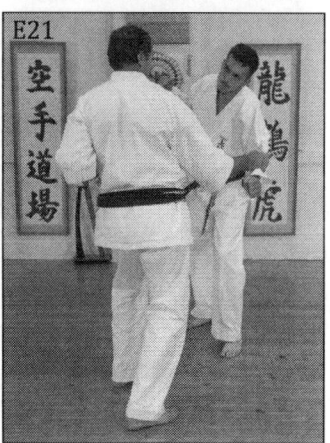

E11-14 The defender sees an attack coming from the rear and performs a 180° turn (Sanchin turn). He then performs a circle block against the attacker's right punch, and counter-attacks with a hook punch to the head.
E15-18 The attacker strikes from the right. The defender pivots 90° to the right while stopping the attacker's punch with a circle block and counterattacks with a hook punch.

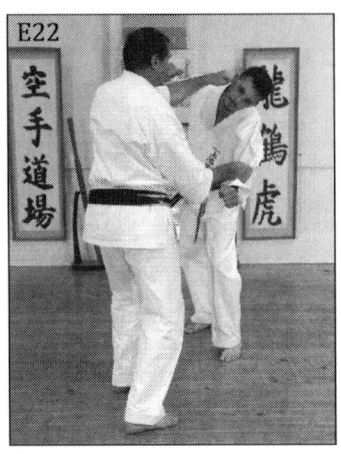
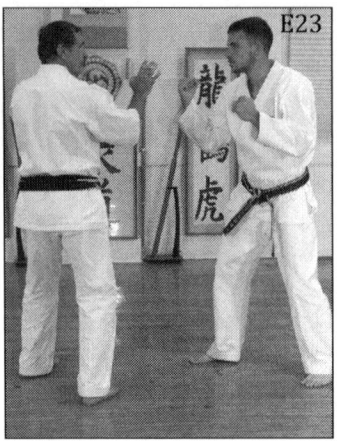
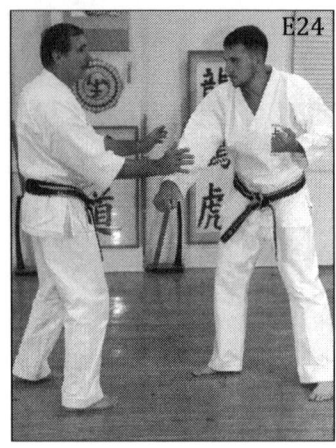

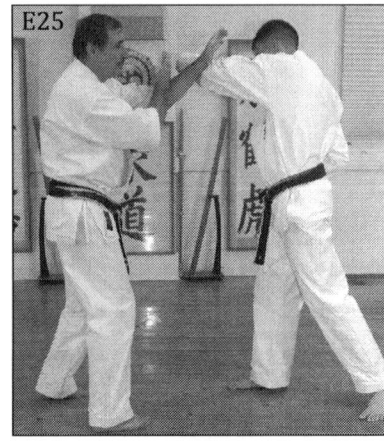

E19-22 The defender sees an attacker coming from behind to punch. The defender pivots 180° (Sanchin turn) and performs a circle block against the attacker's punch. The defender then counter-attacks with a hook punch.

E23-25 The attacker comes in from the right to deliver a combination punch. The defender pivots 90° to the right and stops the attacker's right punch with a right pressing block. The defender next uses a left circle block against the attacker's left punch and finishes with a hook punch to the temple (Note: Finishing punch is not shown).

Conclusion

It is not often that one can add a simple but unique twist to a system or style that has already proven itself and met the test of time. I am pleased to have introduced and shared with you my special way of practicing hojoundo, for the advanced students. Often, over the years, advanced students have complained that they were bored with the same routine, or just needed something more to challenge them. These were the few students that just did not appreciate the effectiveness of simplicity. The belief was that the magic for effective self-defense applications was hidden in complex motor skills. And yet, these were the same students that could not move in any direction without losing some control of the basics. Students learn what is expected of them, and today we must expect more from our students. Not only are they the future of Uechi-ryu, they are responsible for its survival in a very competitive world. Uechi-ryu training has to evolve to meet the demands and needs of a society that is becoming more cognizant of the importance of self preservation. Uechi-ryu karate will survive as long as there is a need for a formidable

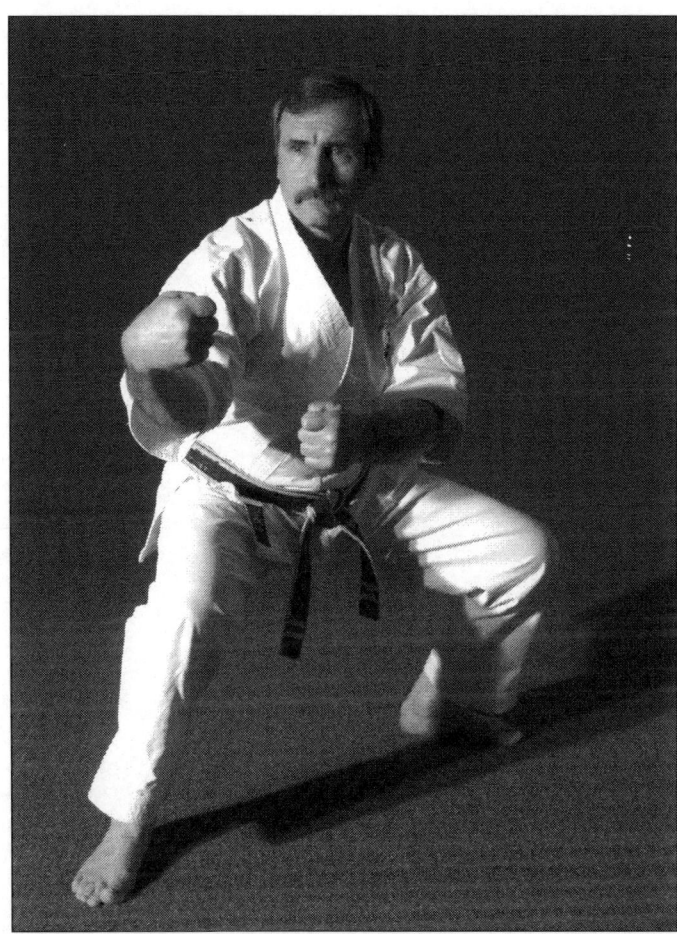

SPECIAL THANKS TO Jennifer Rymaruk for editing support and photography, Justin Rymaruk for being my demonstration partner, and Amber Vosko for technical support.

system of self-defense. A student who is truly gaining mastery of Uechi-ryu will certainly welcome and handle the challenge to raise his/her training to a new dimension. It is like a dart player who can always hit the bull's-eye looking for a challenge by way of putting the dart board in motion. The expert suddenly becomes a beginner.

I have taken my Uechi-ryu from stationary practice, to moving forward and back, to moving to the four cardinal directions. That first step I took years ago in making my Uechi practice more practical has led to the many steps and changes in directions that have given birth to a much more realistic work-out routine for the senior student. While students must first learn certain moves and develop timing, distancing, and proper reflexes appropriate to a given situation in a safe and constructive manner, there comes a time when the developed skills must be set in motion.

Hojoundo is often practiced as a separate entity, relegated to being a warm up for the next phase of skill building. It just makes sense to work the drills that have been practiced the most, get deeper into the style, and continue to build on them, and put them to more practical use. "Defending to the Four Directions" builds on traditional teachings and adds new dimensions and challenges for advanced practitioners of Uechiryu, yet its simplicity makes it highly adaptable for use in other martial arts. It is said "a high tide raises all ships in the harbor." Therefore, if my simple modifications have merit, are accepted and become widely used by my fellow teachers, then I have contributed in furthering our knowledge of the depths of Uechi-ryu.

chapter 55

Kata and Bunkai: A Study in Theme and Variations in Karate's Solo Practice Routines

by Giles Hopkins, M.A.

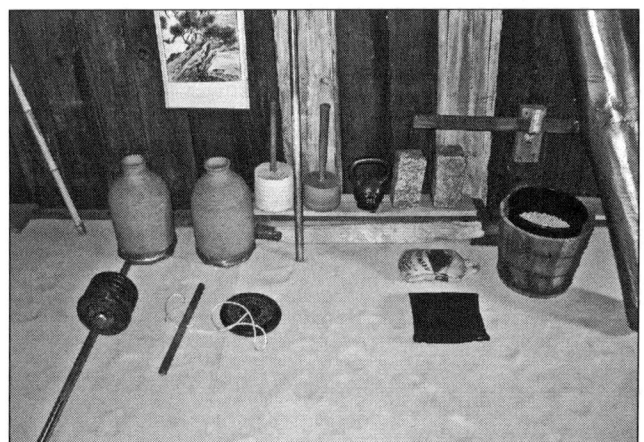
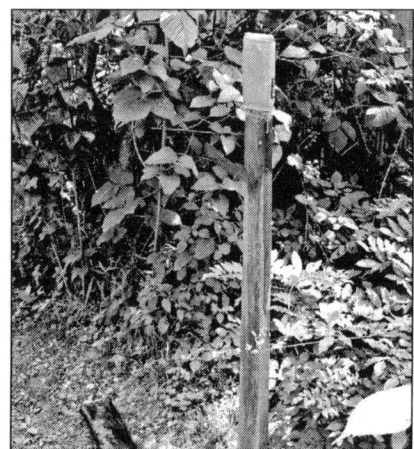

Training implements in the dojo. All photos courtesy of G. Hopkins.

Introduction

Late arrivals had simply kicked off their shoes, thinking no one would notice such a small breech of etiquette. Shoes were piled on top of shoes—mostly sandals and sneakers broken down at the heel. As the children's class came to an end, more and more children jostled their way through the entrance, deftly slipping on shoes and running off into the evening. Adult students were arriving, more serious than their young counterparts, their shoes forming neat rows, each pair facing out towards the street.

Inside, adults were silently stretching and warming up. One was doing exercises with the stone weights (*chishi*), while another was walking up and down the floor with the gripping jars (*nigirigame*). I was familiar with the gripping jars: how the hands spread across the openings of the jars, the sides of the thumbs just catching the lip of the opening. But it was on that first trip to Okinawa in 1986 where I realized that training with the jars, more than just an exercise in posture and stance work or even hand and finger strength, was a silent reminder of how important the grasping hand is to Okinawan karate. Like the tiger—one of the animals that the Goju-ryu katas are said to be based on—once the prey is within his grasp, the Goju-ryu practitioner doesn't let go until the opponent is down and no longer a threat. The techniques of the katas, I began to realize, were meant to show these grabs and controlling hands. But as is so often the case, we see the movements and the hand positions in katas without knowing what we're seeing. Like everyone else, we had studied katas, but we hadn't really seen them.

That first summer in Okinawa we saw a lot we didn't fully understand; in fact, it raised more questions than it answered. The Okinawans seemed to move differently; everything was less rigid. Stances were generally higher. There were even noticeable differences in the classical katas. Why did one dojo start Kururunfa kata on the right and another dojo start it on the left? What we had practiced as a back-knuckle strike (*uraken*) in Sepai now looked more like a downward elbow or forearm strike. Where we did a front kick (*maegeri*) in Sanseiru, the Okinawans merely used a knee kick (*hizageri*). There seemed to be endless examples of these differences, and not just differences between what we had practiced in America and what was being done in Okinawa. There were also considerable differences between the various Okinawan schools.

When I asked Gibo Seki why the Higa dojo (Shodokan) started Kururunfa to the right and the Miyazato dojo (Jundokan) started it to the left, he merely replied, "Why not?" It was as if to say these were insignificant differences, leaving me with the feeling that I had asked not a stupid question but the wrong question. On yet another occasion, I asked him why there were so many apparent differences between the Shodokan (the school of Goju-ryu founded by Higa Seko) version of Sanseiru and the Shoreikan (the school of Goju-ryu founded by Toguchi Seikichi) version. Both teachers, after all, had studied with Miyagi Chojun (as, of course, had Miyazato Ei'ichi). How could the same kata look so different? But again Gibo seemed to brush off my question with a laugh. "I know seven different versions of Sanseiru," he said.[1]

There are numerous examples to illustrate this rather perplexing conundrum—that the same classical Goju-ryu katas are done differently by different schools and dojos even within Okinawa. While some of these differences are certainly important and may lead one to vastly different interpretations of kata applications (*bunkai*), many are rather inconsequential. It is, in fact, easy to get distracted by differences that are really insignificant. Even old-school karate practitioners engage in seemingly endless discussions generated by superficial observations of differences in individual katas—this school starts to the left and that one starts to the right; they use basic stance (*sanchin dachi*) while this other school uses front stance (*zenkutsu dachi*); this school goes straight back and that one goes at an angle.

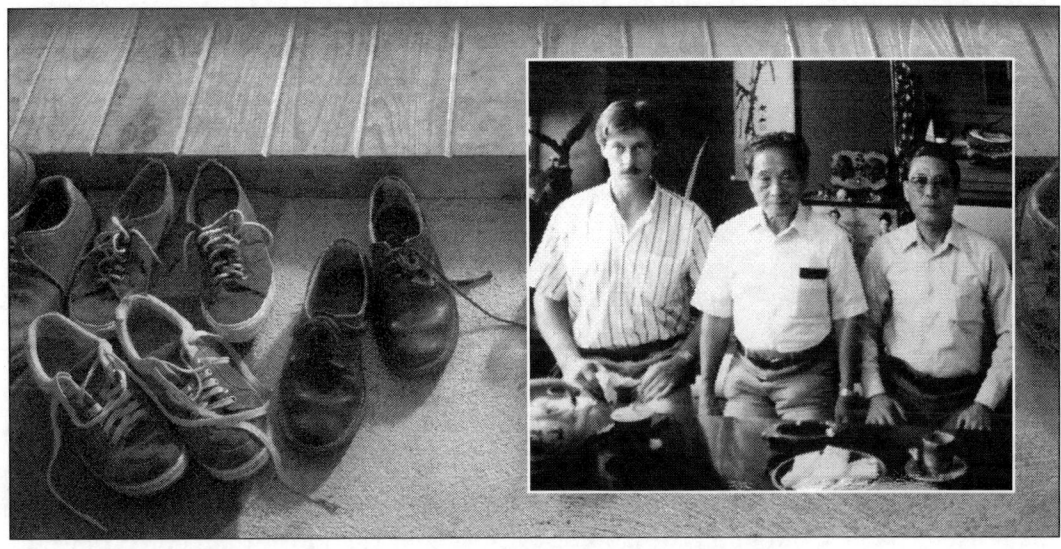

Shoes lining the dojo enterance. Giles Hopkins with
Takamine Chobuku and Higa Seiko at Higa's home in 1986.

More often than not, one of my teacher's teachers, Matayoshi Shinpo (a master of Kingai-ryu, Shorin-ryu, Goju-ryu, and kobudo), would meet these differences with a simple, "Yeah, okay." Most of these differences didn't seem to surprise him. But the journey to Okinawa for any student of karate must be at least in part a confirmation, a journey to make sure one is on the right path. If we are not meant to get answers to all of our questions, we may at least hope that there are enough signs to tell us that we're headed in the right direction. Of course it's in the nature of the martial arts itself that nothing is given away without hard work; there are no short cuts, and no easy answers. Perhaps the only surprise nowadays is that there aren't as many shoes piled up outside the entrance to the dojo—after all, this is the birthplace of karate. But the kids are off playing baseball on dirt playgrounds behind the schools, and the adults are often too busy.

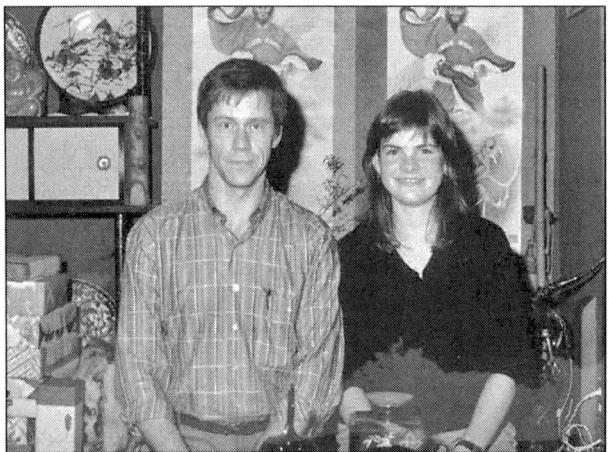

Katas	
Kururunfa	久留頓破
Saifa	砕破
Sanchin	三戦
Sanseiru	三十六(手)
Seipai	十八(手)
Seisan	十三(手)
Seiunchin	制引戦
Shisochin	四向戦
Suparinpei	壱百零八
Tensho	転掌

Giles Hopkins and his wife Martha at Matayoshi's.

Questioning Kata

In Okinawa that summer, I may have been the only one disturbed by these differences. It seemed to me at the time that the classical Goju-ryu katas should be done the same no matter what branch of Goju-ryu one practiced, since all of the founding teachers had studied with Miyagi Chojun or at least with someone who had learned from him. Furthermore, if applications (*bunkai*) are clearly predicated on a kata's movements, one would think that any alteration of the kata's movements would affect one's understanding of application. Katas, after all, should dictate the applications, not the other way round. In some schools, the katas' movements seem to have been informed by someone's personal and perhaps idiosyncratic ideas for application. It is the nature of applications (*bunkai*), however, to be taken from a strict interpretation of the kata's movements. So it is probably still important to find "authentic" katas—what underscores the importance of lineage—but whose lineage?

Additionally, I suspect, logic should provide another sort of barometer since one would expect how one interprets the movements of kata to reinforce the principles found throughout the system; many techniques, after all, show similarity though not necessarily sameness. This, of course, begs the question: If a technique seems to have no other references in other katas is it therefore suspect? Or is it simply unique? Or has it been changed out of either ignorance or a teacher's individual interpretation? But such a debate about which school is right and which is wrong, which kata is more authentic or which has been changed, is really unresolvable at this point.

It is far more instructive to compare similarities between the different katas of a system like Goju-ryu than to compare the differences between different schools. This is a key point. Let me reiterate this. It is often more useful to examine the similarities between movements in different katas than it is to emphasize the differences of how one school and another school perform the same kata. By this I don't mean superficial differences such as which katas end in cat stance (*neko ashi dachi*)—Saifa, Seiunchin, Shisochin, Sepai, Sesan, and Kururunfa—or which katas begin with repetitions of three identical techniques —Saifa, Seiunchin, Shisochin, Sanseiru, Sesan, and Suparimpei. Much has been made of this sort of individual technique analysis.[2] But to suggest that certain katas are unrelated or have a different origin based on a "cluster analysis" of techniques depends largely on what data one inputs into the analysis or the parameters one sets, not to mention the size of the sample or the limited number of techniques one has chosen to analyze. While a focus on some techniques might imply that the Sanseiru and Sepai katas derive from different origins—one begins with a repetition of three techniques and the other doesn't—the similarity of the double-handed techniques illustrated below, for example, would seem to argue for a common source or at the very least that they are indeed forms from the same system (see illustrations 3a and 3b on page 680). Furthermore, to argue differences to support a theory that the original system taught by Higaonna Kanryo was comprised only of Sanchin, Sesan, Sanseiru, and Suparimpei katas seems purely academic; that is, it doesn't seem to get one's practice very far, unless, of course, there is a less than obvious political agenda for such an assertion. While this is not to discount the rather nebulous feeling that Kururunfa exhibits more affinity to Sepai and Saifa than it does to either Sesan or Sanseiru, there may be any number of explanations. Since there is really no definitive way to know the origins of any of the Goju-ryu classical katas, or the myth-shrouded origins of any Chinese-based forms for that matter, it would seem to me to be a better use of one's time and effort to focus on similarities in techniques of the generally accepted canon of Goju-ryu katas.

VARIATIONS ON A THEME

When we compare the similarities between techniques in the different Goju-ryu katas, what we see are variations on a theme. In looking at katas in this way, we start to see each of the katas as a part of a system—that is, related. We can then begin to examine the variations and question when it might be preferable to use one variation rather than another. We can also begin to examine the principles that different variations have in common. This is really the essence of kata study and should be the focus of any study of a particular martial art. So often, students see an art as an infinite collection of techniques, as if we are meant to draw from this collection in the split-second of a life-threatening encounter. Those who advocate this sort of collection theory, or encyclopedic use of katas, argue that one simply needs to practice more if this seems overwhelming. This only serves to highlight the oft-repeated dojo admonition that one needs to practice a kata at least a thousand times before one understands it.

But this is, perhaps, a misunderstanding of what it means to practice. While there is certainly some truth to the idea that we practice so that our responses become second-nature, more importantly we practice in order to understand the principles behind the seemingly infinite variety of techniques. The system, then, becomes much more manageable. We begin to see not only how the system is put together, but also how we can effectively use it as a system of self-defense, and not merely resort to the same two or three techniques that we so often see in tournament sparring matches. For example:

We start to see (and feel) similarities between the opening move of Sepai kata and the "hammer-fist strike" in Saifa kata (see illustrations, 1a Sepai and 1b Saifa).

Or, we begin to see a similarity between the closed-hand two-handed blocking technique of Seiunchin kata and the open-hand double-hand blocks of Saifa (see illustration 2a Seiunchin and 2b Saifa).

Or, we notice that the two-handed technique from Sepai kata is very similar to the two-handed technique from Sanseiru kata (see illustrations 3a Sepai and 3b Sanseiru).

Or, we start to feel that the entry technique in the leaning-away stance followed by the front kick in Sepai kata (the beginning of the second sequence) is very much like the high-low horse stance blocking position in Seiunchin kata (see illustrations 4a Sepai and 4b Seiunchin).

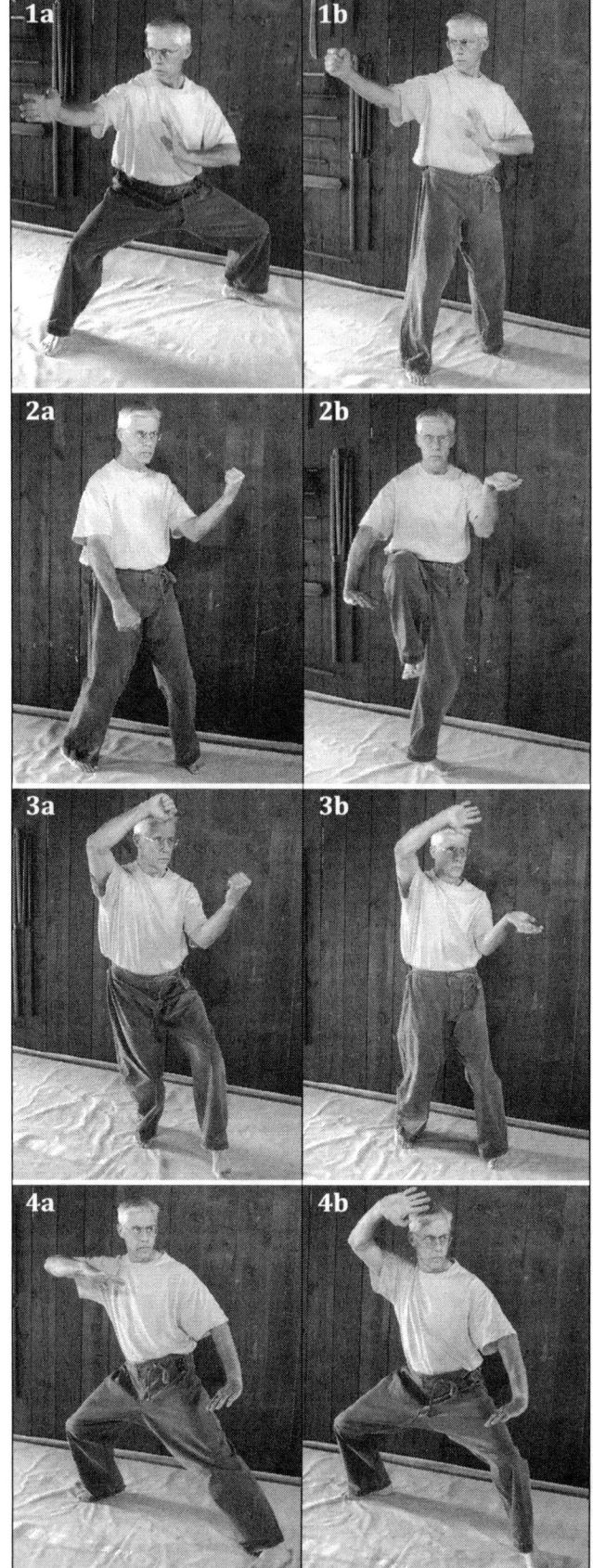

Or, we notice that the grab and finger thrust (*nukite*) from Suparimpei looks the same as the grab and open hand technique from Seiunchin except one is in basic stance (*sanchin dachi*) and the other is done in horse stance (*shiko dachi*) (see illustrations Suparimpei 5a and Seiunchin 5b).

The question is: What does one do with the system once one begins to see the similarities between apparently different techniques from different katas? Might this simply be a case of redundancy? In the first example cited above (the opening move of Sepai kata and the hammer-fist strike from Saifa kata, see illustrations 1a and 1b), the techniques that follow also exhibit a certain similarity. One (Saifa) is followed by a closed-hand undercut punch, while the other (Sepai) is followed by an open hand coming under to the opponent's chin (see illustrations 6a and 6b).

However, even though they are similar, they are not the same; they each illustrate different responses depending on the circumstances of the attack or what follows. But, this similarity is the whole point of variations. Since the Saifa and Sepai sequences begin with the same "block" or receiving technique—and the techniques that follow also show a degree of similarity— one might continue the response initiated by the Saifa block and hammer-fist strike with the open hand to the chin, followed by the neck twist, of Sepai kata (see illustrations 7a thru 7d).

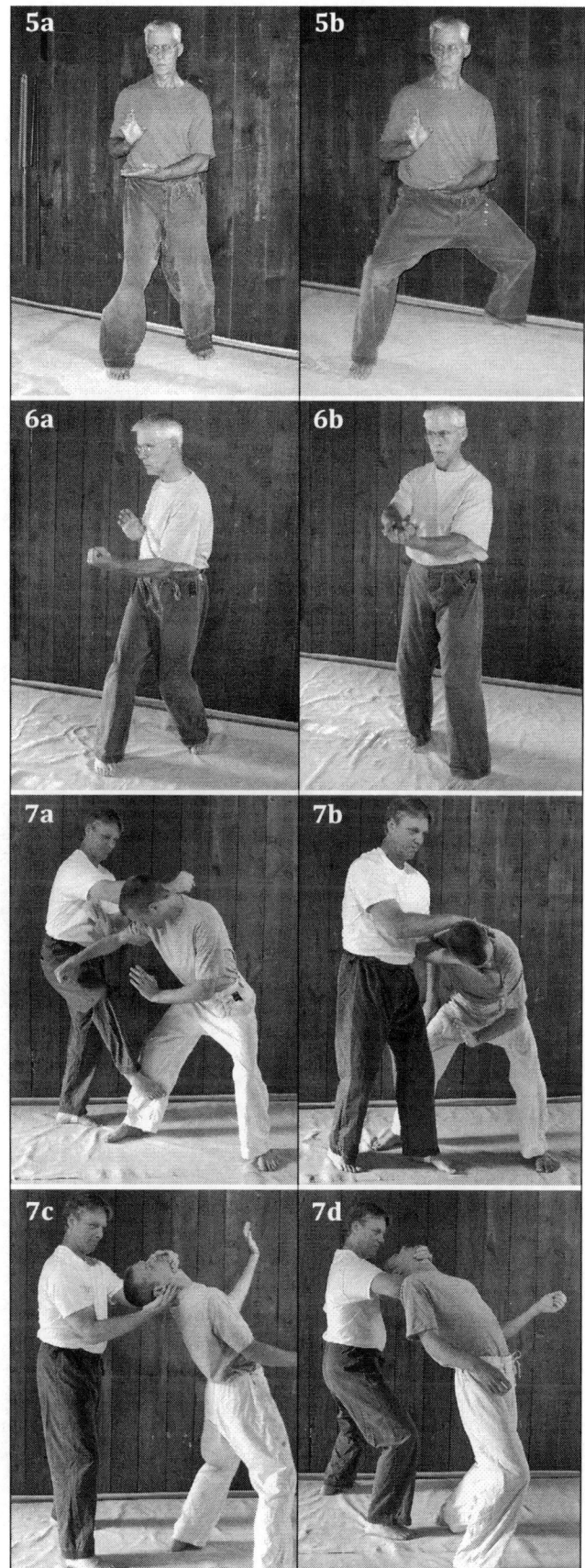

681

Alternatively, one might begin by "receiving" (*uke*) the opponent with the opening technique from Sepai kata—blocking with the left hand and striking with a downward knife-edge, while stepping back into horse stance (*shiko-dachi*). From here, one could continue moving into the controlling technique of this sequence from Sepai kata (see illustrations above, 7b and 7d) or, depending on how the opponent moves, tack on the finishing technique of Seiunchin kata (see illustrations 8b thru 8e).

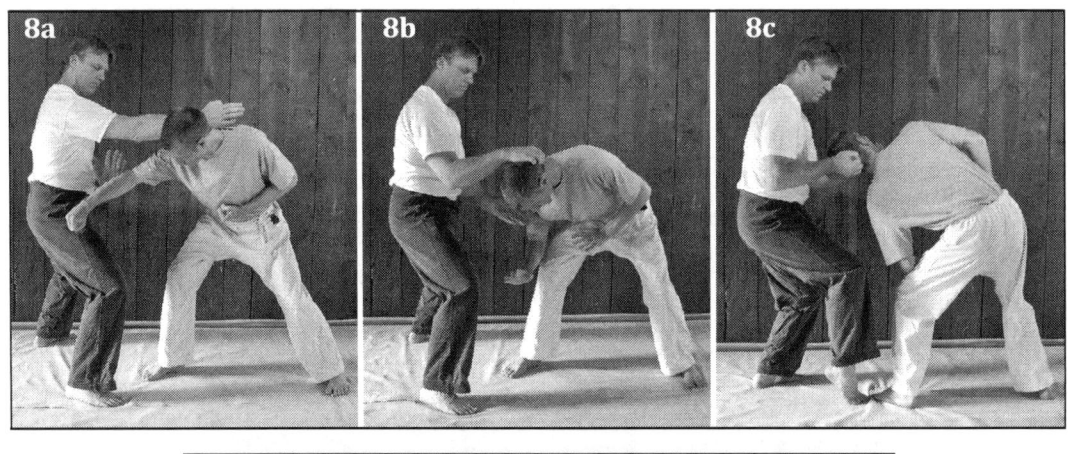

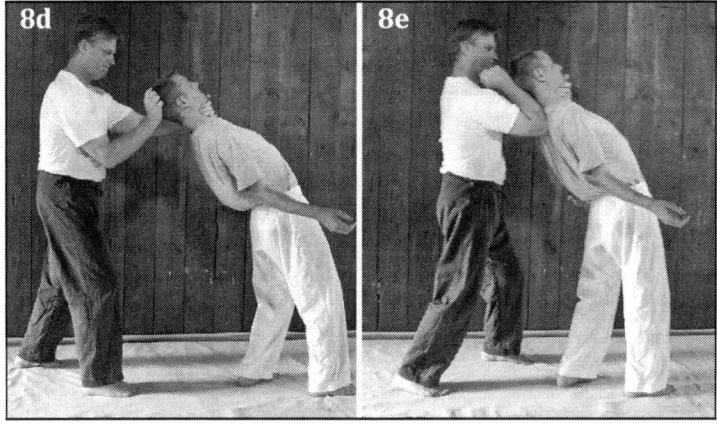

If the opponent begins to stand up, for whatever reason, one can change to the knee kicks which open Kururunfa kata (see illustrations 9a–9b–9c).

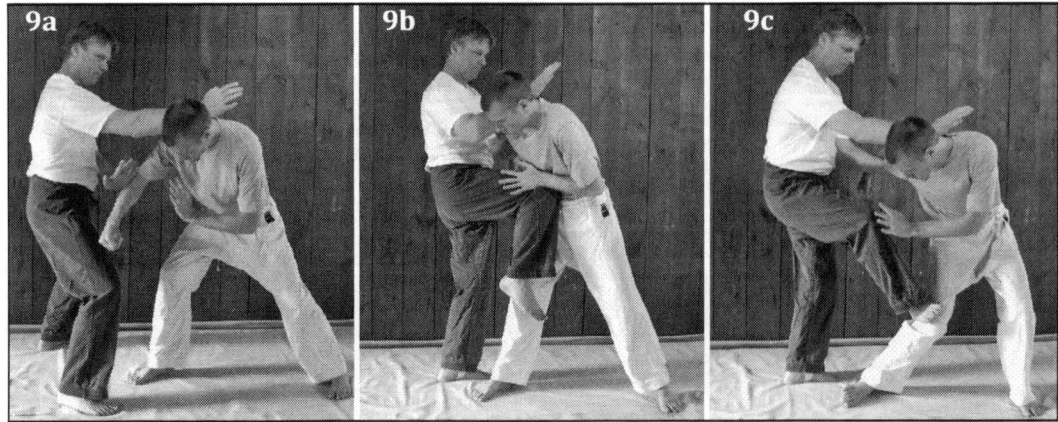

Or, if the opponent begins to move in, one might step back and continue with the throw from Sepai kata (see illustrations 10a–10b–10c). Each of these is just an example to illustrate the way one can employ kata variations.

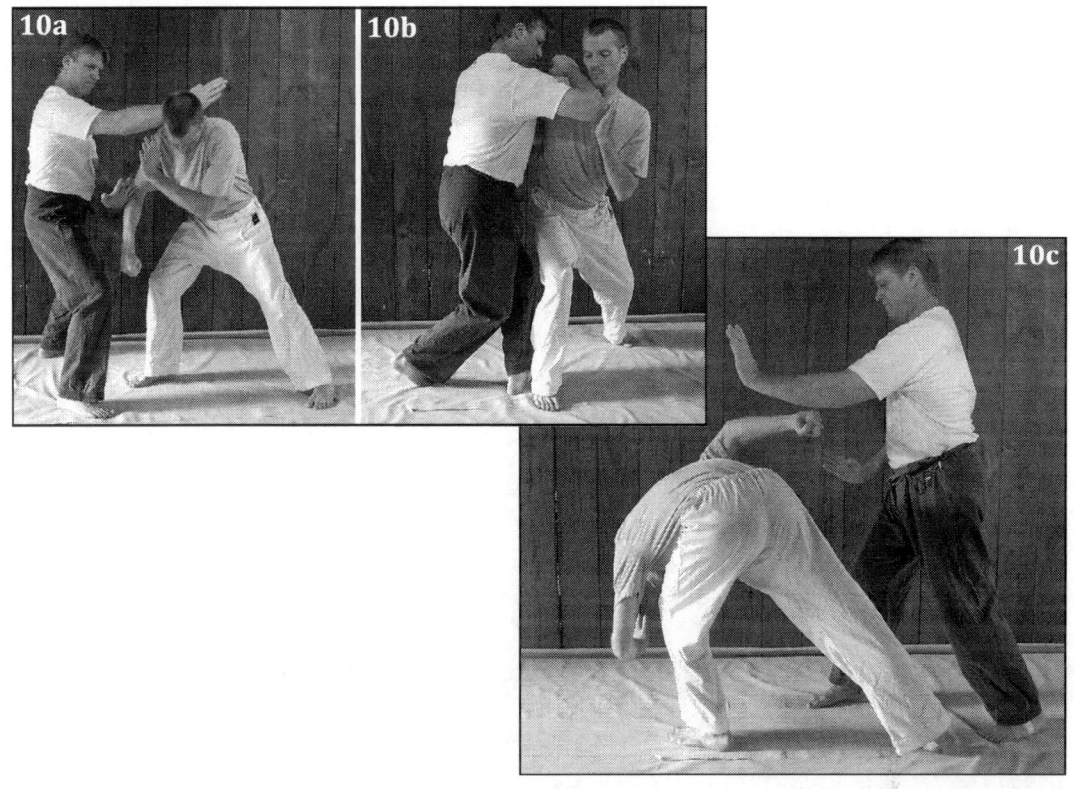

What quickly becomes apparent is that each kata within this "system" is composed of combinations or sequences (Hopkins, 2002). Some, of course, have argued that there is no way one can be sure that this is correct. I would be the first to admit that not all systems of traditional Asian martial arts seem to have preserved their forms with the same intent—showing application combinations. Some systems seem much more guarded, in a way, showing only techniques, like basics, that must be accompanied by the explanations of a knowledgeable teacher. And, of course, we don't have anyone around who was there at the beginning to ask. But neither did Copernicus or Galileo or Darwin. Scientific inquiry demands that we find other proof, and I would suggest three "proofs:" one, the techniques within the katas are self-referential, meaning they show variations within the larger system; two, when looked at in this way, the techniques are more deadly (effective), which is, of course, the whole point of a martial art; and three, in application, there is no disengagement from the opponent, reinforcing the Okinawan concept of sticking (*muchimi*) or ippon kumite—that is, allowing the opponent only one attack—and consequently more realistic.[3]

If we accept this initial premise then—that the Goju-ryu katas are composed of combinations or sequences of techniques—it is easy to see that each combination can be broken down into entering or receiving techniques, bridging or controlling techniques, and finishing techniques.

The entry or receiving (*uke*) techniques depend on a variety of factors: the position of the defender, the speed and angle of the attack, and the direction of the attack, for example (see illustrations of opening or entry techniques, 11a thru 11j).

Examples of Opening or Entry Techniques

Each sequence begins with a block or receiving (*uke*) technique and generally an attack. Off-line movement or stepping accompanies each entry technique. There are a finite number of entry techniques (though more than are depicted here). The greater percentage of techniques in the Goju-ryu classical katas is comprised of finishing techniques.

The receiving techniques (*uke*) of Goju-ryu are almost always accompanied by a nearly simultaneous attack with the other hand, and generally to the opponent's head or neck. This can be seen in the final block and attack of Saifa kata, for instance (see illustration 11a). The defender is responding to a right punch, blocking with the left hand or forearm, and attacking the opponent's left-side head (or outside) with the right open hand.

Alternatively, in the final sequence of the Sepai kata, the defender is also responding to a right punch, blocking again with the left hand or forearm, but in this case attacking

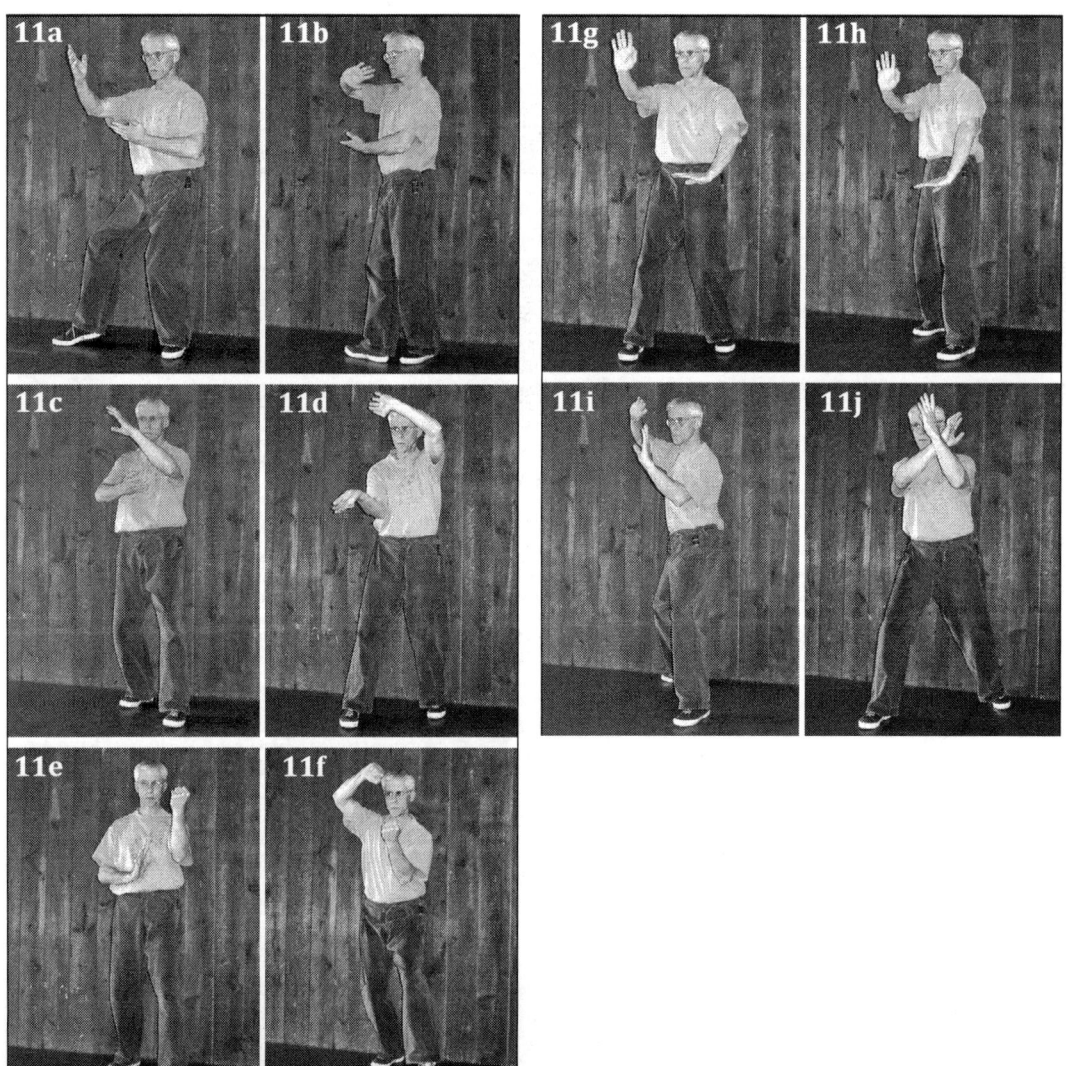

the opponent's right-side head or neck (or inside) with the right open hand (see illustration 11b). This technique is very similar to the opening technique of the Kururunfa kata—both attack the opponent's neck (inside) on the same side as the blocked attack (see illustration 11c).

The entry or receiving techniques then dictate to a large degree what necessarily follows—that is, the controlling and finishing techniques. If one begins with this last entry technique from Saifa kata (illustration 11a)—though one may, of course, continue with the same sequence that is shown in the kata,[4] one might also change the response to any of the techniques in any of the other kata that also begin with a block and opposite-side head attack. For example, one might shift into the kicking sequence of Saifa and stay within the same kata (see illustrations 12a–12b–12c), or one might draw the head down and attack to the back of the neck as in Suparimpei kata (see illustrations 12a–13b–13c).

One might even turn to face the attacker, step back into a right-foot-forward cat stance (*neko-ashi-dachi*), grab the head, and use the knee to attack the opponent's face, as in Seiunchin kata (see illustrations 12a–14b–14c). The variations—or how and when one changes from one sequence of techniques to another—are dictated by the opponent's responses and the ever-changing circumstances of a self-defense scenario.

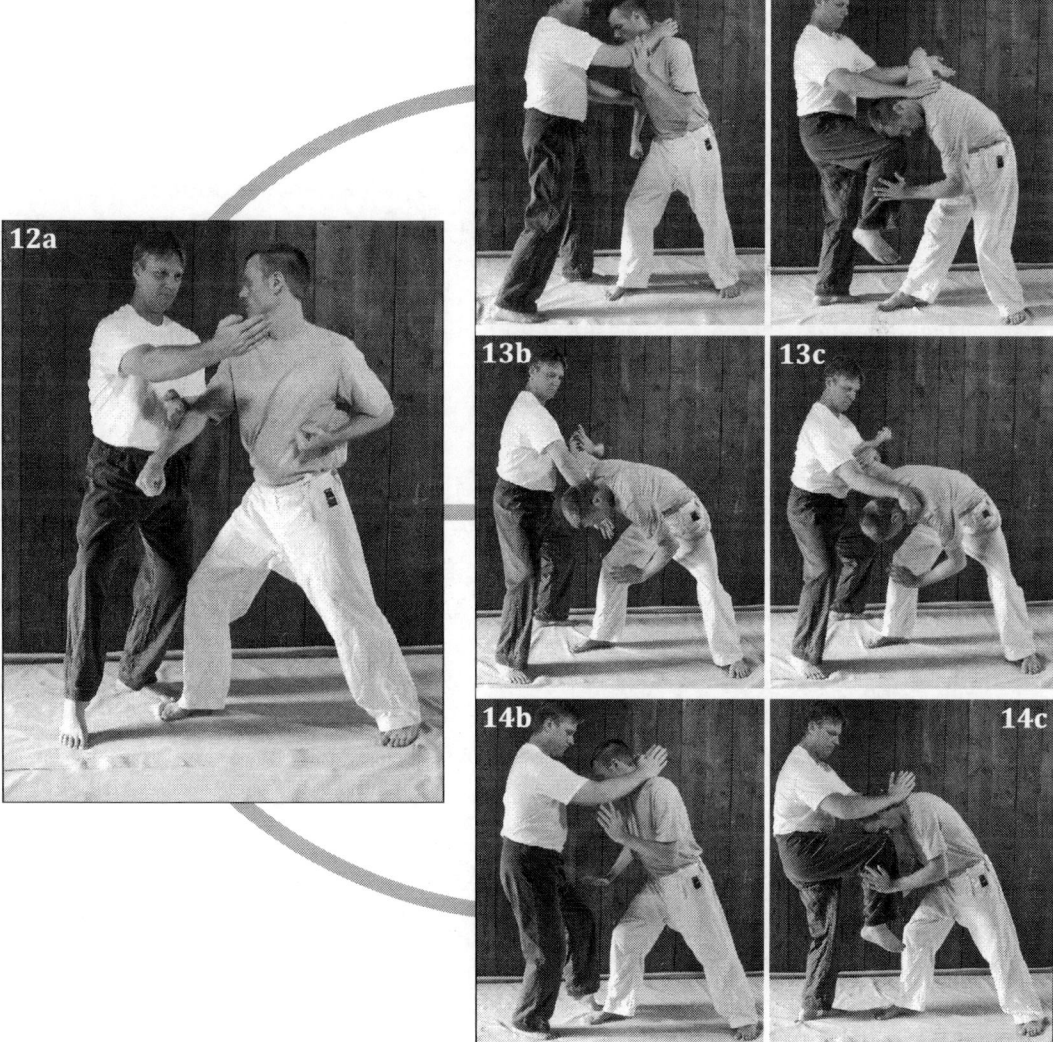

This is particularly true of the bridging or controlling techniques—techniques that generally involve grasping or holding the opponent—that depend largely on the response of the attacker to the defender's initial move. There are any number of different controlling and finishing techniques. So, what we see as possible responses in a situation actually multiply. One could, for instance, begin with the receiving or entry technique from the Sepai kata and tack on the controlling and finishing techniques from the Saifa kata, or vice-versa, as in the illustration above. It all depends on how fluent or practiced one is with the whole system. Or one might continue from the Sepai opening technique (a block and nearly simultaneous attack to the back of the opponent's neck) to the controlling and finishing techniques found in a later sequence from the Sepai kata (see illustrations 15a–15b–15c).

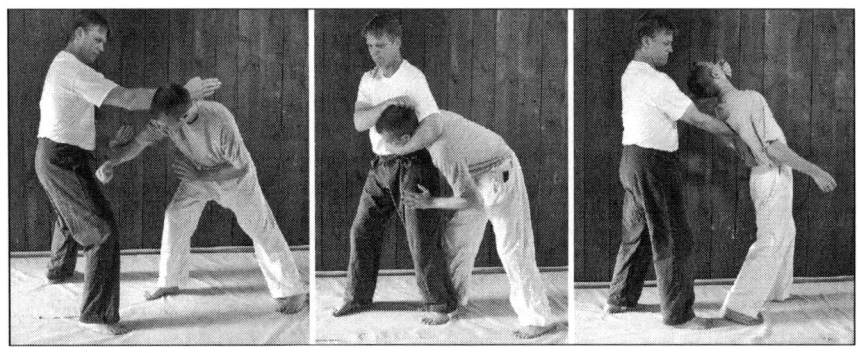

There are, after all, only a limited number of ways to receive (*uke*) or block an opponent's attack. But once one has "blocked" or intercepted the opponent's attack, there is a wide range of controlling techniques or finishing techniques to draw from. And at any point in the sequence one might move between the techniques of different katas. The variations seem to branch out almost like a spider web. It's analogous to a jazz musician who practices scales and familiar melodies endlessly, so that he or she can seem to "improvise" effortlessly.

It should be emphasized here that one changes in response to the opponent's movements; one doesn't merely disengage and start over again, trying something else, if the initial response doesn't work. After one receives or blocks the opponent's initial attack, the idea is to adhere or stick to the opponent, following his movement, as one counterattacks.

Any one kata then, it might be assumed, shows only one possible scenario out of many. Other katas show variations or, in other words, other possible scenarios. (Of course, these themes and variations are shown within the same kata as well.) One might, in fact, go further along these lines and suggest what may seem blasphemous to some: that katas are not, in one sense at least, sacrosanct. This is not to suggest that the katas themselves should be changed, but that in practicing, in seeking to understand katas, one should be able to disconnect techniques within the katas and reconnect them in different ways. This sort of exploration gives one the flexibility to apply the kata techniques in response to self-defense situations that are fluid and changing. For example: one might respond to an attacker's push by moving diagonally, blocking with both hands, as done in Saifa, and kicking. But instead of stepping up and using the second knee or kick, as in a continuation of this sequence in Saifa, one might step back, drawing the head down, and use the forearm to attack the opponent's neck, as in Seiunchin kata (see illustrations 16a thru 16d).

Or, one might begin with the double-handed entry technique from Sanseiru, and then step around and throw the attacker as one does in Sepai kata (see illustrations 17a thru 17d).

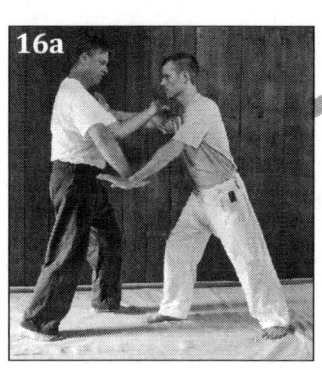
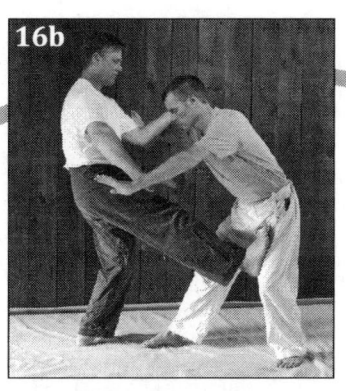
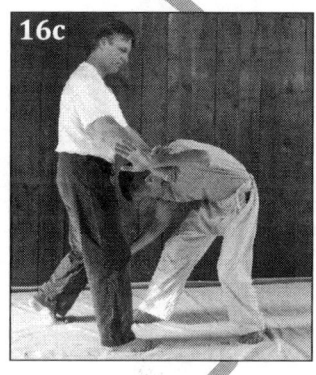
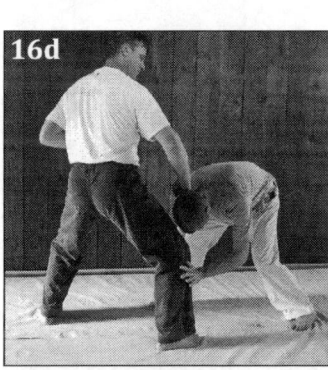

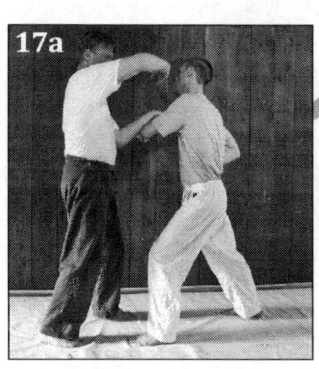
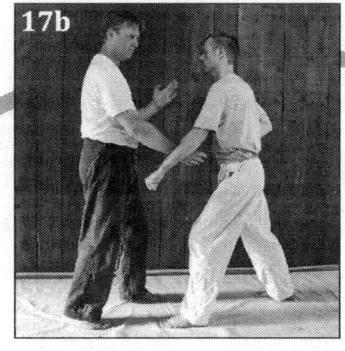
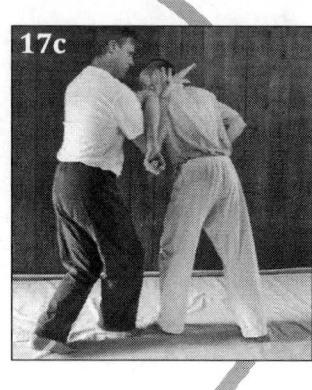
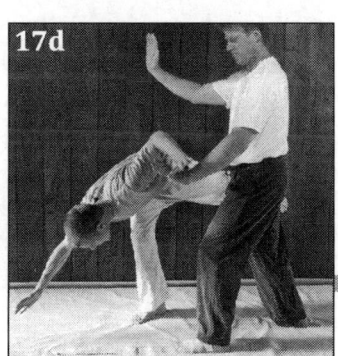

Listening Points

In these illustrations, the defender is initially responding with the entry technique at the beginning of the Kururunfa kata (18a). The initial block and entry can then easily change into a host of controlling and finishing techniques taken from other katas: the continuation of the initial sequence in the Kururunfa kata (18b–c); next, Shisochin kata (18d–e); the final technique from the Suparimpei kata (18f–g); and the ending of the Sepai kata (18h–i).

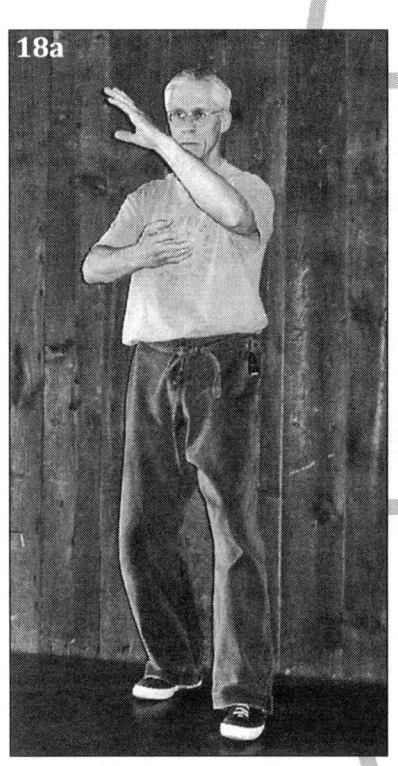

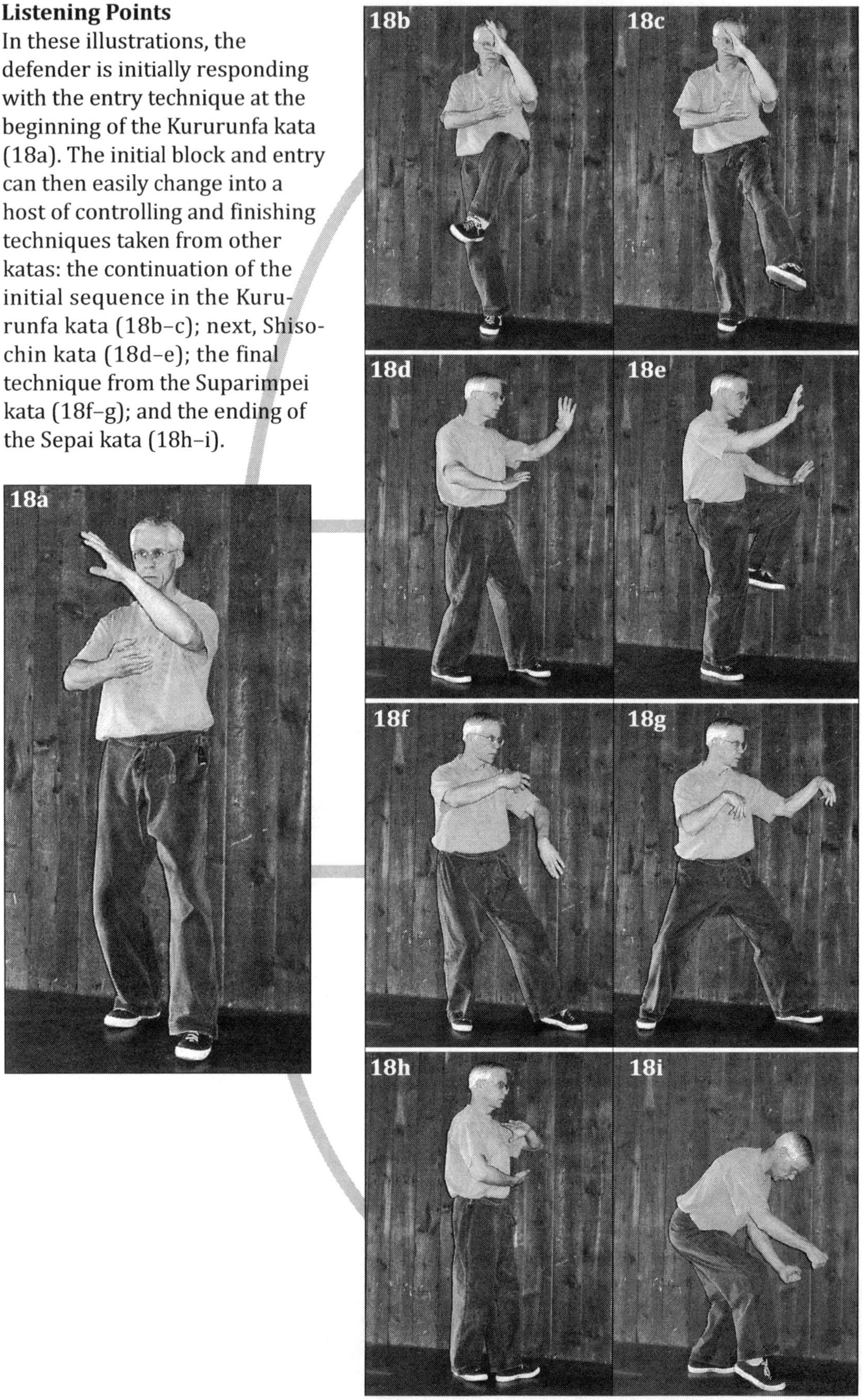

Listening Points

Changing one's response to an attack or when to employ variations generally occurs at the point of contact with the opponent's attack. The initial blocking position of the hands occurs in a number of places in different katas, but at the point of initial contact the defender's movement is incomplete. The hand position here (19a) is showing the point at which the defender's hands contact the hands of the attacker.

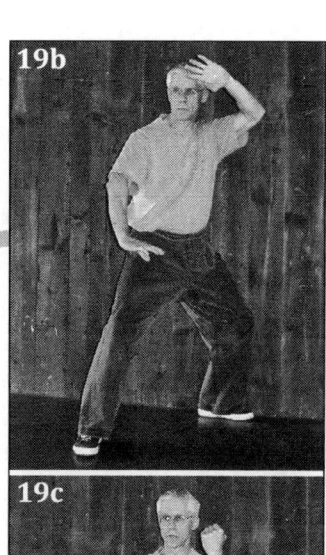

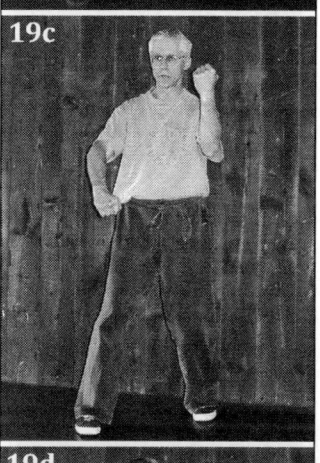

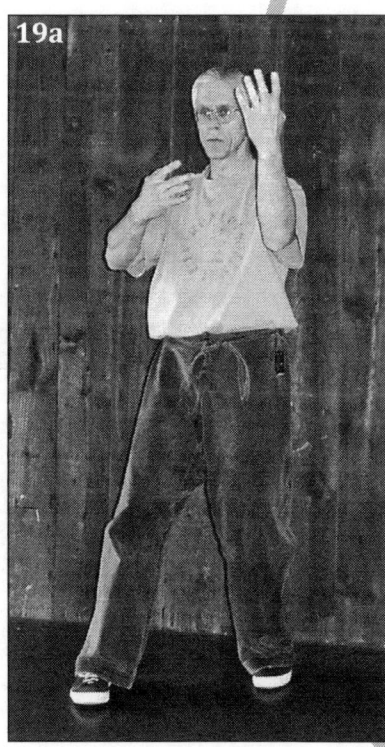

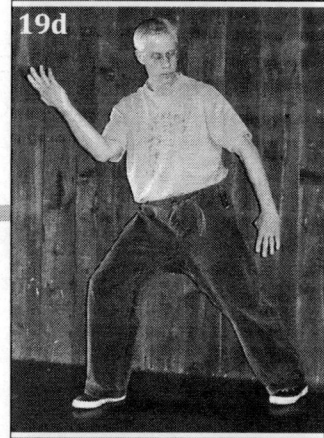

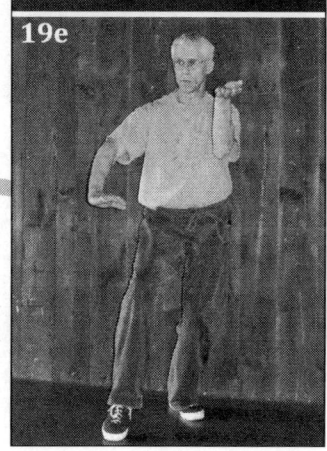

It is at this point of contact that the defender "listens" to the attack and responds appropriately. This is the point at which one might change to any of the entry techniques illustrated from various katas (19b, or 19c, or 19d,

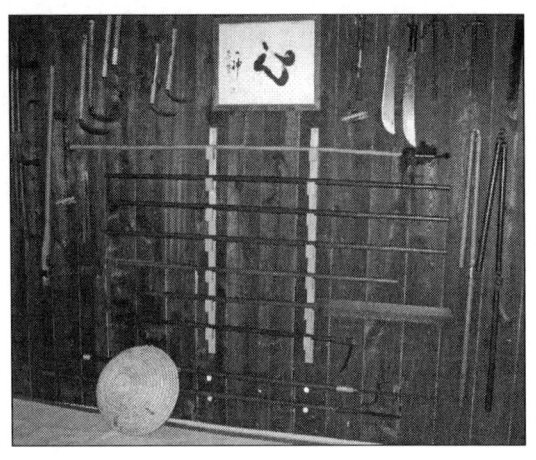 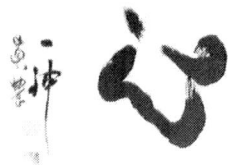

Brush script by Matayoshi of "*kokoro*" (spirit) displayed in the author's dojo.

What I am suggesting is another, perhaps new, way of training: studying katas and their applications (*bunkai*), not individually but in their relationship to other katas and similar applications. It's also a way of training what the Chinese martial arts refer to as sensitivity—being able to instantaneously change one's technique in response to the opponent's movements. We take, for instance, one entry technique (usually a "block" or uke and simultaneous attack with the other hand) and see where we can go from there, how many variations we can tack on to the end of it. In the process, we move sometimes within the same kata—because katas have themes—and sometimes between similar techniques in other katas, but we learn and begin to use a system of self-defense as it was meant to be used.

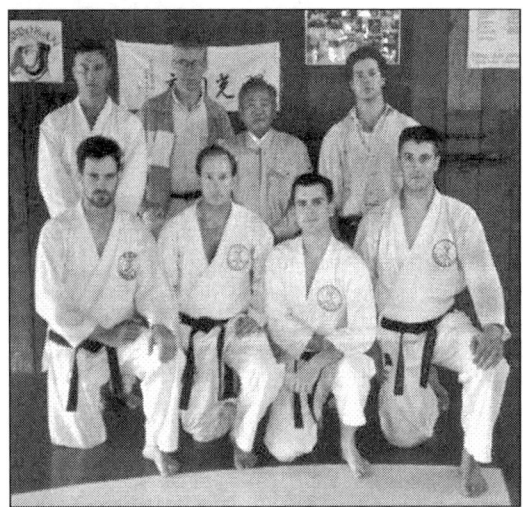 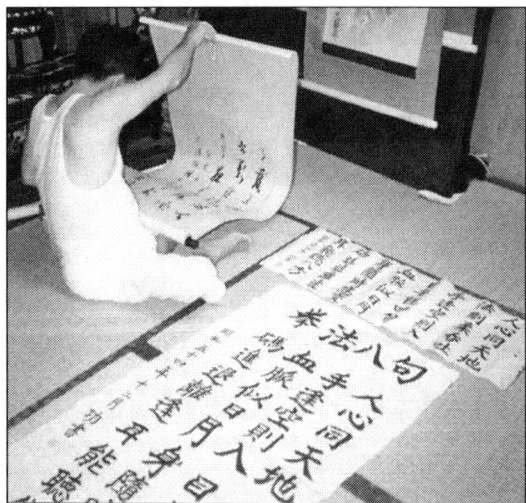

Matayoshi, with some of the author's senior students,
visiting the author's dojo in 1995.
Matayoshi showing author scrolls at his home in 1986.

Conclusion

It is difficult to argue that the different Goju-ryu katas come from independent sources or the polyglot nature of a system that seems to be so self-referential. There is a lot of argument nowadays that Miyagi Chojun either created many katas of his own or brought them back from China, but that in any case these katas—Saifa, Seiunchin, Shishochin, Sepai, Kururunfa among them—were not part of the original system taught by Higaonna Kanryo. This theory suggests that these katas have a separate origin, distinct and perhaps unrelated to the origins of Sanchin, Sanseiru, Sesan, and Suparimpei. I would suggest, however, the very fact that techniques seem to reference other techniques in other katas—that is, they appear to be variations on a theme, if you will, we should accept the Goju canon as it has been passed down, as a system—and it is the whole Goju-ryu system that one must be conversant with in order to employ the katas' techniques in the way that they were originally intended, not merely one or two or even three katas.[5] It is an oft-repeated story that in the old days teachers like Miyagi Chojun taught Sanchin kata and only one or two other katas to each student, depending on the student's ability or body type. From this, authors Lawrence Kane and Kris Wilder conclude that "each kata contains a complete, integrated fighting system." In fact, they go a step further to suggest that in modern times, when each "practitioner is given a lot more material to digest"—all eight classical subjects of the Goju-ryu canon, for instance—"it is quite understandable for their level of comprehension to be somewhat less" (Kane and Wilder, 2005:21). But we don't want to extrapolate from legend—we know that there were many that learned the whole system, all the katas. And we should recognize that any one kata is not complete in itself, nor should we necessarily have a favorite kata. There is no playing of favorites; one must invest in the whole system.

I am reminded of something that Matayoshi once said that summer so long ago. One evening, he invited us to his house for dinner. After dinner, he started to show us different examples of calligraphy, taking them down from a shelf where he had them stored away and spreading them out on the floor. Some were wonderful scrolls of the *Goju Happo* (Eight Laws), some were charts of lineage, others were single character sayings. Many of them had been given to him as presents. One was a particularly beautiful example of free-form brush work (*sosho* or grass writing). This one was the kanji script for "*kokoro*," or spirit, though that is perhaps a rather limited translation. In any case, Matayoshi took out a brush and wrote his name on the side, stamped it with his seal, and handed it to me. He stressed the importance of spirit in training, and that the exercise of karate trained not just the body but the spirit as well.

Many of these lessons, of course, come to mind when I enter the dojo and see this piece of calligraphy hanging on the wall. It also reminds me of what George Donahue talks about in his article, "Kata, Bunkai and Calligraphy"—how kata may start off at the beginner stage, like calligraphy, stiff and formal, but that over time, it becomes more fluid, like the "grass writing" of Japanese calligraphy. I once sat in on a writing class on a visit to a Japanese high school in Hokkaido, the northern most province of Japan, a long way from Okinawa. We spent an enjoyable hour laughing and practicing calligraphy alongside a class full of giggling high schoolers, filling in large-squared graph paper with basic brush strokes. Each of 10,000 or so pictographic characters is made up of only a very few different strokes—they're just arranged differently on the paper. To me, this is like katas. If one understands the system as a whole, one can take the techniques, or characters, apart and rearrange them in different combinations until one's self-defense is fluid, changing, and almost limitless. The only thing that may prevent

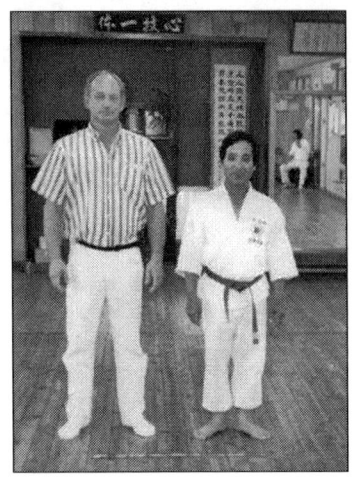

Kimo Wall and Gibo Seki in Japan, 1986.

us from discovering these themes and variations within katas is a rigid and ritualistic adherence to mindless regimentation. Perhaps as Matayoshi often suggested —and as my own teacher, Kimo Wall, passed on to me, after a rigorous training session, where each technique in the katas was corrected and perfected, we would be well advised to tell our students to "go play."

Notes

[1] Many of the teachers who studied under Miyagi Chojun have formed different schools or branches of Goju-ryu (Higa Seko's Shodokan, Yagi Meitoku's Meibukan, Toguchi Seikichi's Shoreikan, Miyazato Ei'ichi's Jundokan) and there are often slight or not-so-slight differences in katas. Gibo Seki is a senior teacher in the Shodokan.

[2] See F. Camara and M. McKenna, who have suggested that a "cluster analysis" of techniques within the Goju-ryu kata may "prove" that there are really two strains or sources of the katas that form the Goju-ryu system: one group that Higaonna taught, comprised of Sanchin, Sanseiru, Sesan, and Suparimpei; and the other group added to the system by Miyagi, comprised of Saifa, Seiunchin, Shisochin, Sepai, Kururunfa, and Tensho. It may be worth noting here that even if the structure of various katas differ, implying a different kata origin, the techniques within the kata may not necessarily be from a different source. Also see M. Ravignat, elaborating on an earlier article by Charles Swift, who suggests that the katas that comprise the accepted Goju-ryu canon were not all taught by Higaonna to Miyagi Chojun, but may have come from different sources. He bases his ideas on, among other things, a perception of symmetry and asymmetry in various katas—the Higaonna katas being asymmetrical and the Miyagi katas being symmetrical. But even the most superficial analysis would suggest that this may be an over-simplification.

[3] Dan Smith, a noted Shorin-ryu teacher, has suggested that this idea of "one punch, one kill" has been misunderstood. Smith writes: "All Okinawan karate has the same objective and that is to stop an attack and survive without being hurt. We call this *ippon kumite* or one technique fighting. Many people think that ippon kumite is a promised fight that only allows one attack from the opponent, but this is not what the Okinawans intended. The meaning is that if you move out of the way and block effectively, the opponent will only have the chance to make one attack. Your counterattack follows the practice of only allowing one attack."

[4] To see the standard application for this last technique of Saifa kata, see article: Hopkins (2004).

[5] Compare to what Burgar sets out to do in his oft-cited book, *Five Years, One Kata*. While an admirable expression of perseverance, unless one is imaginative enough to find the rest of the system within a single kata, such a practice seems of little practical use, notwithstanding the Thoreau-like analogy: "I have traveled much in Concord."

Bibliography

Burgar, B. (2003). *Five years, one kata*. Hemel Hempstead, UK: Martial Arts Publishing.

Camara, F. and McKenna, M. (2007). A preliminary analysis of Goju-ryu kata structure. *Journal of Asian Martial Arts, 16*(4), 46–53.

Donahue, G. (2003, April 1). Kata, bunkai and calligraphy. http://www.fightingarts.com/ reading/article.php?id=154

Hopkins, G. (2002). The lost secrets of Goju-ryu: What the kata shows. *Journal of Asian Martial Arts, 11*(4), 54–77.

Hopkins, G. (2004). The shape of kata: An enigma of pattern. *Journal of Asian Martial Arts, 13*(1), 64–77.

and Wilder, K. (2005). *The way of kata: a comprehensive guide to deciphering martial applications*. Boston: YMAA Publication Center.

Ravignat, M. (2004). The history of Goju-ryu karate: New ideas on Goju-ryu's direct Chinese ancestors. www. Meibukanmagazine.org

Smith, D. (2002). From a private correspondence, March 10, 2002.

Swift, C. (2003). The kenpo of Kume village. *Dragon Times*, (23):10–12 and 34.

Glossary

Bunkai	分解
Chi shi	力石
Goju-ryu	剛柔流
Higa Seiko	比嘉 世幸
Higashionna Kanryo	東恩納 寛量
Jundokan	順道館
Kata	型, 形
Kingai-ryu	金硬流
Kobudo	古武道
Meibukan	明武館
Miyagi Chojun	宮城 長順
Miyazato Ei'ichi	榮一宮里
Nigiri game	にぎりがめ
Shodokan	尚道館
Shoreikan	昭霊館
Shorin-ryu	小林流
Yagi Meitoku	明德八木

Acknowledgements

A special thanks to my students, Bill and Lucas Diggle, for demonstrating applications. Also, thanks to my wife, Martha, for her editorial assistance and patience, and the teachers who have helped me along the way: Kimo Wall, Matayoshi Shinpo, and Gibo Seki.

chapter 56

Evaluating Makiwara Punching Board Performance

by Paul K. Smith, Ph.D., Timothy Niiler, Ph.D., and Peter W. McCullough, B.S.

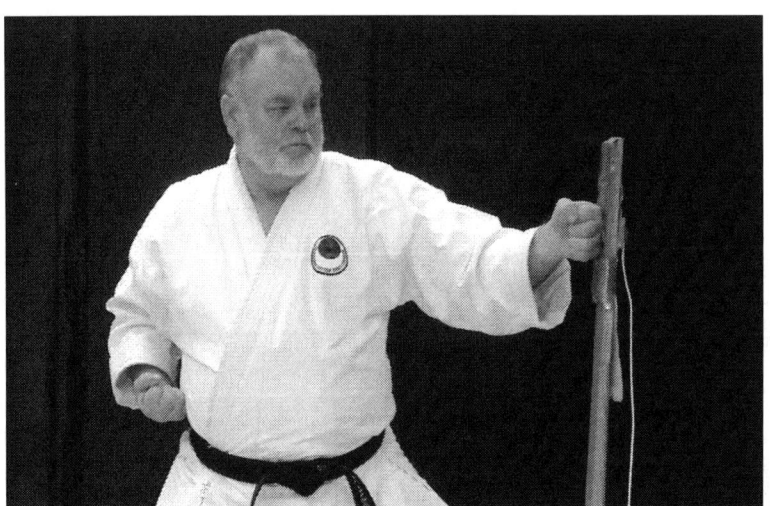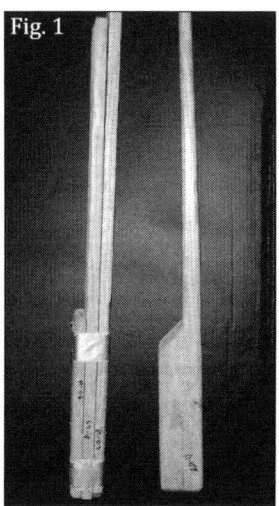

Dr. Paul Smith punching the makiwara board.
Figure 1: Photos of stacked and tapered makiwara boards. The stacked makiwara design is comprised of several boards that are secured together, whereas the tapered makiwara design is comprised of a single molded piece of wood. Illustrations courtesy of P. Smith except where noted.

Introduction

Karate is a Japanese martial art offering the benefits of self-defense training for the practitioner, in addition to health-related, psychomotor, cognitive, and affective domain areas of development. As such, it is an excellent medium for physical education, plus the added value of learning practical skills. In karate training, punching and kicking are the two most often used techniques utilized to overcome an opponent. Characteristic of karate punching and kicking is the principle of "one blow, one kill" (*ikken hitsatsu*), a Japanese concept which means that the practitioner should be capable of disabling an attacker with one blow (Okazaki and Stricevic, 1984)—not necessarily to "kill" the opponent. Of the estimated fifty million persons involved with karate training (Smith, 1984), it is probable that every participant will, at some point, be exposed to the phenomena of punching some type of device to enhance his/her skill and "get a feel" for what it is like to impact an object. *Makiwara* ("coiled straw," punching board) training is considered by many proponents of this traditional martial art to be an integral part of the development of proper karate punching technique to the necessary standards (Okazaki and Stricevic, 1984).

The makiwara board is a vertically mounted device, attached or buried at one end

(Figure 1), which is used to develop punching effectiveness through repeatedly punching or striking a pad attached to the free end of the board. The pad is generally of some variety of foam, rope, straw, or textile material used to soften the impact on the knuckles. The board's shape may be tapered or stacked, and its dimensions are generally about 8.89 cm (3.5 in.) width by 127.00 cm (50.00 in.) height above the floor. General physical principles imply that the type of wood used, its length, and the board's degree of taper should determine the strength of the "spring" of the device. Another popular design consists of various lengths of boards stacked in descending order of length to create a leaf-spring configuration. Several species of hardwoods or softwoods have been used. Usually, the student selects the boards to train with on the basis of personal preference or what boards are available in the training hall (Okazaki, 1998).

The mechanism by which the board helps develop punching proficiency involves the coordination of the body's movements such that the "force" or "energy" is concentrated, or focused, at a particular point within the impacted target. This is usually about 5.08-15.24 cm (2 to 6 inches) deep to the target surface and requires timing the puncher's segmental motions to impact the target with his weapon mass, body inertia connected to the fist or foot, moving at an optimum velocity at the time of impact. Impacts of varying characteristics are required to stop an assailant dependent on which part of the body is involved. Impacts can be characterized both in terms of mass-velocity relationships, such as "high velocity/low mass" or "low velocity/high mass," and the nature of the movement of the impacting weapon in applying force, e.g., linear or angular application of force. Punching is considered a relatively low velocity/high mass technique in which the force is applied in a linear fashion (Smith, et al., 1993). The fist and forearm are thrust in a "push-like" manner into the target, rather than whipped or snapped into the target in a "throw-like" action (Kreighbaum and Barthels, 1996). This type of technique is better used for impacting the opponent's trunk, where a deeper penetration into relatively soft tissue or vulnerable bone is needed to break, accelerate, or lacerate the bones, nerves and tissues of the body. The throw-like action, commonly known as a strike or snapping technique, is used to attack harder or more fragile areas of the body, such as the nose or joints, and "shock" the impacted tissues beneath the surface or break the relatively fragile bone or joint harder tissues.

According to Smith (1999), the appropriate technique for punching or striking the makiwara would be to stand directly in front of the board in a stance of your choice and applying the force of the technique by "punching through" the pad on the board and holding the full penetration momentarily to allow the body to train the muscles and "focus," or concentrate the body's energy, at the end of the movement. Punching force should be mildly applied in the beginning and progress to harder punches as experienced is gained. The body would be adapting to the reaction forces, or load, of the board. Care should be used in driving through the surface of the target toward full extension of the technique and not "slapping" the board. This would allow the body to coordinate and develop the neuromuscular system for more effective execution of the techniques.

No specific training sequences, or periodization of training, have been published (Smith, 1999) for the number of sets and number of repetitions in each set for makiwara training. Based on the training principles of progression (McArdle, Katch, and Katch, 2001) and practical experience of the authors, it would seem reasonable to begin with a low number of sets and repetitions when impacting the makiwara board and progress to higher numbers of repetitions and loads. Similar progressive resistance training has been shown to be effective in improving kicking performance in taekwondo athletes (Jakubiak and Saunders, 2008).

Methods

A first step in determining the efficacy of makiwara boards for resistance training is to evaluate the stiffness characteristics of the board itself without human intervention. This may be done via the load-deflection technique in which the makiwara board is loaded with a series of known weights while measuring the resultant deflection. The load may be plotted versus the deflection to visualize stiffness which is defined as the slope of this curve. As a result, materials with steeper load-deflection curves are stiffer and resist deformation more easily. Understanding this, it is tempting to go and look up the stiffness of a given wood and draw conclusions as to which wood might be more appropriate to one's training level. An expert makiwara user might choose a stiffer wood than a beginner. However, this overlooks some key issues. First, the stiffness by itself says nothing about the amount of force it takes to deflect a board of a given shape or construction. An expert will have just as much trouble punching a fixed 4"x4" wooden beam as the layman regardless of wood type since this geometry has little flexibility. Thus, real testing of the shapes in question are needed to establish force benchmarks by wood and design. Second, it is necessary to test multiple instances of a type of wood and design to ensure reliability of results. Wood is quite variable by its nature, and its age, grain, and other factors can cause differences in stiffness.

Therefore, five replications each of northern white ash, Pennsylvania cherry, red oak, and Douglas fir makiwara boards of the tapered and stacked board designs were constructed for testing in a base/loading mechanism specifically designed for this purpose (Figure 2). Boards were tested by loading each with weights and recording deflection values at 111.2 N (25 lbs) increments of weight ranging from 111.2 N to 1000.8 N (25– 225 lbs) in counterbalanced order to distribute any cumulative stress effects throughout the study. Force-deflection data were plotted for each board specie and design. Furthermore, lines of best fit that showed the average trends in stiffness for each board type were plotted to ease visual comparison between both specie and design.

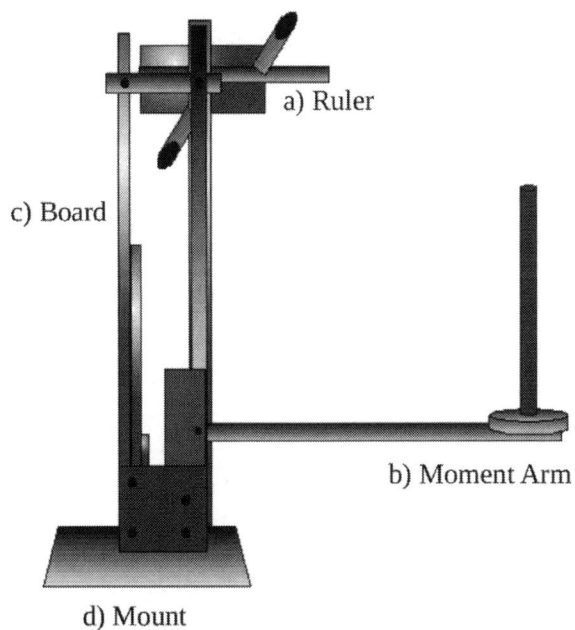

Figure 2: The makiwara device. A ruler (a) was clipped perpendicular to the makiwara board (c) to determine deflection. The loading device consisted of a moment arm (b) where weights could be placed to deflect the board. The mount (d) was set in concrete using lag bolts to ensure immobility of the base.

This method of viewing results has one drawback from a scientific perspective: despite visual trends one cannot tell whether differences in the slopes are the curves are significant or not. When we say that there is a significant difference between two groups, we are indicating that any differences observed between the groups is not a result of random chance alone. Without statistical significance, we often say that the result is anecdotal and we have no confidence that the results are repeatable. The statistical tool that is used in cases like this is the analysis of variance (ANOVA) which will determine if any significant differences exist among the designs or the species of wood. Given that such a difference exists, a post-hoc test identifies specifically which groups are different from one another.

Results

General results are summarized in Tables 1, 2, and 3. Table 1 presents results in the form of combined makiwara board deflection means (mm) of ash, cherry, fir, and oak species for stacked (ST) and tapered (TA) board types (BDTYP). Deflection means (mm) for stacked makiwara boards are shown by specie in Table 2 while those for tapered boards are shown in Table 3. Specie of wood is abbreviated as ash (A), cherry (C), fir (F) and oak (O). The differences in numbers of boards of each specie are due to breakage. Our use of a 2x4 ANOVA (two types of boards by four types of wood) with a Neuman-Keuls post-hoc tests indicated that there was, in fact, a significant difference between force-deflection properties of all groups except for the tapered ash and cherry boards.

Discussion of Trends

Further examination of results indicated a number of noteworthy trends. Tapered boards showed significantly less flexure upon loading than did stacked boards (Table 1). This is not surprising since there is no horizontal binding force other than friction in between the stacked boards. This allows the stacked boards to slide with respect to one another under loading unlike the tapered boards that do not have this degree of freedom. As such, there is a greater mobility of the striking surface in the stacked board design. A consequence of this mobility is that the stacked boards will more readily approach their elastic limit in deflection after which they will either not return to their original shape or experience fracture. In actual fact, breakage occurred quite frequently in the more compliant stacked

TABLE 1

Wood	N	Mean	Std Dev
ST	156	102	68*
TA	180	65	46

* $p < 0.05$

TABLE 2

Wood	N	Mean	Std Dev
C	41	118	74*
A	36	106	71*
F	34	94	64*
O	45	90	59

* $p < 0.05$

TABLE 3

Wood	N	Mean	Std Dev
C	45	78	54*
A	45	76	52*
F	45	55	36*
O	45	50	33

* $p < 0.05$

TABLE 4

Wood	Board Type	
	Tapered (N/m)	Stacked (N/m)
C	5389 ± 10	3907 ± 19
A	5253 ± 9	3245 ± 6
F	8096 ± 4	3985 ± 11
O	8653 ± 7	4882 ± 13

boards. Specifically, four of the stacked fir boards broke (80%), all five of the stacked ash boards broke (100%), and two of the stacked cherry boards broke (40%). None of the oak boards broke and none of the boards broke at the lowest load (111.2 N).

When boards were analyzed according to specie, for both tapered and stacked board types, oak had the least average deflection followed by fir, cherry, and ash (Tables 2-3). This is inconsistent with average impact bending parameters from the material data sheets in that one would expect ash to be stiffer and fir to be more compliant (Green, et al., 1999). However, since the impact bending parameter may vary as much as 25% for a given board type, the results are realistic. Furthermore, the similarity of results from board to board of the same specie is due to these boards having been made from the same tree. Stiffness calculated from the best fit load/deflection lines (Figures 3-4) show the same trends as with average deflections with oak being the stiffest wood and ash being the most compliant (Table 4).

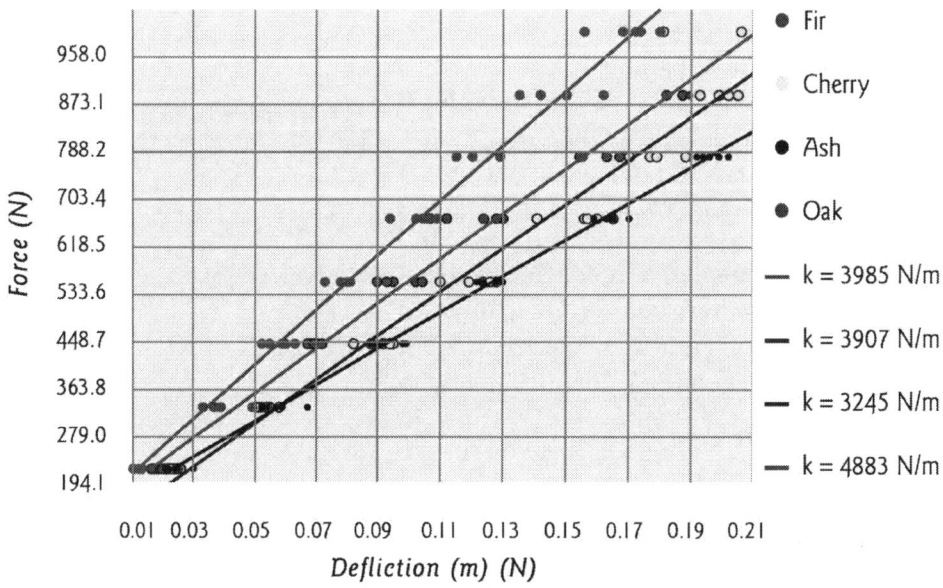

Figure 3:
Force-deflection curves for stacked boards. Boards that deflect less under a given load are considered to be stiffer. Significant differences in average force and average deflection were detected between each type of stacked board.

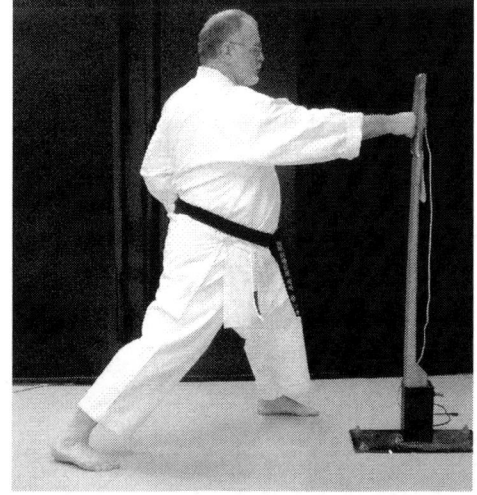

Dr. Paul Smith punching the makiwara board.

Implications for Training

When viewed in light of the well-known recommendations of progressive overload in sports training (McArdle, Katch, and Katch 2001), this study's results are suggestive of a facility for the progression of training for appropriate development. The lower stiffness (by a factor of two) of stacked boards implies a greater suitability for novice practitioner as these will offer less resistance and lower reaction forces to the punch. For truly progressive training, one could start with the most compliant wood type (ash) and move up toward the stiffest (oak). However, in consideration of the breakage of all wood types of stacked boards except oak, perhaps only oak should be considered as a material for this design. Although oak has a higher stiffness, this could be modulated by varying the thickness of the boards or the addition of extra padding at the striking surface. More advanced practitioners could then move to the tapered design for increased resistance training.

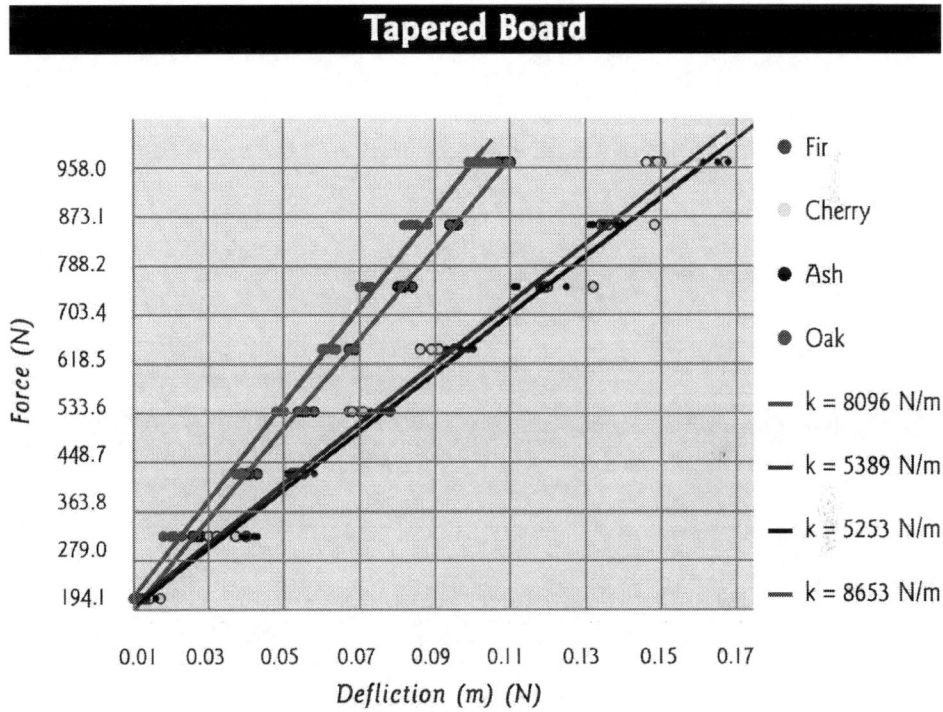

Figure 4:
Force-deflection curve for tapered boards. Significant differences were detected between each type of tapered board except between ash and cherry ($P < 0.05$).

This study also provides, by means of the quantification of makiwara board force-deflection curves, a standards-based way to estimate the workload associated with a given practice regimen. The American College of Sports Medicine (ACSM) regularly publishes a paper titled "Progression Models in Resistance Training" that is a summary of current best practice in designing strength training workouts. According to this document's the most recent update (ACSM, 2009), resistance training for beginners should be 60-70% of the one repetition maximum (1RM) of a given exercise. A standard exercise that is similar to the reverse punch is the bench press. If one could press 225 lbs for ones 1RM (using two arms), half of this is 112.5 lbs. Seventy percent of the one arm maximum load is 78.75 lbs or 351 N. So, if one were using the more compliant stacked cherry makiwara, the deflection corresponding to this load would be about 6 cm or about 2.3 inches. Considering that the punch is actually dynamic, a greater deflection would probably occur; but this estimation sets the lower limit of what would be expected of such a person. Alternatively, this calculation could be reversed to determine the most appropriate makiwara board for an individual based on their 1RM bench press.

Having established a way to estimate the workload, it is then possible to apply ACSM guidelines regarding repetitions for progressive training. Although many different protocols exist, the generally cited 8-12 repetitions with multiple sets still seems to be the standard for beginners (ACSM, 2009). Recent meta-analysis of 37 strength training studies indicates that gains in strength are optimized at eight sets per muscle group (Peterson, et al., 2005). However, because no studies of the efficacy of such an exercise protocol with respect to the makiwara board have been conducted, it may be that increased repetitions per set and fewer sets may be equally productive.

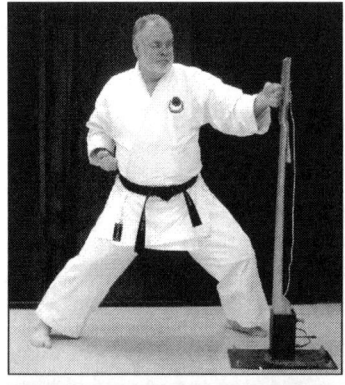

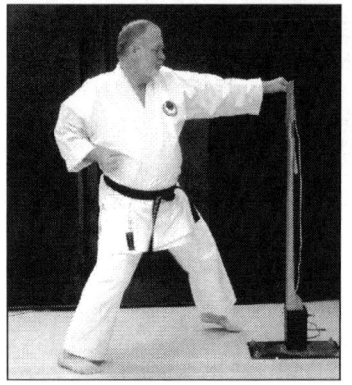

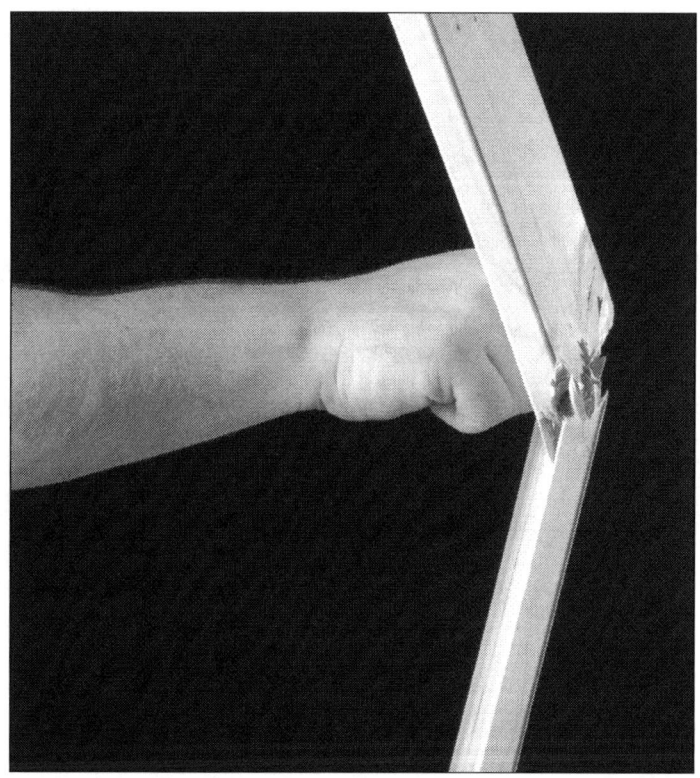

Conclusions

It can be concluded from our findings that there were differences between the makiwara designs and differences among the wood types tested. The tapered board design was stiffer than the stacked configuration; however there was no difference between the cherry and ash makiwara with the tapered design. Makiwara stiffness was progressively less from oak to fir to ash to cherry wood boards. A logical progression for training would be to begin with the stacked design of one of the lesser stiff woods to makiwara made in the tapered design of one of the stiffer woods. Based on the force-deflection curves, it is also possible to roughly estimate workload and thereby design an effective resistance training program.

一拳必殺	*ikken hitsatsu*	"one blow, one kill"
卷藁	*makiwara*	"coiled straw"

References

American College of Sports Medicine (2009 March). American College of Sports Medicine position stand. Progression models in resistance training for healthy adults. *Medicine and Science in Sports and Exercise, 41*(3): 687-708.

Green, D., Winandy, J., and Kretschmann, D. (1999). *Wood handbook: Wood as an engineering material.* Madison, WI: USDA Forest Service, Forest Products Laboratory. General technical report FPL; GTR-113: Pages 4.1-4.45.

Kreighbaum, E., and Barthels, K. (1996). *Biomechanics: A qualitative approach for studying human movement* (4th Ed.). Needham Heights, MA: Allyn and Bacon.

McArdle, W., Katch F., and Katch V. (2001). *Exercise physiology: Energy, nutrition and human performance.* Baltimore, MA: Lippincott, Williams & Wilkins.

Okazaki, T. (1998). Personal communication. ISKF Headquarters Dojo, 222 S. 45th St., Philadelphia, PA, 19104.

Okazaki, T., and Stricevic, M. (1984). *Textbook of modern karate.* Tokyo: Kodansha International.

Peterson, M., Rhea, M., and Alvar, B. (2005). Applications of the dose response for muscular strength development: A review of metaanalytic efficacy and reliability for designing training prescription. *Journal of Strength and Conditioning Research*, 19: 950-8.

Stricevic, M., Dacic, D., Miyazaki, T., and Anderson, G. (1989). *Modern karate: A scientific approach to conditioning and training.* Rockville Centre, NY: Miroto Karate Publishing Co.

Smith, P., Viano, D., Faust, D., and Faust, L. (1993). Thoracic injury effects of linear and angular karate impact. In *Biomechanics in Sports XI.*, Hamill, J., Derrick, T., and Elliott, E. (Eds.), Amherst, MA: International Society of Biomechanics in Sports.

Smith, P. (1984). Selected impact characteristics of karate and boxing gloves. Unpublished doctoral dissertation. Southern Illinois University at Carbondale, Carbondale, IL.

chapter 57

Attention, Sit, Meditate, Bow, Ready Position: Ritualized Dojo Pattern or Character Training?

by Marvin Labbate

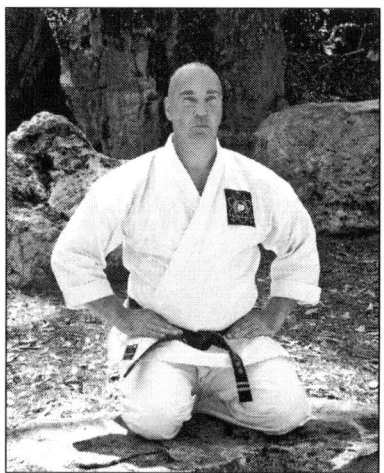

Photography courtesy of M. Labbate.

The Ritualized Pattern at the Start of Class

The *dojo*, literally translated, means "Way place." It is the place to learn the Way. An explanation of the Way is a topic deserving of its own paper, but for our dojo it is the development of mind, body, and spirit through the study of traditional Okinawan Goju-ryu karatedo. The dojo reflects the philosophy of our past and present masters who are peaceful, loving, spiritual people. The environment of the dojo is extremely influential on the spiritual and focused mind-set of the students. We do not want to walk into a chaotic environment that is distracting and adds to the anxiety of our day. The dojo should be serene, stark, and clean. The dojo is our sanctuary for learning and developing our total being.

The white uniform, which was adopted from judo, founded by Kano Jigoro (1860-1938), is a symbol of purity, perfection, and equality. Students and instructors should dress in clean, crisp uniforms. Changing into a clean uniform is a physical, outward expression of the mental, spiritual, and physical development we are striving for through our karate training. We are shedding our "old" clothes and cleansing ourselves of anxieties and events that can distract us during training. Putting on a clean uniform is rejuvenating and helps prepare us for training.

The preclass period at the dojo is a time for talking to fellow students, stretching, and mentally unwinding. There is a Chinese proverb that says, "Empty your cup before you fill it." We can't come to class with a full cup. We must leave our egos outside the dojo and put our day behind us if we are to approach our training and each other with humility, openness, and willingness to learn. It is very difficult to teach and to learn if we have inflated egos, are closed minded, or are distracted by life outside of the dojo.

At the start of class, students are instructed to shugo, which translates as "to gather around" but is used to mean "line up." Shugo, as well as the other elements of the ritualized pattern, can be broken down into physical and mental components. Physically, the students are simply lining up in rows. It is the transition from the free-flowing preclass time to the structured class time. After the students have properly lined up, they immediately stand in a ready position (*yoi*). The students are standing with their feet firmly planted in a parallel stance (*heiko dachi*), their eyes looking forward, and hands clenched by their sides (figure 1). Lining up in a ready position sends the mental signal to the students that class is beginning and it is time to prepare. When the students are lining up, they are mentally aware of and adhering to the tradition of lining up by rank, designated by belt color. The ranking system, also developed by Kano Jigoro, was adopted with the systemization of karate. The higher-ranking students line up in the front of the class, followed by intermediate and beginner students. A student's position in the line places responsibilities on him or her. For example, a student in the middle of the group must show the proper respect and etiquette to the senior students, be responsible for his own training, and be an example to the junior students who are watching. Maintaining neat, orderly lines throughout class enhances the nonchaotic, concise atmosphere of the dojo. The instructor then tells the students to come to attention (*kiotsuke*) (figure 2). *Kiotsuke*, when broken down, literally means, "Take your ki, or energy, and bring your full attention to the training and the present moment" (Opdam, 2007). Physically, the students are in a stance with heels together (*masubi dachi*), toes pointing out at a 45-degree angle, and their hands are open by their sides. The back is straight, the chin is pulled in, and the eyes are focused straight ahead toward the *shomen* wall (the wall of honor within a dojo). This phase of class is extremely important because the physical posture just described is conducive to listening, focusing, and committing students' full attention to the instructor. The students are engaged at a heightened level of awareness, bringing mind and body to attention.

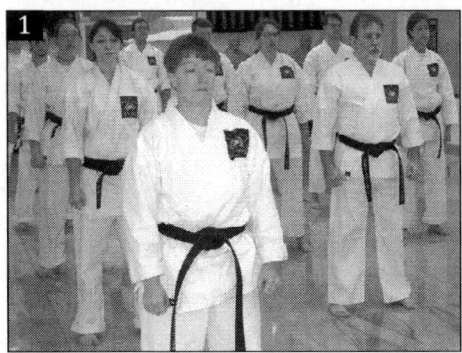
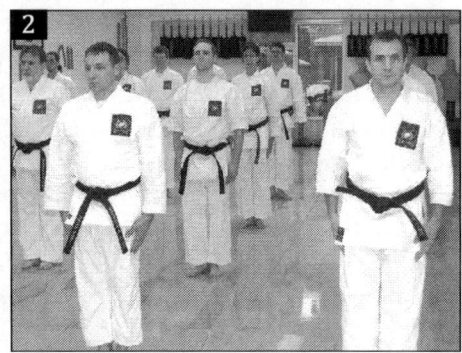

Still at attention (*kiotsuke*), the students and instructor do a standing bow (*rei*), bending from the waist and keeping their backs straight. This bow is a common courtesy to show respect to our fellow companions. It is a general greeting and a show of good manners likened to the western custom of shaking hands and saying hello. After bowing, everyone returns to attention. The students are then instructed to sit (*seiza*), which was once the respectful, formal way of sitting adopted by the warrior class in Japan. The instructor and students lower themselves to their left knee, then their right, to a kneeling position seated back on their heels (figure 3). Their backs are straight, chins pulled in; their tongues are on the hard upper palate, and their hands are resting on their legs. The instructor will then say, "*mokuso*" (meditate), which can be thought of as the mental component of seiza sitting. When the instructor says *mokuso*, the students close their eyes and begin to meditate or "clear one's mind," breathing in deeply through the nose, drawing in energy, and moving this energy to their physical center (*tanden*) (figure 4). Alternatively, students may choose to reflect on their training by asking themselves some of the following questions. What corrections did I receive last class? Have I tried to incorporate these corrections into my training? Have I improved? Do I need to focus on the same corrections again? Students may choose to use this time to reflect on their spiritual development or to pray. Yagi Meitoku (1912–2003; 10th-degree ranking in Goju-ryu Meibukan) had many dojo rules that he taught his students as part of their spiritual training. One of the many is "*Oku myo zai ren shin*," which means, "The secret techniques come from having a good heart," or "Train your spirit to be a good person" (Yagi, et al., 1998). A student may want to reflect on his or her responsibilities as a karate practitioner. Does he set a good example to other students? Does he live by the dojo principles and treat family, neighbors, co-workers, and strangers with respect and humility? Just as putting on a clean white uniform is an act of outward cleansing, meditating (*mokuso*) is an act of inner cleansing. Students can also choose to reflect on or pray for any particular need they may have on that day.

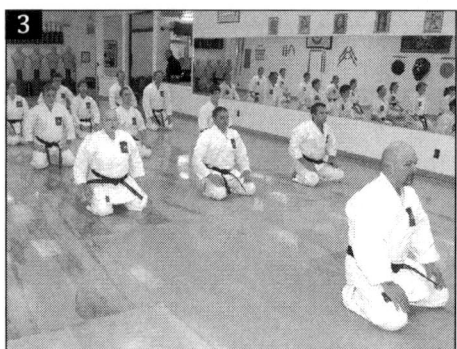
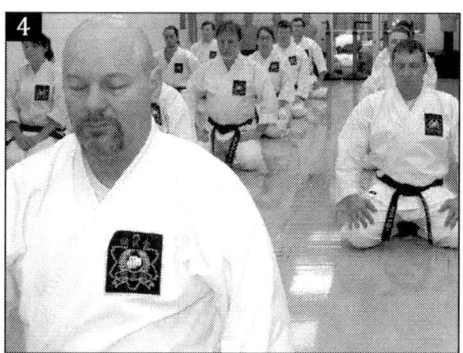

For the class instructor, this can be a time to reflect on the class he or she is about to teach and how to best communicate with the students. When I am teaching class, I pray to God as my personal form of reflection. I pray for my students. I pray that I can teach them techniques in the most effective yet safe way so that no one is injured. In viewing myself as a servant, I pray that the students will benefit from training, be it physically, mentally, or spiritually. I use this time to reflect on my character. Am I a good role model? Do I demonstrate good moral character through my teaching? Am I teaching to be a blessing to my students, or am I teaching to satisfy my ego? Many of us may not have the self-discipline to spiritually "work out" on our own, so this can be the perfect time to reshape our inner being through meditation and reflection.

Several aspects of meditation (*mokuso*), when considered together, can be overwhelming to a student. One does not have to reflect on every aspect of his mental, physical, and spiritual development every class. What one reflects on specifically may change with the day. What is important, then, is to find and reflect on weaknesses you are feeling at a given moment and ask yourself what you need to do to improve and strengthen your inner self. A minimum of three to five minutes of meditation is crucial in preparing for training and should not be skimmed over. By the time the instructor says, "*Mokuso yame*" (stop meditating), each student should have a clear connection between mind and body. Students and the instructor are now fully engaged in a learning mind-set, ready to continue with their physical training.

The final element of the ritualized pattern goes back to the bow (*rei*), but with different physical and mental components. Bowing is done from sitting in the seiza posture. Facing the shomen wall, the instructor says, "Shomen ni rei," which means, "Bow to the wall of honor." The instructor and students bow by bringing their left then right hands together on the floor directly in front of them (figure 5), then lowering their heads to their hands (figure 6).

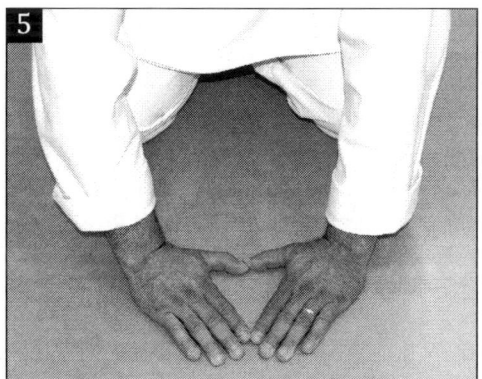
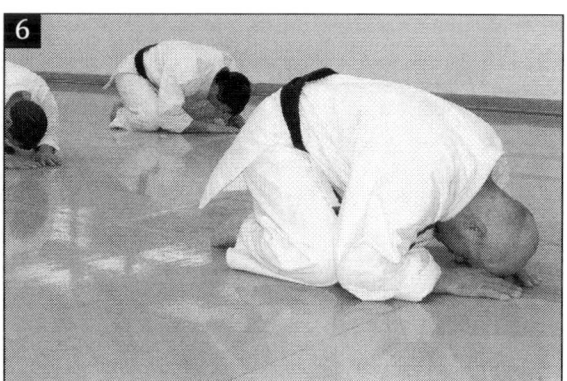

The simple physical act of bowing encompasses a wealth of meaning. Bowing to the shomen wall is a sign of respect, not worship, for past and current masters. Mentally, we are acknowledging the traditions, wisdom, and insight the masters have passed on to us. Traditional karate can be likened to our parents, grandparents, and great grandparents who have shared traditions, family history, and wisdom with successive generations. This natural family model is the basis for the karate family that has developed over many, many years. The early karate masters believed in the family unit and considered their karate students as family and as the means for passing on coveted knowledge to future generations. Traditional Okinawan karate has survived the centuries because our past masters believed in its value and were committed to sharing karate in its entirety.

There is a spiritual aspect of bowing to the shomen wall as well. Each dojo has a unique shomen wall, usually containing some element of spirituality. At my dojo, there is a cross representing Christianity on the shomen wall. If I have been praying, I am humbling myself and bowing to the Lord when I bow to the shomen wall. Bowing to the shomen wall is a private exercise, and the intent of the individual's bow depends on his or her faith, beliefs, and mind-set. Bowing is also a sign of respect for the dojo. It is an outward expression of an inward responsibility. Students and instructors alike are responsible for maintaining an environment conducive to learning by reflecting on their surroundings. Does the dojo reflect the traditions and philosophy of Okinawan karate? Is the dojo clean, tidy, stark, and serene? Paying attention to such details trains us to be visually aware of our surroundings, which will carry over to our everyday life. Adherence to the rules of the dojo is an effective yet subtle way to cultivate responsibility and self-discipline both inside and outside of the dojo.

After the instructor and students have bowed to the shomen wall, the instructor turns to face the students, and the highest-ranking students say, "*Rei*" (bow). The instructor and students bow to each other, saying, "Onegai shimasu," meaning, "Please teach me" (figure 7). Learning is a mutual process for the instructor and the students.

The instructor enters training humble, empty, willing to learn through teaching, and showing the utmost respect to his or her students. The students bow to the instructor as a sign of respect. As we get to know our instructors, we gain a sincere respect for their knowledge, insight of the art, and their overall character. In this regard, when the students bow to the instructor and he to them, it is at a deeper, more personal level. Everyone now stands up and goes back to the ready position (*yoi*). The students are now physically, mentally, and spiritually prepared to train.

Students are frequently brought back to the ready position between drills and exercises. This is a time to reconnect the body and mind through focus and deep breathing. When students get tired, they are often easily distracted, making it important to draw them back to a learning mind-set and to refocus on the lesson.

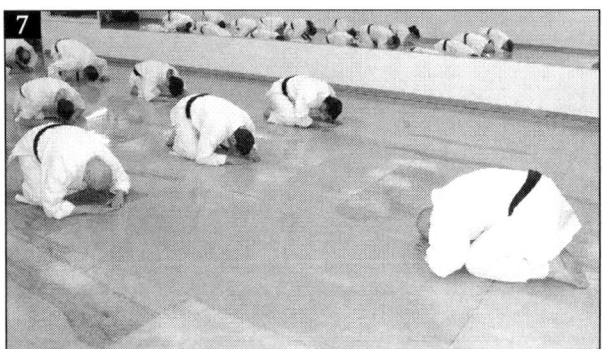
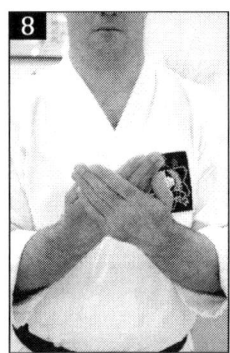

The Ritualized Pattern as it Applies to Solo Training

The next segment of class is the lesson the instructor has planned, which may focus on solo training, partner training, or both. Before the lesson begins, the instructor and students will perform a ritualized pattern that differs somewhat from the one done at the beginning of class. It is, however, made up of the same elements: ready posture, attention, bow, meditate, and back to the ready posture. It is essential that this routine be incorporated into your karate training, whether you are practicing alone or as an individual in a group. Performing this routine at the start and conclusion of kata, drills, or partner drills helps establish the mind-set of learning. Training at the dojo is done in the context of learning, often through self-discovery, and developing mentally, physically, and spiritually.

A kata is a formalized sequence of martial self-defense moves performed like a dance or shadow boxing, often done solo. At the start of kata training, the students are in a ready position while respectfully waiting for instructions (figure 8). When the instructor announces *kiotsuke* (attention), the students physically move to an attention stance, as previously described (figure 9). Mentally, each student is focused, actively listening and visually aware. Next the instructor and class do a standing bow, again saying, "*Onegai shimasu*" (Please teach me) (figure 10). Similar to the bow at the beginning of class, the students perform this bow as an act of respect for the instructor, but it also holds a deeper meaning. The instructor and the students alike are acknowledging a level of seriousness for their karate training. The students engage their minds and bodies in a serious, introspective approach to analyze principles, movement, and self-defense applications. Before performing the kata, the students center their energy (*mokuso*), in a standing position. The students bring both hands up to approximately chest level, with fingers pointing up, and breathe in deeply through the nose, gathering their energy (figure 11). The palm of the left hand is placed on the back of the right hand so that the knuckle of the right middle finger presses against the *laogong* pressure point (PC8), located between the second and third metacarpal bones of the left palm (figure 12) (Montaigue and Simpson, 1998). While exhaling and with the hands maintaining contact, the hands are rotated so that the fingers point downward. At the same time, the hands are moved down to the center of the body (*tanden* 丹田) (figure 13). The rotation of the knuckle against the *laogong* point of the palm activates an energy channel. Air, breath, and mind move to the center, and from this point forward, our mind and movement remain at our center. The final component of the ritualized pattern for solo training is what I refer to as a heightened ready position (*yoi*)—an "I'm ready" position of confidence.

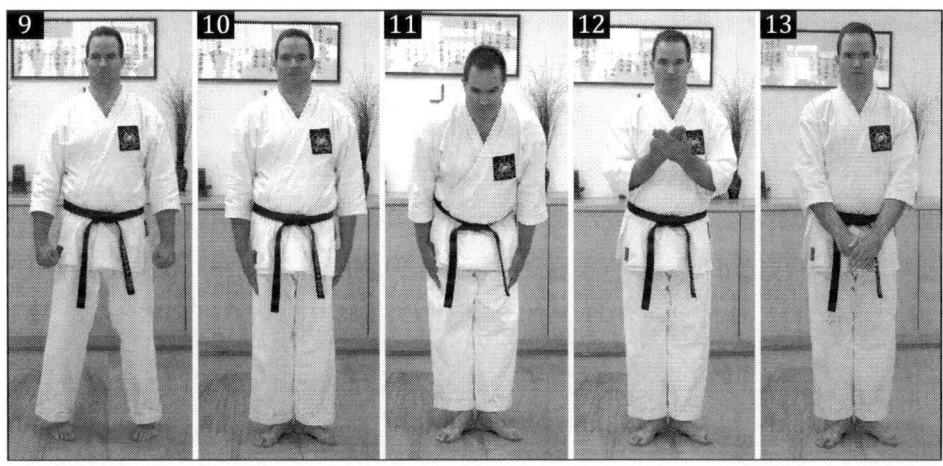

While the foundation of training rests in respect and courtesy, the practice of harmonizing mind, body, and breath is also critical to training. Learning to harmonize each element follows the same process as learning a kata. As novices, we learn gross motor movements and concentrate on memorizing the routine. As we advance in our training, we start thinking about the Sanchin kata principles of structure and movement and begin to incorporate them into our kata training (Labbate, 1999). Likewise, the ritualized pattern advances to a higher level in which static meditation transitions to moving meditation. Breathing and centering remain the same, but we now harmonize our breathing with movement.

Upon completion of the kata, the students meditate again to gather and center their energy, calm down, and reestablish the mind-body connection through deep breathing. They bring their hands to their sides, do a standing bow, and say, "*Domo arigato gozaimasu*," which means "Thank you," and is an outward expression of gratitude for the lessons learned and what they have discovered about their kata. A student's level of mental endurance will dictate the number of repetitions of a kata that can be done during a training session. Performing a kata or any drill at one hundred percent effort is mentally tiring, but mental endurance will develop with consistent training, just as with physical endurance.

The Ritualized Pattern and Partner Training

The physical, mental, and spiritual aspects of solo training also apply to partner training with an added layer of complexity as a result of working with another person. Training with a partner is advanced and takes on new principles on all three levels. Partners line up facing each other in the ready position and perform the same ritualized

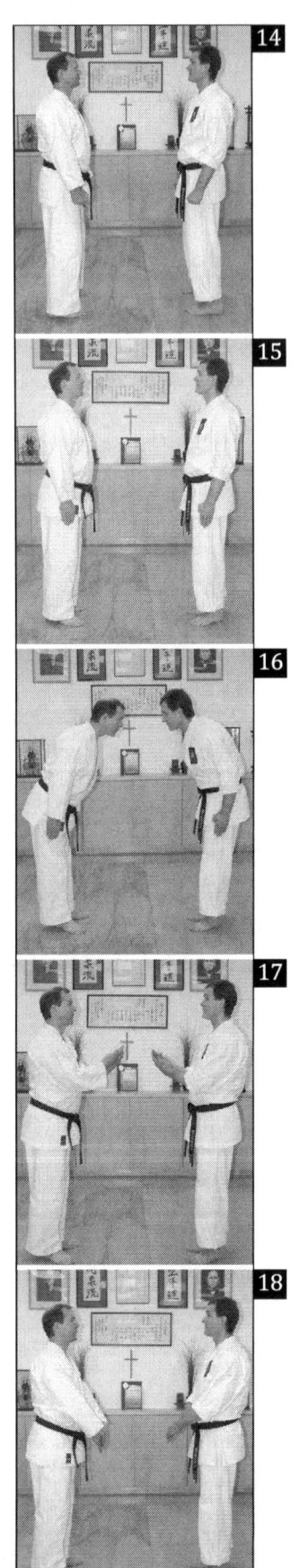

pattern of coming to attention, bowing, meditating, and returning to a ready position before starting the drill (figure 14). This is the point when partners make eye contact with each other. Eye contact is critical in partner training because it is the initial way to create and fully engage in a connection between partners. After coming to attention, each partner is alert and focused on the other person (figure 15). This is a time to "size up" your partner. How do your height, weight, and reach compare? What kind of adjustments might you have to make to compensate for physical differences? What is your partner's skill level? These are all important observations to consider.

The next component of the ritualized pattern is the bow (figure 16). Unlike the other bows, the bow in partner training is unique and specific. Partners bow to each other to demonstrate mutual respect, modesty, humility, and harmony. When the students say, "*Onegai shimasu*" to each other, they are saying, "Please trust that I will care for you." There is a maxim that accurately describes the essence of partner training: *jita kyoei*, 自他共栄—mutual welfare and benefit (Watanabe, et al., 1972). Partners are entering into a level of training with high regard for each other's progress and safety so that each will benefit. Partner training is never one sided, even between beginner and advanced students. The higher-skill-level student takes on a mentoring role and will learn through teaching, whereas the lower-skill-level student will learn from one-on-one time with his or her partner. Neither student is a punching bag or a target for the other's ego. After bowing, the students remain in the bow position. The instructor announces the drill and says, "mokuso" (meditate). The students perform mokuso as they would kata training, drawing in and centering their energy and concentrating on connecting with their partner (figures 17–18). The mind-body connection between partners is much more complicated than the mind-body connection an individual develops within him- or herself. There is a physical, mental, and spiritual awareness between partners that develops with repeated partner training.

We discussed the physical awareness partners have of each other and went into a bit more detail discussing the spiritual aspects of partner training; now let us explore mental awareness. This refers to a mutual understanding partners have of each other's emotional state and the effect partners have on each other. For example, failing to shed anxiety during meditation can be distracting to the person you are working with. It is important to give 100 percent of your attention and effort to your partner. Sense your partner's mental and emotional state. Is he or she approaching this training with the same level of seriousness, intensity, and humility as you? Is your partner nervous or anxious? Awareness and sensitivity to your partner's emotional and mental status is paramount in partner training. Ultimately, students will develop the sense of mental control needed for physical control.

Dialogue between partners during drills is a unique aspect of partner training that is mutually beneficial. If partners perceive there is a disconnect between them, they can stop, determine the reason, and then concentrate on reestablishing the connection. Partner training will expose each other's weaknesses. Through honest, humble dialogue, the students can help each other correct and understand techniques. This not only elevates each other's skill development but also aids in building a bond of trust between partners.

During partner training and upon completion of the formal partner drills, the students come back to the ready posture to re-establish the mind-body connection as individuals and as partners. When partner training ends, the students maintain eye contact, come to attention, and then bow, saying, "*Domo arigato gozaimasu.*" The students are offering a genuine "thank you" for the time spent with each other, the mutual benefits each received through this training, and for the positive impact the partners have on each other because of their humble, respectful attitude.

The Ritualized Pattern at the End of Class

At the end of class, the same ritualized pattern as that done at the beginning of class is performed. The students and instructor line up in a ready position, move to the seated position, and meditate. As with the beginning of class, the students can use this time for meditation, reflection, or prayer. When I am the class instructor, I pray that the students have benefited from the class and are leaving feeling better in some way, be it mentally or physically. Perhaps something a student had been struggling to understand or perform became clear and achievable. Students should reflect on the class they just participated in. Some questions they might ask themselves include the following: Did I remember the corrections from last class and try to improve? Did I receive any new corrections or new information to incorporate into my training? After meditation, the instructor and students bow to the shomen wall. Again, as at the beginning of class, they are honoring the past karate masters. Additionally, this bow serves as a reminder that as students and instructors we have the responsibility to pass down the knowledge that has been given to us. The price we pay for studying karate is to share this knowledge in its original form and meaning. It is through the giving/receiving relationships of instructors to students and students to students that this knowledge is passed on. The instructor then faces the students. They bow to each other, offering a mutual, genuine thank you by saying, "*Domo arigato gozaimasu.*" The students should be thanking the instructor for the time he or she has donated. The gift of time is priceless in and of itself and it is through this gift that the art of karate is passed on from generation to generation. Students may not know and appreciate this at first, but as they get to know the instructors, *domo arigato gozai-masu* will come to mean much more than thank you for the karate lesson. As the instructor, I am thanking the students for the knowledge I have gained through teaching and for allowing me to touch their hearts in some way. For as many people as I teach on any day, I have the responsibility to be pure of heart and to impact people in a positive way. Funakoshi Gichin (1868–1957) wrote in the first of the Twenty Precepts: "Karate-do begins with courtesy and ends with a bow." Ultimately, we will learn that it is this higher level of thankfulness and gratitude that keeps us humble. Being humble drives us to constantly strive to learn and improve.

• • •

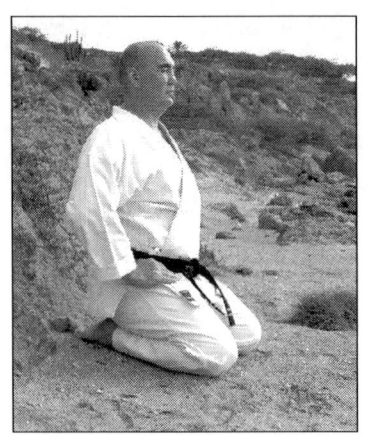

We have explored the origin and meaning of each component of the ritualized pattern and why it is performed at the beginning of class, during solo and partner training, and at the end of class. We've also explained that there are physical, mental, and spiritual aspects to each component that develop and deepen in meaning with practice. The ritual in and of itself is training, which, with a full understanding and continuous practice, will further enhance the student's skill level. It is my hope that you now have a better understanding of the significance of the exercise that appears to be a simple ritual.

References

Labbate, M. (1999). Elements of advanced karate technique. *Journal of Asian Martial Arts, 8*(2):80-95.

Montaigue, E., and Simpson, W. (1997). *The encyclopedia of dim-mak.* Boulder, CO: Paladin Press.

Opdam, L. (2007). *Karate Goju Ryu Meibukan.* Los Angeles, CA: Empire Books.

Watanabe, J., and Avakian, L. (1972). *The secrets of judo: A text for instructors and students.* Rutland, VT: Charles E. Tuttle Co.

Yagi, M., Wheeler, C., and Vickerson, B. (1998). *Okinawan Karate-Do Gojyu-ryu Meibu-Kan.* Charlottetown, PE, Canada: Action Press.

chapter 58

Nahate: The Old-School Okinawan Martial Art and Its Original Four-Kata Curriculum, Part I

by Mario McKenna, M.S.

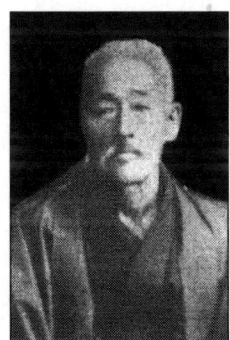
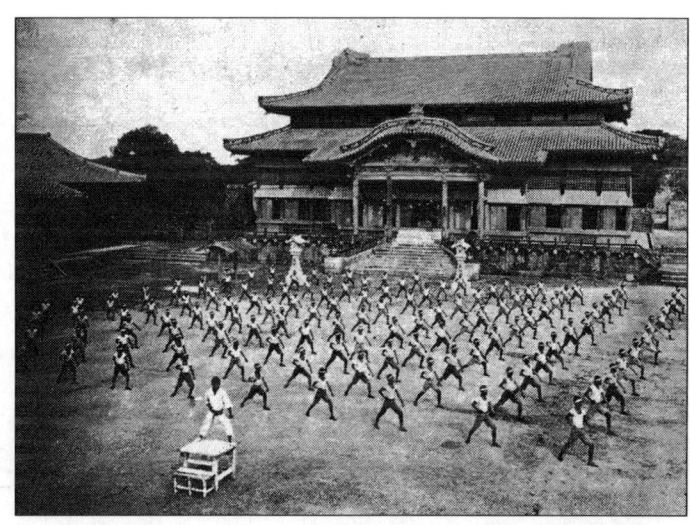

Karate practice at Shuri Castle, c. 1938.
Inset photograph of Higaonna Kanryo (1850–1915).

Nahate

Nahate (那覇手), along with Shurite and Tomarite, was an important boxing culture practiced in and around the Kumemura area of Naha (Kumemura, Wikipedia), Okinawa. For several generations it was passed down until the late nineteenth century, when its popularity began to wane. Its resurgence is most often ascribed to Higaonna Kanryo (1850–1915). Folklore tells us that Higaonna traveled to Fuzhou city in China's Fujian province and remained there for up to fifteen years, studying Chinese boxing from a teacher called Ryu Ryu Ko (aka., Ru Ru Ko, 1852–1930). Who Ryu Ryu Ko was and what he taught Higaonna is a point of debate among karate historians that has yet to be satisfactorily resolved (Kinjo, 1999; Tokashiki, 1991).

Be that as it may, Higaonna eventually returned to Okinawa and began teaching his system to a small group of students in Naha. Orthodox history states that he taught nine katas: Sanchin, Saifa, Seiunchin, Sanseru, Sepai, Shisochin, Sesan, Kururunfa, and Suparimpei/Pechurin, which were then passed down by his most prolific student, and founder of Goju-ryu, Miyagi Chojun (1888–1952). However, my own contention is that the original Nahate curriculum consisted of four katas: Sanchin, Sesan, Sanseru, and Suparimpei/Pechurin (Câmara and McKenna, 2007; McKenna and Swift, 2002; McKenna, 2001; McKenna, 2000a, 2000b).

That said, I would like to discuss the content of these four Nahate katas—Sanchin, Sesan, Sanseru, and Suparimpei/Pechurin—in more detail in order to provide the reader with a better understanding of the rich techniques each of them contains. To do this, I will compare and contrast the two major lineages of Nahate with respect to these kata that originated from Higaonna Kanryo: Goju-ryu (剛柔流) and Tou'on-ryu (東恩流). Throughout these essays I will briefly explain the main techniques found in each kata and their applications, along with some of the verbal explanations that descended with these traditions, and finally the importance of hidden meaning in katas.

Sanchin Kata 三戦

The Sanchin kata forms the basis for Nahate techniques. Although there are many superficially different versions of this kata, essentially all of them can trace their origin to Higaonna Kanryo, or, to a lesser extent, Uechi Kanbun.[1] Regardless of the version practiced, the technical content of the kata is largely the same:

1) stance,
2) midlevel blocks and thrusts,
3) turning,
4) grasping hands and fingertip thrusts, and
5) the circle block.

Let's examine each of these parts one by one.

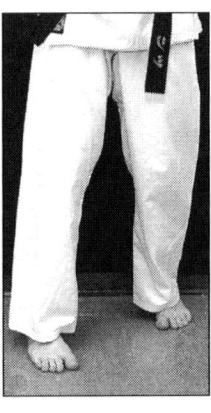

(1) Stance.

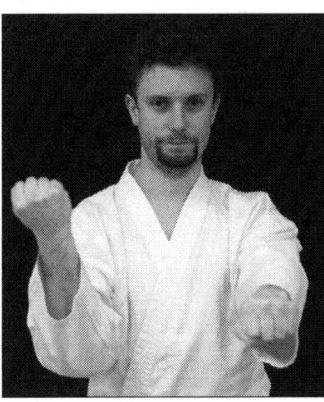

(2)   Left: Sanchin midlevel block/punch, Goju.
Right: Sanchin midlevel block/punch, Tou'on.

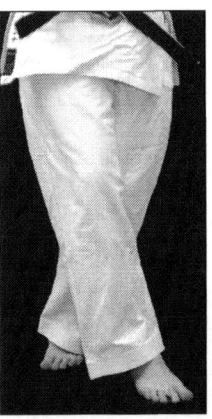

(3) Sanchin turn.

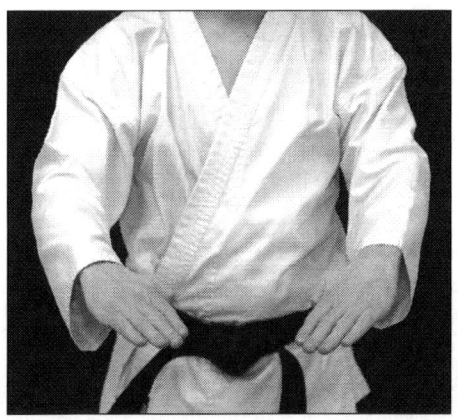

(4) Spear hand thurst.

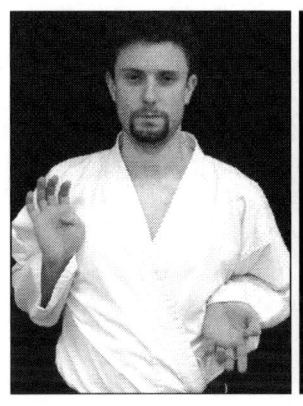 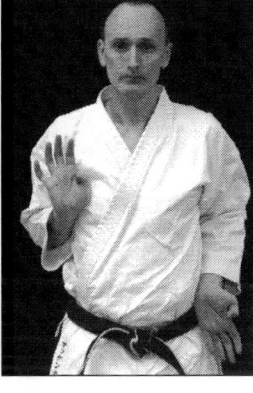

(5) Left: Sanchin circle block, Goju.
Right: Sanchin circle block, Tou'on.

Sanchin Kata and Combative Concepts

When two people face each other during a modern, sport free-fighting exchange, they will start at quite a distance from each other. As a result, the percentage of strikes that land is quite low, and those that do land are not target specific. In general, we could say that modern free-fighting practice tends to be inaccurate in its strikes. We can also observe that the striking distance is closed quite rapidly—only after a few strikes have been exchanged.

When we contrast this method to the older Nahate practices and techniques as embodied in the Sanchin kata, we can see some very interesting differences: A) the engagement distance (*maai*) is much closer; B) body position, alignment, and placement are extremely important; C) seizing (*tuidi*), locking (*chigedi*), and entangling (*karamidi*) techniques followed by strikes dominate.

These types of techniques have a number of advantages, two of which are increased precision and power when striking. Nahate's seizing, locking, and entangling techniques secure an opponent, which allows a greater possibility of striking smaller and potentially more effective targets with greater accuracy and with more effective tools (e.g., one-knuckle fist [*ippon ken*]). These are techniques you would never see used in a free-fighting exchange because they are quite literally too dangerous. Therefore, when we think about the training methods used in the past, we should consider them not as methods of fighting per se, but as methods of self-protection.

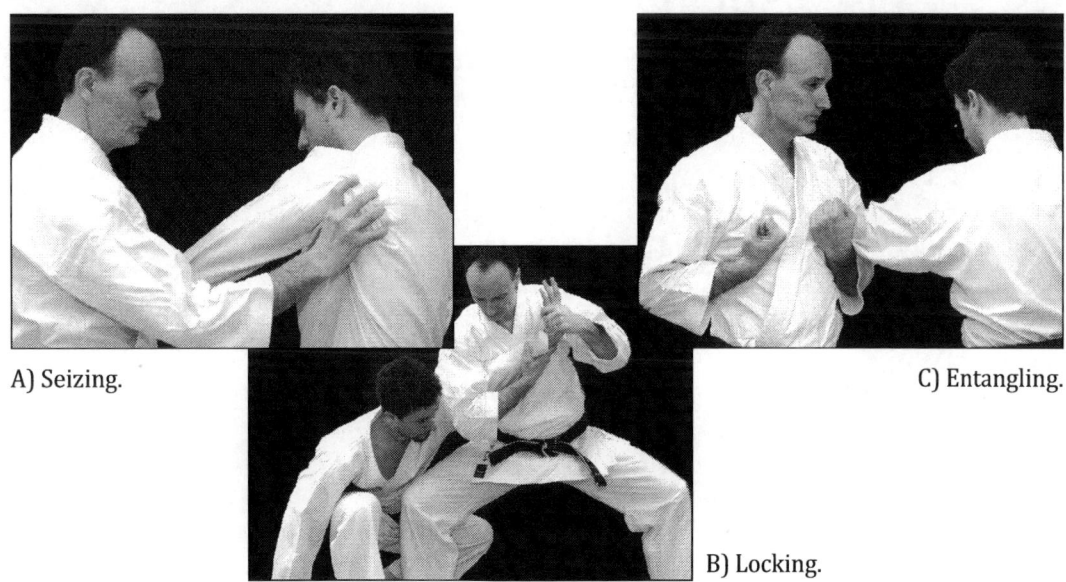

A) Seizing.

C) Entangling.

B) Locking.

Sanchin Stance

At the heart of the Sanchin kata is the Sanchin stance. According to Hirakami Nobuyuki, this stance is very rare in mainland Japanese martial culture, with the possible exception of old-style sumo (Hirakami, 2000). Indeed, Sanchin stance appears unique to Okinawan martial culture and emphasizes a natural posture with the weight evenly distributed on both legs with the toes of the lead foot slightly turned to the inside. The importance of Sanchin stance is in teaching the student how to generate, store, and release energy when striking. This explosive type of energy is commonly referred to as *fajing* in Chinese martial culture (發勁; Japanese: *hakkei*). Therefore, we can think of Sanchin stance as allowing for the efficient transfer of energy generated by the body and delivered through the arms.

Midlevel Block and Thrust

Sanchin's midlevel block is performed on the same side as the lead leg. In contrast, the punch is delivered with the opposite hand of the lead leg, and is therefore commonly referred to as a reverse punch (*gyaku tsuki*). There are a few minor differences between Tou'on-ryu and Goju-ryu with respect to these techniques. The two most noticeable ones are chambering the fist at the chest versus the hip, and thrusting straight out versus to the centerline. Putting aside these differences for the moment, the most common applications of these techniques are to deflect an incoming strike (either to the inside or outside) and to counter with a punch to the opponent's body. Although acceptable for teaching beginning students, this is a very crude explanation of this technique and grossly simplifies many of its deeper applications, which include the aforementioned seizing, grabbing, and locking techniques.

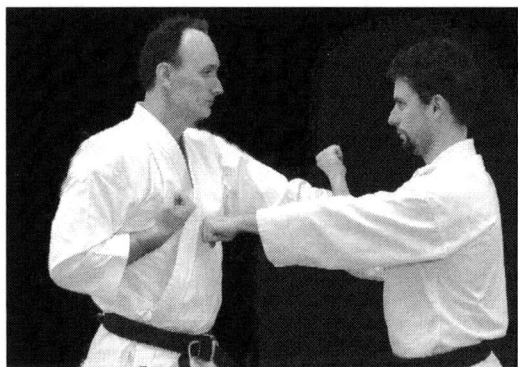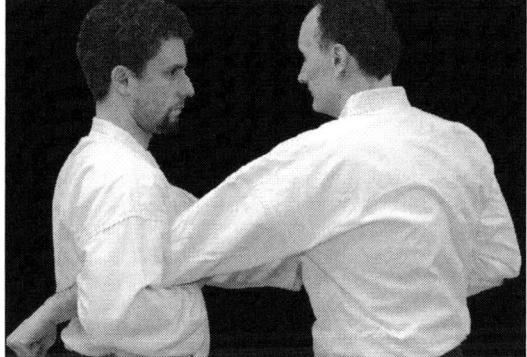

Left: Sanchin midlevel block and punch. Right: Sanchin entangled arm.

Not only do these sorts of rudimentary explanations obfuscate many of the more jujutsu-like applications found in Sanchin and in other katas, but they also create the idea that kata techniques cannot be used in an actual confrontation (which, ironically, is often described in the context of modern sport competition, such as sport karate, mixed martial arts, wrestling, or boxing). Some modern karate styles have attempted to overcome this perceived weakness by creating various forms of arranged sparring, such as one-step or three-step sparring, but these methods are modern creations, with the oldest known being published by Funakoshi Gichin (1868–1957) in *The Karatedo Instruction Book* (Karatedo Kyohan). Furthermore, they are largely divorced from actual kata technique. The solution is that function does not always follow form in old karate (Okinawan: *toudi*) katas (Hirakami, 2000).

As I mentioned earlier, when we think about the combination of Sanchin stance, midlevel block, and reverse punch, we see it is never used in modern, sport-based karate competition. In contrast, lunging forward stances and reverse punches between contestants who are meters apart are more commonly seen. Why is it we do not see the former? The answer is surprisingly simple: because that technique is far too dangerous to be used in competition. It is quite literally meant to destroy the attacker (Hirakami, 2000). One simple example of its use in downing an attacker is to use entangling techniques (*karamidi*), in which the "blocking" arm wraps the opponent's arm and the reverse punch is used to attack the centerline.[2] This technique would lead to disqualification in a tournament, but when used as a self-protection method, it is clearly an effective and powerful technique.

Fingertip Thrust and Grasping Hands

Near the end of the Sanchin kata there are three clenching pulls and three open-hand fingertip thrusts. These are essentially performed the same in Goju-ryu and Tou'on-ryu. The full sequence consists of grasping with both hands, closing them into fists, and pulling them back to the waist or chest, followed by opening the hands, turning them over, and thrusting with the fingertips. Let's examine the use of the fingertip thrusts by looking at a historical example.

In An Overview of Karatedo (1938), Shiroma Shimpan describes the formation and use of fingertip thrusts in his chapter called "Karatedo Kata and Their Meaning." Shiroma first describes the technique: "If the back of the hand is facing upwards and the fingers are held horizontally then it is known as horizontal fingertip thrusts [sic]. Horizontal fingertip thrusts can be seen in the kata Sanchin. In Sanchin kata both hands are held at midlevel and simultaneously strike using horizontal fingertip thrusts" (Nakasone, 2009: 97).

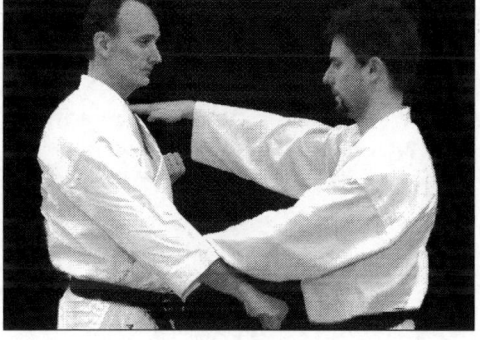

Sanchin finger tip strike to the throat.

Shiroma (Nakasone, 2009:98) explains the use of this technique:

If an opponent fixes his eyes on your solar plexus and launches an attack, we use the principle of simultaneous attack and defense as I have previously explained by using double horizontal fingertip thrusts to both attack and defend. This double sided fingertip thrusts [sic] is a very effective technique. If however, the opponent strikes at your face you can perform an open hand side block and with the same hand you can strike your opponent's face with either horizontal or vertical fingertip thrusts. Therefore high and midlevel fingertip thrusts are both an effective and advantageous means of attack and defense.

Circle Block

The final sequence of Sanchin kata in both Goju-ryu and Tou'on-ryu consists of stepping back one step in Sanchin stance and performing a circle block. In Goju-ryu it is referred to as "circle block" (*mawashi uke*), while in Tou'on-ryu it is referred to as "comma block" (*tomoe uke*). There is a noticeable difference how the block is performed between the sister styles, but we will get to this important difference a little bit later.

The circle block is an extremely powerful technique that is often applied as a strike. This is a completely valid application of the technique, but it expresses only one dimension of it. An alternate name for this technique is *tora guchi*—the mouth of the tiger. The choice of name is quite interesting, as it evokes the frightening image of a tiger consuming its prey. But why this name? As you are probably aware, there are superficial (*omote*) and deeper (*ura*) applications of techniques in karate (*toudi*), and this includes the circle block. In this light, the striking application can be seen as a superficial application, but a deeper application would be the use of tora guchi in some other manner.

I think most people who practice Sanchin have thought of this and may even have stumbled onto a few alternative uses for tora guchi during their practices, but I would encourage you to continue to delve deeper into its study. There are countless applications for tora guchi: locks, throws, sweeps, traps, etc. I suspect that if your background is sports-based karate, then these applications may not be readily apparent, but with a little effort and experimentation outside of a sports context, they will reveal themselves to you little by little. Of course, it helps if your teacher is knowledgeable with these techniques, but it is not essential—at least not in the beginning.

Now let's return to the differences between Tou'on-ryu and Goju-ryu and how they perform the circle block at the end of Sanchin kata. In it, the arms are not extended out to project energy as you would as if trying to strike (this is more apparent in the Uechi-ryu interpretation and less so in the Goju-ryu version but still present). Instead the arms (especially the elbows) are kept close to the body. Also the position of the palms is quite different, with the upper hand in front of the collarbone and the lower hand in front of the groin. From this position one can easily "devour" an opponent. In closing I will leave the reader with the following image to contemplate the meaning of the circle block: "[T]he tiger always catches its prey" (Hirakami, 2000:pt. VI, 63).

Psychological Aspects to Sanchin

Not only does Sanchin kata provide deep technical and physical training; it also provides profound training for the spirit and mind. This is expressed very eloquently by Dr. Takamiyagi Shigeru, a high-ranking Uechi-ryu teacher of the Okikukai (Okinawan Karatedo Association) in his essay entitled "Sanchin and its Five Cardinal Points" (Takamiyagi, 1996:158).

> The practice of Sanchin, the foundation kata of Okikukai, develops the student in five ways that reach beyond the basic needs of exercise or self-defense. Properly understood, Sanchin is a philosophical statement. The five benefits of Sanchin are as follows:
>
> 1) Sanchin integrates all parts of the stance;
> 2) Sanchin corrects the breathing;
> 3) Sanchin develops penetrating eyes;
> 4) Sanchin cultivates spiritual concentration;
> 5) Sanchin strengthens the body.

The key for understanding Sanchin is "integration." Proper stance anchors the student to the floor; while proper concentration and breathing integrates all body movements. Proper eye contact demonstrates uninterrupted awareness, focusing the mind on every area of attack of the opponent. To develop a strong and integrated Sanchin kata is to forge a well-honed and ordered self.

Comments on Sanchin

There are a few expressions that have been passed down in karate (*toudi*) about the importance of Sanchin kata, such as, "Sanchin is the beginning and the end," or, "Three years of study for Sanchin kata." These expressions tell us that although a short kata, Sanchin formed the backbone of Nahate upon which subsequent technique and understanding were built. In the next part of this chapter I will discuss the Sesan kata.

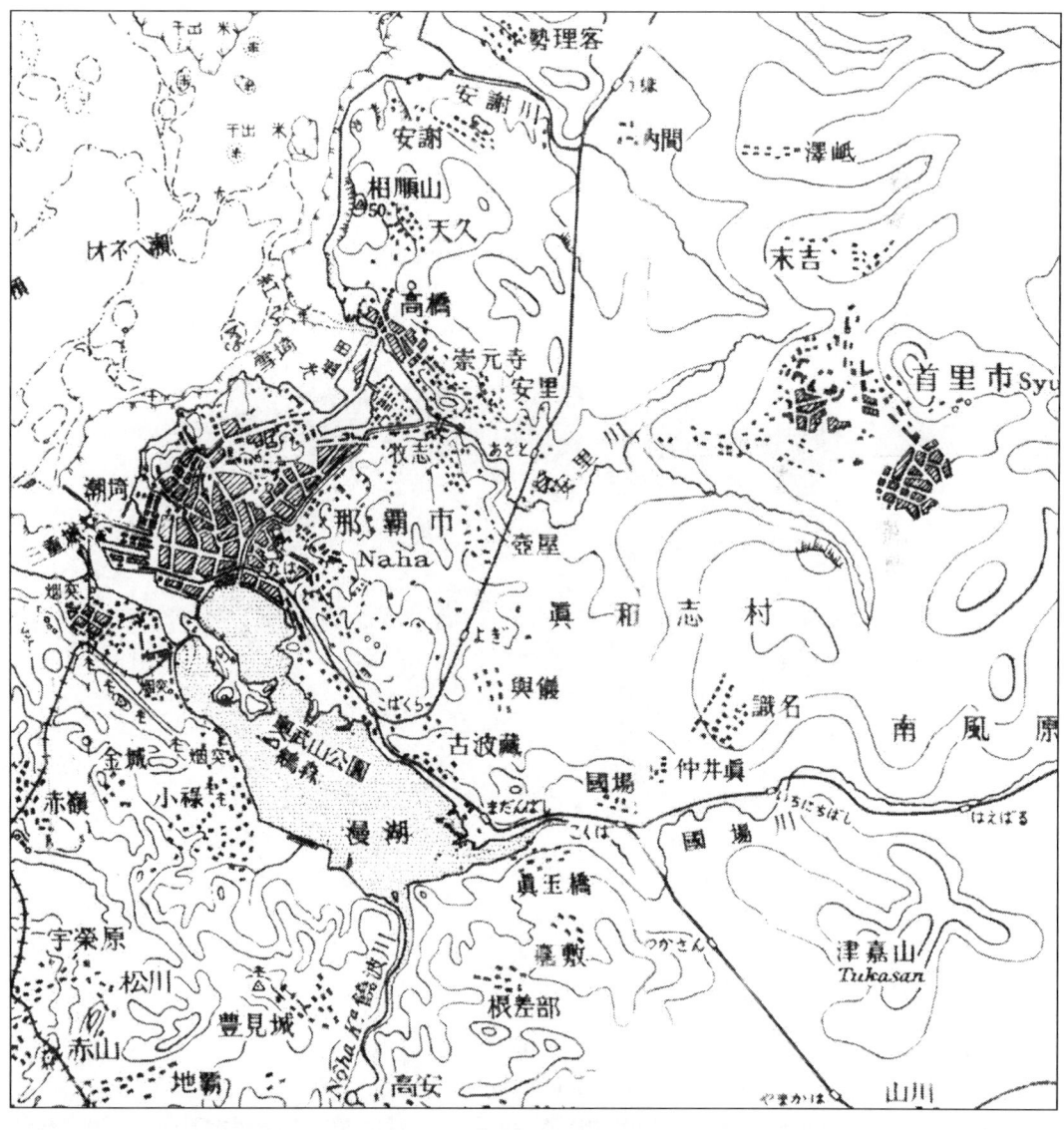

Detail from a 1937 nautical chart showing the area around
Naha city. Naha to Shuri (Syuri) is about three miles.
From the Library of Congress print collection.

Sesan Kata 十三手

The next kata in the Nahate curriculum we will discuss is Sesan, which is typically viewed as an intermediate-level kata.[3] Sesan is written as the number "13" but the reason for this is not entirely clear. Some teachers have stated that Sesan refers to the number of individual or composite techniques in the kata, while others state that it refers to the number of steps in the kata. For some, these methods sum to thirteen, leading them to believe that this is the meaning of Sesan (see Tokashiki, 1991; Kinjo, 1999). However, overall these methods of defining Sesan are unsatisfactory because of their inconsistency when applied across the different lineages of Sesan found in karate (*toudi*). What we can say with some certainty is that Sesan builds upon the techniques learned from Sanchin.

For this portion, I will only be examining the Sesan taught by Higaonna Kanryo (1850–1915), which, unfortunately, was not passed down in Tou'on-ryu. Therefore a cross-comparison within the same lineage of kata cannot be done. Tou'on-ryu uses a version of Sesan, which originates from Higaonna Kanyu (1849–1922) and differs quite markedly in comparison to the Kanryo version. With that said, let's take a look at some of the techniques found in the Higaonna Kanryo version of Sesan.

Sword-Hand Strike and Continuous Block

Like Sanchin kata, Sesan opens with three steps forward in Sanchin stance in conjunction with three midlevel blocks and punches. As this was already discussed in the Sanchin section, I'll move on to the next major set of techniques: a sword-hand strike followed by three rapid blocks and three double fingertip thrusts and knee strikes in succession.

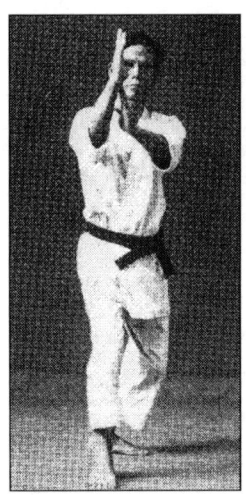 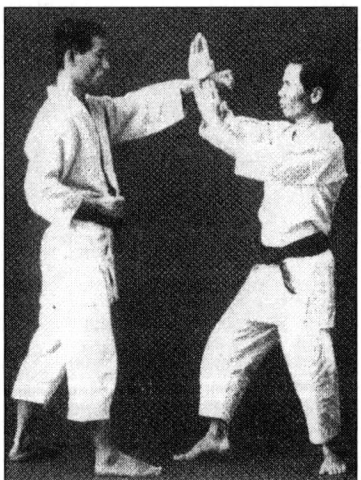

Left: Shiroma Renzoku Uke. Right: Shiroma Renzoku Uke Applied.

First, let's examine the continuous block. These are unique to Sesan kata and are a solid example of a practical self-defense technique. They are excellent for a number of reasons, but let's highlight two of them. First, they are executed toward the centerline of the opponent's body while simultaneously protecting your own, and second, they can be used to deflect an attack and simultaneously counter toward vulnerable parts of the throat and head. This series of blocks is referred to as *renzoku uke* in Japanese and is described in An *Outline of Karatedo* by Shiroma Shimpan in his chapter called "Karate Kata and their Meaning" (Nakasone, 1938:104):

When your opponent punches with his right fist, you block his attack with your left forearm (the right forearm is then held ready). However if your opponent attacks again with his left fist, you can quickly raise your right forearm to block his attack. [This technique is illustrated in figures 1 and 2.] *Renzoku-uke* is intended to block multiple strikes from an opponent, but during an actual fight it is not enough to simply block the attack; this is meaningless. It is vital to quickly strike your opponent's oncoming blow with your right or left hand chambered in front of you (since in karatedo kata double or triple punches are executed).

When shifting from defense to offense with renzoku-uke, either in kata or in actual fighting, a useful technique is nukite.... For example, after executing the third *renzoku-uke* you can strike your opponent with a right *tate nukite* (or *yoko nukite*). Even if your opponent simultaneously punches at you with his right fist, you will have the advantage because your right hand is on the inside.

Low-Level Side Kick and Turn

In Sanchin kata there are no kicks, but in Sesan the first kick a student learns through this kata is the low-level side kick. This kick is typically taught to attack the opponent's knee and is an adequate (albeit limited) explanation of its application. Other applications can include sweeps to the front or back of the knee or ankle, and are dangerous. In addition, the turn in Sesan can be used to throw an opponent. The Sesan rendition is to prop the opponent's foot and use the turn to trip him—an exceedingly simple technique, and one that is more reminiscent of jujutsu than modern judo (Hirakami, 2000).

These kinds of simple sweeps can be found in Takenouchi-ryu jujutsu and are well suited to real combat, as they allow the defender to maintain a stable position while being able to throw an opponent to the ground with minimal effort (Hirakami, 2000). Unfortunately, in some modern dojos, practice takes place on hard floors, making it difficult to use such techniques safely. As a result, the low-level side kick is usually literally applied as a kick to the knee as described earlier. Even more discouraging is that the practice of these kinds of throwing techniques has mostly disappeared in modern karate training.

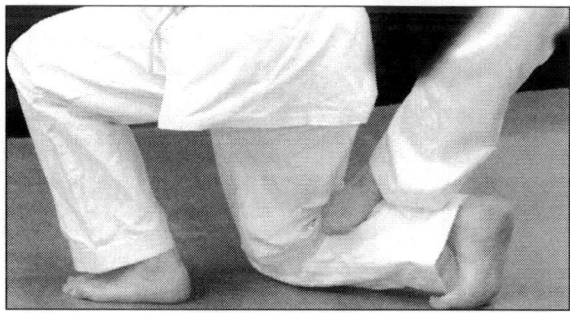

Sesan low-level side kick, applied.

Scooping Block

The next section of Sesan introduces a new technique, the scooping block, which resembles open-hand mid- and low-level blocks. A typical application of the scooping block is to deflect an opponent's attack with one hand, and hook and pull as the other hand strikes the face. This is a surface-level application and is adequate for beginning students, but intermediate students should be thinking of deeper applications. To give you an example of a deeper meaning of scooping block, Tou'on-ryu students are taught that this technique can be an entangling technique (*karamidi*), and they should think along these lines when applying the technique to an opponent. For example, using the block's low-level portion to deflect and seize an attack, and the midlevel portion of the block to entangle the opponent's arm at the elbow and force him down.

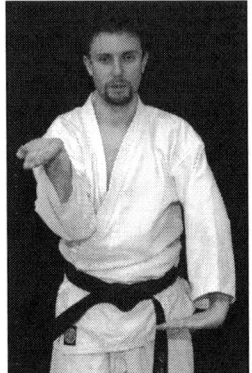 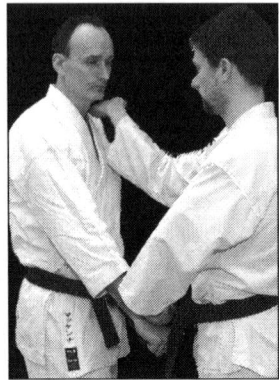 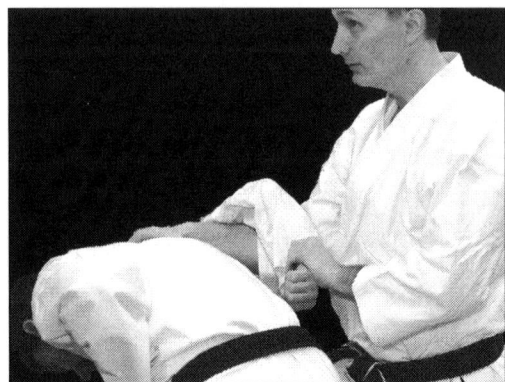

Sesan scoop block and applications.

Combination Punches and Low Side Kick

The next main technique sequence that we'll look at is the combination punches found in Sesan that are performed to the right and left.[4] After blocking the opponent's attack, the defender enters and strikes the opponent with a combination of punches. Although simple in appearance, this technique is very dynamic and powerful. This sort of aggressive punching technique is very rare in mainland Japanese jujutsu, and it is perhaps one reason why there might have been such a strong interest in karate (*toudi*) when it was demonstrated on Okinawa to judo founder Kano Jigoro, and later on the Japanese mainland at the Kodokan. Be that as it may, the combination punch in Sesan is a simple but elegant technique intended to down an opponent quickly.

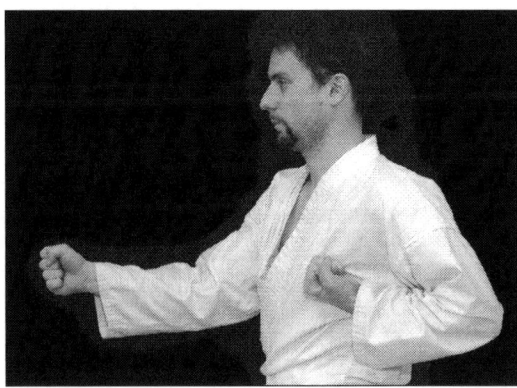

Sesan vertical fist.

The first series of punches consists of a vertical-fist punch followed by two rapid twisting punches. The vertical-fist punch is very important, as it introduces the concept of short power (*chinkuchi*). This image may draw to mind the idea of a "one-inch punch" delivered in Bruce Lee's style (Jeet Kune Do), but instead the idea is to generate maximal force in a swift and relatively short distance. This requires a strong base, which should have been previously developed when practicing Sanchin kata—relaxing the shoulders, elbows in, coordination of the breath, and continuity of reaction forces from the ground through the leg, hips, back, arms, and into the target. This is one reason we traditionally see the progression of the kata as Sanchin to Sesan. After the vertical-fist punch, the two twisting punches are delivered, followed by a low-level block and low-level side kick. We have already discussed this type of punch in the section on Sanchin kata.

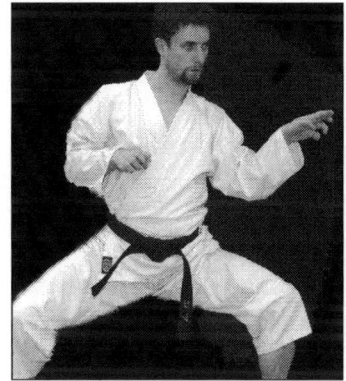
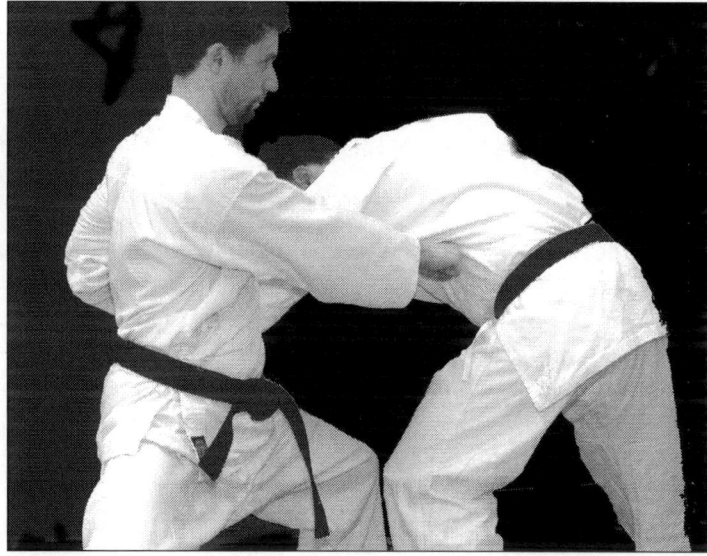

Sesan hooking block and application.

The next punching sequence is three twisting punches performed to the opposite side. Before we discuss this sequence, let's spend a few moments looking at the movement just before the punches. It consists of sliding forward, dropping into a horse stance, and performing a hooking block. A rather nice analogy for this technique is to think of a tiger pouncing on its prey and grasping it with its claws. With the attacker temporarily immobilized, three rapid-fire punches are delivered. The rhythm of these punches may vary, but they are all delivered with a heavy feel to them, and with a slight downward trajectory.

Uppercut, Backfist, Dropping Elbow Strike, Low-Level Block, Hook Punch, and Low Side Kick

Following the combination punches is a long and complex sequence of techniques delivered in rapid succession. Most of these techniques are encountered in Sesan kata for the first time and introduce a novel set of tools to be learned and mastered. Although there are a bewildering number of uses of these techniques, we will just focus on a few of the less obvious ones to show their utility. The first one we will look at incorporates locking and throwing techniques and was popularized by the late Goju-ryu Shoreikan founder, Toguchi Seikichi (1917–1998) (see, Toguchi, Wikipedia). It involves seizing the attacker's right arm, delivering the uppercut and backfist to the face, and then using the dropping elbow to lock and secure the arm. The low-level block is then used to prop the inside knee, and the attacker is rolled forward, somewhat like the judo throws *tomoenage* (circle throw) or *taniotoshi* (valley drop).

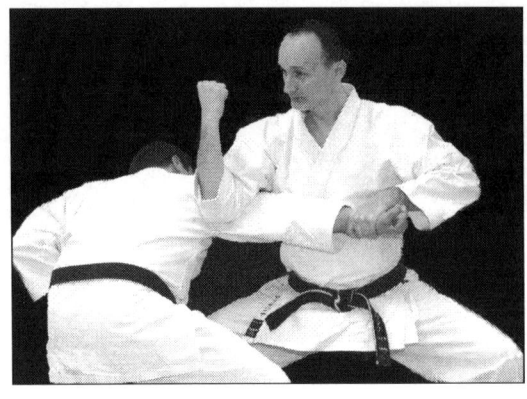 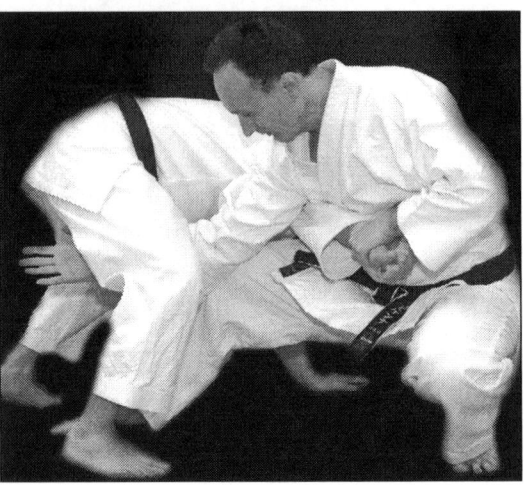

Sesan throwing progression.

The next application we will look at is less spectacular, but perhaps a bit more practical, especially since it incorporates the idea of karamidi. Like the previous example, it starts with seizing the attacker's arm, but from the outside, and then delivering the uppercut and backfist strikes to the face. The dropping elbow strike is used to bend the attacker's arm at the elbow, while the low-level block strikes the groin and then encircles the attacker's arm to lock it. With the attacker secured, the hook punch delivers a strike to the face, and the low side kick is used to kick or throw the attacker to the ground.

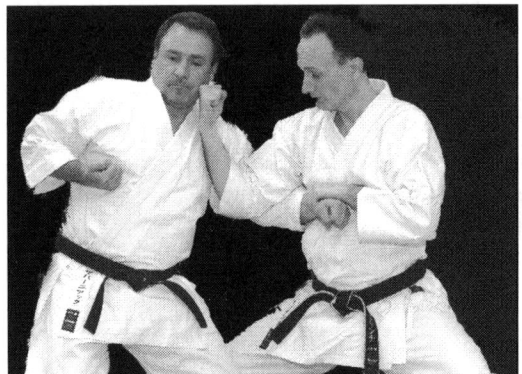 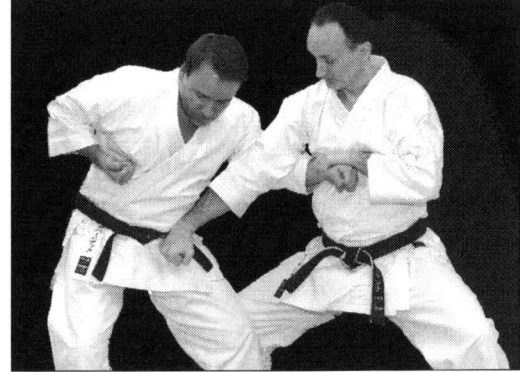

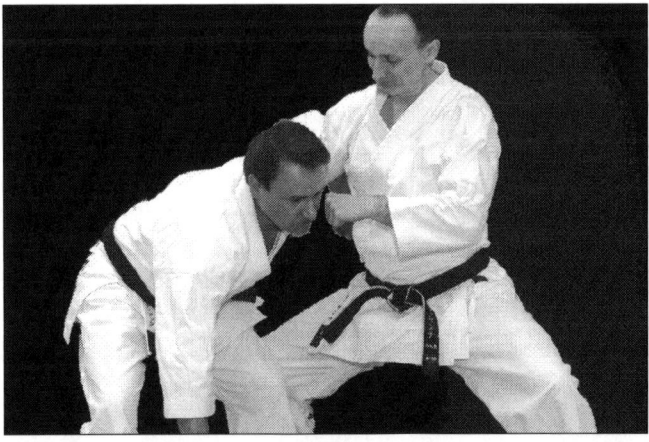

Sesan backfist and entangled.

Front Kick and Reverse Punch

The next segment of Sesan we'll look at is the front kick and reverse punch combination. The front kick is the second kick introduced in Sesan after the low-level side kick. It is executed by seizing the opponent and kicking directly into his body. The next technique after the front kick is the reverse punch. Previously, this punch was taught using Sanchin stance, but now it is performed in a forward stance while the other hand simultaneously does a palm block. At face value, this technique is quite simple and brutally effective, but, as with other techniques, there are various levels to applying it.

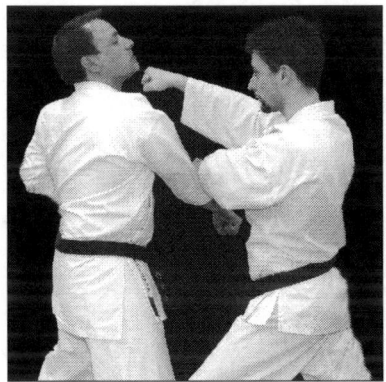
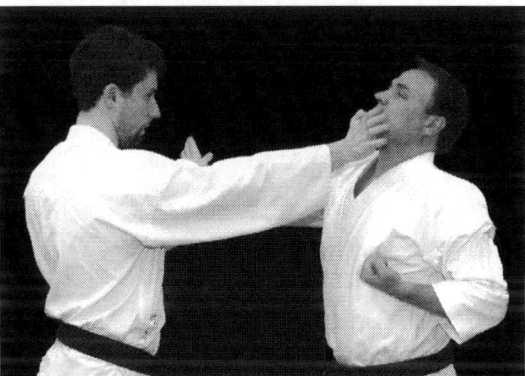

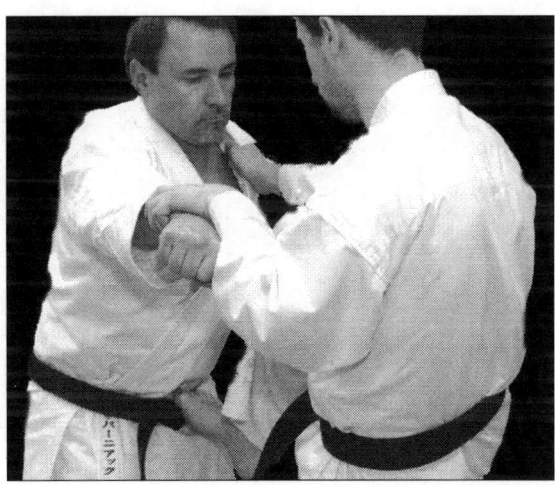

Sesan applications: 1) sweeping block/strike 2) palm-heel 3) front kick.

Cat Stance and Circle Block

Sesan ends by performing a circle block from the cat stance. As I have already talked about the circle block, I won't discuss it here, but I will touch upon the importance of the cat stance. The cat stance provides the defender with a new protective strategy. In modern karate, it is typically explained as a fighting posture, but this runs counter to old-style karate (*toudi*), which does not use static postures (Nakasone, 1938: 86). Although there are many uses for the cat stance, in Sesan kata it is used in conjunction with a circle block. In this context, tora guchi is used to capture and ensnare (*karamidi*) the opponent's arms, and the cat stance is used to move the defender's center of gravity in order to drop the opponent to the ground. It also allows the quick delivery of a kick with the lead leg.

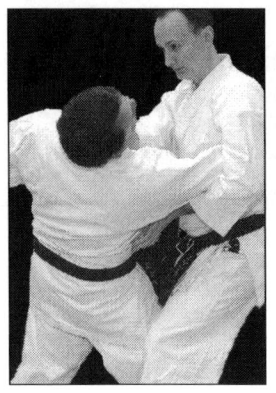 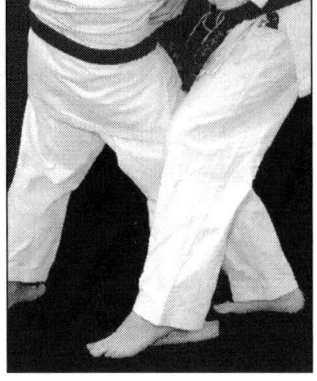

Left: Sesan circle block application.

Right: applied with leg sweep.

Notes

1. There are other variations that exist (e.g., Okinawa Kenpo, Motobu-ryu, etc.), but these are minor katas and will not be considered for the purpose of this article, as they follow essentially the same form and have the same technical content.
2. This same technique is overtly shown in the Uechi-ryu kata Sanseru, but in place of a regular fist, a one-knuckle fist is used.
3. Interestingly enough, in Tou'on-ryu and Uechi-ryu, Sesan is taught before Sanseru.
4. Of note are the twisting combination punches that are only found in Sesan, and not seen in Sanchin, Sanseru, or Suparimpei/Pechurin. Likewise, they are also not found in Saifa, Seiunchin, Sepai, Shisochin, or Kururunfa.

Acknowledgments

I would like to extend my sincerest thanks to Mr. Maik Hassel for taking the photographs that illustrate this article, and to Mr. Olivier Riche and Mr. Brent Zaparniuk for posing for the photographs.

Bibliography

Câmara, F. and McKenna, M. (2007). A preliminary analysis of Goju-ryu kata structure. *Journal of Asian Martial Arts*, 16 (4), 46–53.

Hirakami, N. (2001). Koden Ryukyu Kenpo: Nahate no Himitsu. *Gekkan Hiden*: Issues 1–10.

Kinjo, A. (1999). Karate denshin roku. Okinawa: Tosho Center.

Kumemura. http://en.wikipedia.org/wiki/Kumemura

McKenna, M. & Swift, C. (2002). Etmology of Goju Ryu kata. *Dragon Times*: 21: 12–13, 35.

McKenna, M. (2001). Chinese boxing master Go Ken Ki: Okinawan karate. *Dragon Times*, 20, 13–15.

McKenna, M. (2000a). To-on-ryu: A glimpse into karate-do's roots. *Journal of Asian Martial Arts*, 9(3), 32–43.

McKenna, M. (2000b). Exploring Goju Ryu's past, part 1 and 2. *Dragon Times*, 19: 18–19; 15–17.

Nakasone, G. (2009). *An overview of karatedo–English Translation and Commentary by Mario McKenna*. Raleigh, N.C.: Lulu Press.

Takamiyagi, S. (1996). Sanchin and its five cardinal points (pg. 158). publisher?

Toguchi. http://en.wikipedia.org/wiki/Seikichi_Toguchi

Tokashiki, I. (1991). *Gohaku-kai nenkanshi*. Naha: Published privately.

chapter 59

Nahate: The Old-School Okinawan Martial Art and Its Original Four-Kata Curriculum, Part II

Mario McKenna, M.S.

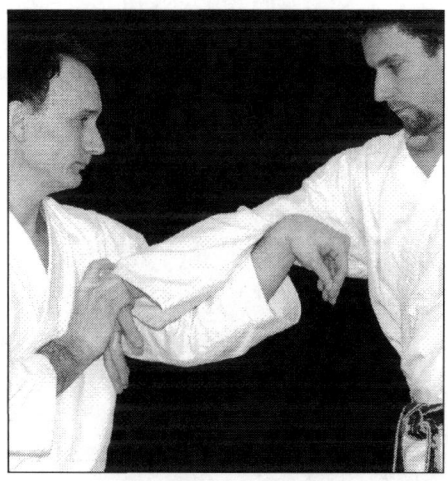

Photographs courtesy of Mario McKenna.

Sanseru Kata 三十六

If you were to ask a Nahate student what is one of the most notable techniques of Sanseru, he would probably answer that it is the use of the elbow. The elbow strike is referred to as *enpiuchi* or *hijiate* in Japanese, and is a powerful technique in the old karate (Okinawan: *toudi*) arsenal. Compared to the fist, the elbow is much stronger, larger, and closer to the body, which allows it to concentrate more energy into a strike. It also requires less impact training (e.g., makiwara) compared to the fist, and is less prone to injury. Perhaps a better saying than the traditional karate maxim of "One punch, one kill" would be "One elbow, one kill." Before examining the elbow strike and other techniques in Sanseru, let's review a little bit of Sanseru's and its different versions.

Odd Man Out
Sanseru is the odd man out in Nahate katas. Compared to the other main Nahate katas, it seems like a kata with multiple personalities. When we examine the Higaonna Kanryo (1850–1915) lineage of Sanseru, we can see three main versions:[1]

1) Miyagi Chojun (宮城長順 1888–1952) version,
2) Kyoda Juhatsu (許田 重発 1887–1968) version, and
3) Higa Seko (比嘉 世幸 1898–1966) version.

I must admit my bias at this point and feel that the Kyoda version is probably the closest to the original that Higaonna taught. There is enough anecdotal evidence to argue for this. There are stories of Miyagi's being upset when he returned from his military duty to find out that Kyoda had learned Sanseru; Kyoda's being noted as an expert in this kata and performing it at many festivals and demonstrations; Miyagi's deferring to Kyoda with respect to Sanseru kata among his students; the presence of the midlevel block, front kick, and elbow strike—which are signature techniques of Miyagi found in his version of Sanseru—and Miyagi katas Gekisai I and II; and the statement from Miyagi Kei (1919–2009) (Miyagi Chojun's son) that his father learned this kata from Kyoda. Ironically, however, compared to the Kyoda, the Miyagi version is now the most common version taught in the majority of Goju-ryu dojos around the world.

The Higa version of Sanseru is a bit of a conundrum in that it seems to mix the Miyagi and Kyoda versions. We shouldn't really be surprised at this given the dual influence of Miyagi and Higaonna on Higa Seko.[2] This alone might be enough reason to explain the hybrid nature of the Higa Sanseru.[3] The Higa Sanseru has many techniques mixed from the Miyagi and Kyoda versions, as well as its own unique techniques. For example, like the Kyoda version, there is a knee strike in place of the double kick at the beginning. Like the Miyagi version, it uses the midlevel block, front kick, and elbow combination. And uniquely it turns in the opposite direction when performing the final crane posture.

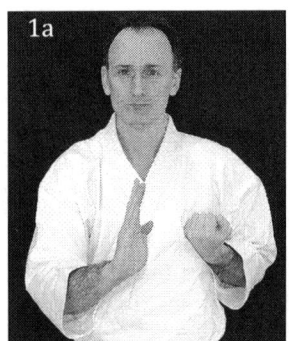
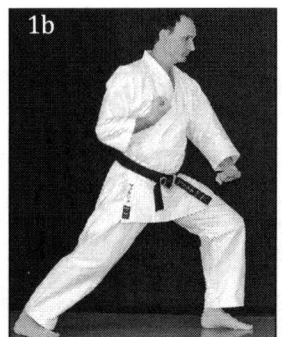
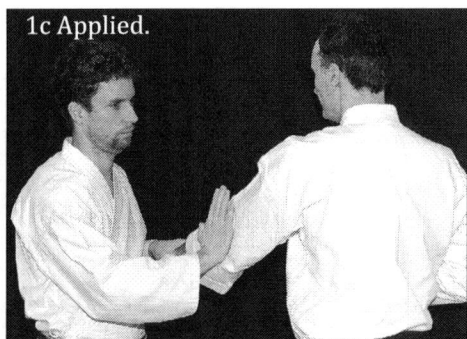

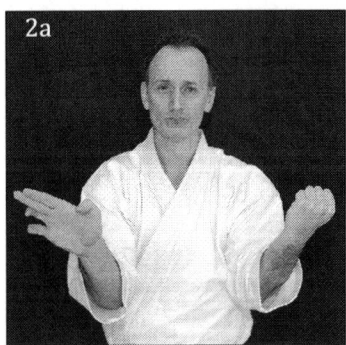
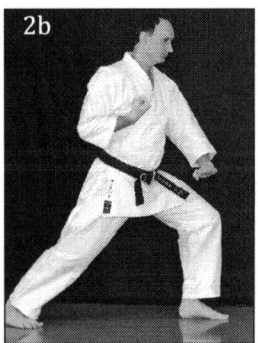
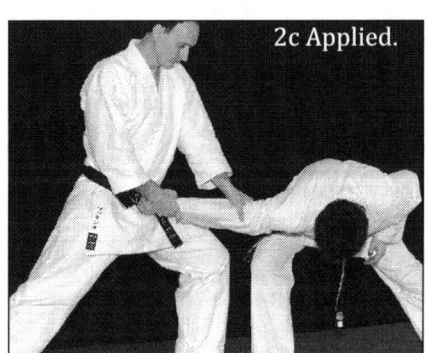

1a-c: Sanseru Goju escape and lock.   2a-c: Sanseru Tou'on escape and lock.

Escape Technique and Joint Lock

Like Sanchin and Sesan earlier, Sanseru kata begins with three steps in Sanchin stance in combination with three reverse punches and three midlevel blocks. The first major technique after this sequence is an escape and joint lock technique akin to the aikijujutsu wristlock (*nikkajo*), although there are some differences in how the technique is performed in the Kyoda, Miyagi, and Higa versions. The seized wrist is used to secure the opponent's hand, while the other hand locks the opponent's elbow. The opponent's balance is broken by stepping back into a forward stance, which also provides additional leverage.

Elbow Strike, Hook Punch, and Low Side Kick

Sanseru introduces the vertical elbow strike in conjunction with a forward stance. The forward stance deserves a bit of discussion at this point. One of the first things we should notice is that the forward stance appears often in the Sanseru kata, is absent in the Sanchin kata, and only appears once in the Sesan kata. We should stop and ask ourselves why that is. As we saw earlier in the opening segment of Sanseru, the forward stance provides greater leverage and the ability to break the opponent's balance when we execute the escape and joint lock technique. However, there is much more to the forward stance than this. In Sanseru, the forward stance is used as a means of moving quickly forward to enter and occupy an opponent's space, and to transfer body weight into the strike. When this is combined with the use of the vertical elbow, the result is a technique that can crush an opponent.

At this point we should note that there are substantial differences among the three versions with respect to the techniques performed before the vertical elbow strike. In the Higa and Miyagi versions, a midlevel block and front kick are performed in Sanchin stance, while in the Kyoda version, an inverted rising block in Sesan stance is performed with no kick. These are very important differences that need to be considered when examining the evolution of Sanseru kata—or any Nahate kata, for that matter. It provides a sort of a DNA signature, if you will. At any rate, this difference in the stances and techniques performed prior to the execution of the vertical elbow strike is important, as it changes the dynamics and functionality of the technique quite drastically. The Kyoda version teaches much more clearly the importance of entering straight into a technique (*irimi*).

Sanseru Goju-ryu elbow sequence and application.

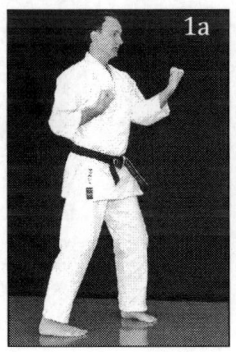
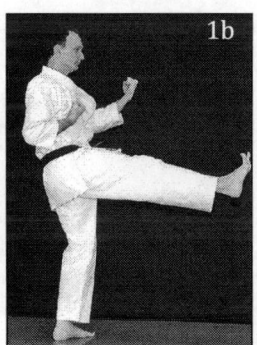
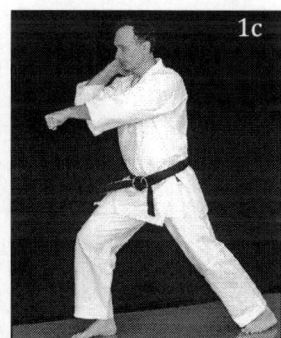
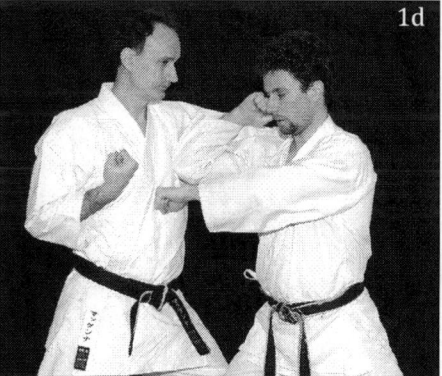

Following the vertical elbow strike, a left punch is delivered. Here there are some minor variations, with the Higa and Kyoda versions remaining in a half-facing (*hanmi*) forward stance before delivering the punch, while the Miyagi version squares the waist and performs the punch. Functionally the technique is the same in all the versions and is typically used as a quick follow-up strike to the elbow strike.

The final portion of this sequence is the low side kick, and here we can see differences among the different versions. In the Miyagi and Higa versions, the leg is drawn back slowly, then the kick is delivered quickly, and then retracted quickly and placed on the ground. In the Kyoda version, the leg is pulled back rapidly, the kick delivered quickly, but the leg is left extended, and then placed on the ground. Regardless of how the technique is performed, there are many interesting uses for the low side kick. At a superficial level, much like Sesan earlier, the kick can be delivered directly to the knee with very dangerous consequences. However, as I discussed in the Sesan portion, there are many other interesting uses for this technique, some of which include throws and sweeps, and Sanseru introduces a new perspective on how to use them.

Sanseru Tou'on-ryu elbow sequence and application.

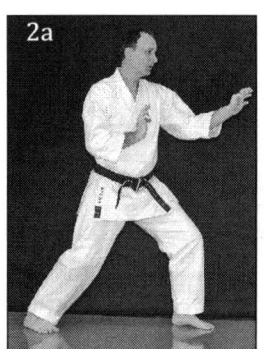
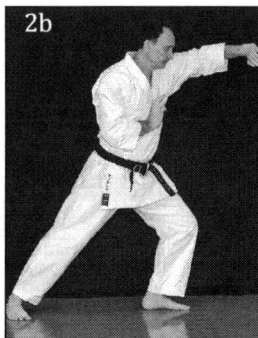
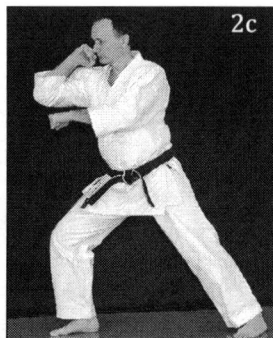
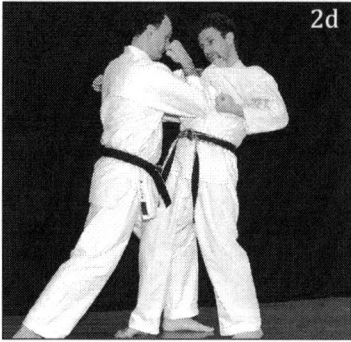

Below: Sanseru elbow sequence variation applied.

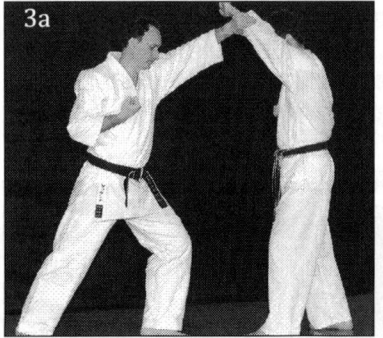
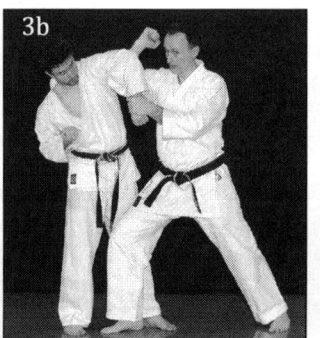
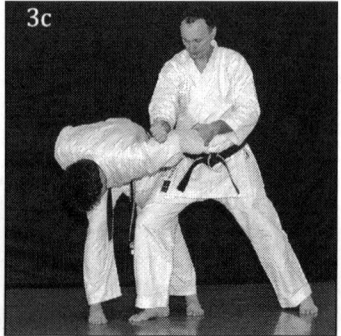

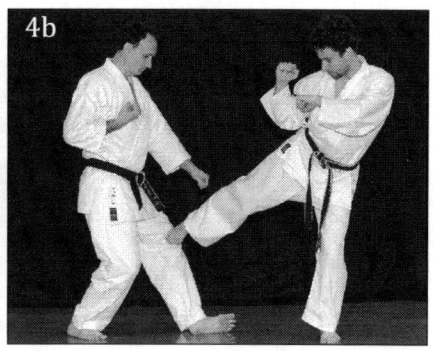

Sanseru
Goju-ryu
Tou'on-ryu
low side kick.

Low Cross Block

The next portion of the kata has the performer execute two separate low cross blocks in succession: one with open hands and one with fists, in a horse stance. The sequence in the Miyagi and Higa versions is with an open-hand block first, followed by a fist block, while in the Kyoda version, the sequence is reversed. Regardless of the sequence of open to closed block or vice versa, the low cross block is an interesting technique. On the surface this technique could be interpreted literally as a low block, perhaps against a kick, but, as I stated previously, form does not always follow function. Of course with a little experimentation it is also soon apparent that this is a very superficial and potentially dangerous technique to use by the defender. Instead we should remember that karate has many jujutsu-like applications found in its katas, and a key concept is the use of entangling techniques (*karamidi*). This gives us a clue to decipher its meaning. For example, in the Kyoda version of Sanseru, this section of the kata is taught as a joint lock and rotary throw, somewhat similar to aikido's rotary throw (*kaiten nage*).

SANSERU X-BLOCKS

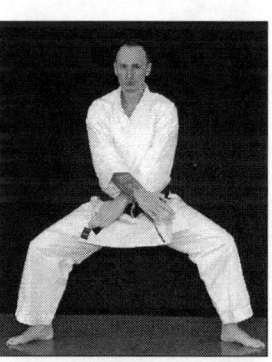

Sanseru
X-block sequence.

1A–C) Sanseru
Goju-ryu.

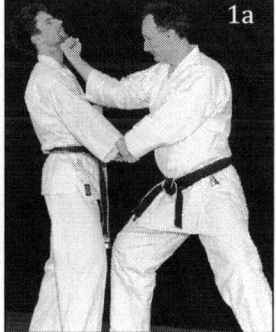
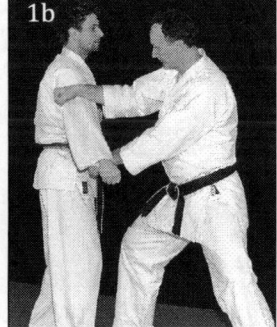
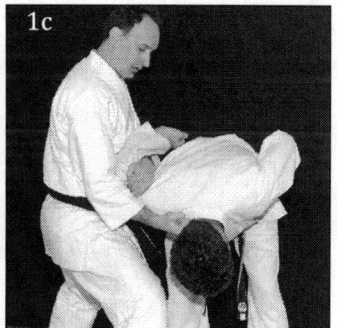

Sanseru
X-block sequence.

2a–c) Sanseru Tou'on-ryu.

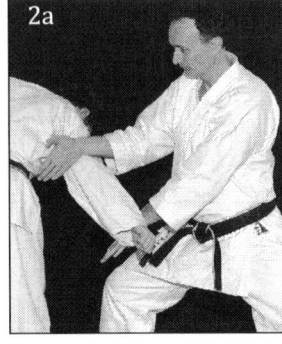
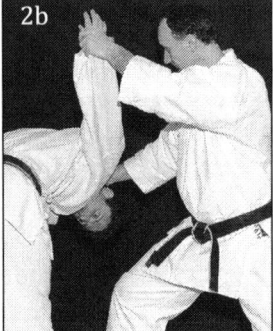
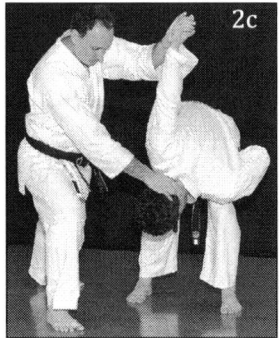

Double Block and Double Punch

The next technique that we will look at is the double block and double punch combination found near the end of Sanseru. Here again the three versions of Sanseru differ in their execution of the technique, with the Miyagi version transitioning from a horse stance to a Sanchin stance, the Higa version transitioning from a rooted stance to a natural stance, and the Kyoda version transitioning from a cat stance to a forward stance. The differences in stances are important because they dictate the position of the hands in the double block. In the Miyagi version, which uses a horse stance, the hips are turned in, and therefore the arms are held close to the body. In contrast, the Higa and Kyoda versions use a natural stance and a forward stance so the hips are turned out, and therefore the arms are extended. This changes the function of the technique somewhat, but at its heart it is a technique for seizing control of the opponent.

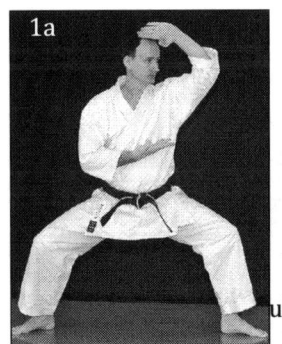
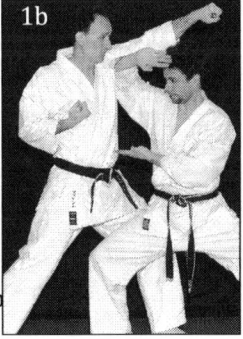
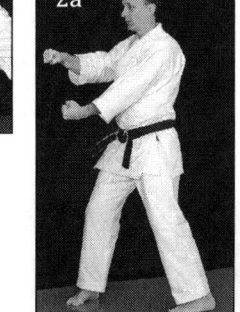
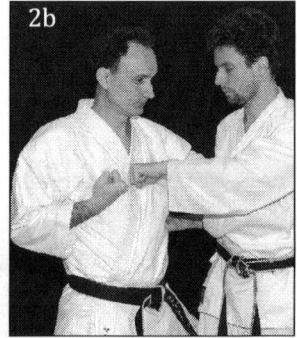

1A) Sanseru Goju-ryu double block. 1B) Applied.

2A) Sanseru Goju-ryu double block. 2B) Applied.

The double block is followed by a double punch, which is a new technique and was not found in the Sanchin or Sesan kata. Interestingly the double punch is also a technique rarely found in Japanese jujutsu, and we can say that it is unique to karate (Hirakami, 2000). There are various applications based on different instructors' teachings, the most rudimentary of which is to use this technique to deflect an opponent's attack and simultaneously strike the body. Of course, there are more interesting and dangerous techniques, especially when linked to the previous double block technique and the entangling technique concept (*karamidi*) is incorporated into it.

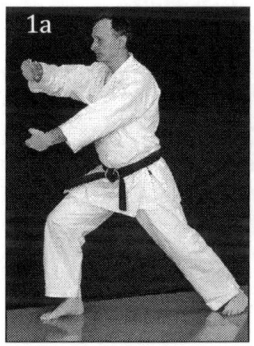 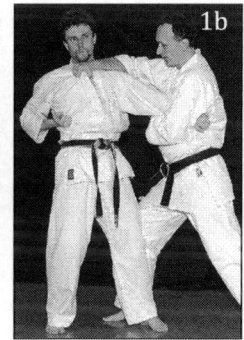 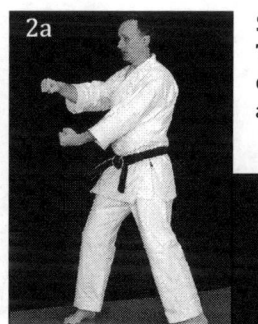

Sanseru Tou'on-ryu double blocks and applications.

Crane Posture

At the end of Sanseru the performer executes the crane posture. This posture consists of one arm extended and the other held close to the body with the wrists of both hands bent and the fingers bunched together. In Sanseru, the crane posture is performed with a turning movement, with the performer finishing in a horse stance. Here again the three versions of Sanseru differ in the direction and the number of degrees they turn. The Miyagi version turns approximately 220° to the right, the Higa version turns to the left approximately 50°, and the Kyoda version turns 90° to the right. The direction and number of degrees of the turn are important, as they dictate the angle and direction of entry. However, if we apply the entangling principle (*karamidi*), we can see that one use of this technique is to lock the opponent's arm and drop him to the ground.

With the progression from Sanchin to Sesan, and now to Sanseru, an interesting observation begins to emerge. All three Nahate katas begin with the fundamental midlevel deflection, and punch from Sanchin stance repeated three times, then introduce an escape technique, followed by a new impact technique, before then finishing with a grappling technique—a pedagogically sound progression.

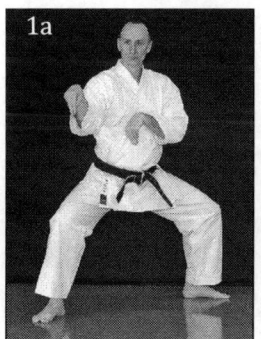 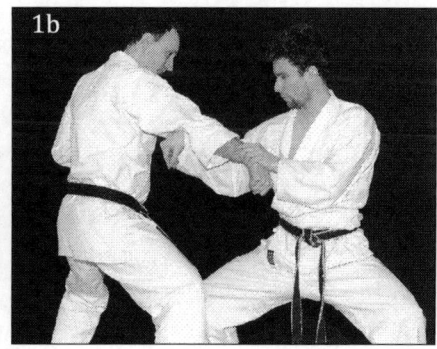

1A) Sanseru Goju crane posture.
1B) Application.

There is a reason this final posture is referred to as the crane posture, much like why a circle block is sometimes referred to as "tiger mouth" (*tora guchi*), but to explain this might be giving too much away. So I will leave it up to the readers to ponder this by themselves, but not without providing a hint. Sanchin and Sesan katas end with the tiger-mouth posture, while Sanseru and Suparimpei end with the crane posture (*tsuru no kamae*). In other words, the tiger and the crane combine to create a synergy of karate techniques. This is expressed in the Chinese idiom, "Like a tiger growing wings" (Hirakami, 2000).

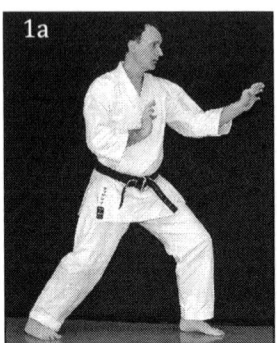
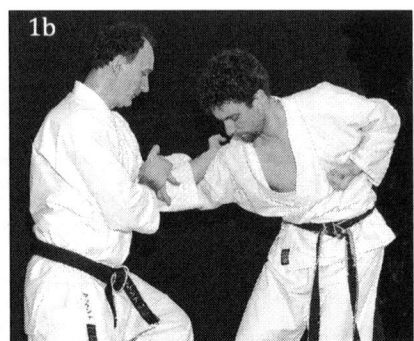

1a) Sanseru Tou'on-ryu crane posture; 2b) Application.

壱百歩連 Pechurin/Bechurin • Suparimpei 壱百零八

After learning the Sanchin, Sesan, and Sanseru katas and coming to an understanding of their techniques, we arrive at the final kata to be learned. But what do we call it? In Goju-ryu it is typically referred to as Suparimpei (and occasionally Pechurin Jo), while in Tou'on-ryu it is called Bechurin or Pechurin (both pronunciations are considered acceptable). There has been much theorizing as to the origin of the names and with respect to which name is correct, but this is beyond the scope of this essay. For those interested in this topic, I would recommend reading the work of Kinjo Akio and Tokashiki Iken. Both researchers present some excellent historical and linguistic research into its possible origins. That said, for the remainder of this part of the series I will use the name Suparimpei to refer to the kata used in Goju-ryu, and Bechurin as the kata used in Tou'on-ryu.

In traditional dojos, from the time a person learns Sanchin to the time he or she learns Suparimpei, it is a very long apprenticeship. But nowadays we see junior high school children performing this kata at regional, national, or international competitions, on DVDs by different instructors, or on the internet, where we are subjected to varying levels of competence. Regardless of the medium, I am inclined to think, as Hirakami Nobuyuki stated, that you cannot help but feel a bit sad because the sense of appreciation toward the opportunity to learn this kata is all but gone (Hirakami, 2000).

Double Palm Strike to the Sides

Like the katas learned before, both Bechurin and Suparimpei use the same base techniques for their opening sequence: advancing three times in Sanchin stance along with three reverse punches and three midlevel blocks. From here the palms are brought in front of the chest and then extended to the right and left in a slow and deliberate manner. In Suparimpei there is a distinct lowering and rising of the body when performing this technique, which is absent from Tou'on-ryu. In addition, Tou'on-ryu uses a thumb strike identical to the one used in Uechi-ryu in place of the palm strike found in Goju-ryu.

An application for this technique is an escape from a double hand grab that simultaneously pulls the opponent and positions him for the next technique. Tou'on-ryu's use of the thumb strike opens up some different applications, especially when we consider the attacker trying to grab hold of you. In Tou'on-ryu the power of the thumb strike is passed down through the story of Yabu Kentsu (屋部 憲通 1866–1937). In their version of the story, during his military days as a sergeant in the Japanese army, Yabu faced court martial for striking and severely injuring a superior officer. An inquiry exonerated him, since Yabu apparently only used his palm to strike the man. However in Tou'on-ryu the damage inflicted was the result of a well-placed thumb strike.

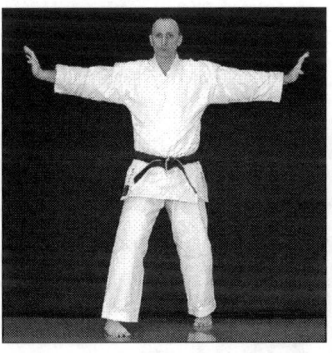

Suparimpei Bechurin Goju-ryu Tou'on-ryu, right and left palm strikes.

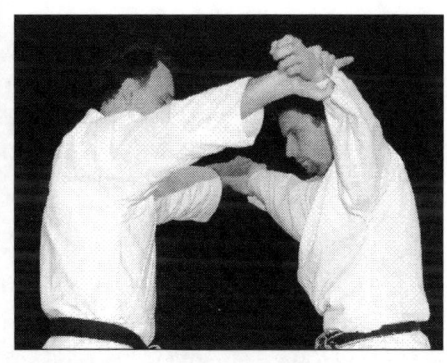

Suparimpei double "palm strike" applied.

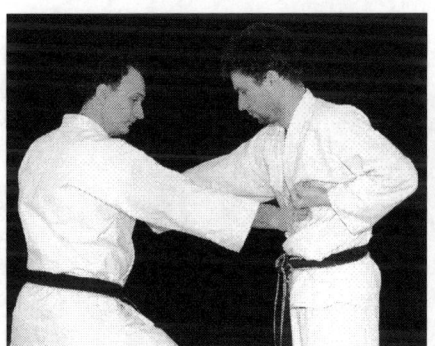

Bechurin double palm strike applied.

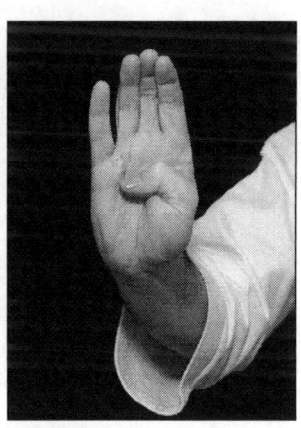

Bechurin Tou'on-ryu thumb strike.

Circle Block, Hooking Block, and Sword-Hand Strike

Following the double palm strike, two circle blocks are performed while moving forward. These are followed by a hooking block and a sword-hand strike. There are some minor differences here between Suparimpei and Bechurin in how the hooking block and sword-hand strike are performed, but the techniques are essentially analogous. Both sets of techniques are repeated to the four compass points. As I mentioned earlier, the circle block has many jujutsu-like applications contained within it. As most of us know, trying to apply any sort of locking technique on a resisting opponent can be very difficult. Performing the circle block twice is one way of overcoming an opponent's resistance by reversing direction and collapsing the opponent backward with an entering throw akin to aikido's iriminage, Tenjin Shinryo-ryu jujutsu's tengusho, or Shotokan's kubiwa. Using two circle blocks in succession is akin to saying that the tiger bites twice (Hirakami, 2000).

After the two circle blocks comes the hooking block and sword-hand strike sequence. There are many different explanations for this technique depending on the teacher and the respective school, but the superficial explanation is to parry, seize an attacker's arm, and to follow up with a strike of your own to the torso. Of course, there is nothing wrong with this explanation, but there are other, more dangerous uses of it. A simple variation would be to hook the head and use the sword-hand to strike the neck.

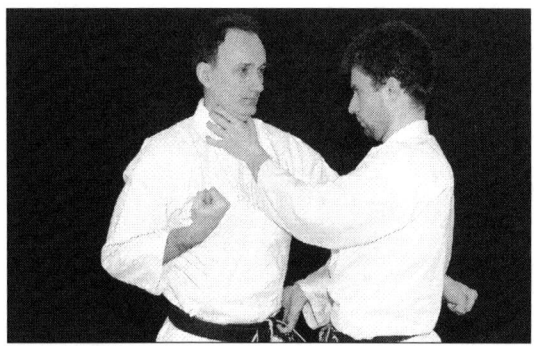

Suparimpei Bechurin circle block applied.

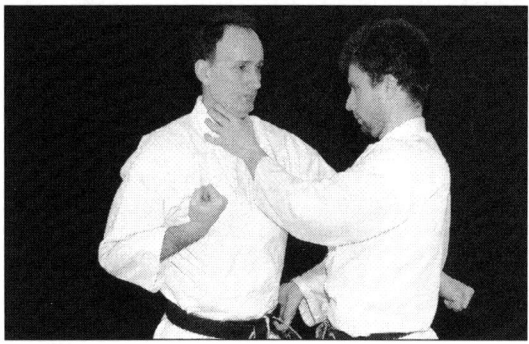

Suparimpei Bechurin finger tip strike applied.

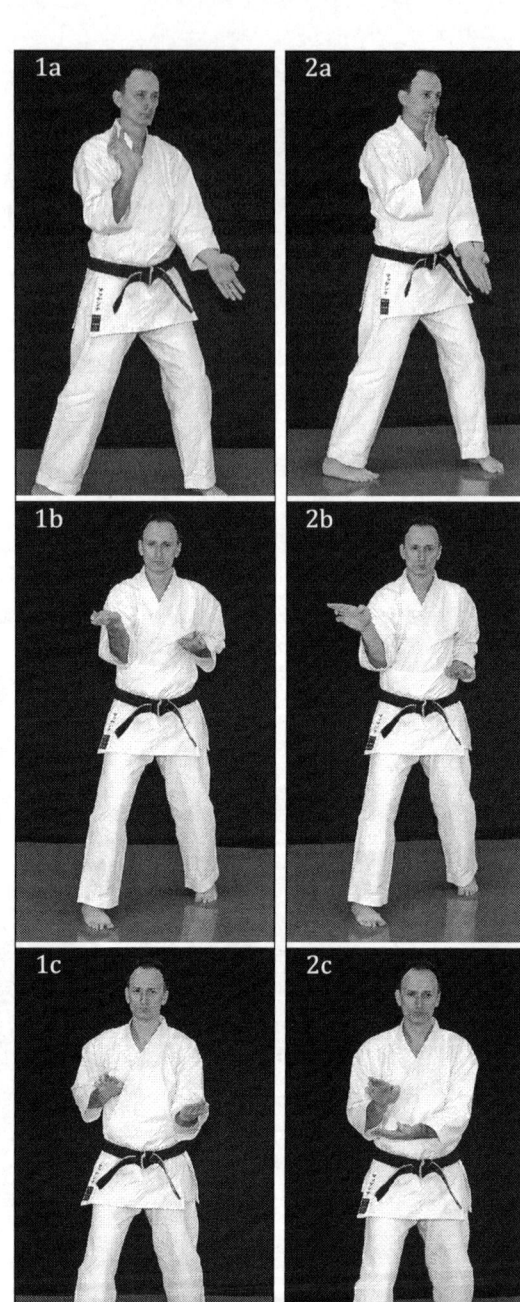

Suparimpei:
1a) circle block,
1b) hook block,
1c) fingertip strike.

Bechurin:
2a) circle block,
2b) hook block,
2c) sword-hand strike.

Circle Block/Backhand Block

The next sequence differs quite markedly between Bechurin and Suparimpei. In Suparimpei there is a series of three circle blocks performed in a cat stance, a pairing of techniques that we have encountered before in the Sesan kata. In Tou'on-ryu we find the use of a backhand block (*ura uke*) performed in a high cat stance. We know from our earlier discussion of Sesan when the cat stance and circle block were introduced, the intention was to entangle an attacker's arms and then drop him to the ground, but since Tou'on-ryu does not use a circle block in this part of the kata, what is the purpose of the backhand block? The answer may lie in an old anecdote provided by the late Matsubayashi-ryu founder Nagamine Shoshin's book. Nagamine (1986:100) describes a technique used in an altercation that involved Higaonna Kanryo. The original Japanese translation reads as follows:

> Kanryo quickly slid back as the punch came towards him and at the
> same time used his right wrist to strike the man's forearm down.[4]

The reference to using the wrist suggests that Higaonna used a backhand block to defend himself. This is the same application that is taught in Tou'on-ryu for this portion of Bechurin kata. Essentially the technique is used to either strike or to seize the limb of the attacker in a fast, whipping action.

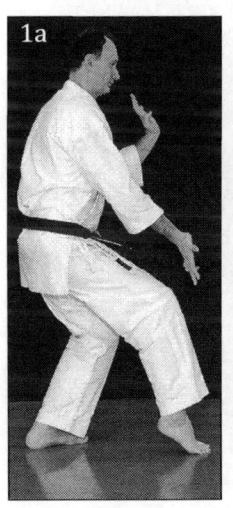
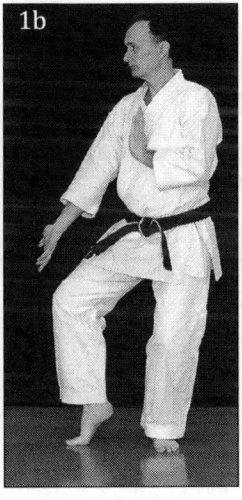
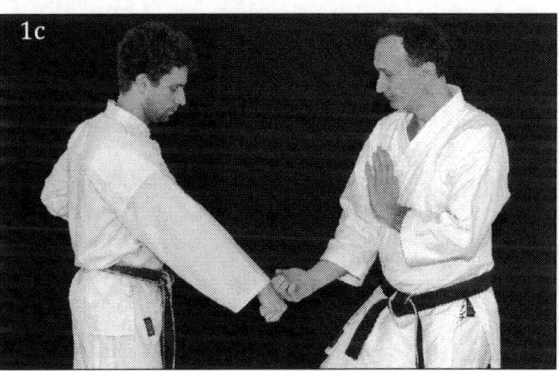

1a) Suparimpei cat stance and circle block.
1b) Bechurin cat stance and back hand block.
1c) Bechurin back of hand block applied.

Entering the Gate

An important characteristic of both Bechurin and Suparimpei is the use of the eight gates or directions. In Sanchin kata the student learns to execute techniques toward the east and west. In Sesan and Sanseru karate this is expanded and students repeat techniques to the four cardinal points of east, west, south, and north.[5] These are expanded upon in the last Nahate kata to include an additional four points on a diagonal plane, so that now techniques are performed to all eight compass points. There are two main reasons for the introduction of these additional four points in Bechurin and Suparimpei. The first is that it brings a very strong sense of spatial awareness that teaches the performer to let loose techniques at will in any direction. The second is that karate is a method of self-protection and as such it is necessary to be able to receive an attack from any direction. Therefore Bechurin and Suparimpei teach the student these concepts in a systematic way.

Double Punch, Low Block, and Reverse Punch

The next sequence we'll look at is the double punch/low bock/reverse punch combination. Here again we see differences between Suparimpei and Bechurin in how these techniques are performed, but we can consider them analogous for the purpose of our discussion. In the previous kata, Sanseru, we saw the introduction of the double punch, but in Bechurin and Suparimpei we have the addition of the low block and reverse punch. The double punch is most often applied as a simultaneous block and counter. However, if we remember the principle of karamidi, then the double punch can entangle the opponent's arms, while the block can also be used to apply a joint lock followed by a reverse punch to finish the opponent. Indeed, there is an overt wrapping motion in the Tou'on-ryu Bechurin kata that clearly shows this technique.

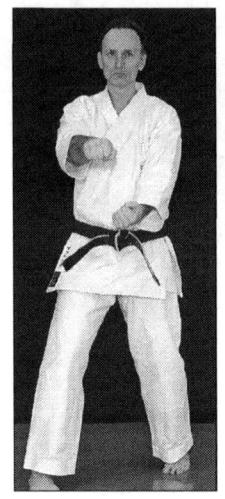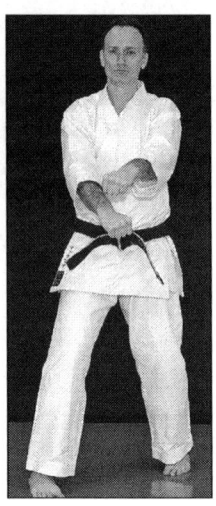

Suparimpei double punch.

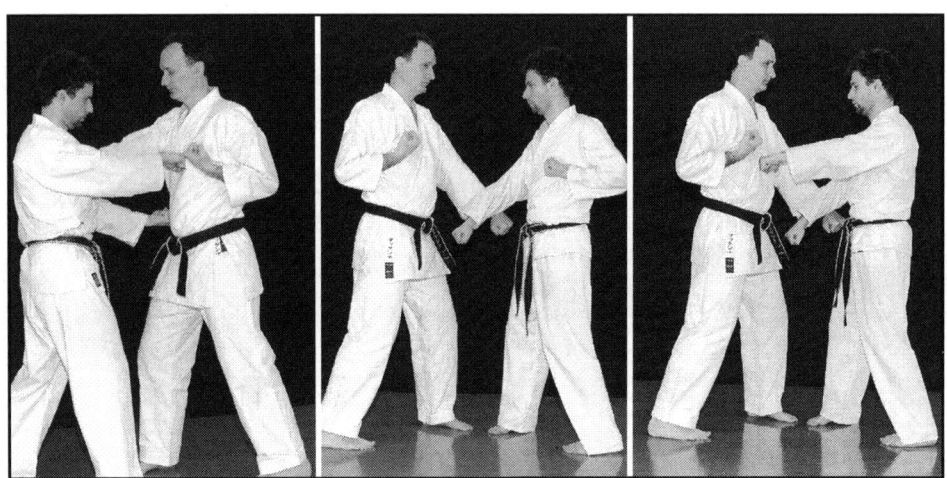

Suparimpei double punch applied.

Uppercut, One-Knuckle Thrust, or Single-Finger Thrust, and Double Low Block

The next sequence also differs between Bechurin and Suparimpei. In Bechurin the performer takes a double guard position with the arms and stands in a forward stance. In this instance, the forward stance is unique in that the upper body is bent forward. In contrast, Suparimpei uses a horse stance and also assumes a double guard position, but the hands are held either in a one-knuckle fist or a single-finger hand.[6] The one-knuckle fist is formed by protruding the first joint of the index finger and supporting it with the thumb. The single-finger hand is formed by extending the index finger, bending the remaining fingers at the first joint, and tightly squeezing the fingers together.

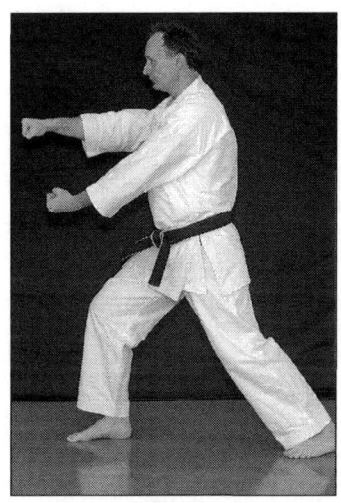
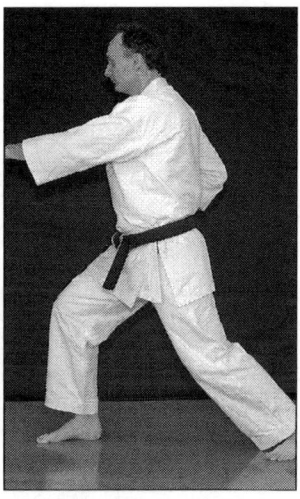

Bechurin double punch.

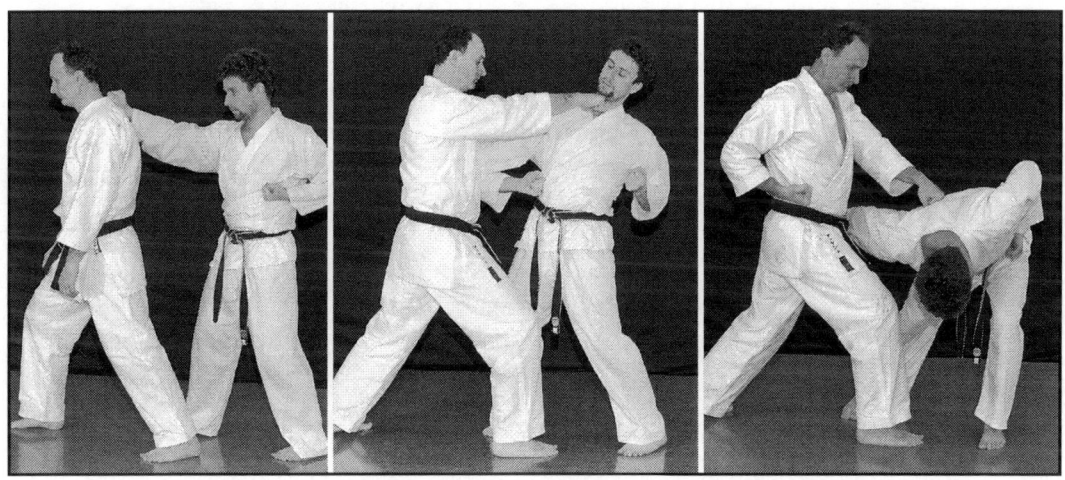

Bechurin double punch applied.

From these respective stances and hand postures, both katas deliver strikes, but again there is an apparent difference in the target area. In Bechurin the uppercut is directed toward the head. Suparimpei, on the other hand, appears to direct its strike to the torso from a horse stance. This is a very interesting difference and somewhat paradoxical. Both the one-knuckle fist and the single-finger hand lack strength in directly attacking the torso, but are excellent tools for attacking the face or other vital points. Yet only Bechurin overtly attacks the face. This is something I would ask the reader to consider.

The next movement in both Bechurin and Suparimpei involves dropping down into a horse stance and executing a double low block. At face value, this technique is a little difficult to understand, but if we remember that entangling, seizing, and locking techniques are part of all the Nahate katas, then we can work out the meaning of this technique. This would imply that the initial double guard position is used to grab or entangle the attacker's arm, and then stepping through to strike redoubles its power. This also allows the defender to transition into the horse stance, where the double low block makes more sense. A simple example would be to use the double low block to not only apply a joint lock, but also to use it as a hammer strike.

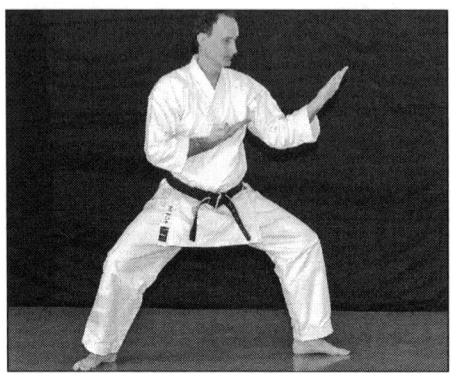
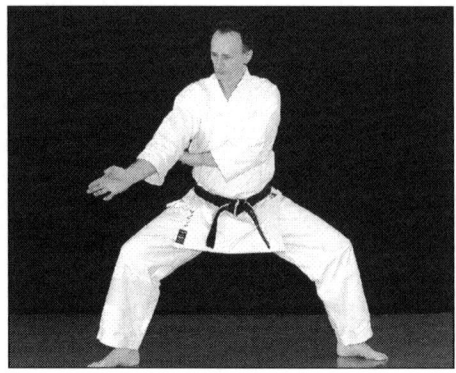

Left: Suparimpei Higa double guard.   Right: Suparimpei Higa hand strike.

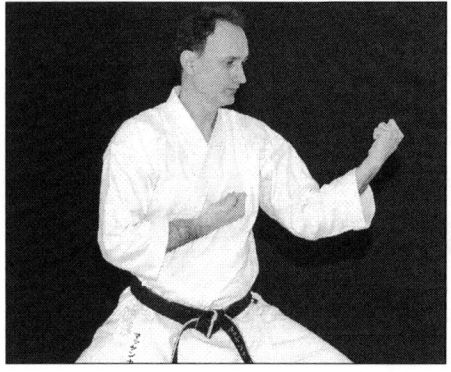
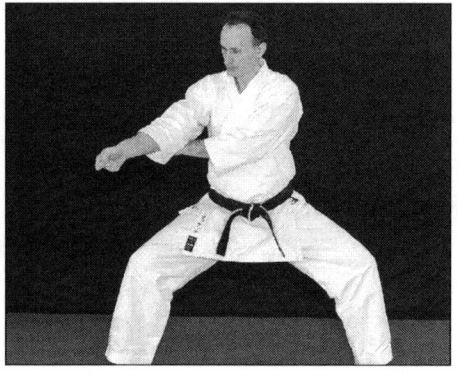

Left: Suparimpei Miyagi double guard.   Right: Suparimpei Miyagi hand strike.

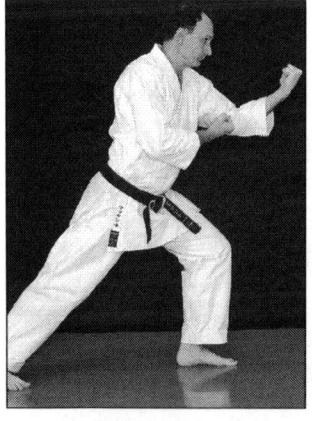
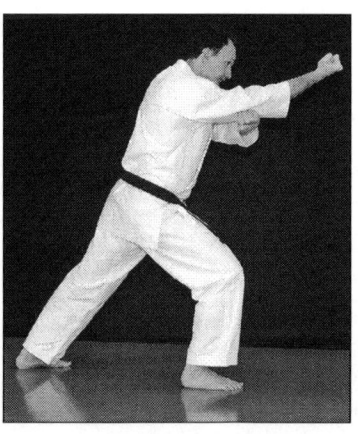

Left: Bechurin double guard.   Right: Bechurin upper cut.

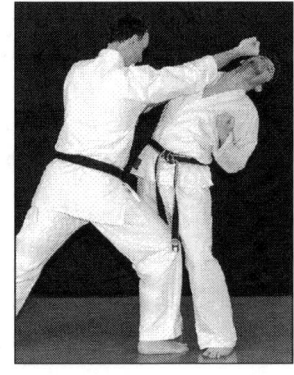 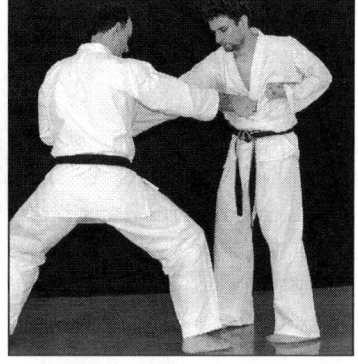

Left: Bechurin double guard applied.   Right: Suparimpei double guard applied.

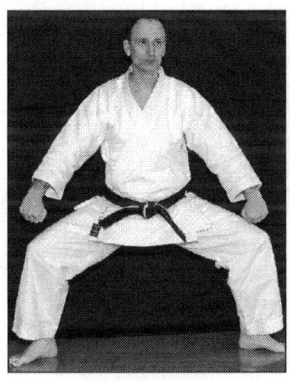 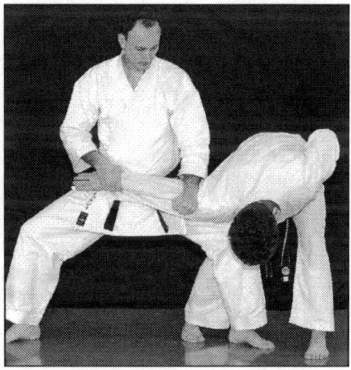

Left: Suparimpei Bechurin double low block. Right: Suparimpei Bechurin double low block applied.

Divergence

After the double low block, there is a divergence in the techniques performed between Suparimpei and Bechurin. Bechurin lacks the pressing block, front kick, horizontal elbow strike, backfist strike, and hand escape; the follow-up elbow strike, backfist strike; and the final finger-tip strike before the crane posture.[7] Therefore, for the remaining part of this discussion I will focus on the techniques common in both katas.

Crescent Kick

The crescent kick in Suparimpei is preceded by a 360° turn, whereas in Bechurin it is preceded by an 180° turn. The kick in both katas is performed at head height, with the right leg into the palm of the left hand. This technique is commonly seen as a wrist escape in Goju-ryu, or as a kick to the opponent's face in both Tou'on-ryu and Goju-ryu. In Tou'on-ryu the crescent kick is also sometimes applied as a flying kick followed by a low sweep, similar to some Northern Chinese gongfu systems. Regardless, these are surface-level applications and not very satisfying. When examining this technique, it is vital to remember that karate is a method of self-protection and applications must be applied in this context.

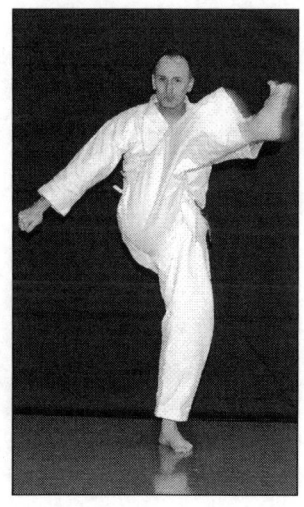

Suparimpei Bechurin crescent kick.

Double Kick

Immediately after the crescent kick, a double kick is performed in both katas. In Suparimpei this takes the form of two consecutive snapping front kicks delivered after jumping vertically. The Tou'on-ryu method is quite different in that the performer also leaps vertically, but the kick is executed with the legs straight, giving the outward appearance of a vertical scissor kick. Each of these methods has its own unique applications, but at a rudimentary level the double kick is used to finish an attacker after controlling his body. For the Suparimpei kata, one of the more interesting applications that I learned from Tokashiki Iken (founder of the Goju-ryu Tomarite Association) could be described as a bando-style knee strike, in which you place one foot on the opponent's hip and use it to launch a knee strike with the other leg to the head.

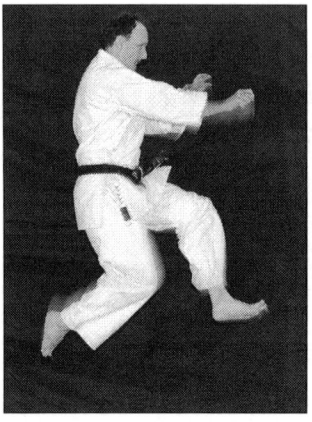 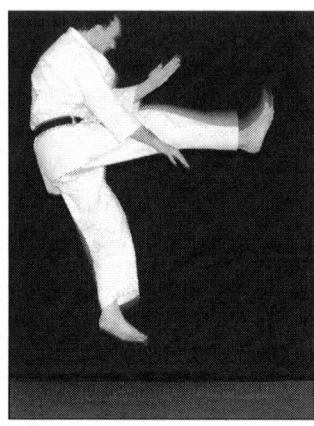

Left: Suparimpei double kick.   Right: Bechurin double kick.

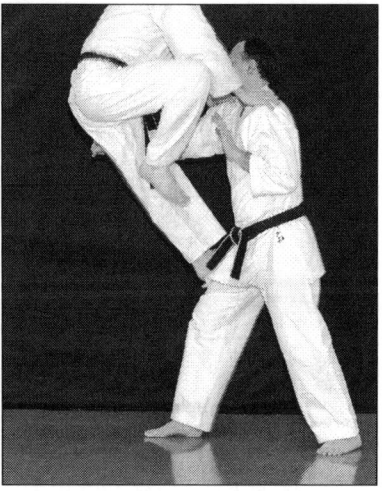

Suparimpei Bechurin double kick applied.

Crane Posture

As with Sanseru, this is the final combative posture, and here also differences emerge between Suparimpei and Bechurin. In Suparimpei the performer does not spin as much compared to Sanseru, but still ends in a horse stance. There are also some minor intergroup differences between the Miyagi and Higa versions, with the hands forming the crane posture traveling from high to middle in the Higa version and from low to middle in the Miyagi version. In Bechurin there is no turning at all, and the performer simply steps back and assumes the crane posture with the hands. But interestingly this is immediately followed by a hooking block. This difference may be the result of the *kuden* (spoken lessons) handed down in Tou'on-ryu, which says that the final combative posture of any kata is not fixed once the kata is learned and understood. As we have already discussed the crane posture and its use in the section on Sanseru kata, I will not explain it here, but would encourage the reader to think about her own applications—especially when applying the principle of *tuidi* (grappling), *karamidi* (entangling), *chugedi* (locking), and other ideas that have been introduced in this article.

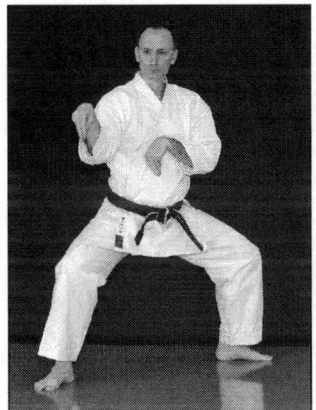 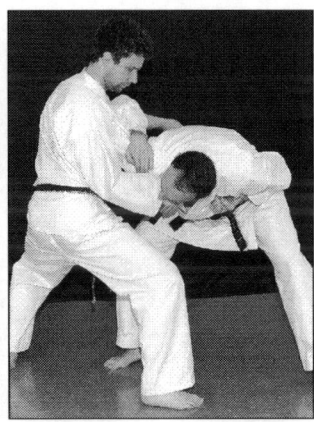

Left: Suparimpei crane posture. Right: Suparimpei crane posture applied.

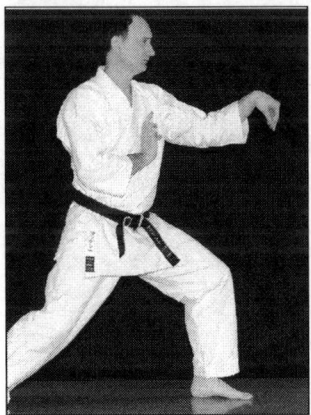 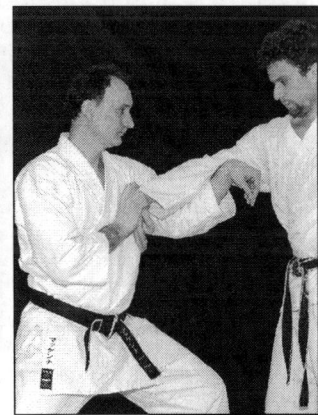

Left: Bechurin crane posture.
Right: Bechurin crane posture applied.

Right: Bechurin crane posture applied.

Notes

1. Though historically important, we will limit our discussion to the Higaonna Sanseru kata and exclude the Uechi-ryu version of the same kata.
2. See http://en.wikipedia.org/wiki/Seko_Higa.
3. As an aside, many of Higa Seko's students know and teach the Miyagi version of Sanseru, as well as the Higa version of the same kata. More recently, the main Higa lineage group, the International Karatedo Kobudo Federation, emphasizes the Miyagi version to more freely interact with other Goju-ryu associations and events with respect to kata.
4. This translation was done by the author of this article, Mario McKenna.
5. Traditionally, katas were started facing the east, and this direction is commonly noted in many earlier karate books from the 1920s and 1930s.
6. The single-finger hand is also called the "blade of grass" hand and is illustrated in the *Bubishi*. This hand formation is more commonly found in the Higa lineage of Suparimpei.
7. As an aside, this is one possible explanation that I would put forward regarding the difference in names between Suparimpei and Bechurin.

Bibliography

Hirakami, N. (2001). Koden Ryukyu kenpo: Nahate no himitsu (The ancient transmission of Ryukyu boxing: The secret of Nahate). *Gekkan Hiden* ([Martial] Secrets Monthly): Issues 1–10.

Kinjo, A. (1999). *Karate denshin roku* (A true record of the transmission of karate). Okinawa: Tosho Center.

Nagamine, S. (1986). *Okinawa karate sumo meijin-den* (Tales of Okinawa's karate and sumo masters). Tokyo: Ouraisha.

Tokashiki, I. (1991). *Gohaku-kai nenkanshi* (Gohaku-kai yearbook), Vol. 4. Naha: Published privately.

Acknowledgments

I would like to extend my sincerest thanks to Mr. Maik Hassel for taking the photographs that illustrate this article, and to Mr. Olivier Riche for posing for the photographs.

chapter 60

Issues Concerning Board Breaking

by Phil Davison, M.A.

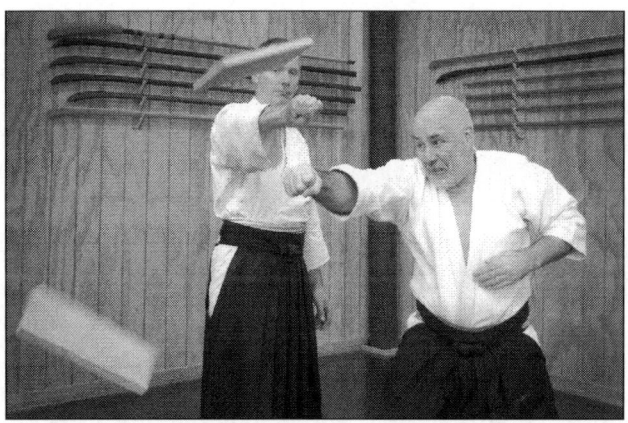

The author breaking an unsupported board.
Photographs courtesy of P. Davison.

Once when Kyuzo Mifune visited a karate dojo, he was shown a demonstration of tile-breaking by one of the karate men. After the karate man had smashed a number of tiles piled on top of each other, he asked Mifune, "Can a Judo man do this?"

"Yes, it is very easy," Mifune replied.

"Is that so? Can we see what kind of technique a Judo man uses?" the karate man challenged.

"Of course. Please set up the tiles. I'll be back in a minute," Mifune instructed. Mifune returned with a hammer he had brought along in his bag.

"You are not going to use that to break the tiles, are you?" the karate man protested.

"Yes. I told you it was easy. Efficient use of energy is a key principle of Judo."

— John Stevens, 2001:107

Arthritis

It has become clear that osteoarthritis is not an inevitable disease of aging: osteoarthritis is associated with some occupations more than others. For example, a 2003 Quebec study demonstrated clear links between occupations involving manual labour and the onset of osteoarthritis (Rossignol, 2004). What we do to our limbs may return to haunt us in later life. The aforementioned study showed the peak prevalence of symptoms in men was in the 70-to-79-year age bracket.

There are few longitudinal studies focusing on the relation of injury to development of osteoarthritis. One study, the Johns Hopkins Precursors Study, followed a large cohort from young adulthood into old age, and was able to demonstrate a relationship between injury and the onset of arthritis (Gelber, 2000). In this study 1,321 medical students were tracked over several decades, and it was shown that an injury to the knee in youth or middle age resulted in nearly three times (the actual figure is 2.95) the likelihood of developing osteoarthritis in later life.

However, the Johns Hopkins study focused on easily measureable injuries, such as dislocation or fracture. The sort of injury sustained in breaking boards is less severe, but more repeated. One does not break a leg regularly, yet some people will perform *tamashiwari* (testing one's combat skills by breaking objects) as often as monthly. The effects of repeated low-level trauma are more difficult to assess outside of a martial arts environment—ethics committee approval to get a cohort to regularly smash their limbs into hard objects is not easily forthcoming—and outside of a martial arts environment it is hard to conceive of people who could be persuaded to act in such a way.

To further complicate matters, there are a surprising variety of results concerning exercise and the risk of osteoarthritis, showing both increased and decreased risk. Heesch et al. found that light exercise tended to lessen the risk of arthritis in older women but not in middle aged women (Heesch, 2007).[1] Other studies, such as that by Carol Teitz, have shown an increased risk of developing osteoarthritis in elite athletes and dancers (Teitz, 1998). Chakravarty (2008) found little difference in the risk of developing arthritis between long-distance runners and a control group over a period of twenty years.

Differences among individuals should also be taken into account, especially in regard to the difficulty of board breaks. Women have significantly lower bone mass and density. Van der Sluis (2002) measured the total bone mineral content of women at the age of twenty-two to have a mean of 2,790 g, compared with 3,515 g for men of the same age. Moreover, the difference between the largest male total bone mineral content is much more than twice that of the smallest female: around 4,700 g for the largest male compared with around 1,800 for the smallest female.

The Physics of Striking

Angelo Armenti has analyzed the force needed to break bone and concluded that there is significantly less force involved in breaking bone than in one of the standard boards used today (Armenti, 1992). In Ameneti's analysis it takes 3,111 N to break a pine board 300 mm x 200 mm x 10 mm. A board like this would be much easier to break than the standard boards in common use (300 mm x 300 mm x 20 mm—probably around twice as hard to break, if not harder). In Armenti's analysis he claims that breaking a bone with a 10 mm radius, 200 mm long, supported at both ends, should take 3,142 N.

Unfortunately, Armenti's analysis is seriously flawed. John Currey describes the difficulty in measuring Young's modulus of rupture for bone in a laboratory setting (Currey, 2002). This is compounded by the fact that the bone in vivo is surrounded by muscle, usually in motion, and definitely not supported at both ends. Bone is composed of different materials (compact and cancellous), which respond to forces differently and, in particular, cancellous bone responds to force differently at the ends compared to the middle of the bone. "The assumption [of fracture mechanics] is that any part of the material will behave linearly elastic until it ruptures. This is certainly not true for bone."

Since it is not possible to define accurately the amount of force required to break living bone, it is not possible to state that the force required to break a board is greater (or less) than that required to break a bone, but rather that the force required to break bone is highly unpredictable. This is borne out by anecdotal evidence from sparring accidents in the dojo: a blow with tremendous force can land on someone, knock him over, and yet cause no injury, yet a light blow at the correct angle on a vulnerable target is capable of causing serious injury.

To analyze an effective strike, from a power point of view, it is an oversimplification to use the kinetic energy equation (1/2 mv2). We must look at the momentum of the striking arm, the mass of the limb, the degree of connectedness the limb has to the rest of the body, the momentum of the body, and the degree of connectedness the body has with the ground, the hardness of the limb, and finally the momentum of the target. If we label the degree of connectedness as "transference," we can say that the key factors are mass, transference, velocity, hardness, and the momentum of the target.

Mass is not a straightforward item to measure in regard to punching. The weight of the limb striking is not really relevant to measure—measuring just the limb would only be appropriate if measuring a severed limb thrown at the target. A skilled striker is able to transfer energy from the body to the striking limb, effectively putting more mass into the strike (i.e., he has greater skill at transference). A skilled striker is able to generate considerably more transference than an unskilled person. In everyday language we could say someone is putting his or her whole body into the strike.

A second form of transference is the ability of the striker to brace himself against the ground when striking. Since, in Newtonian physics, every action has an equal and opposite reaction, it is essential that the striker be grounded to propel him- or herself into the punch. For example, someone standing on a slippery surface will have a great deal of difficulty in propelling himself into a strike.

Velocity is an important variable in that the equation for kinetic energy reveals it to be squared—a small increase in velocity results in a big increase in power. Certainly there is a difference of velocity between skilled and unskilled strikers, yet the difference between the slowest and fastest punch of people with at least a little training is probably not enough to make a large difference in the force applied to the board.

For example, a typical skilled person can punch at around 9 meters per second. Assuming that an unskilled person's punch travels as slow as 7 meters per second[2] and, although perhaps unrealistically, that a person could put 100% of his body weight behind a punch[3], we can calculate the energy produced by slow and fast punches from people of different body weights.

Mass (halved)	Velocity (squared)	Resulting Energy
90 kg	9 mps	3645 j
90 kg	7 mps	2205 j
50 kg	9 mps	2025 j
50 kg	7 mps	1225 j

As can be seen in the table above, the difference between a fast and slow punch is less than the difference created by people of different body weights. If we compare the differences between 9 mps punches and 7 mps punches the results are 1,400 j at 90 kg (3,645 j less 2,205 j) and 800 j at 50 kg (2,025 j less 1,225 j). By contrast, the difference between the resulting energy figures between different body weights is 1,620 j at 9 mps (3,645 less 2,025 j), and 980 j at 7 mps (2205 j less 1,225 j).

The hardness of the objects being struck together determines which will be damaged by the impact. A one-kilogram sledgehammer striking a brick wall will damage the wall. A blob of jelly of the same weight, striking at the same velocity, will itself be damaged, leaving the wall undamaged. In punching terms this relates to the support of the muscular structures and to the density of the skeletal structures in the hand. Tensing the muscles on impact is one of the first skills learned from punching bags or focus mitts, but due to their lower bone density (Van der Sluis, 2002) women's bones are not as hard as men's and therefore are more at risk of injury when board breaking.

The momentum of the target is not really an issue in board breaking—the board is stationary and the mass is standardized. However, in self-defense situations the momentum of the target is a crucial factor in the impact delivered in a strike. A person who walks into a punch suffers a great deal more than someone who rolls with it.

We can see that, with training, a person can improve transference to get more mass behind the strike, and can increase punching velocity. Also with skill one can learn to adapt to situations where a punch is delivered when the opponent's momentum is optimal. This can enable a small person to "punch above her weight," i.e., to punch much harder than would be expected for a smaller person. However, purely in terms of power, the slightly built person is at a serious disadvantage when compared to a person with significantly more mass. A smaller person will never be able to match the power of a larger person who has similar skills.

This is not to say that smaller people cannot defend themselves. A smaller person may not be able to match the power of a larger person, but may have significant advantages in agility, and the many advantages of a better skill set gained through training far outweigh the advantage of being born with a larger body. Furthermore, breaking boards is an activity only tangentially connected to practical self-defense, in that boards do not move, do not fight back, and do not defend themselves—perhaps the primary skill in combat is the ability to overcome the opponent's defenses, and, in terms of striking, the primary skill is to delver the most appropriate strike for a given target, rather than the most powerful. The focus should not be on who is the most powerful, but rather on who can best deliver enough impact to the appropriate target to gain the desired effect.

It must also be said that a focus on power is misleading: the best punch is not the most powerful; it is the most appropriate. The ability to deliver a powerful punch is not useful if the punch elicits a defensive response from the enemy that means the punch does not land: a strike that is too powerful will not land, as it is more likely to provoke a defensive response. A light tap that does land on a vulnerable target can be effective in itself, and open the way (*suki*) by causing a momentary breach in the opponent's concentration, allowing more effective strikes.

Discussion

In the section on arthritis we can see that there is a link between injury and late-life arthritis. From the studies of risk of arthritis arising from different occupations we can see that repeated minor injury can also contribute to increased risk. Therefore, we can see that board breaking will cause some increase in risk, although it is not possible to say how much. We need to carefully weigh the unknown amount of risk of late-life arthritis with the benefits of breaking boards.

From the discussion of different body weights and bone densities we can see that board breaking is most certainly not a level playing field. A slightly built woman is likely to have a significantly harder time breaking boards than a strongly built man.

This raises the problem of a "standards based" approach to board breaking, if board breaking is included in a school's grading syllabus. Should we be saying that a person merits a certain grade because he can do a certain break (i.e., smaller people require a lot more skill than larger); or should we say that people of comparable skill level merit the grade (i.e., the breaking difficulty is adjusted to meet the body mass and/or gender of the student)?

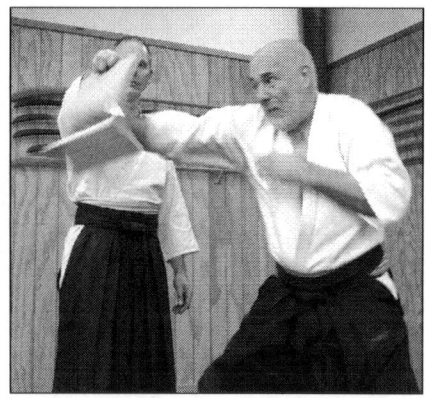

The risk of a break failing is far greater for a slightly built person (regardless of gender) simply because of the lower mass striking the target. Should the break fail, the risk of injury, and of consequent late-life osteo-arthritis, is far greater than if the break is successful. Women, with lower bone density are more at risk of injury than men, and doubly so because there is a greater element of risk of the break failing due to (on average) less lean body mass.

Given the difference of skill levels required to perform the same break from people of widely different body weights and the increased risk of late-life arthritis, it would seem to me that any breaking syllabus should not be "one size fits all," and that the syllabus should change to meet individual needs.

There is a danger in emphasizing powerful strikes in that students come to regard power generation as more important than it really is for self-defense. Anyone should be able to knock an opponent down if that opponent stands still and does not defend him- or herself; a more significant skill is striking someone without raising his defenses. My concern is that excessive emphasis on power may hinder the ability to strike effectively (i.e., appropriately), and may actually reduce a student's fighting ability.

A partial solution could be the breaking of unsupported, lightly held boards. To break an unsupported board requires more skill, and especially more velocity, meaning there is less advantage in a higher body mass. Brute strength cannot break an unsupported board. Furthermore, the risk of injury is less, since a board that is not broken simply flies away with much less impact on the practitioner's hand. Repeated striking of unsupported boards, whether they break or not, may cause bruising, but is less likely to cause injury.

Appendix: Survey

In preparation for this essay I conducted an informal survey of people fifty years old or older who had been involved in board breaking in their youth. Unfortunately, there were only four respondents, meaning the sample size is too small to be anything other than anecdotal. Of the four respondents only one reported no issues with arthritis, two reported significant problems with arthritis that appeared to have no direct connection to board breaking, and the fourth reported issues with arthritis that could possibly have been related to board breaking. Given that in all cases the people had lived active lives, it is not really possible to pinpoint any direct link, or lack of direct link, between board breaking and late-life osteoarthritis. Perhaps the only conclusion that can be drawn from this survey is how difficult it is to obtain enough data to draw meaningful conclusions on the subject.

Notes

[1] The authors suggested that mid-aged women were mostly in paid employment and were therefore more active than their older counterparts. Very likely the mid-aged women reported no exercise as such, yet were leading more active lives than their older counterparts.

[2] I think this is very conservative, but I have been unable to find reliable figures for the punching velocity of typical untrained people. Perhaps 8mps is more likely.

[3] This is a function of transference. A downward strike could have 100%, or close to it, of body mass transferred to the striking limb. Conceivably, a person skilled in keying into the ground could even transfer more than 100% of his mass, using his feet to brace his mass against the ground, effectively transferring the ground mass into the striking limb.

References

Armenti, A. (1992). *The physics of sports*. College Park, Maryland: American Institute of Physics.

Chakravarty, E. (2008). Long distance running and knee osteoarthritis: A prospective study. *American Journal of Preventive Medicine, 35*(2):133–138.

Cooper, C. (2003). Occupational activity and arthritis of the knee. *Annals of the Rheumatic Diseases, 53*(2):90–93.

Currey, J. (2002). *Bones: Structure and mechanics*. Princeton, NJ: Princeton University Press.

Gelber, A. (2000). Joint injury in young adults and risk for subsequent knee and hip osteoarthritis. *Annals of Internal Medicine, 133*(5):321–328.

Heesch, K. (2007). Relationship between physical activity and stiff or painful joints in mid-aged and older women: A 3-year prospective study. *Arthritis and Therapy, 9*:R34.

Rossignol, M. (2004). Primary osteoarthritis and occupation in the Quebec national health and social survey. *Occupational and Environmental Medicine; 61*(9):729–735

Stevens, J. (2001). *Budo secrets: Teachings of the martial arts masters*. Boston: Shambhala Publications.

Teitz, C. (1998). Premature osteoarthritis in professional dancers. *Clinical Journal of Sports Medicine, 8*(4):255–259.

Van der Sluis, I. (2002, October). Reference data for bone density and body composition measured with dual energy x ray absorptiometry in white children and young adults. *Archives of Disease in Childhood, 87*(4):341–347.

Acknowledgment

Special thanks to those who helped with the photography:
Gary Wilkins, who bravely suspended the boards,
and to photographers Wally Seccombe and
Marilyn Jankowska for capturing the moments.

chapter 61

Ryukyu Kempo and Small Circle Jujitsu

by Will Higginbotham, B.A.

Where I Learned These Techniques

As a strong proponent of the value of classical kata practice, I stress that applications for techniques can be derived directly from traditional katas. Further, karate and jujutsu techniques work wonderfully well together to "fill in the gaps" in seeking ways to maintain control of an attacker.

The particular sets of techniques or "flows" presented in this chapter are variations on—and combinations of—well-known and commonly practiced individual techniques. The reason these sets are among my favorites is that they illustrate the importance of preventing the practitioner from simply "stalling out" after performing a single counter to a given attack.

The first set deals with a takedown to a prone position from a hammerlock, using a finger lock for maximum stability and control. Here I credit Leon Jay (Small Circle Jujitsu) for sharing his expertise in joint manipulation.

The second set involves a series of defenses from a right-left punch combination delivered by a determined assailant. At each step the defender aims to control his opponent and deter further aggression, using force proportionate to the nature and duration of the attack. By aiming blocks and strikes at specific pressure points, the defender hopes to injure or disable the attacking arm, stun the attacker, and finally subdue him altogether by taking him to the ground in a controlled fashion. Here I credit George Dillman (Ryukyu Kempo) for sharing his expertise with pressure-point techniques.

Memorable Incidents Involving These Techniques

The hammerlock is sometimes taught as a static technique, leaving the defender holding the attacker in a somewhat precarious standing position from which a number of counters and escapes can be performed. A common follow-up is the application of additional torque to the shoulder, forcing the opponent to the prone position on the floor. One problem with this follow-up is that the defender is often forced to slam the opponent downward in order to maintain control. The version presented here shows how the defender can maintain a higher degree of control throughout the encounter.

One of my senior students—sixth dan Anthony Everett—is the agent in charge of training on the national level for the Department of Veterans Affairs. Because of the superior control afforded by the takedown from the hammerlock presented herein, the agency has adopted this particular technique as part of its combatives training in controlling and handcuffing.

The defense for the right-left combination attack is similarly controlled, but equally powerful and adaptable. One sensible goal is to use the minimum force required to prevent the attack and keep oneself safe. This is important for ethical as well as legal reasons.

In the sequence illustrating the defense against the right-left punch combination, the defender reacts to protect himself and control the situation with escalating force, making sure the response at each stage is proportionate to the increasing intensity of the attack.

This technique is also highly adaptable. For example, when working this technique with a Muay Thai stylist at a European seminar in 2008, the attacker had the good sense and training to retract his left fist to guard his jaw after I had blocked his second attack. Luckily, force can be easily transferred through a solid object, and I was able to complete the technique perfectly simply by palming the attacker's own guard into the intended target.

Tips on Practicing These Techniques

In applying the controlled takedown from the hammerlock, the free hand is used to control the shoulder, preventing the opponent from turning counterclockwise to spin out of the hold. As the right hand slides down and behind the opponent to grasp his fingers, the left hand snakes around the elbow to create a base and prevent a spinning or turning counter to the finger lock. As the defender applies controlled pressure to the fingers, the left hand strokes the carotid sinus to force the opponent to the ground.

In the defense against the right and left punch sequence, the defender begins with a guard position that is intended to be relatively nonthreatening. When the attacker punches, the defender parries and simultaneously "stings" the sensitive points on the inside of the wrist with his other hand, so as to deter any further attack if possible. If the attacker continues with a left punch, the defender clears the parried right punch down and to the side while simultaneously parrying the incoming attack with his rising, right ridge hand. If these two defenses have not ended the confrontation, the defender is now inside the attacker's guard and has a clear shot at neck and head targets. Finally, by cupping the back of the attacker's neck with the right hand while leaving the left hand

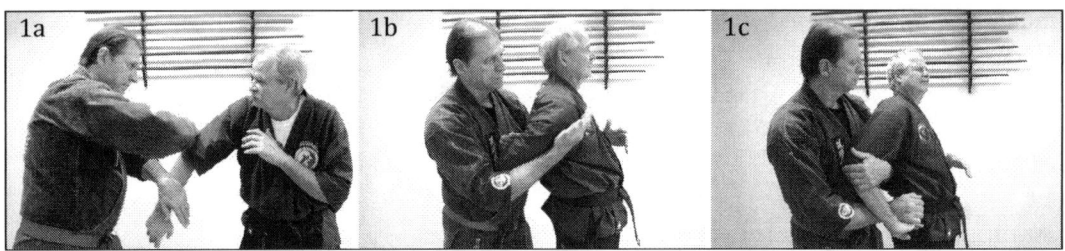

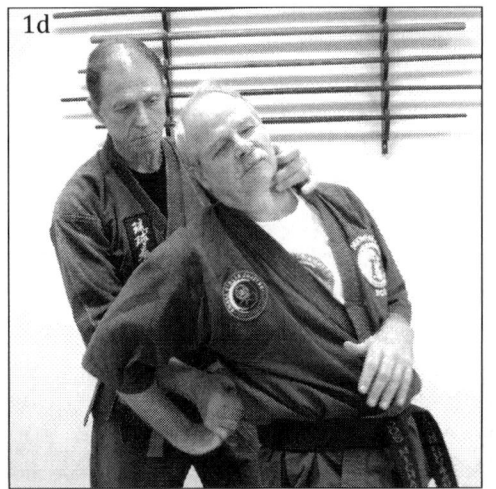

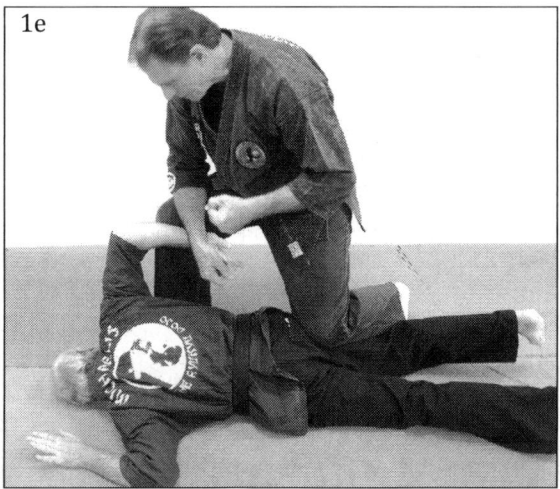

free, the defender can apply as little or as much force as is needed to take the attacker down and can control his fall to boot.

Technique 1: Controlled Takedown from the Hammerlock
1a) The defender slaps the opponent's attacking right forearm down with his left palm, then shoots his right hand across and behind the attacker's elbow. 1b) The defender continues around the forearm with his left hand and pulls with his right to rotate the opponent. He "tightens" the hammerlock by stroking the right palm up. 1c) The defender slides his right hand down and behind to grasp his opponent's ring and pinky fingers. His left hand wraps the elbow from inside to prevent twisting out of the finger lock. 1d) Once the finger lock is secure with the right hand alone, the middle finger of the left hand strokes up the sternocleidomastoid muscle, forcing the assailant to fall on his back. The reverse two-finger lock is then used to flip him over on his face, using his left hand to cup his head for safety. 1e) The defender can now base the finger lock with his leg for more intense control while kneeling on the opponent's sciatic nerve to stabilize him.

Technique 2: Escalating Defense from Right and Left Punches
2a) When confronted, the defender assumes a hands-up, palm-open "don't hurt me" type of posture. 2b) If the attacker strikes, the defender parries down with a left open-palm slap while striking to the inside of the wrist with a right punch. 2c) If the attack continues with the free left hand, the defender's parrying hand continues its arc to clear the opponent's right arm. The defender's right ridge hand parries up, striking. 2d) The defender is now inside his attacker's guard and in a position to strike simultaneously to the neck and jaw. 2e) The defender's right hand snakes around to cup the attacker's neck, while his left hand can press or strike the forehead as needed to subdue the attacker with minimum damage and maximum control.

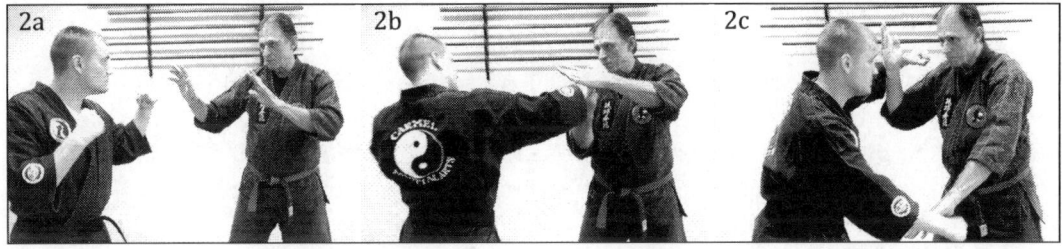

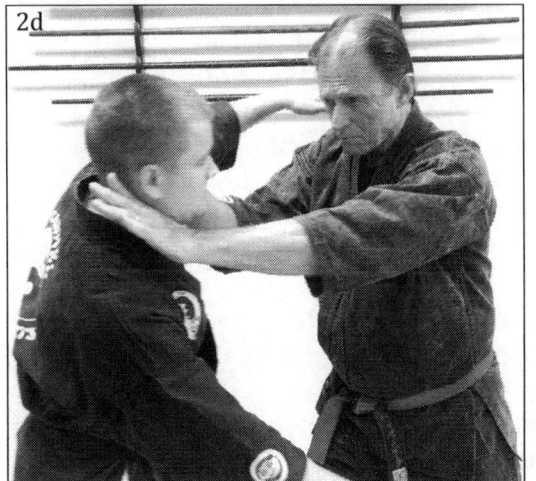

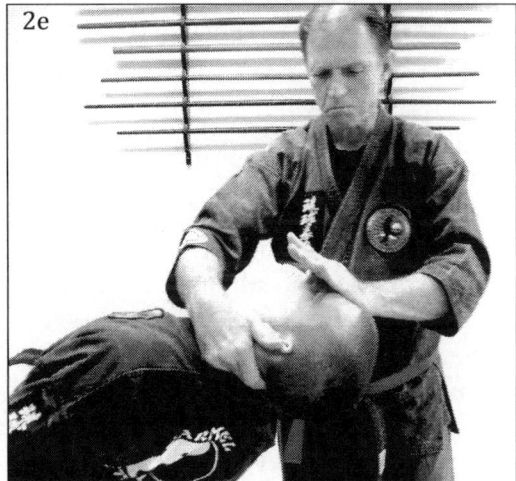

chapter 62

Kata-Based Training of Goju-ryu Karate

by Marvin Labbate

This short piece presents Okinawan Goju-ryu karatedo as a kata-based training system. It brings together kata-based training elements for various levels of understanding and application, combining solo principles and partner-based training principles. At its most basic level, a kata is a form or pattern of movements that train various fighting scenarios and responses. At the most advanced level, for which katas serve as the encyclopedia of the entire martial art, katas provide a sequence of dangerous to deadly techniques. Between the two extremes are levels of development to which masters have historically controlled access. While these restrictions were to ensure that only those with appropriate moral, spiritual, and physical preparation were able to use and teach these ideas, in modern times these restrictions have been relaxed for commercial gain. Thus, it is more important than ever to address responsible training and use of these principles.

As this chapter will discuss, the art of Goju-ryu is also a system. While karate training can be "performance based" for showy applications such as tournaments, traditional training for self-defense is kata based, and thus the center of the Goju-ryu system is also kata-based training. Each series of kata movements has a translation—the basic form and pattern—but it has many applications. Thus, while "practicing" a kata provides a first step, if the karate practitioner wishes to fully grasp a kata's richness, he or she will explore these applications. Furthermore, while the understandings and applications of the kata will vary, the basic system applies to any and all katas. As I will describe below, this system includes familiarizing oneself with the background of the kata, working through solo and partner training, and developing a self-defense repertoire based on traditional kumite sets.

It is helpful to approach any kata by familiarizing oneself with some historical and technical background. One combines a general awareness of karate-related culture, philosophy, etiquette, and language with kata-specific information, such as the name of the kata, its definition or meaning, and its history or origins (such as why and how it was developed, when, where, and with whom). By studying the background of a kata, the karate practitioner gains insight that can help develop the kata and its applications. He understands that historically there have been various levels of kata application: obvious techniques; intermediate-level applications that must be taught; individual interpretations through which the black belt ranks are able to become artists; and *okuden*, or hidden techniques and principles that historically masters did not transmit except to select individuals with sufficient merit. Through this background, a kata is understood as a deep, meaningful source of martial knowledge. Then the practitioner moves on to training in the kata itself.

Kata-based training has two major components: solo and partner training. In solo training, one begins with memorizing the pattern of a kata, its basic steps and movements. Once the pattern is mastered, principles are layered over and integrated with the movements. Among others, key principles include the Sanchin kata's principles of structure, movement, and breathing, and karate drum principles of generating close-range power. Thus, the elementary movements of the kata are broken into parts that are drilled in order to internalize the basics and develop the specific kata. This layered solo training gives basic body mechanics and allows the kata to evolve. Solo movement is then further developed by moving with a partner. Partner training adds elements such as distancing, timing of entering and exiting, and awareness. This phase includes practices such as *tai sabaki* (body shifting, or giving up space without giving up ground) and *kakie* (push-hands, or sensitivity training, which teaches how the partner will move without having to watch).

In order to practice and develop kata-based training (whether novice, intermediate, or advanced) into a fighting or self-defense repertoire of techniques, one then follows a formula based on traditional sparring sets, some of which are presented here in the diagrams below. These kumite sets can include the following: basic *bunkai*, or one-step attacks with defense and counter taken from kata sequences; advanced bunkai that combine the basic moves with takedowns; flow drills that teach how to flow from one move to another with a partner; basic grappling; advanced grappling with the application of choking techniques; two-person katas; freestyle drills; and other variations. Together, these elements develop any kata at any level as an effective means of self-defense.

The steps for the kata-based training system are the same for any kata. A single step, sweep, and shuto technique—from a novice Goju-ryu kata called Gekisai-Dai-Ichi—is presented here in order to illustrate the fact that when combining the principles and formula, the basics are the best techniques. By following the system, one can defend oneself even with a basic kata. As part of individual karate practice, however, the practitioner will apply the training system to different katas based on his or her individual body, skills, and gifts.

Basic Tegumi (Grappling) Kumite
1a) The attacker and defender are in traditional grappling stances.
1b) The defender throws a right slap to the left side of the attacker's neck.
1c) The defender follows through with his right hand and sweeps the attacker's front leg.
1d) The defender throws a right shuto to the right side of the attacker's neck.
1e) The defender's arm continues around the attacker's neck, forcing him down.
1f) The defender applies a choke.

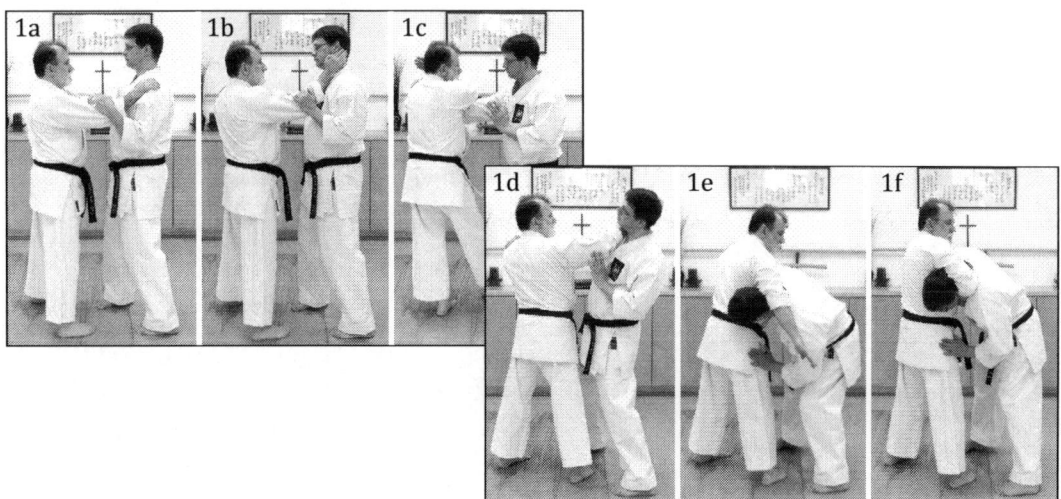

Jiyu Kumite (Freestyle Sparring)

2a) The attacker and defender pair off in sparring stances.
2b) The defender grabs the attacker's leading hand and chambers.
2c) The defender steps in and sweeps the attacker's leading leg.
2d) The defender throws a shuto across the attacker's neck.

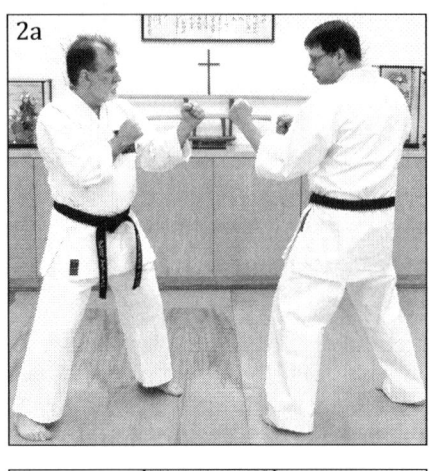
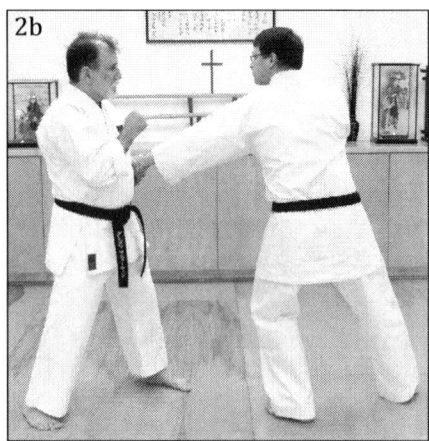
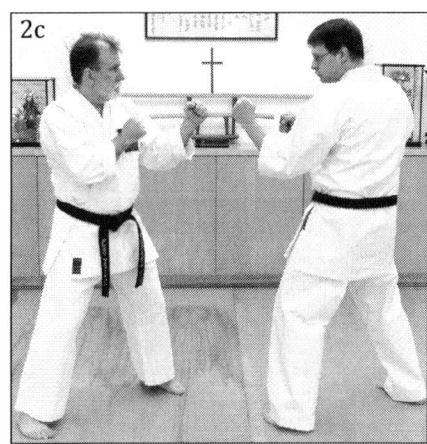
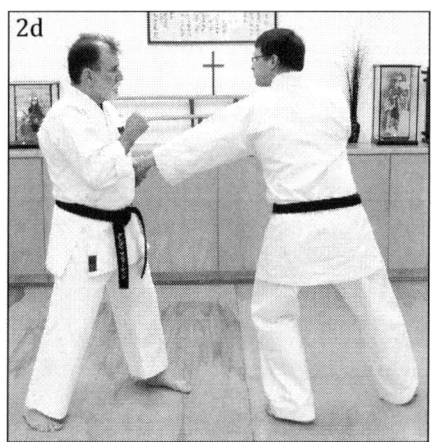

Acknowledgments
to Greg Macedin and John Nelson for help
with the demonstrations; Jill Petersen Adams,
assistant; and Scott Gardner, photography.

chapter 63

Tekko: Ryukyu Kobudo Shinkokai's Knuckle Duster

by Mario McKenna, M.Sc.

Where I Learned These Techniques

Most karate practitioners are familiar with the tonfa, bo, sai, and nunchaku as they are practiced in many karatedo dojos around the world, but Ryukyu Kobudo, the weapons tradition of Okinawa, encompasses a wider range of weaponry than just these four. This was the extent of my knowledge until I moved to Japan and began studying Ryukyu Kobudo formally with Minowa Katsuhiko and Yoshimura Hiroshi. Under their tutelage I learned that Ryukyu Kobudo uses a plethora of different weapons that are supported by multiple katas and two-person sets. One of those weapons I was introduced to is the *tekko*, or *tikko*, as Minowa preferred to call it.

It was during my second year of practice that I first encountered the tekko, and my initial thought was that it resembles a "knuckle duster." After being handed a pair, it was obvious that this weapon was much "meatier" than a "knuckle duster"; it was thicker, denser, and heavier—it clearly had intent. Yoshimura told me the tekko was a *kakushi buki*, or concealed weapon, that was popular for self-defense in old Okinawa, since it is relatively small and easy to conceal.

For several months I was drilled in Maezato no tekko, the kata that supports the techniques for the tekko. This kata is named after its creator, Minowa sensei's teacher, Taira Shinken (1897–1970). Once I had gained some proficiency with the tekko, I was slowly introduced to the two-person fighting set.

Memorable Incidents Involving These Techniques

I had been practicing both the kata and two-person set for a year and was starting to feel more comfortable with them. Along the way there were the usual mishaps, mostly self-inflicted, but not always. Yoshimura sensed my surge in confidence and, like any good teacher, decided to push the boundaries a little. The next time we practiced the two-person fighting set, he went a little harder and a little faster. Tekko in hand, I was the defender, but I struggled to keep up and it was obvious my technique wasn't good enough yet. Minowa looked over and said, "*Mada desu*"; you don't have it right yet.

A few months later I was facing Yoshimura again, but this time I was the attacker. Bo in hand, I delivered the strikes with all the vigor and stupidity of youth. A few sequences into the set, I felt a sharp pain on my fingers and dropped the bo to the floor. Yoshimura had given me a light tap with the tekko. Nothing was broken, no blood, but that light tap taught me how dangerous and debilitating this weapon can be in the proper hands. It is a lesson I never forgot.

Tips on Practicing These Techniques

Although the original two-person set has the attacker using a bo, the techniques are not limited to countering only that weapon. They can be applied equally against empty-hand attacks or bladed weapons. To that end, it is important to become accustomed to different combative engagement distances and their associated timing (*maai*). When practicing these techniques, I recommend progressing through different ranges and weapons until proficiency is reached:

1) close range (e.g., empty hand)
2) short range (e.g., knife or stick)
3) midrange (e.g., four-foot staff), and
4) long range (e.g., six-foot staff)

When using the tekko as a weapon of self-defense, there are two key points you should bear in mind. The first is to not become trapped in a block-and-counter paradigm. This is not only slow and unrealistic, but also potentially dangerous to the defender. Instead, attack and defense are to be used simultaneously. That is, the tekko must be used to strike vulnerable parts of the opponent's body as he attacks. Strikes should be aimed at the joints of the body, as this inhibits or stops the attacker from using his own weapons. The second point is that footwork (*taisabaki*) is extremely important for fist-loaded weapons like the tekko. You must not only avoid the attack, but place yourself in an advantageous position to deliver your own. The following photographs illustrate the use of the tekko against the empty hand.

Technique 1: Overhead Deflection and Low Strike

1a) Face your opponent with your left foot forward in a natural stance. Both hands are in front of your torso with the left hand leading. 1b) As the opponent moves forward to punch, step forward with the right foot, and raise both hands to catch the opponent's arm at the elbow. **Key point:** Take a deep step forward into the opponent; palms are open when performing the over-head deflection with the right hand on top of the left hand (see tekko detail). 1c) Shift your weight onto your lead leg and press up with both palms to unbalance the opponent. **Key point:** To clear the attack, spring the hands up and away. 1d) Shift your weight onto your right leg, bend your torso, and strike down in front of you with both hands on the opponent's knee. **Key point:** Use the handles of the tekko to strike the opponent. The thumbs apply pressure to the top of the tekko for stability.

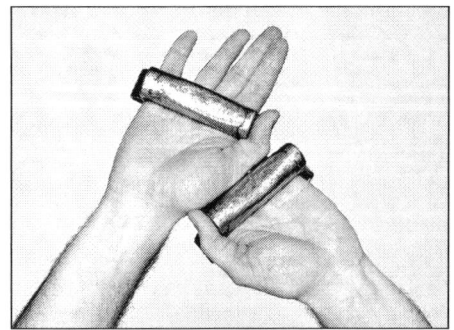

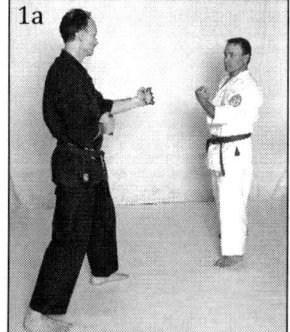

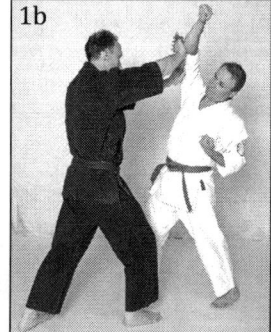

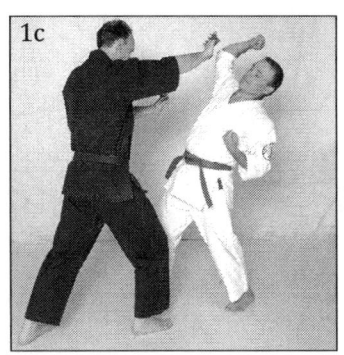
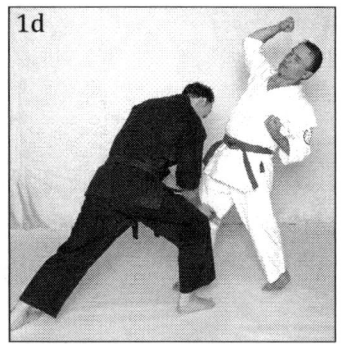

Technique 2: Midlevel Counterstrike

2a) Face your opponent with your right foot forward in a natural stance. Both hands are in front of your torso with the right hand leading. 2b) Pivot to the right, step in with your right foot and deliver a left vertical punch. **Key points:** Shift your weight to your rear leg as you pivot; stabilize the tekko by pressing down with your thumb on top of the handle; the counterstrike is aimed at the opponent's arm (i.e., elbow, wrist, or hand—see detail shown above). 2c) Press with the right tekko to unbalance the opponent and move his arm away. **Key point:** When you press with the tekko make sure to do it in a snapping action. 2d) Shift your weight onto your right leg, slide in and deliver a high, left vertical punch. Key point: The punch must be performed vertically with the thumb stabilizing the tekko.

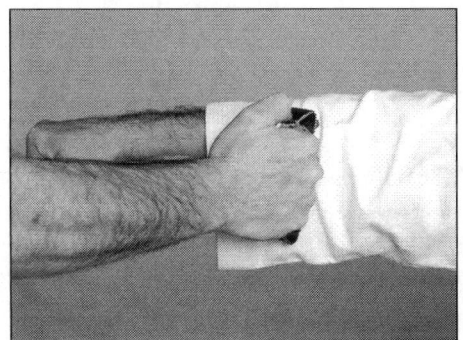
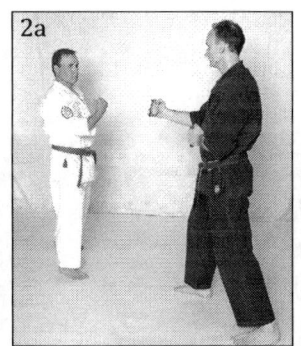
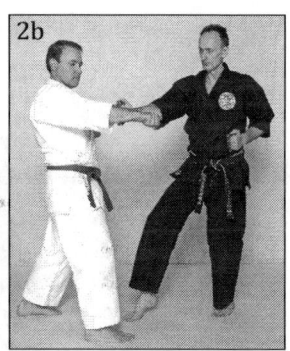
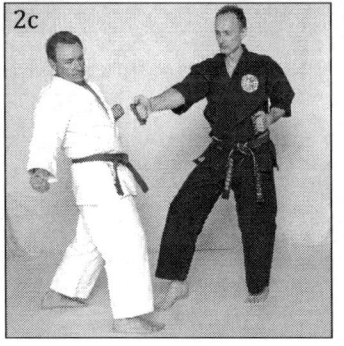
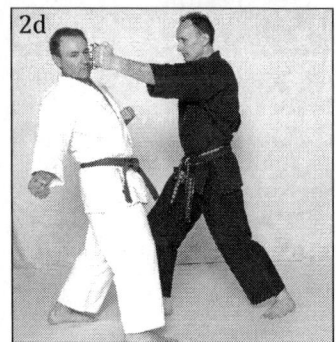

Acknowledgements

I would like to extend my sincerest thanks to Maik Hassel
for the fine photography work, and Brent Zarparniuk
for posing as the *kosha* (opponent) in the photographs.

Sources of Original Publication

Articles in this anthology were originally published in Via Media Publishing's *Journal of Asian Martial Arts,* and from the book titled *Asian Marital Arts: Constructive Thoughts and Practical Applications.* Listed according to original date of publication:

Manyak, A. and Silvan, J. (1992)	Vol. 1 No. 4, pp. 100–111
Harrison-Pepper, S. (1993)	Vol. 2 No. 2, pp. 90–103
Wingate, C. (1993)	Vol. 2 No. 3, pp. 10–35
Bolz, M. (1993)	Vol. 2 No. 3, pp. 82–93
Stebbins, J. (1993)	Vol. 2 No. 3, pp. 94–101
McCarthy, P. (1994)	Vol. 3 No. 2, pp. 90–99
Hershey, L. (1994)	Vol. 3 No. 3, pp. 52–61
Porta, J. and McCabe, J. (1994)	Vol. 3 No. 3, pp. 62–71
Yokoyama, K. (1994)	Vol. 3 No. 3, pp. 72–83
Bolz, M. (1995)	Vol. 4 No. 1, pp. 84–99
Wolfe, R. (1995)	Vol. 4 No. 3, pp. 76–99
Boudreau, F., et al. (1995)	Vol. 4 No. 4, pp. 50–69
Taylor, J. (1996)	Vol. 5 No. 1, pp. 78–85
Porta, J. and McCabe, J. (1996)	Vol. 5 No. 2, pp. 60–73
Freund, R. (1996)	Vol. 5 No. 3, pp. 40–43
Florence, R. (1996)	Vol. 5 No. 3, pp. 66–89
Lorden, M. (1997)	Vol. 6 No. 3, pp. 60–70
Pieter, W. and Van Ryssegem, G. (1998)	Vol. 7 No. 1, pp. 10–27
Bluming, J. (1998)	Vol. 7 No. 2, pp. 74–85
Silvan, J. (1998)	Vol. 7 No. 3, pp. 72–95
Bolz, M. (1998)	Vol. 7 No. 3, pp. 42–55
Van Horne, W. (1998)	Vol. 7 No. 4, pp. 82–99
Neide, J. (1999)	Vol. 8 No. 1, pp. 44–49
McKenna, M. (1999)	Vol. 8 No. 1, pp. 74–91
Labatte, M. (1999)	Vol. 8 No. 2, pp. 80–95
McKenna, M. (1999)	Vol. 8 No. 4, pp. 28–47
Labatte, M. (2000)	Vol. 9 No. 1, pp. 56–69
Flanagan, S. (2000)	Vol. 9 No. 1, pp. 82–92
McKenna, M. (2000)	Vol. 9 No. 3, pp. 32–43

McKenna, M. (2000)	Vol. 9 No. 3, pp. 44–57
Paz-y-Miño, G. (2000)	Vol. 9 No. 4, pp. 22–35
Labbate, M. (2001)	Vol. 10 No. 1, pp. 84–99
Svinth, J. (2001)	Vol. 10 No. 2, pp. 8–17
Toth, R. (2001)	Vol. 10 No. 3, pp. 84–91
Goedecke, C. (2001)	Vol. 10 No. 3, pp. 36–63
Florence, R. (2001)	Vol. 10 No. 4, pp. 20–43
Labatte, M. (2002)	Vol. 11 No. 1, pp. 80–95
Bolz, M. (2002)	Vol. 11 No. 2, pp. 80–91
Toth, R. (2002)	Vol. 11 No. 3, pp. 84–93
Hopkins, G. (2002)	Vol. 11 No. 4, pp. 54–77
Toth, O. and Toth, R. (2003)	Vol. 12 No. 4, pp. 66–81
Hopkins, G. (2003)	Vol. 12 No. 4, pp. 64–77
Toth, R. (2004)	Vol. 13 No. 4, pp. 60–71
Noble, G. (2005)	Vol. 14 No. 1, pp. 52–73
Hopkins, G. (2005)	Vol. 14 No. 2, pp. 52–69
Campbell, P. (2005)	Vol. 14 No. 4, pp. 62–73
Toth, R. (2006)	Vol. 15 No. 1, pp. 62–75
Hobert, P. (2006)	Vol. 15 No. 2, pp. 50–59
Donohue, J. (2006)	Vol. 15 No. 3, pp. 8–19
Toth, R. (2006)	Vol. 15 No. 4, pp. 54–71
Toth, R. (2007)	Vol. 16 No. 2, pp. 48–61
Hopkins, G. (2007)	Vol. 16 No. 3, pp. 30–49
Câmara, F.P., and McKenna, M. (2007)	Vol. 16 No. 4, pp. 46–53
Rymaruk, I. (2007)	Vol. 16 No. 4, pp. 66–77
Hopkins, G. (2009)	Vol. 18 No. 4, pp. 28–45
Smith, P., et al. (2010)	Vol. 19 No. 2, pp. 34–45
Labatte, M. (2011)	Vol. 20 No. 1, pp. 82–93
McKenna, M. (2011)	Vol. 20 No. 2, pp. 82–103
McKenna, M. (2011)	Vol. 20 No. 3, pp. 38–61
Davison, P. (2011)	Vol. 20 No. 3, pp. 22–31
Higginbotham, W. (2012)	*Asian Martial Arts*, pp. 70–73
Labatte, M. (2012)	*Asian Martial Arts*, pp. 98–101
McKenna, M. (2012)	*Asian Martial Arts*, pp. 110–113

INDEX

A
active breaking, 7–8, 34, 45, 58, 141–146, 186, 190–191, 224–225, 476, 540, 743–747
Adams, Hamish, 549
Ahagon, Naonobu
aikido, 254, 256, 428, 610, 729, 733
air compression theory, 88–89
Akamine, Eisuke, 267, 270, 301–302
All-Japan Karatedo Association, 141
All-Japan Karatedo Federation (Zen Nihon Karatedo Renmei), 352
All-Okinawan Goju-Kai, 81–82, 512
All-Okinawa Karate and Kobudo Combined (United) Association, 168, 433
All-Okinawan Karate Federation, 530 note 3
All-Okinawa Karatedo League, 232
archery (*kyudo*), 1, 25, 29, 389
arm toughening drills (*koteikitai*), 355, 487
Arakaki, Ankichi, 172, 580
Arakaki, Ryuko, 76, 148–149, 522, 625
Aragaki, Seisho, 511, 523, 659, 660 note 4
Arneil, Steve, 532–553
artifacts, 11–14
Asayama Ichiden-ryu, 299–300, 304–305
Ashihara, Hideyuki, 535, 541
Association for the Martial Virtues of Great Japan (Dai Nippon Butokukai), 79, 481 note 12, 487, 497, 523
Azama, Kasai (Nanjo Kiju), 550, 569

B
back-fist (*uraken*), 108, 118, 121, 360, 362–363, 365, 367–368, 494, 537, 677
Backhus, Bill, 220–221, 224
baguaquan, 77, 299–300, 304, 310, 481 note 13, 581
basic karate fist (*seiken*), 49, 143, 171, 201
basic techniques (*kihon waza*), 33, 71, 257, 269, 485, 538, 645–646, 649, 651
Battle of Okinawa, 80, 340, 524
Bechurin, 659, 732–741, 742 note 7
Black Turtle (*Genbu*), 403 note 2, 568, 571–576
Blue Dragon (*Seiryu*), 403 note 2, 568, 571–572, 575–576
Bluming, Jon, 219–227
boat oar (*kai eku, iyeku*), 16, 95, 250, 271, 308, 349, 482
bola (*suruchin*), 15, 17, 95, 257
Bolton, Bob, 533
Book of Five Rings (Go Rin No Sho), 24
"brass knuckles" (*tekko*), 95, 271–273, 275, 755–757

breathing methods, 6, 27, 77, 87–88, 143–144, 194, 285, 288, 290, 293–295, 316, 329, 339, 341, 372, 374, 536, 598
British Karate Control Commission, 548
British Kyokushinkai, 532
Bryner, Robert, 184 note 21
Bubishi, 11, 14, 28, 79, 302, 341, 344, 346 note 7, 353, 398, 432, 440, 459–460, 521 note 3, 523, 628, 635 note 8, 646, 742 note 6
budo, 20–41, 64, 125–127, 253, 257–259, 299, 304, 306–307, 410, 599, 601, 645
Bugeikan, 175, 444 note 10
bujutsu, 22, 24–26, 29, 35–36, 40, 165, 167–168, 600–601
bull fighting, 187–189, 203, 224, 230
bunkai, 46, 96, 97, 152, 155, 246, 251–253, 257, 270, 339, 483, 514, 556, 562, 566 note 4, 604, 643–644, 677–678, 690, 753
bunkai kumite, 556
bushido, 23–24, 28, 33–35, 40
Byakko see White Tiger, 403 note 2, 568, 571–572, 575–576

C
Cauley, Thomas, 253–266
Chandler, Chuck, 435, 441, 445 note 18
Chatan Yara no Kusanku (*kata*), 235, 656
Chen, Panling, 304
challenge match (*kakidameshi*), 169, 180
Chibana, Choshin, 64, 80–81, 229–231, 233, 242, 299–307, 339–340, 393, 654
Chinen, Masami, 301, 435
Chinen Shichiyanaka no Kon, 62, 310
Chinese kenpo, 12, 61, 174, 186, 191, 241, 243, 304, 306, 338, 411, 525
Chinese hand (*tode*), 22, 27, 166, 169–170, 181, 182 note 6, 241, 391, 430–431, 628
Chinto kata, 304, 410–411, 440, 596, 618, 620–621
chishi (weights), 18, 76, 148, 152–157, 292, 339, 355, 625, 631, 676
Chito-ryu, 473, 476, 480 note 3, 503–505, 511 note 3
Chitose, Tsuyoshi, 480 note 3, 500, 502, 504, 506, 511 note 3
Collins, Howard, 548–549
Confucianism, 23, 26, 60–62, 601–602
cross power theory, 85–90

D
Dai Ni Seisan, 248
Dai Nippon Butokukai, 79–81, 481 note 13, 487, 497, 523, 612, 622 note 6, 641
Daito-ryu, 580–581

Daoism, 26, 295
DeBacario, Luis, 583
Dillman, George, 591–598, 749
dojo, 13, 21, 31–34, 37, 56, 61, 67, 76, 78, 80–82, 106–107, 124, 149, 166, 168–169, 174–176, 180–181, 188, 190–191, 194, 196–197, 199, 201–202, 221, 255–256, 258–259, 268–270, 299, 301, 303, 306–307, 340, 556, 570, 583, 585, 592, 594, 601, 603, 627–629, 631, 637, 646, 661–662, 676–679, 690–691, 702–710, 719, 726, 732, 743, 745, 755
dojo ethics (*dojo kun*), 29, 197
Donovan, Ticky, 548–459
Draeger, Donn, 25, 219–222, 225, 227, 533–535

E

Enoeda, Keinosuke, 542, 548
entangling technique (*karamidi*), 713, 715, 720, 722–723, 729, 731, 736, 741
European Kyokushin Kaikan, 226
Evans, Gerald, 20
Exhibit Hall of Okinawan Karate, 11–19

F

Federation of Okinawan Karate and Kobudo Organizations, 168
fencing (*kendo*), 24, 29, 80, 94, 174, 254, 299, 502–503, 590 note 3, 603, 610, 618, 632, 641
Fitkin, Brian, 548–549
Five Ancestors Fist (*wuzuquan*), 646, 655
focus (*kime*), 145
folklore, 11, 228–229, 240–241
Fong, Leo, 593–594, 596
foot fist (*sokusen*), 50
forearm training (*kotekitae*), 355, 487
forward stance (*zenkutsu dachi*), 193, 195, 248, 490, 517, 677
fracture, 162–163, 330, 332, 453, 455–457, 459, 697, 744
Free sparring (*kumite*), 33, 71, 89, 110–111, 114, 121, 147, 190, 195–196, 220, 229, 243, 257–258, 270–271, 276, 339, 358–370, 408, 411, 440–441, 485, 502, 513, 533, 538–540, 544–546, 556, 566, 662, 683, 692 note 3, 752–753
Fujian Province, 27, 76–77, 174, 282 note 4, 241, 338, 341, 430, 511 note 5, 523, 626, 635 note 8, 655, 711
Fujian White Crane boxing (*baihequan*), 77, 339, 344, 357 note 5, 432, 435, 438, 440, 521 note 4, 655

Fujihira, Akio, 541, 546–547
Fujita, Seiko, 300–301, 304
Fukuchi, Seiko, 236–237, 243
Fukuda, Shoen, 254
Fukyu kata, 514, 556
Fukyugata kata, 398
full-contact training (*jissen*), 188, 196, 199, 202, 358, 434
Funakoshi, Gichin, 1–2, 21–23, 28–30, 33–36, 38–39, 64, 72–73, 173, 186–187, 256, 353, 357 note 6, 388–389, 429, 480 note 12, 506, 511 note 2, 512 note 7, 603, 612–613, 616, 622 note 4, 654, 709, 714
fundamentals (*kihon*), 257, 269, 442, 485, 538, 645–647, 649, 651
Fushinomiya Prince, 62
Fuzhou city, 76–77, 338–339, 341, 346 note 6, 353, 357 notes 4 and 5, 397–398, 429, 431–432, 438, 441–442, 445 note 20, 635 note 8, 711

G

Garyu kata, 194
Gaviola, Frank, 583, 590 note 5
Geesink, Anton, 222–223, 543
Gekiha, 556
Gekisai kata, 78, 194, 302, 398, 485–486, 498, 514, 528, 556, 566 note 3, 653 note 1, 655, 657, 726, 753
Gekisaisho kata, 194
Gibo, Seiki, 516, 677, 692, 692 note 1
Go, Kenki (Wu Xianhui), 339, 353, 357 note 5, 433, 443, 646
Goju-ryu/Gojyu-ryu, 13, 18, 45, 65, 75–82, 148–150, 152, 157–159, 165, 187, 236, 238, 243, 251, 256, 285, 294, 302, 316, 320, 329, 337, 340–341, 346 notes 1, 2 and 5, 348, 351–352, 354, 372, 387, 397–398, 402, 405, 430, 444 notes 9 and 10, 447, 449, 473–477, 480, 482–487, 497–498, 505, 511 note 7, 513–517, 521, 521 note 2, 522–525, 530, 530 note 4, 554–567, 590 notes 1 and 3, 624–625, 627, 629, 632, 634, 634 note 1, 643–652, 653 note 3, 654–660, 676–692, 692 notes 1 and 2, 702, 704, 712, 714, 716, 721, 727, 729–733, 740, 752–754
Goju-ryu Keishin-kai, 13, 251
Goju-ryu Shinko-kai, 80–81, 755
Goju-ryu Tomari-te Association, 740
Goshin-do Karate Association, 405
grappling (*tuite, torite, tuidi*), 17, 148, 220, 239, 243–244, 741, 753, 751–752
gripping jars (*nigirigame*), 76, 148, 156, 158, 303, 339–340, 355, 513, 637, 676

H

hakkei, see issuing power.
Hakko-ryu, 254
Hakutsuruken, see White Crane.
Hanashiro, Chomo, 58, 62, 64, 67 note 1, 80, 242, 590 note 2, 655
Hanko-ryu, 435, 523
Harada, Mitsusuke, 391
Hatsumi, Yoshiaki (Hatsumi Masaaki), 305
Hawai'i, 243, 388, 392–394, 481 note 13, 580–581
Hawai'i Karate Kodanshakai, 581
Heaven and Earth (Tenshi), 403 note, 568, 571, 577
Hirakami, Nobuyuki, 714, 732
Higa, Seiko, 78, 80–81, 236–237, 243, 482, 653 note 3, 677
Higa, Seitoku, 175, 299–302, 304, 433, 444 note 10
Higaonna, Morio, 286, 398, 486
Higaonna/Higashionna, Kanryo, 61, 76, 78, 82, 148–149, 300, 302, 337–340, 342–343, 345, 348, 351, 3454, 357 note 1, 397–398, 403 note 1, 432, 443, 444 note 10, 445 note 19, 511 notes 3 and 5, 522, 655, 660 note 2
Higashionna, Tanmei, 351, 357 note 3
Hirohito Crown Prince, 28, 79, 242, 639
hoe (*kuwa*), 95
Hokama, Tetsuhiro, 11, 13–16, 18–19, 229, 236, 241 note, 389, 656
Hollander, Loek, 225–227

I

iaido, 29, 51, 353
Ikeda, Horitoshi, 176
injury, 33, 53–54, 57, 114, 117, 143, 147, 151, 159, 161, 163–164, 170, 193, 195, 204–214, 330–331, 334, 455, 457–459, 472, 506
International Budokaikan, 225
International Karate and Kobudo Federation, 81
International Karate Organization, 203, 474, 537
Inoue, Motokatsu, 254, 273, 299–302, 304, 307
Inoue, Takekatsu, 254
International Koei-Kan Karatedo Federation, 141–143
International Okinawa Kobudo Association, 95, 252
International Seibukan Karate Association, 233
ippon kumite, 692 note 3
Iraha, Choko, 345
Irei, Tadashiki, 251

Irimaji, Seiji, 431, 433–436, 440–443, 445 notes 18 and 21
iron clogs (*geta*), 18, 237
Ishibashi, Masami, 540–541
Ishikawa, Masanobu, 176
Isshin-ryu, 120, 165, 330–331, 334, 351, 404–425
issuing power (Chinese *fajing*; Japanese *hakkei*), 296–297, 714
Itokazu, Seiki, 245
Itosu, Anko/Ankoh (Yasutsune), 28, 59–62, 67 note 2, 168, 230–231, 242–243, 254, 304, 338–340, 389–391, 485, 654–655, 660 note 1
Itosu's Ten Lessons, 61–64
Itto-ryu, 117
Iwah, 431–432, 440, 443, 445 notes 16 and 20

J

Japan Karate Association, 353
Japan Kobudo Association, 168
Jana, Teido, 524
Jay, Wally, 593–596
Jigen-ryu, 59
Ji'in kata, 272
Jion kata, 272, 339 note
Jo-ryu Mai Te Gassen Karatekai, 175
judo, 25, 28–29, 32, 39, 79–80, 149, 177, 180, 187, 219–223, 227, 237, 240, 254, 281, 299, 388, 408, 430, 444 note 8, 474, 481 note 13, 502–503, 505, 528, 533, 542–543, 547, 580, 582, 601, 603, 610–611, 630, 641, 702, 719–721
Jundokan, 81, 677, 692 note 1

K

kaho, 600, 602–605
kakie, see push-hands
Kakuho kata, 482, 484, 556
Kamiunten, Fumiko, 176, 178, 184 note 20
Kanazawa, Hirokazu, 542, 549
Kanchin kata, 248
Kanegawa, Gibu, 272
Kaneshima, Shinyei, 169
Kanku kata, 186, 194
Kano, Jigoro, 28, 32, 79, 149, 430, 528, 702–703, 720
Kanshiwa kata, 248
Kanzaki, Shigekazu, 303, 337, 340, 342, 345, 348–357, 398, 655
karate drum, 318–319, 372, 380, 387, 451, 753
Karate Research Society (Karatedo Kenkyu Kai), 339, 344, 353, 357 note 5
kata, 6, 33, 45, 65–66, 253–254, 256–257,

269–273, 276, 285–286, 290–294, 296–297, 300–310, 316–317, 319, 329, 339–344, 346 notes 1, 3 and 6, 349–355, 357 note 6, 359, 372–387, 391, 394, 397–403, 404, 406, 408, 410–414, 416, 418, 432–433, 435–438, 440–443, 444 note 9, 447–460, 476–479, 482–499, 513–521, 524–526, 528–530, 538–540, 542, 548, 554–578, 583, 585, 592–593, 596–600, 602–605, 612–613, 616–621, 622 note 5, 624, 627, 629–632, 639, 641, 643–652, 653 note 1, 654–662, 676–692, 706–708, 711– 742, 749, 752–753, 755

kata's floor pattern (*embusen*), 514

kendo, 24, 29, 80, 94, 174, 254, 299, 502, 590 note 3, 603, 610, 618, 632, 641

kenjutsu, 24, 59, 108, 114, 117, 142, 301, 339, 628

Kenkyu-kai, 339, 344, 353, 357 note 5, 644, 646

Kihongata I and II, 340

Kim, Richard, 58, 66, 270, 390–391, 398, 474–475, 481 note 13, 579–590

Kimura, Mits, 220

Kingai-ryu, 482, 484, 678

Kinjo, Akio, 341, 344, 732

Kinjo, Hiroshi, 58–62, 64–67, 398, 581, 590 note 2, 655

Kinjo, Kazufumi, 267

Kinjo, Masahiko, 252

Kinjo, Takashi, 51, 245–252, 435

knife-hand (*shuto*), 143, 146, 201, 203, 225, 373, 376–377, 381–385, 425, 453, 457, 459, 489, 648, 651, 653 note 2, 753–654

Knighton, Stan, 549

Ko, Ryuryu (aka. Ru Ru, Ryuru), 76–77, 238–239, 397–398, 432, 443, 445 notes 15 and 19, 523, 626–627, 646, 711

Kobayashi-kan Kyokai, 299

Kobayashi-ryu, 242, 270, 299–300

Kobayashi Shorin-ryu, 230, 233

Kobu no Ti Naka, 251

kobudo, 28, 51, 94–97, 105, 174, 245–246, 249, 252, 254, 257, 267–271, 273, 275–276, 278, 299–302, 304, 306–307, 434, 462–463, 472, 475, 482, 653 note 3, 678

Kobukai Konan-ryu, 245, 248, 435

Kobuken ("Kinjo's Martial Fist"), 248

Kobuzai (sai kata), 249

Kochinda, Saburo, 435

Kodokan, 28, 220–223, 533, 542, 601, 720

Koga-ryu, 304

Kogusuku, 432, 444 note 11

Kojo, Isei, 431–433

Kojo, Koho, 431–434, 440–442

Kojo, Saikyo, 431–432, 433 note 21

Kojo, Saisho, 431–432, 442

Kojo, Shigeru, 433–436, 440–441

Kojo, Shinpo, 431, 445 note 13

Kojo, Shinunjo, 431

Kojo, Taite, 338, 397, 431–433, 523

Kojo, Yoshiakam, 431, 433–434, 436

Kojo, Yoshitomi, 433–436, 440–441, 443, 445 note 21

Kojo-ryu, 182 note 4, 428–443, 445 note 21

Konan-ryu, 245–246, 248–249, 251, 435

Kongo no Ko (bo kata), 301

Konishi, Yasuhiro (aka Konishi Koyu), 169, 254, 256, 300, 304

Koshin-ryu, 428, 434–436, 442–443

Koshin-ryu Kohokan Karate and Kobudo Organization, 434–435

Koshiro, Shuren, 433, 445 note 20

Kumemura village, 167, 432, 523, 711

Kurosaki, Kenji, 224–225, 533–534, 539, 541, 545–547

Kururunfa kata, 78, 398, 486, 521 note 1, 566 note 3, 569, 631, 645, 655, 657–659, 677, 679, 682, 685, 688, 691–692, 711, 724 note 4

Kusanku kata, 121–122, 231, 235, 656

Kuwae, Ryosei, 59, 61

Kyan, Chofu, 242

Kyan, Chotoku (nickname: Chan Migwa), 64, 166, 231–235, 242, 340, 393, 511 note 3

Kyoda, Juhatsu, 59, 299–300, 302–304, 306–307, 337–341, 343–345, 348–349, 352, 354, 398, 444 note 10, 626–627, 634 note 2, 654–655, 659, 725

Kyoda, Juko, 303, 343–345, 348–350, 355

Kyokushin, 186–203, 225–226, 528, 530 note 4, 532–553, 589 note 1, 601

Kyokushin Kaikan, 203, 219, 221, 223, 226–227

L

Lee, Bruce, 15, 408, 527, 593–594, 596–597, 602, 720

London Judo Society, 547

long staff (*bo*), 16, 97, 99, 103–104, 230, 149, 249–251, 264, 266, 270–271, 273, 275–277, 300–302, 308, 310–313, 354, 583, 585, 618, 756

M

Mabuni, Kenwa, 64, 166, 236, 256, 304, 339, 344, 357 note 6, 613, 616, 622 note 5, 636, 644, 654–655

Maeda, Akira, 227
Maeda, Esai, 530 note 5
Maeshiro, Chaya, 64
Maeshiro, Shusei, 246
Maezato no Nunchaku Sho/Dai, 302
Maezato no Tekko, 269, 272, 755
Makabe, Chan, 231
makiwara, see striking post.
manji sai, 95
martial dance (*moudi*), 170
martial sport, 20–21, 27, 30, 38, 41, 46, 59, 66, 132, 223, 304
Masanobu, Shinjo, 81–82, 150, 486
Matayoshi, Shinpo, 16, 95, 236, 246, 249, 346 note 6, 482–484, 486, 498–499, 637, 652, 653 note 3, 678, 690–692
Matsubayashi-ryu (Shorin), 254, 735
Matsuda, Tokusaburo, 433
Matsugawa no Tecchu, 270, 272–273
Matsumora, Kosaku, 242, 622 note 5
Matsumura, "Bushi' Sokon, 15–16, 28, 59–61, 172, 230–234, 389, 431, 443, 445 note 16, 580
Matsumura Sokon's wife, 230
Matsumura's Precepts on Bu, 60–61
Meibukan, 81, 444 note 10, 524, 528, 530, 556, 571, 624–634, 692, 704
Mie, Junshin, 270
Mifune, Kyuzo, 219–220, 743
Mimoun, Boulahfa, 184 note 21
Minowa, Katsuhiko, 267–278, 301, 755
Minowa no Kon Sho/Dai, 270
Minowa no Sanbon Nunchaku, 270
Minowa no Tecchu, 270
Mirakian, Anthony, 556–567
Miyagi, An'ichi, 568
Miyagi, Chojun, 64–65, 75–82, 148–159, 166, 236–237, 243, 256, 285, 296, 300, 302–303, 337–343, 346 note 5, 348, 351–354, 357 note 4, 372, 393, 397–398, 403 note 2, 474, 485–486, 512 note 7, 513, 515, 522–527, 555, 566 note 1, 568–571, 590 note 3, 625–629, 632, 634, 639, 641, 643, 645–646, 654–655, 657–660, 677–678, 691, 692 notes 1 and 2, 711, 725–726
Miyagi, Kei, 351, 568, 726
Miyagi, Masu (Tsuru), 569
Miyahira, Katsuya, 169, 229–232
Miyashiro, Thomas, 394
Miyazato, Ei'ichi / Eiichi, 75, 78, 568, 677, 692
Monk Fist boxing (*lohanquan*), 655
Moriwasa, Nashimoto (Prince), 80
Moromizato, Shinsuke, 177, 179
Moromizato, Shinzato, 175

Motobu Association, 176
Motobu, Anshi, 244
Motobu, Choki, 80, 166, 256, 391, 612, 616, 622 note 5
Motobu Choyu, 166, 339, 511 note 3
Motobu-ryu, 165, 254, 299–300, 444 note 10, 724 note 1
Murakami, Katsumi, 655–656, 659
Munenori, Yagyu, 21, 108
Mushindo Kempo Association, 406

N

Nagaishi, Fumio, 267
Nagamine, Shoshin, 60, 62, 169, 394, 398, 412, 653 note 1, 735
Naha city, 76–77, 79, 81, 95, 165–166, 173, 182 notes 2 and 3, 236–237, 243, 245, 251, 257, 268–270, 273, 339–340, 343, 397, 429, 433–435, 444 note 7, 551 note 5, 522, 524–525, 568, 626, 629
Naha-te, 76–79, 82, 149, 165, 179, 182 note 4, 243, 353, 430, 503, 511 note 5, 523, 622 note 5, 634 note 3,
Naihanchi/Naifanchi kata, 62, 89, 92–93, 231, 305, 391, 394, 411, 440, 593, 616
Nakama, Chozo, 169, 233
Nakama, Roykin, 394
Nakaima, Genkai, 569
Nakaima, Kenri, 403 note 1, 511 note 5, 569
Nakamoto, Aisho, 357 note 4
Nakamoto, Masahiro, 267, 270, 272, 301
Nakamura, Seigi, 513
Nakamura, Tadashi, 224, 541–543, 545–547, 552
Nakasone, Genwa, 62, 64, 340, 357 note 7, 393, 636, 642–643
Nakasone, Koshin, 267
Nakayama, Masatoshi, 28, 30–31, 34, 221
Nakazato, Joen, 232
Nakazato, Shugoro, 230, 299–301, 307
Nanbansato-ryu, 300–301, 304
Ninomiya, Kojo, 550
Nishiuchi, Mikio, 44, 51, 95, 252
Nishiyama, Hidetaka, 475
"no mind" (*mushin*), 37, 108, 113, 256, 306
Northern Japan Yuishinkai Kobudo, 254, 299
Nozaki, Yukikazu, 175–177
nunchaku (flail), 14–15, 95, 270–271, 273, 302, 308, 354, 462, 466–470, 755

O

oar (*eku/ieku/kai*), 16, 95, 250, 271, 308, 349, 482
Obata, Isao, 221

Ochiai, Hidy, 255
Ogasawara, Jiro, 254–256
Ogasawara, Tokushiro, 254–255
Ohtsuka, Hironori, 304, 512 note 7
Okada, Hirofumi, 540
Okada, Jiro, 254–256, 259
Okazaki, Teruyuki, 30, 36
Okinawa Budo International (OBI), 251
Okinawa Karatejutsu Kenkyu Kai (Okinawa Karatejutsu Research Club/Association), 339, 344
Okinawa Kokusai Budo Karatedo Renmei, 251
Okinawa Konan-ryu Kohokan Karate and Kobudo Kyokai, 435
Okinawa Prefectural Athletic Association, 340
Okinawa Prefectural Karatedo Promotion Society, 340
Okinawa Prefectural Karatedo Federation, 168
Okinawa Tode Research Club, 166, 391
Okinawan dance (*odori*), 15, 172
Okinawan Goju-ryu Shobukan Association, 82, 150, 157
Okinawan Karatedo Association, 237, 716
Okinawan Karate-do Preservation Society, 80
Okinawan Prefectural Karate Association, 168, 229
Okinawan weapons, 15, 637
one-knuckle punch/fist (*shohken-zuki*), 47–50, 713, 724 note 2, 736–737
O'Neill, Terry, 549
Onishi, Eizo, 141–142
oral teachings (*kuden*), 15, 228–229, 235, 241, 254, 405, 433, 460, 655, 741
Oshiro, Chojo, 58, 62, 166, 339, 590 note 2
Oyadomari, Kokan, 242–243
Oyama, Masutatsu, 186–203, 219, 221–227, 474, 530 note 4, 532–553, 581, 589 note 1
Oyama, Shigeru, 541–543, 545–457, 550, 552
Oyama, Yasuhiko, 546
Oyata, Seiyu, 592–594

P

palm strike, 90–91, 118, 143, 398, 648–650, 732–733
passive breaking, 143–144, 146
Pangainoon-ryu/Pwang Gai Noonryu, 44–51, 245–246, 430, 661
Passai kata, 304, 394, 440
Pai, Daniel, 475, 594
Parker, Ed, 594
pechin officials, 67 note 3, 389
Pechurin kata, 339, 343, 346 note 1, 350–353, 655–656, 658–660, 711–712, 724 note 4, 732
Pinan kata, 194, 242, 344, 394, 440, 514, 593, 613, 616–617, 654
police, 80–81, 95–96, 177, 236, 240, 355, 433, 503, 592, 610–611, 618, 625
Poynton, Bob, 549
prearranged sparring (*yakusoku*), 270–271, 276, 339, 354, 513
precepts of *shuhari*, 65
Presas, Remy, 593–594, 598
pressure points (*kyusha*), 14–15, 170–171, 301, 420, 432, 440, 456, 591–592, 594–595, 597–598, 749
protective gear (*bogu*), 174, 258, 408
push-hands (*kakie*), 339, 354, 376, 387, 753

R

ranking, 6–7, 27, 32, 254, 256, 268, 299, 405–407, 414, 430, 443, 480 note 3, 511 note 6, 581, 600–601, 614
Red Sparrow (*Shujakku*), 403 note 2, 568, 571–575
Renbukan, 175
respiration theory, 87–88
reverse punch (*gyaku-zuki*), 86, 109, 118, 248, 319, 359–364, 367–368, 699, 714–715, 723, 726, 732, 736
Ricci, Brian, 579–589
Rikkyo University, 221, 533
Ritsumeikan University, 79–80
rocks in a net (*ishibukro*), 18
rokushaku bo (six-foot staff), 271, 273, 275–276, 308, 431
rokkishu exercise, 525, 530 note 1, 646
Royama, Hatsuo, 550
Ryukyu Kobudo Hozoin Shinkokai (Ryukyu Kobudo Preservation and Promotion Association), 267, 271–273, 300, 571

S

sai, 15, 17, 95–105, 249, 253, 270–271, 308, 442, 571, 584
Saifa/Saiha kata, 78, 194, 517–520, 540, 558, 563, 566 note 3, 569, 645, 648, 655, 657–659, 679–681, 684–687, 691, 692 notes 2 and 4, 711, 724 note 4
Sakiyama, Kitoku, 403 note 1, 511 note 5
Sakihama, Seijiro, 435
Sakiyama, Tatsutoku, 569
Sakugawa, Kanga ("Tode"), 12, 16, 231, 241–242, 431
Sakugawa, Koshiki Shorinji-ryu, 253–259

Sakugawa no Kon Sho, 270, 302
samurai sword (*katana*), 34, 105, 174, 237, 604
sanbon nunchaku (three-section flail), 14–15, 95, 273
Sanchin kata, 18, 45, 77–78, 82, 120, 143, 149, 156, 194, 201, 240, 248, 285–298, 302, 316–320, 329, 339, 341, 343, 346 notes 1 and 3, 349–350, 353, 355, 372–375, 380–385, 398, 409, 412–414, 416, 449, 451, 487, 524–525, 536, 569, 629, 631, 645–646, 648, 655–665, 671, 673–674, 677, 679, 681, 691, 692 note 2, 707, 711–719, 721, 723, 724 note 4, 726–727, 730–732, 735, 753
Sancho Zai (three-sai kata), 96, 249
Sanseiryu kata, 78, 248, 302, 343, 569
Sato, Katsuko, 549
Sato, Kinbei , 299, 304–305
school clothing (*gi*), 32, 81, 285
Seibukan Shorin-ryu, 233–234
Seichin kata, 248
Seido style, 175, 184 note 21, 552
Seienchin kata, 78, 194
Seipai kata, 78, 194, 350, 526, 630, 645, 648, 655–659
Seiro, Iju, 237
Seiryu kata, 248, 403 note 2, 568, 571, 575–576
Seisan kata, 78, 248, 302, 339, 342–343, 346 note 1, 349–351, 353, 411, 416, 418, 524, 526, 629, 632, 645, 648, 655–657, 659
Seiunchin kata, 398, 447–452, 486, 521 note 1, 524, 554, 558–560, 562–565, 566 note 3, 567 note 5, 569, 629, 645, 655, 657–659, 679–682, 685–687, 691, 692 note 2, 711, 724 note 4
self-development, 21–24, 37–40, 126
Sepai, 487–497, 419, 519, 677, 679 689, 691, 692 note 2, 711, 724 note 4
Sesan, 569, 659, 679, 717–724, 724 note 3, 726–728, 731–732, 735
shield (*timbei*), 95
Shikiyanaka, Chinen, 62
Shimabukuro, Takashi, 176, 179
Shimabukuro, Zenpo, 233–234
Shimabukuro, Zenryu, 233
Shindo, 607, 614–615, 618–621
Shindo Jinen-ryu, 254, 256, 300, 304
Shindo Yoshin-ryu, 512 note 7, 612, 616, 622 note 2
Shindo-kan Shorin-ryu, 230
Shinjo, Masanobu, 81–82, 150, 155, 486
Shinpan, Shiroma (Gusukuma), 80, 237, 340, 393, 715, 718

Shinshukai (Association for True Study), 268
Shinto, 23, 26, 602, 635 note 9
Shinzato, Jinan, 79–81, 523–524, 628, 634
Shinzato, Katsuhiko, 229
Shiroma, Masahige, 626, 634 note 3, 715
Shiroma, Seihan, 175
Shirotaru no Kon, 302
Shisochin kata, 78, 354, 484, 486, 521 note 1, 558, 566 note 3, 569, 645, 655–659, 679, 688, 692, 711, 724 note 4
Shito-ryu, 64, 165, 236, 256, 344–345, 474, 622 note 5
Sho Ko (king), 169, 230, 233
Sho Shin-O (king), 183 notes 10, 12 and 15, 308, 430
Sho Tai (king), 166, 244
Shorei-ryu, 357 note 6
Shorin-ryu, 634 note 3, 653 note 1, 678, 692 note 3
Shorinji-ryu, 253–259, 270, 408, 580
short spear (*tinbe, yari*), 338, 581, 585
Shudokan, 299
Shotokan, 254–256, 444 note 4, 475–476, 480 note 12, 505, 533, 538, 582–583, 589 note 1, 601, 616, 733
Shukokai, 538
Shuri city, 257, 271, 308, 339, 389–390, 393, 393 note 7, 430, 444 note 7, 524, 622 note 5, 641, 656, 717
Shuri Castle, 389, 523, 641–643, 645, 659, 660 note 5, 711
Shuri-te, 304, 339, 344, 353–354, 357, 430–431, 440, 475, 503, 511 note 5, 622 note 7, 711
shuriken, 300–301
Shushi no Kon kata, 301, 304
sickles (*kama*), 269, 275
Small Circle Jujitsu, 593–594, 749
Sochin kata, 344, 558, 566 note 3
social behaviors, 281, 599–600, 638–639
Soeishi no Kon (bo kata), 302
Soeno, Yoshiji, 550
Soken, Hohan, 435, 592–593, 596
Sokudai katas
spear (*yari*), 172, 174, 178, 245, 338–339, 432, 581, 585
spear-hand, 187, 398, 436, 448, 450, 530 note 1, 650, 720
sport karate, 30, 41, 528, 714
sports competition 20–21, 30, 68, 71, 84, 108, 118, 121, 174, 199, 592–593
staff (*bo*), 16, 79, 95, 97, 99–105, 149, 170, 264, 271, 308–310, 354, 431–432, 442, 463–465, 468–469, 583, 585, 618, 756

sticking (*muchimi*), 320, 322, 376, 378–379, 486, 489, 683
striking post (*makiwara*), 49, 52–57, 76, 143, 148, 303, 340, 354, 513, 523, 570, 625, 629–630, 694–700, 725
stone lever weight (*chishi*), 18, 76, 148, 152–159, 292, 339–340, 355, 625, 631, 676
stone padlocks (*sushi*), 18
stone weight (*sashiishi*), 18, 149
sumo, 299, 388, 391–392, 450, 714
Sunsu kata, 120, 351, 411
Supairenpei kata, 78, 81
Suparinpei kata, 398, 486, 521 note 1, 645, 648
suruchin (weighted chain), 15, 17, 95
Sushiho kata, 194
swordsmanship (*kenjutsu*), 24, 59, 108, 114, 117, 142, 339, 481 note 13, 513, 613, 635 note 7

T

Taba, Seiichi, 175
taijiquan, 79, 304, 306, 311, 408, 428, 561, 581
Taikyoku katas, 194
Taira, Shinken, 254, 267–268, 271–273, 300–302, 571, 753, 755
taisabaki (body movement), 256, 323, 612–614, 617, 756
Takahara Peichin, 241
Takamatsu, Sumisuke, 305
Takamine Choboku, 677
Takamiyagi Shigeru, 445 note 22, 716
Takeda, Sokato, 581
Takenouchi-ryu, 719
Takushoku University Karate Club, 30, 186
tameshiwari (breaking), 7–8, 34, 45, 58 141–147, 186, 190–191, 200–201, 224–225, 476, 540, 743–747
Tanaka, Masahiko, 20
tanden, 63, 87–90, 92, 107, 143–144, 285, 290–291, 293–295, 297, 381, 451, 507, 704, 707
te, 165, 169, 174, 180, 182, 243, 246, 429–430, 611, 616, 628, 642
tecchu/tetchu/tekko (palm size stick-like weapon), 95, 246, 251, 270–276, 278, 755–757
Tenjin Shinryo-ryu, 733
Tenshi (Heaven and Earth), 403 note 2, 568, 571, 577
Tensho kata, 77–78, 194, 302, 341, 354, 372–387, 398, 411, 524–525, 569, 572, 644–651, 655–657, 692 note 2
Teruya, Rinko, 349
theory of opposites, 85
three-sectional staff (*sansetsukon*), 95
Tiger boxing (*huquan*), 655
Toguchi, Seiichi, 75, 78, 80–82, 486, 555–557, 569, 630, 677, 692 note 1, 721
Tokashiki, Iken, 353, 430, 444 note 9, 732, 740
Tokuda, Anbun, 229
Tokugawa, Ieyasu, 23
Tokumine Pechin, 168–169
Toma, Shian, 175, 184 note 21, 254
Tomari-te, 711, 740
Tomoyose, Ryuko, 237–238
tonfa (*tuifa/tungua/tunkua*), 15–16, 95, 170, 194, 264, 270–271, 308, 555
To'on-ryu, 299–300, 302–303, 337–345, 346 note 2, 348–356, 444 note 10, 634 note 2, 659
toudi (China hand), 61, 429, 642–643, 660 note 1, 714, 716–718, 720, 723, 725
Toyama, Kanken, 299–300, 304, 307
weight transitioning, 372, 381–383, 385–387, 449, 558, 669, 727, 756–757
Trias, Robert, 475, 594
Tsuken Akachu no Ieku De, 250
Tsuken Bo Sho/Dai, 270
Tsukensunakake no Kon Kata, 268
Tsuruoka, Masami, 473, 500–511

U

Udun-di, 165–168, 170–182, 238, 243, 444 note 10
Uechi, Kanbun, 51, 167, 237, 239, 245, 439, 445 notes 19 and 22, 661, 712
Uechi, Kanei, 51, 237–238, 246, 268–269, 661–662
Uechi-ryu, 167, 182 note 4, 237, 245–246, 248, 268, 273, 430, 435, 438–439, 445 note 22, 661–664, 674–675, 716, 724 notes 2 and 3, 732, 742 note 1
Uehara, Hideko, 176
Uehara, Seikichi, 165–182, 239–240, 243
Uehara, Tsuyoshi, 178
Ueki, Masayuki, 255
Ueno, Takashi, 305
Ueshiba, Morihei, 256, 428
United States Karate Association (USKA), 475

V

Ventresca, Peter, 582
vital point striking (*kyushojutsu*), 50, 257, 447, 452, 460, 597, 737

W

Wado-ryu, 223, 304, 512, 538, 612–613, 615, 617–618
Wai, Xinxian, 432, 443, 445 note 15 and 19

Wall, Kimo, 482, 499, 652, 653 note 3, 692
Wang, Shujin, 304
Wang, Xiangzhai, 581
Washin-ryu, 255
weight lifting, 76, 148–159, 168, 221, 625, 676
weapons ban, 12, 94, 271, 308, 430
weapons use (*kobujutsu*), 12, 308–309, 431, 604
White Crane (Hakutsuru Ken), 77, 339, 344, 357 note 5, 432–433, 435, 438, 440, 554, 646, 648, 655
White Dragon, 432, 441, 475, 571
White Tiger (*byakko*), 432, 438, 568, 571–572, 575–576
Whooping Crane boxing, 353
Wing Chun, 330, 334, 476, 646
World Union of Karate Organizations, 548
World War II, 80, 183 note 8, 187, 268, 300, 339–340, 388, 431, 434, 480 note 3, 481 note 12, 485, 500, 524, 581, 627, 634 note 5, 637, 655
wrist roller (*makiage kiga*), 18, 157–158
Wu, Xiangui (Go Kenki), 339, 344, 357 note 5, 646

X
Xie, Zhongxiang, 338

Y
Yabiku, Moden, 254
Yabiku, Takaya, 429, 433–435, 440–442
Yabu, Kentsu, 67 note 1, 80, 304, 339–340, 344, 351, 353, 388–394, 580, 622 note 5, 733
Yagi, Meitatsu, 522–530, 624–632, 634, 634 note 1
Yagi, Meitoku, 75, 78, 82, 403 note 2, 522–530, 555, 568–578, 625, 627–632, 634, 634 note 1, 692 note 1, 704
Yamaguchi, Gogen, 78, 224, 474, 505, 511 note 7, 533, 539, 581, 590 note 3, 628
Yamaguchi Gosei, 474
Yamane no Chinen Sanda, 67 note 2
Yamane-ryu, 299–302, 304, 435, 444 note 10
Yamashita, Yoshikazu, 220
Yamate-ryu, 112
Yamazaki, Masanao, 254
Yantsu kata, 194
Yara, Choui, 299
Yasuda, Eiji, 539–540
Yasuhito Chichibu (Prince), 79
Yogi, Jitsuei, 78
Yonegawa no Kon, 302
Yoshida, Kotaro, 183 note 8, 579–581, 585
Yoshimura, Hiroshi, 267–268, 276–278, 755
Yuishinkai kobudo, 254, 299
Yunigawa no kon kata, 585, 587

Z
Zen Bei Butokukai, 581–582, 584–585, 590 note 4
Zen Buddhism, 1, 23–24, 26, 40, 601
Zen Nihon Kendo Renmei, 94
Zen Okinawa Kobudo Renmei
Zhang, Zhankui, 304

Other Titles by Via Media Publishing

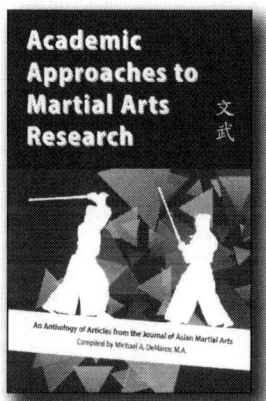
Academic Approaches to Martial Art Research

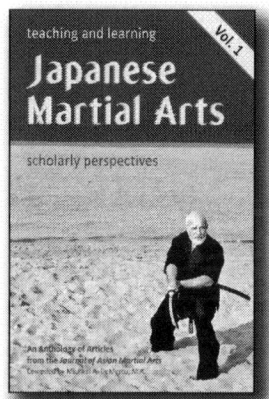
Teaching and Learning Japanese Martial Art Arts Volume I and Volume II

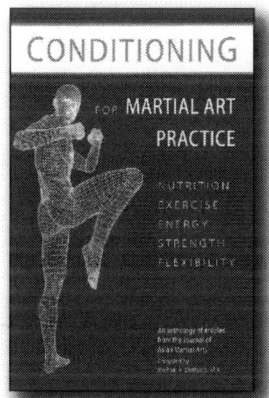
Conditioning for Martial Art Practice

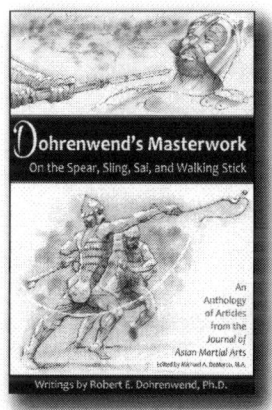
Dohrenwend's Masterwork
spear, sling, sai, walking stick

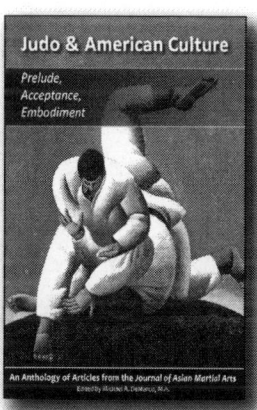
Judo and American Culture

Fiction

Wuxia America - Emergence of a Chinese American Hero

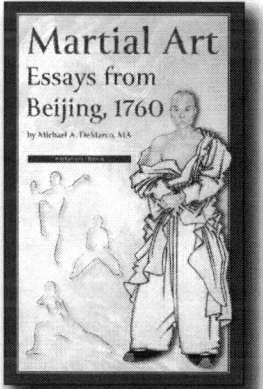
Martial Art Essays from Beijing, 1760

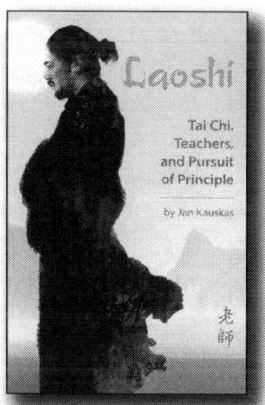
Laoshi: Tai Chi, Teachers, and Pursuit of Principle

www.viamediapublishing.com

Printed in Great Britain
by Amazon

157ffdae-343a-4eb5-aef8-fd8b8eaba1baR01